Science of
Dental Materials
with Clinical Applications

Third Edition

V Shama Bhat MSc
Professor and Head

BT Nandish MSc, PhD
Professor

Jayaprakash K MSc, PhD
Associate Professor

Department of Dental Materials
Yenepoya Dental College
Yenepoya (Deemed to be University)
Mangaluru

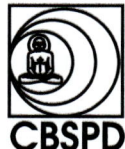

CBSPD

CBS Publishers & Distributors Pvt Ltd

New Delhi • Bengaluru • Chennai • Kochi • Kolkata • Lucknow • Mumbai
Hyderabad • Jharkhand • Nagpur • Patna • Pune • Uttarakhand

Science of
Dental Materials
with Clinical Applications
Third Edition

ISBN: 978-93-88327-57-2

Third Edition: 2019
Reprint: 2024
First Edition: 2006
Second Edition: 2013
Reprint: 2015

Published by Satish Kumar Jain and produced by Varun Jain for
CBS Publishers & Distributors Pvt Ltd
4819/XI Prahlad Street, 24 Ansari Road, Daryaganj, New Delhi 110 002, India
Ph: 011-23289259, 23266861

Website: www.cbspd.com
e-mail: delhi@cbspd.com

Corporate Office: 204 FIE, Industrial Area, Patparganj, Delhi 110 092, India
Ph: 011-4934 4934   Fax: 011-4934 4935   e-mail: publishing@cbspd.com;
                                                                                       publicity@cbspd.com

Branches

• **Bengaluru:** Seema House 2975, 17th Cross, KR Road, Banasankari 2nd Stage, Bengaluru 560 070, Karnataka, India
  Ph: +91-80-26771678/79   Fax: +91-80-26771680   e-mail: bangalore@cbspd.com
• **Chennai:** 7, Subbaraya Street, Shenoy Nagar, Chennai 600 030, Tamil Nadu, India
  Ph: +91-44-26680620, 26681266   Fax: +91-44-42032115   e-mail: chennai@cbspd.com
• **Kochi:** 42/1325, 1326, Power House Road, Opp KSEB, Power House, Ernakulum Kochi 682 018, Kerala, India
  Ph: +91-484-4059061-65,67   Fax: +91-484-4059065   e-mail: kochi@cbspd.com
• **Kolkata:** 147, Hind Ceramics Compound, 1st Floor, Nilgunj Road, Belghoria, Kolkata-700056, West Bengal India
  Ph: +033-25633055, 033-25633056   e-mail: kolkata@cbspd.com
• **Lucknow:** Basement, Khushnuma Complex, 7 Meerabai Marg (Behind Jawahar Bhawan), Lucknow-226001, UP, India
  Ph: +91-522-4000032   e-mail: tiwari.lucknow@cbspd.com
• **Mumbai:** PWD Shed, Gala no 25/26, Ramchandra Bhatt Marg, Next to JJ Hospital Gate no. 2, Opp. Union Bank of India, Noorbaug, Mumbai-400009, Maharashtra, India
  Ph: 022-66661880/89   e-mail: mumbai@cbspd.com

Representatives

• Hyderabad   0-9885175004   • Jharkhand   0-9811541605   • Nagpur   0-8692091830
• Patna   0-9334159340   • Pune   0-9664372571   • Uttarakhand   0-9716462459

Printed at Mudrak, Noida, UP, India

to

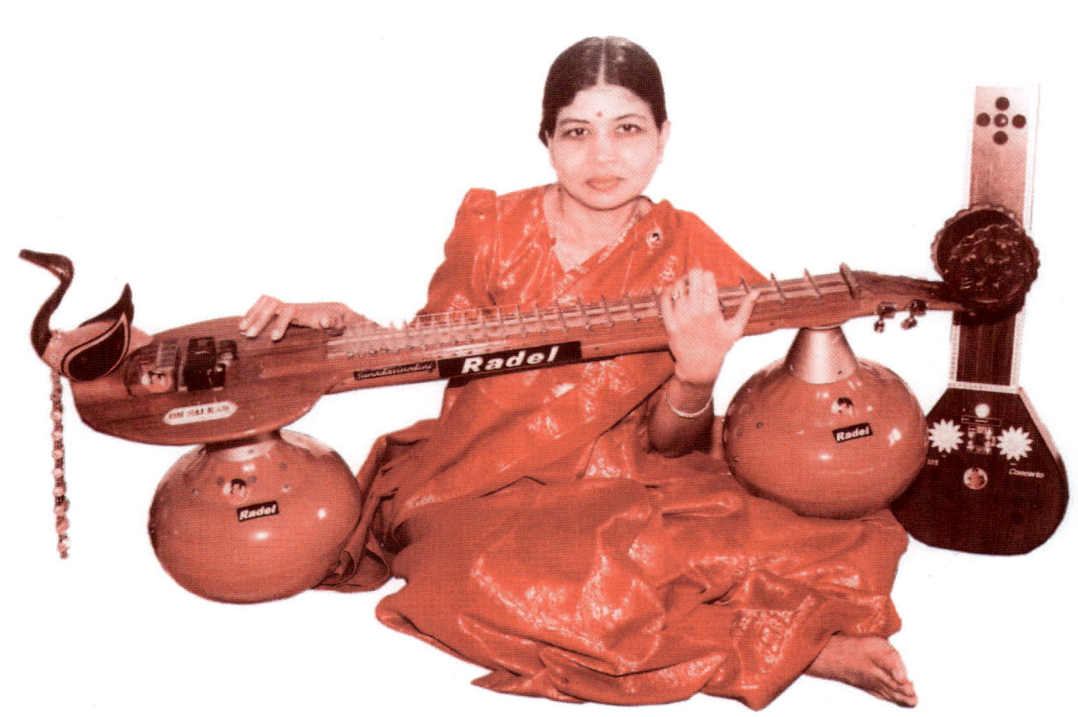

Miss Manipal Aruna Kumari

Veena Vidushi, MA (Sociology)

The extraordinarily-abled challenged lady
she has excelled in Karnataka classical music, vocal,
Veena and Violin recitals

The first-ever "A-Grade" blind veena artist of Prasara Bharathi,
New Delhi, India

Foreword

In recent years, tremendous growth and advancement have taken place in the basic sciences, especially in the field of dental material science which has resulted in numerous innovations and improvements in the clinical procedures of dentistry. This changed scenario warrants the involvement of teachers who are specially qualified in material science, in training the dental students. Through this, the sound knowledge of dental materials will help the qualified dentists to render better treatment for the patients. As a strong believer of this concept, I wanted to implement this in our institution. At that juncture, I was fortunate to get a person like Prof V Shama Bhat who has in-depth knowledge in this field. He has contributed a lot in establishing and developing the department of dental materials along with a museum of high standards. With his constant perseverance, he was instrumental in developing a good curriculum for MSc course in dental materials at MAHE, Manipal. Time has come for all of us to establish the department of material science in every institution with specially qualified teachers. With our constant encouragement, he has come forward to write Third Edition of this book at the age of 87 years. The vast experience of Prof Shama Bhat as a teacher and researcher with great vision and ideas should reach the teachers and student community at large. Seeing the dedication and enthusiasm of the author even at this age and invaluable contributions from his colleagues Dr BT Nandish and Dr Jayaprakash K, I am sure the Third Edition of his textbook will add immense contribution in the progression of dental materials science.

I wish all the success to him and his colleagues in this new venture.

BH Sripathi Rao MDS
Dean/Principal
Yenepoya Dental College
Mangaluru, India
Former Executive Committee Member of DCI, New Delhi
Former Vice Chancellor
Yenepoya (Deemed to be University)

Foreword

The purpose of a good textbook is to provide updated adequate information in a simple, lucid style, for easy understanding to the average students and some challenging advanced topics to the more intelligent class. Excellent presentation with tables, diagrams, question bank, colour plates, etc. make it more attractive and useful to remember.

I am very confident to say that all these requirements have been satisfied by experienced authors in this Third Edition of *Science of Dental Materials Clinical Applications*. I congratulate the authors, very senior professor V Shama Bhat (involved since 1976) and my old student Dr BT Nandish, now faculty and controller of examination and Dr Jayaprakash K, who have excelled in guiding the students in learning and research for the last 20 years. The Yenepoya Dental College has an excellent material research laboratory and a unique museum in dental materials.

Hope the students will appreciate and make use of this.

M Vijayakumar MBBS, DNB, MCh, FRCS
Vice Chancellor
Yenepoya (Deemed to be University)

Preface to the Third Edition

We have received many feedbacks since the publication of the first edition of this work in 2006 and again after the second edition in 2013, expressing its usefulness for UG and PG students as well as the faculties, due to entire coverage of the subject with simple explanations, a method of presentations, model questions, explanatory diagrams, colour plates, etc. Some changes such as reorganizations of tables, figures, colour plates, including corrections, etc. have been incorporated in this Third Edition for updating, as per the feedbacks. We thank, Mrs Sowmya Rao, Assistant Professor, in our department, for the assistance rendered.

We wish to remember Dr Ravindra Kotian of CODS, Mangaluru, Dr Nagaraj Upadhyaya of CODS, Manipal, Dr Kishore Ginjupalli of CODS, Manipal with regard for their valuable contributions to the cause of Dental Materials. We also wish to place on records our thanks to the faculties specially AB Shetty College of Dental Science, Derelakatte, AJ Dental College, Mangaluru, KVG Dental College, Sullia, Srinivas Institute of Dental Sciences, Mukka, Century Dental College, Poinachi-Kasaragod, Educare Institute of Dental Sciences, Chattiparamba, Malappuram, for their encouragement for preparing Third Edition.

We, once again, wish to express our gratitude to his excellency, Yenepoya Abdulla Kunhi, Chancellor, Yenepoya (Deemed to be University) and Dr BH Sripathi Rao, Dean/Principal, Yenepoya Dental College, Mangaluru, for their continued encouragement and support.

V Shama Bhat
BT Nandish
Jayaprakash K

Preface to the First Edition

The *Science of Dental Materials* is an excellent example of a composite applied subject, formed by the interactions between the various basic science subjects and engineering technologies with biological sciences. This science is applied in the clinical procedures of various specialities for the treatments of the dental patients. One cannot think of any dental treatments without applying this science. The dentists have to diagnose, analyse the clinical situations, plan the scheme of treatments, select the most suitable materials and manipulative techniques, to avail the best treatment to the patients. The dental technicians, in turn, have to assist the clinicians in the selection of most suitable materials and fabricate oral appliances with maximum skill and precision. Hence, the technician also should have a thorough knowledge of the methods of controlling the properties of restorative and auxiliary materials, as well as the latest techniques of fabrications and finishing of oral appliances, utilising the sophisticated equipment in the modern laboratories.

To achieve these, the dentists and also the laboratory technicians should have at least an elementary basic knowledge of the following areas, basic sciences, applied sciences, technologies, methods of testing, etc.

In fact, dentists should have a deeper knowledge of the above to give suitable suggestions and guide the laboratory technicians to solve the technical problems related to clinical situations.

At present research and developments can be done in any field, only by a team of research workers. Without adequate knowledge of the above fields, the dentist cannot communicate the clinical problems to his fellow research workers. Perhaps due to this deficiency, research and development in dental materials are at the lowest level, compared to the other fields.

Basic sciences and technologies in recent years are advancing by leaps and bounds and vast research information are communicated to the users, almost immediately. Many research product materials with wonderful properties are entering the market. Present materials become outdated and sometimes obsolete in short times. Dentists have to continuously replenish their knowledge of the developments of materials, techniques and instrumentations to serve the patients' community more effectively.

Unfortunately, many universities and teaching institutions have not yet given the due importance to this basic subject. Very few teaching institutions in India have established separate departments for undergraduate teaching, research and guiding the postgraduate students. Even though the universities and many teaching institutions conduct the postgraduate courses in various specialities, they rarely have basic pieces of equipment required for research and testing of dental materials. In addition, there are no suitably qualified teaching staff, i.e. with postgraduate or MDS qualifications in dental materials and technologies. Perhaps due to all the above situations and deficiencies, adequate research and developments of dental materials and technologies are not progressing in our country. Most of the research papers presented in IDA conferences are related only to clinical studies and applications of dental materials.

Our colleagues, senior professors, and clinicians involved in teaching this subject to undergraduate, postgraduate students, and researchers have experienced the importance of this subject, in the course of dentistry as well as clinical practices. Many teachers also have experienced the difficulties in teaching this complicated subject, specially for undergraduates. That is why in many institutions this subject is taught part-by-part by the staff of different specialities. This prompts the teachers to overemphasize the topics of their specialization which results in imbalance and lack of coordination.

Taking undue advantage of these situations, many authors have oversimplified the subject matter by sacrificing the required scientific explanations, information, technical details and even the clinical orientations. In fact, more complicated scientific explanations and recent developments relevant to dentistry, in many fields, like composite resins, restorative cements, ceramics, metallurgy, etc. are lacking. The new editions of these books have their volumes reduced still further. This oversimplification and reduction in volume is perhaps to please the student population.

There is no clear-cut detailed syllabus. A few universities have slightly modified only a skeleton vague syllabus formed about 50 years back has been slightly modified by a few universities. The syllabus has not defined clearly the extent, details or the depths of the topics to be studied by students of undergraduate and postgraduate courses. Actually the syllabus requires a thorough revision, deleting some obsolete topics and including the modern aspects of this fast developing subject of dental materials. Unfortunately the examination question paper setters and examiners conducting viva voce or practical examinations, many times, expect the beginner students to know everything given in the reference books.

All these situations made us venture in bringing out a textbook of this type to help the students and also teachers, to limit the topics to the undergraduates. The knowledge of basic sciences, acquired by the present students admitted to the first year of BDS course, is taken as the baseline. Care is taken to strike a balance between the basic sciences, technologies and adequate orientation to the clinical applications. A slightly different approach has been adopted as explained in the introduction to dentistry.

This attempt has been made to develop a suitable standard textbook, mainly for the BDS students and also to assist the enthusiastic young teachers to limit the depth of the subject to the level of these students.

Certain topics, like materials used in orthodontia, basic metallurgy, ceramics, etc. have been dealt with slightly greater details, which may help the more intelligent undergraduate students and as an introduction to the postgraduate students of the particular specialties.

V Shama Bhat
BT Nandish

Acknowledgements

This is a copolymerized work of the long experience in teaching the entire syllabus to the undergraduate and postgraduate courses, research publications since 1976 and deep involvements in the new two-year MSc course in dental materials in 1999 at Manipal University. We must acknowledge the persons involved directly or indirectly for their valuable suggestions and encouragements in bringing out the first edition in 2006, second edition in 2013 and as well as Third Edition in 2019 this textbook *Science of Dental Materials with Clinical Applications*. This is a challenging project as the subject is very highly cross-linked by interaction with basic sciences, technologies and dental specialties.

Dr BH Sripathi Rao, Principal, and Professor and Head, Department of Maxillofacial Surgery, earlier Executive Council Member of Dental Council of India and former Vice-Chancellor of Yenepoya (Deemed to be University), was the main initiator. Dr KS Bhat, ex-Dean, CODS, Manipal, who established the separate department of dental materials in 1999, has given us continuous support and suggestions.

Our Respected Chancellor Al Haz Abdulla Kunhi, Dynamic Vice-Chancellor Dr Vijaya Kumar, Late Mr PCM Kunhi, HODs of all dental specialities is our sources of inspirations for us.

Our special thanks to our faculty Mrs Soumya Rao K, Assistant Professor, for her unforgettable help in preparation of this Third Edition, as well as a handbook of Dental Materials (MCQs, viva voce, and spotters).

We wish to place on record our sincere thanks to Mr SK Jain, CMD, and Mr YN Arjuna, SENIOR VICE President—Publishing, Editorial and Publicity, CBS Publishers & Distributors in preparing and setting of the first, second and now for 3rd edition. Our heartfelt thanks go to Dr Hema Nandish and extraordinarily abled musician Miss Manipal Aruna Kumari and late Mrs Hemavathi S Bhat who have helped in releasing our internal stresses by their encouragements.

V Shama Bhat
BT Nandish
Jayaprakash K

Contents

CHAPTER 2: GENERAL PROPERTIES OF MATTER

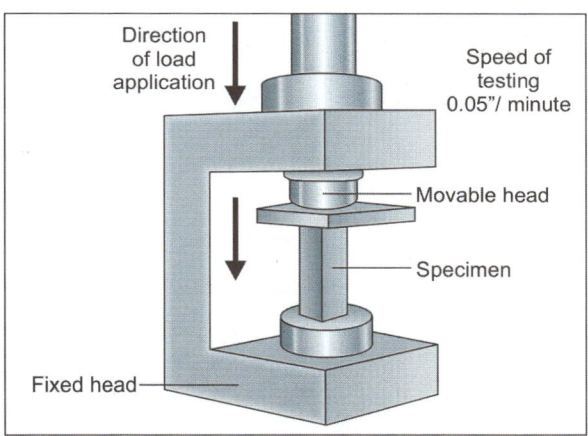

Fig. 2.1: Compression testing

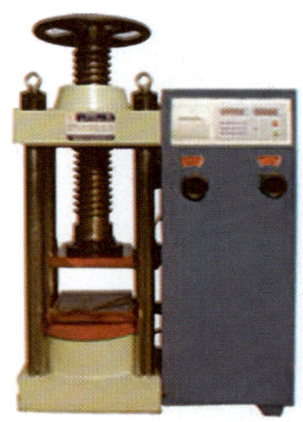

Fig. 2.2: Compression tester

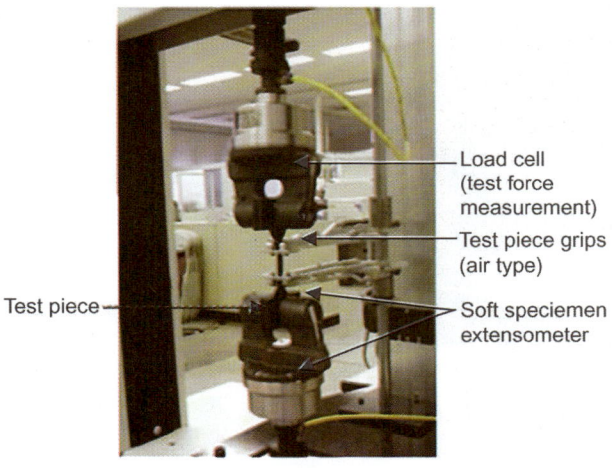

Fig. 2.3: Tension tester

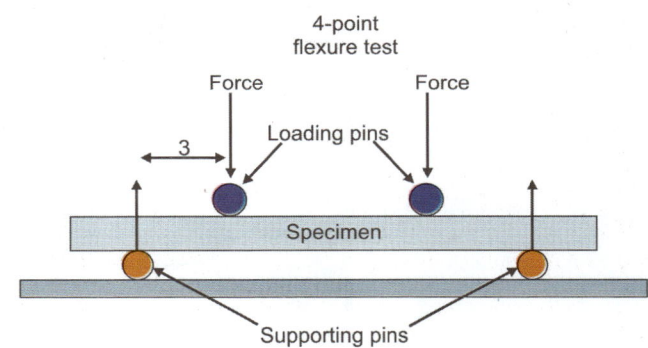

Fig. 2.4: Four-point bending test

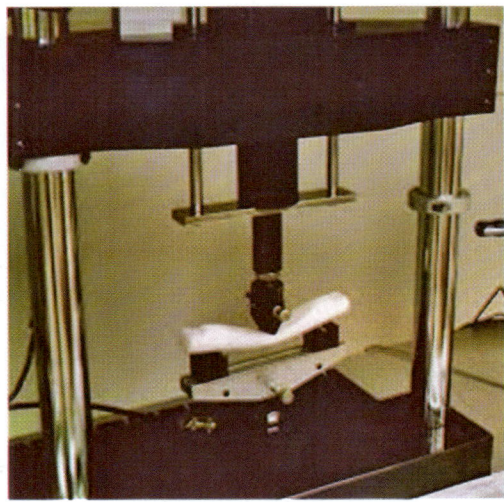

Fig. 2.5: Three-point bending tester

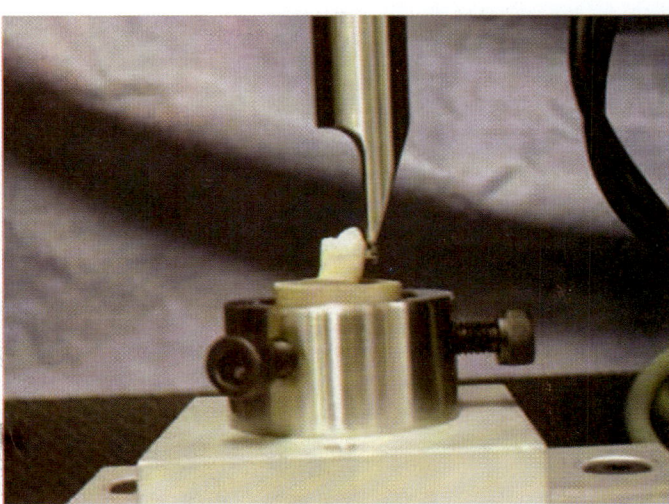

Fig. 2.6: Shear-bond strength

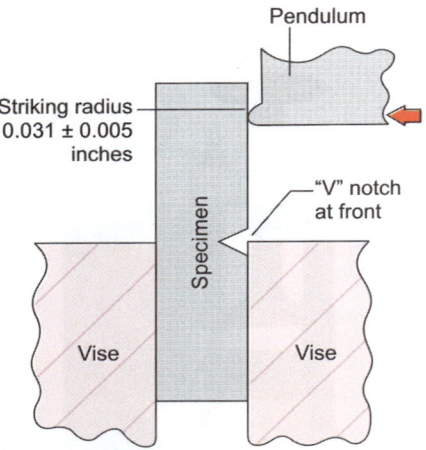

Fig. 2.7: IZOD impact test sample

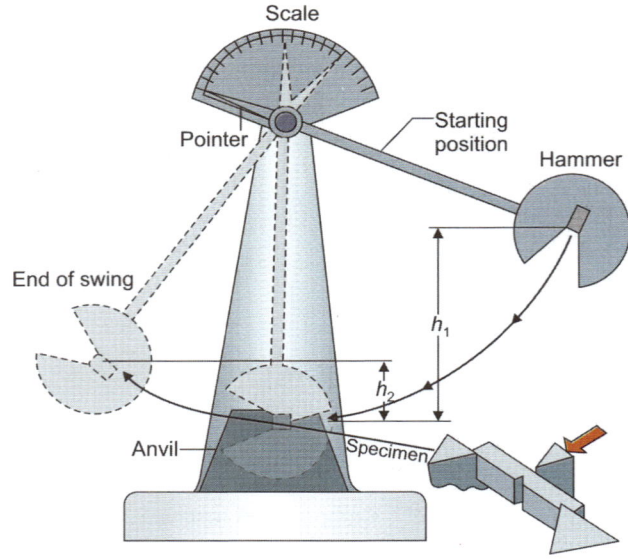

Fig. 2.8: Impact strength tester

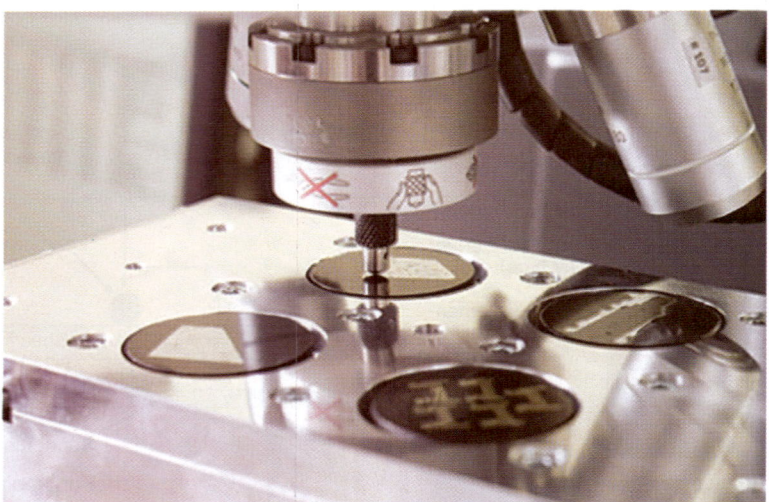

Fig. 2.9: Vicker's hardness tester

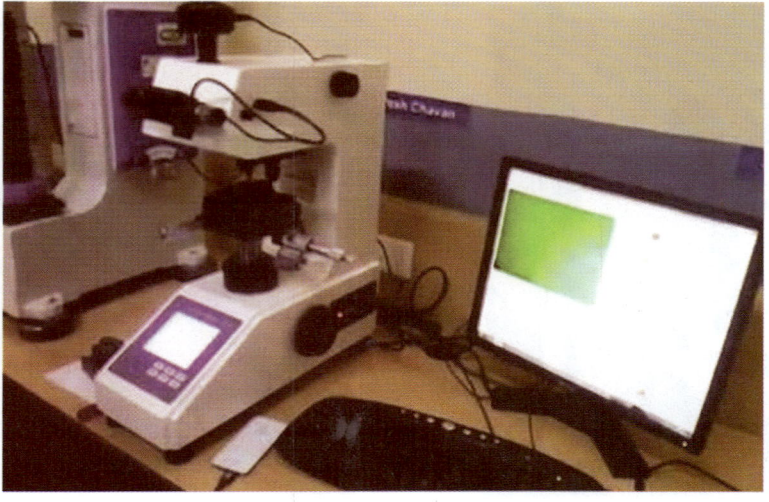

Fig. 2.10: Knoop's hardness test

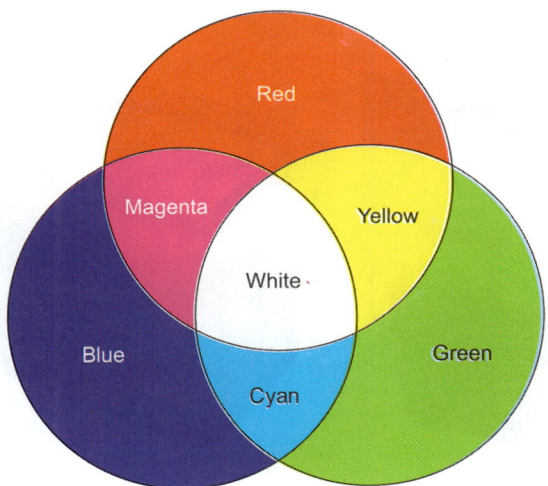

Fig. 2.11: Basic colour additions

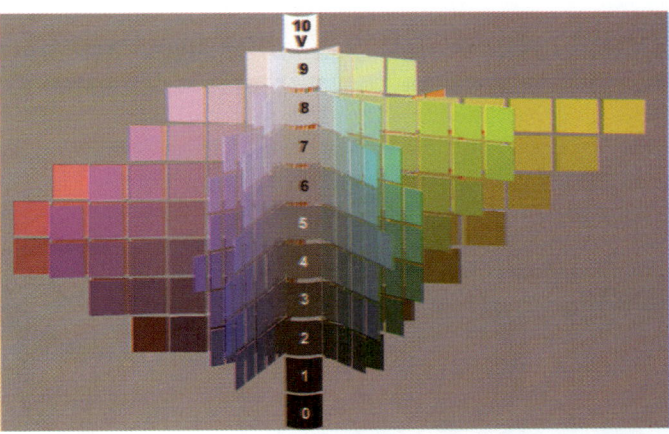

Fig. 2.13: Hue-chroma—values

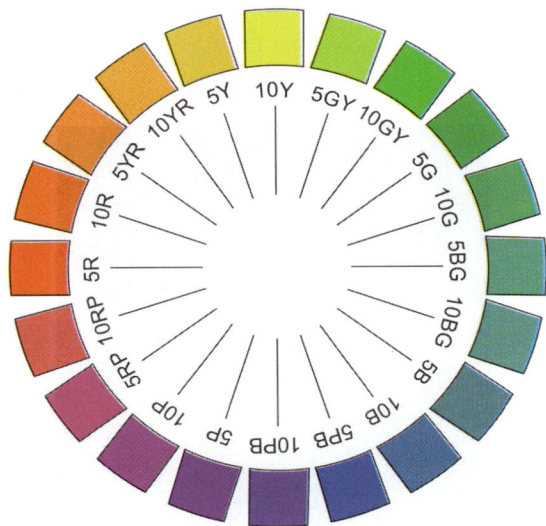

Fig. 2.12: Colour parameter—hue

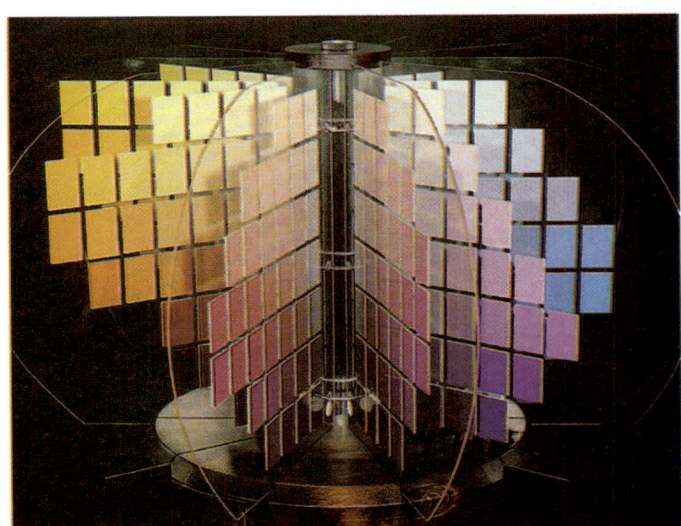

Fig. 2.14: Munsell's colour tree

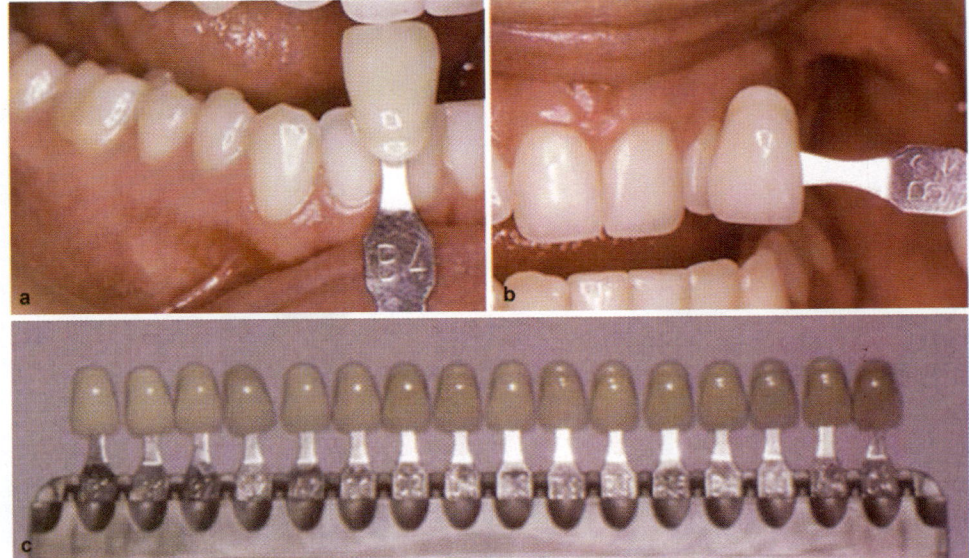

Fig. 2.15: Colour matching, selection, shade guide

CHAPTER 3: IMPRESSION MATERIALS (AUXILIARY MATERIALS)

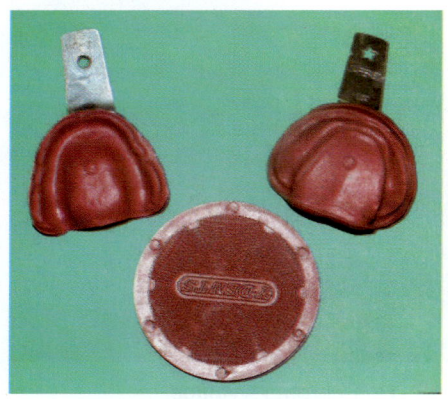

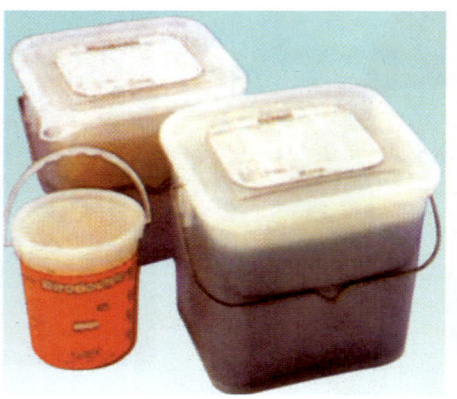

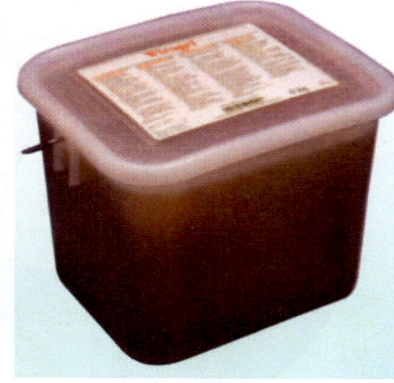

Fig. 3.1: Preliminary impression with impression compound

Fig. 3.2: Agar-agar duplicating materials

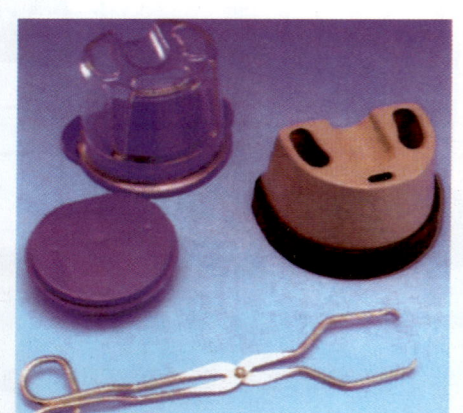

Fig. 3.3a: Agar-agar duplicating flasks

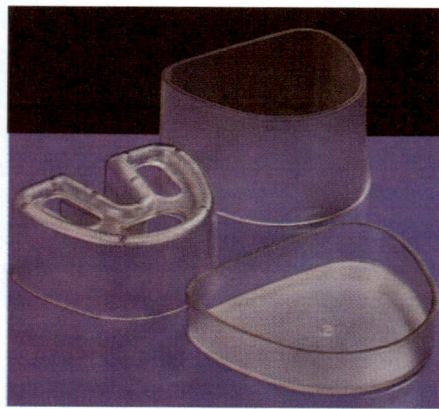

Fig. 3.3b: Silicone duplicating flasks

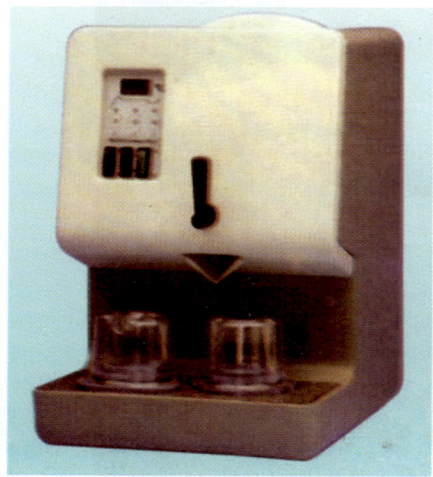

Fig. 3.4a: Agar-agar duplicating unit

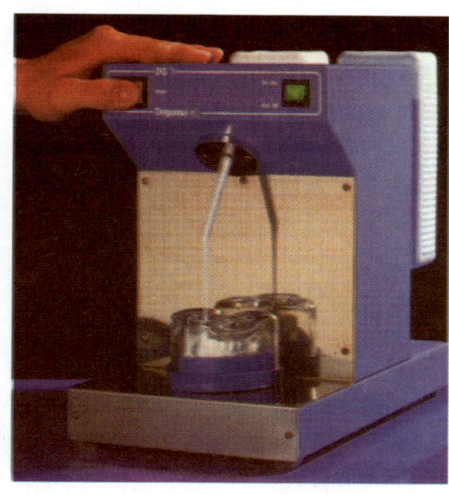

Fig. 3.4b: Silicone duplicating unit

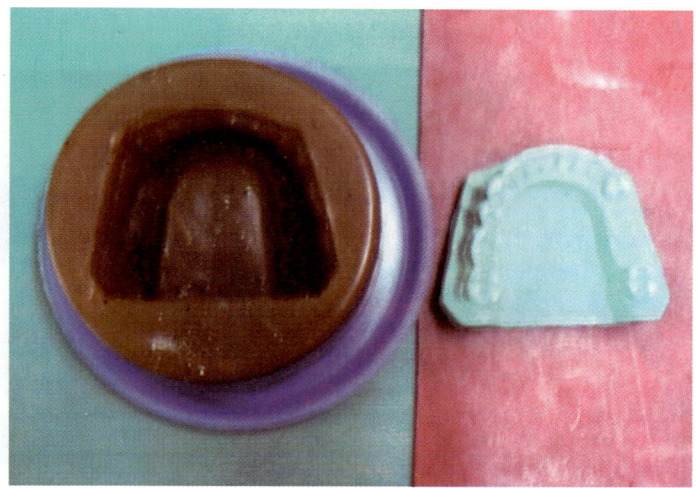

Fig. 3.5: Duplication and cast

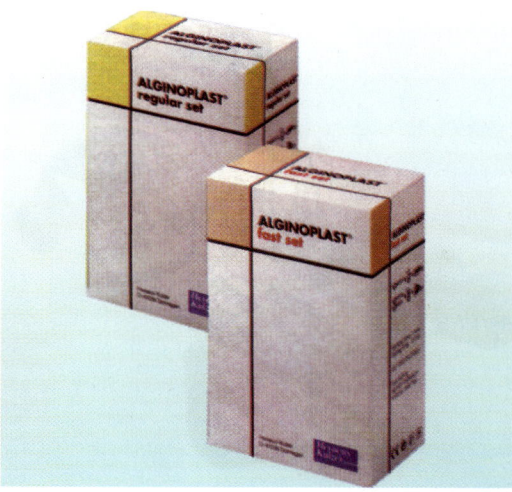

Fig. 3.6: Dust-free alginate

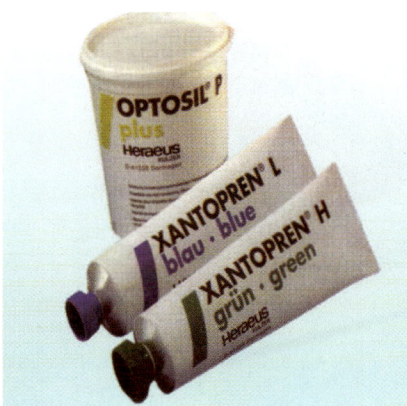

Fig. 3.7a: Condensation polysilicone

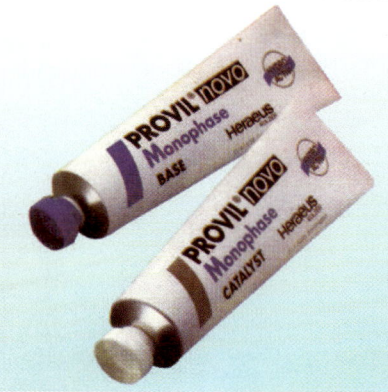

Fig. 3.7b: Addition polysilicone—monophase

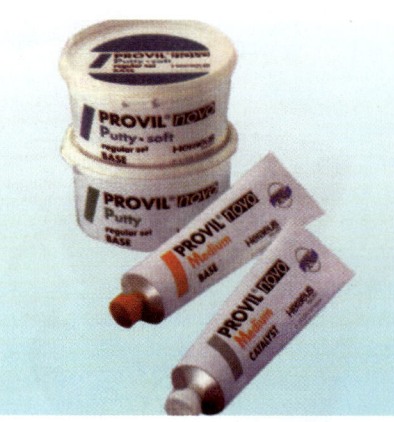

Fig. 3.7c: Addition polysilicone—putty and medium viscosity

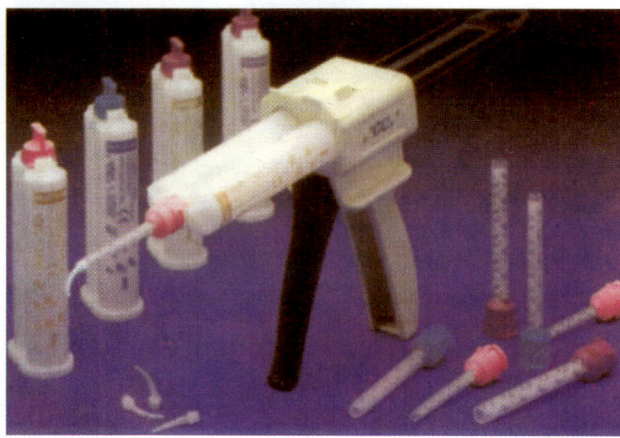

Fig. 3.7d: Elastomer–automixer

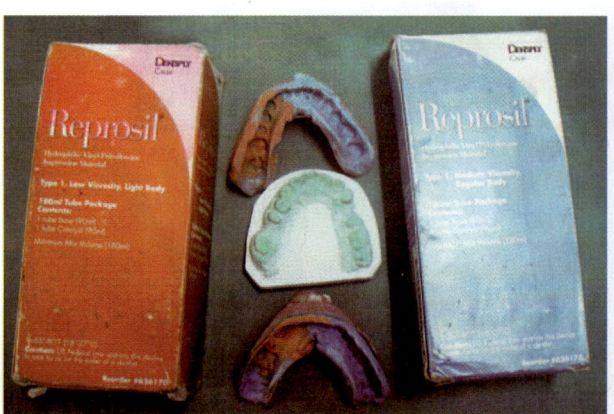

Fig. 3.8: Syringe and medium viscosity double mix—single impression and cast

Polysilicone—putty wash two-step impression technique

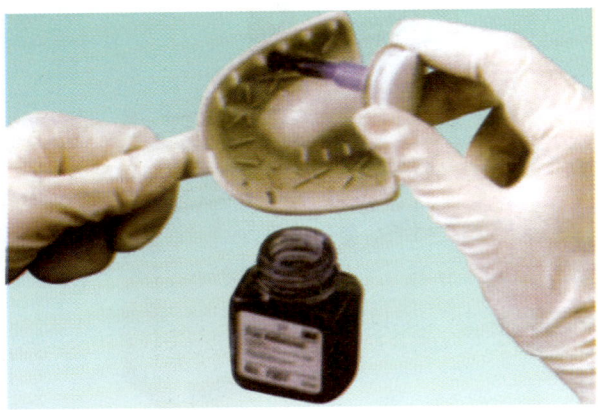

Fig. 3.9a: Apply tray adhesive, allow to dry

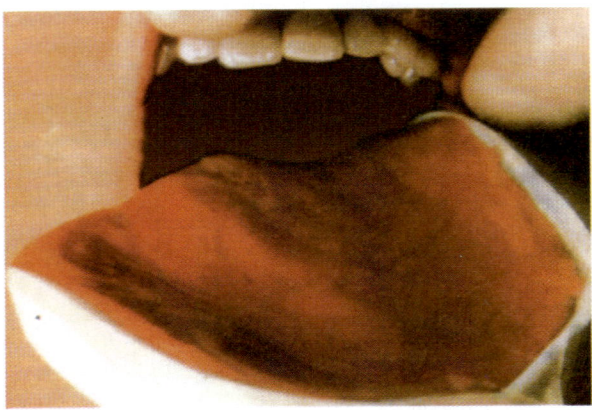

Fig. 3.9b: Needed putty, seated with spacer—preliminary impression

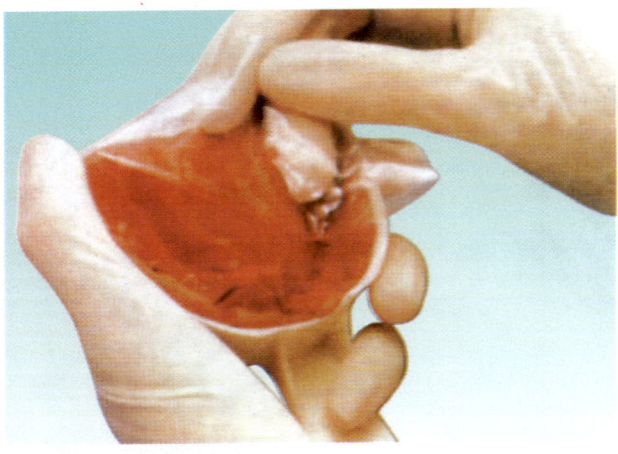

Fig. 3.9c: After setting, remove spacer

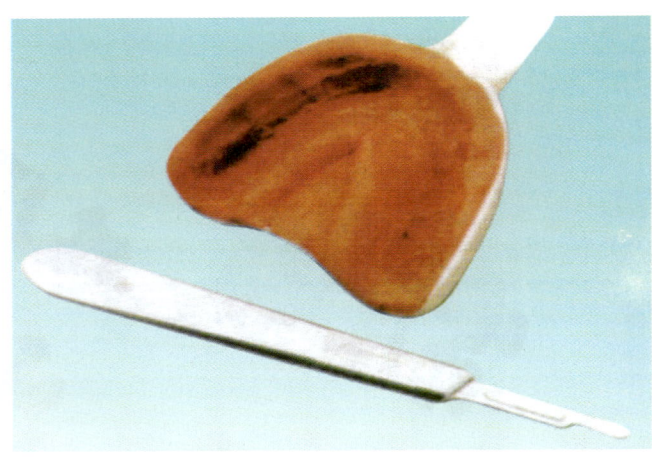

Fig. 3.9d: Provide relief space if required

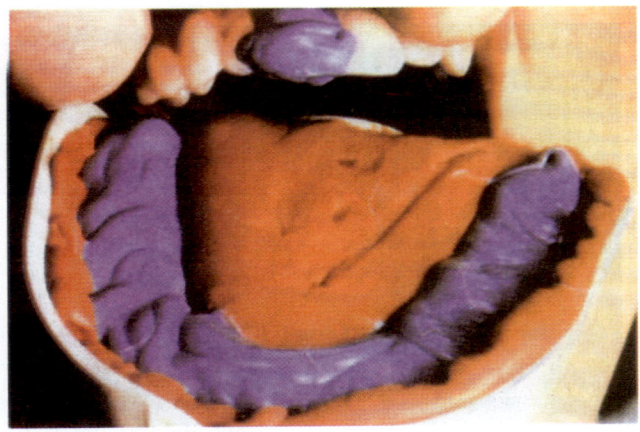

Fig. 3.9e: Load part of syringed material on the tray and apply on teeth

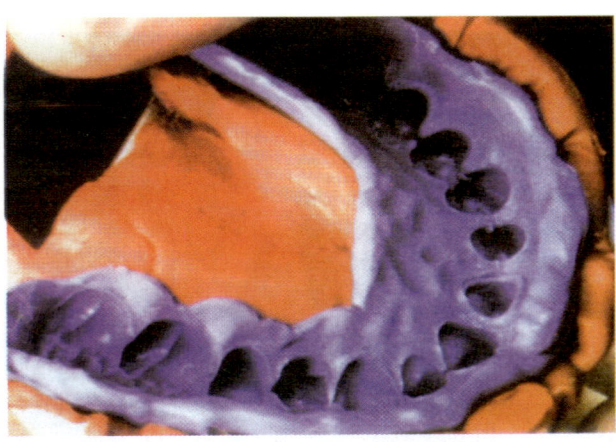

Fig. 3.9f: Final impression

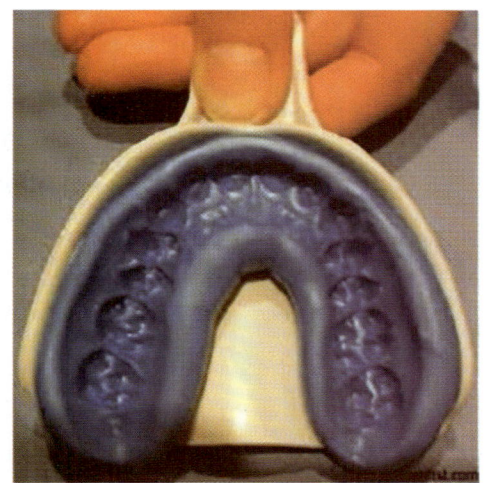

Fig. 3.10: Single elastomer impression

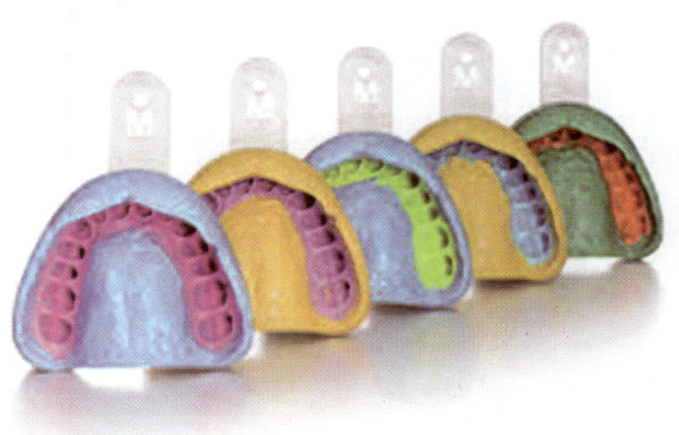

Fig. 3.11: Multiple mix techniques

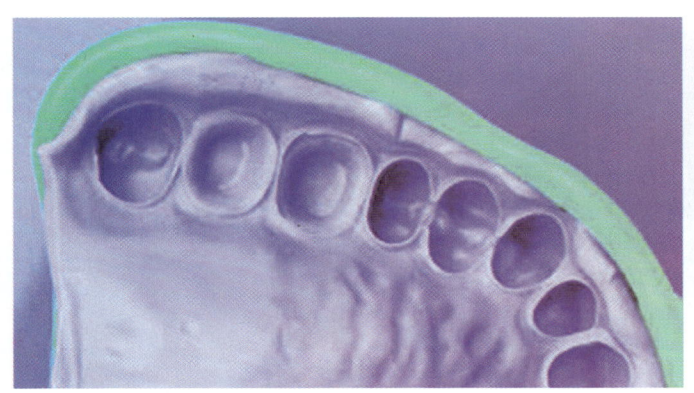

Fig. 3.12: Elastomer part impression

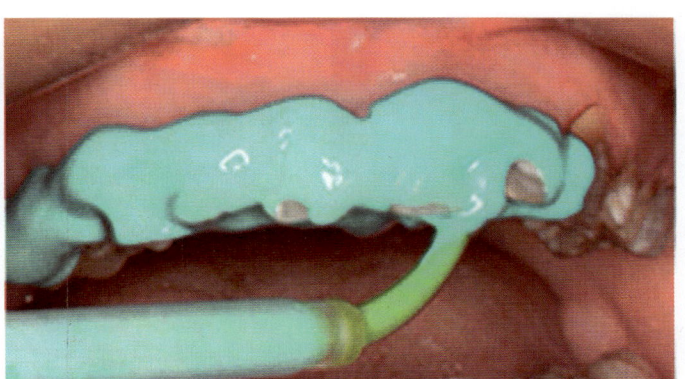

Fig. 3.13: Syringed light body elastomer

CHAPTER 4: GYPSUM PRODUCTS: CAST AND DIE MATERIALS (AUXILIARY MATERIALS)

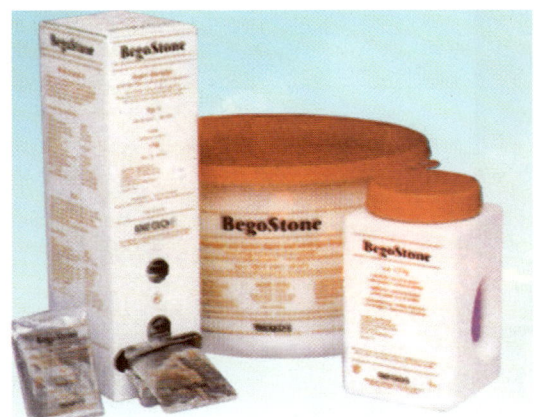

Fig. 4.1: Type IV die stone (NSE = .09%)

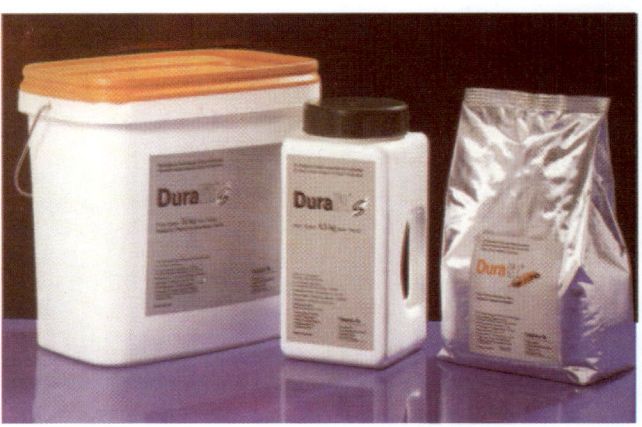

Fig. 4.2: Synthetic gypsum product

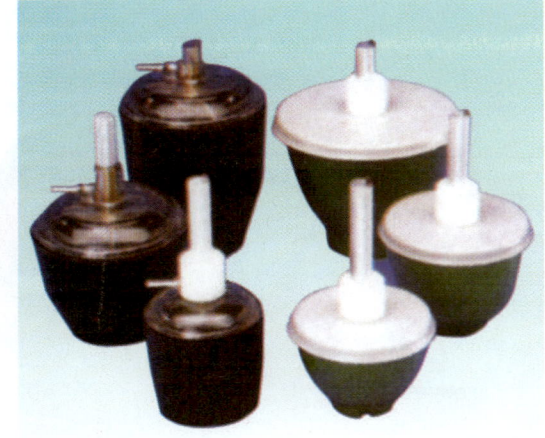

Fig. 4.3a: Vacuum mixer bowls

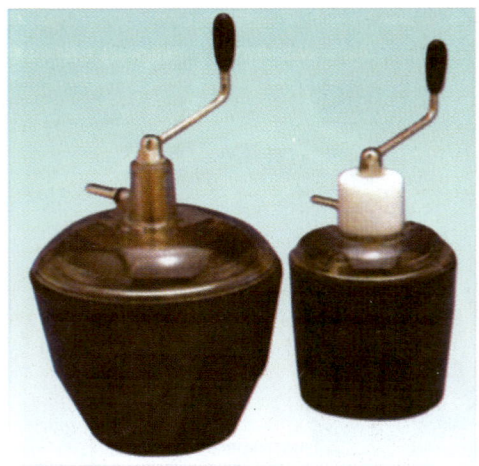

Fig. 4.3b: Vacuum hand mixer

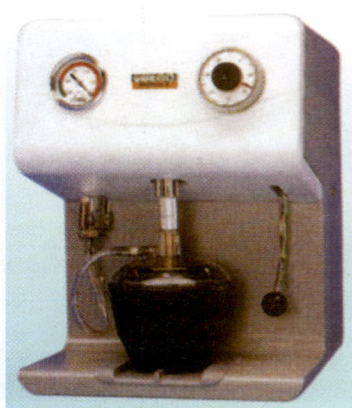

Fig. 4.4: Vacuum electrical mixer with timer, speed controls

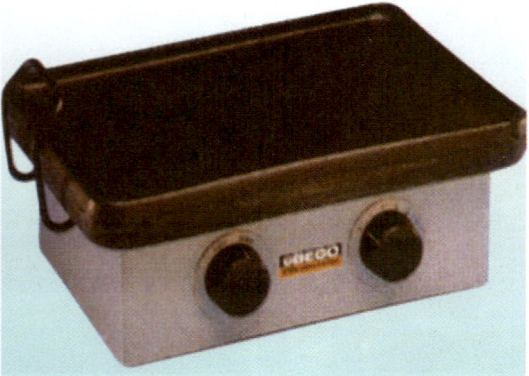

Fig. 4.5: Vibrator

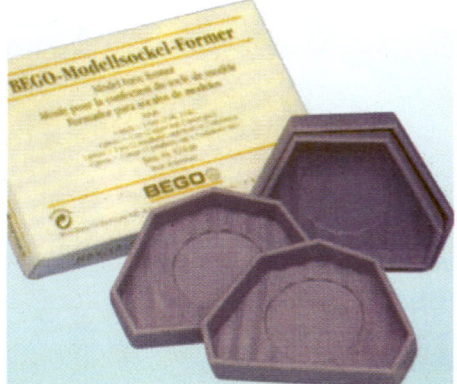

Fig. 4.6: Cast-base former moulds

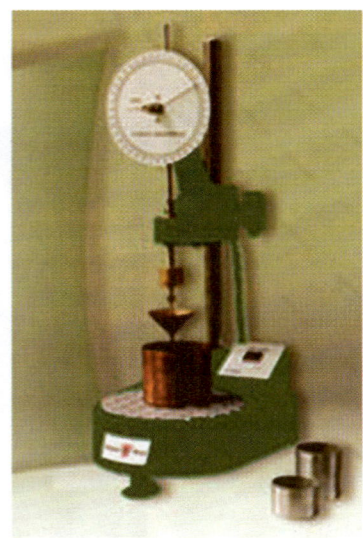

Fig. 4.7: Vicat penetrometer 300 gm wt., 1 mm needle diameter

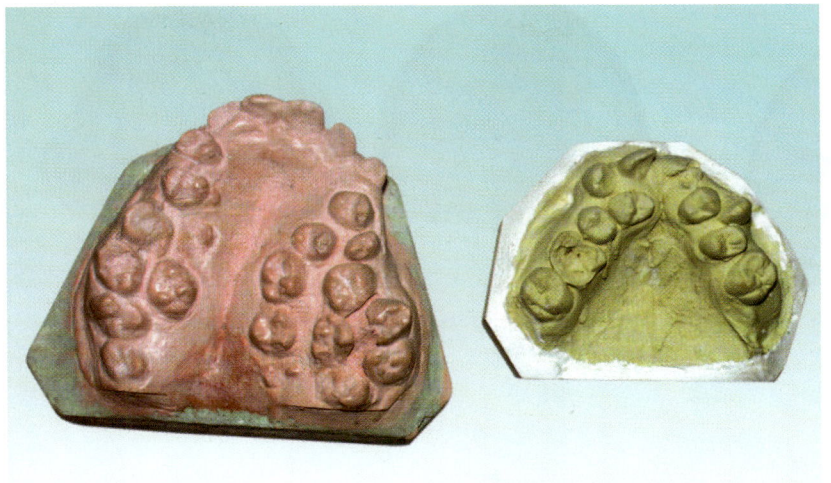

Fig. 4.8: Supernumerary teeth (peculiar cases)

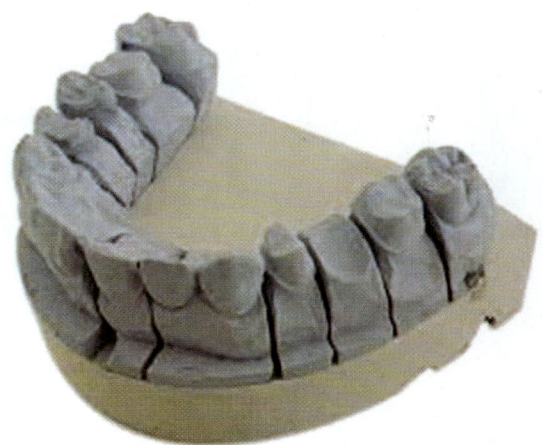

Fig. 4.9: Stone-die preparation

CHAPTER 6: PROSTHETIC APPLICATIONS OF POLYMER RESINS

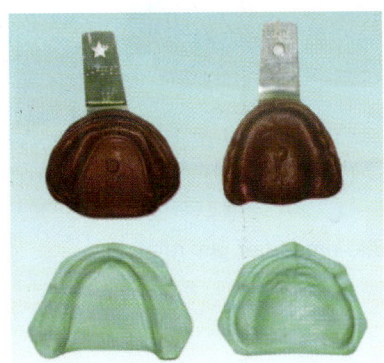

Fig. 6.1: Preliminary impression and casts

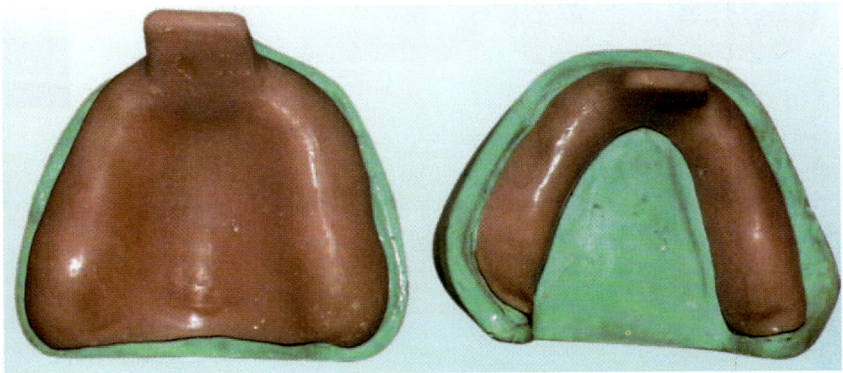

Fig. 6.2: Acrylic special trays

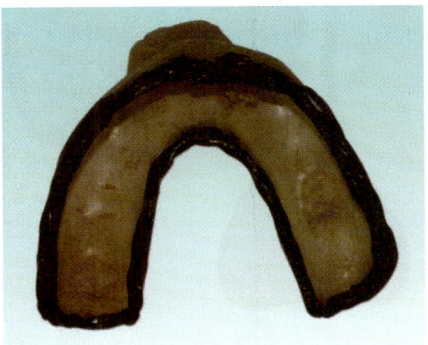

Fig. 6.3: Border moulding—tracing

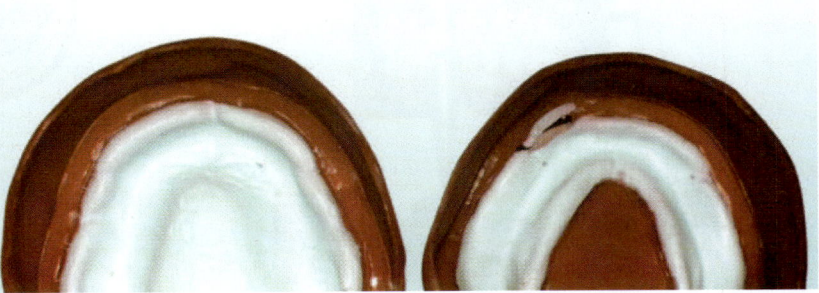

Fig. 6.4: ZnOE wash impression and boxing

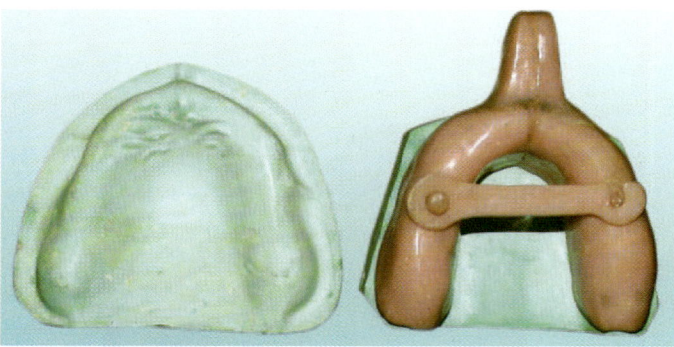

Fig. 6.5: Split cast and split tray

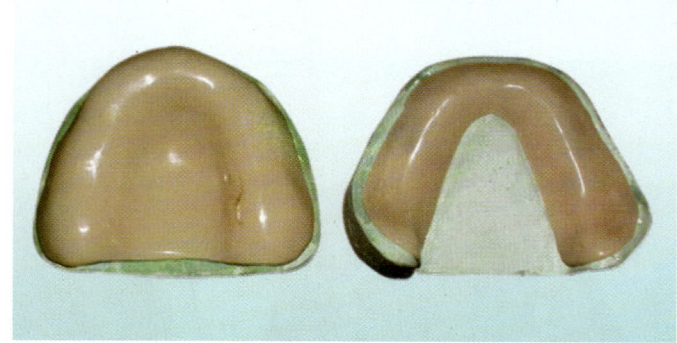

Fig. 6.6: Acrylic record bases

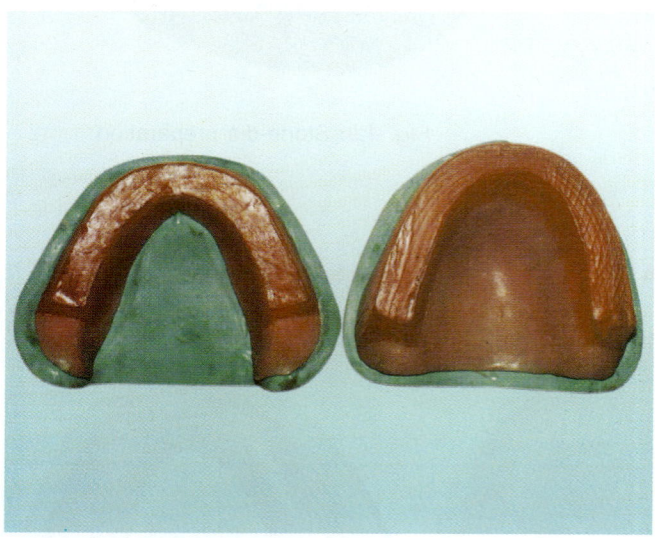

Fig. 6.7: Wax occlusal rims

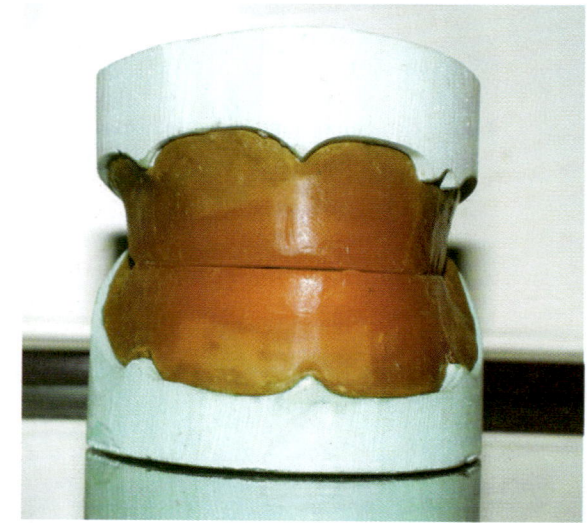

Fig. 6.8: Bite rims after jaw relating

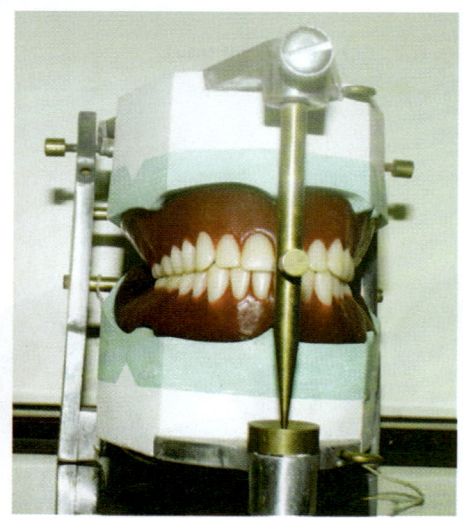

Fig. 6.9: Articulation and teeth setting

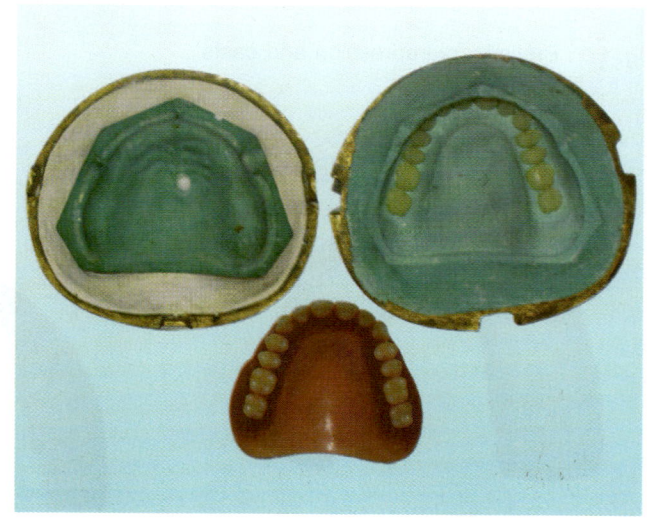

Fig. 6.10: Flasking and dewaxing

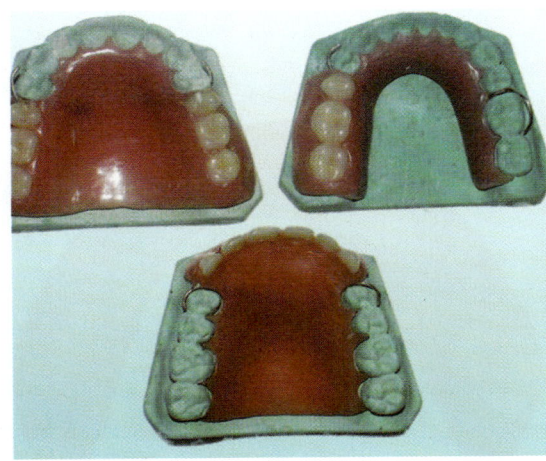

Fig. 6.11: Finished partial dentures

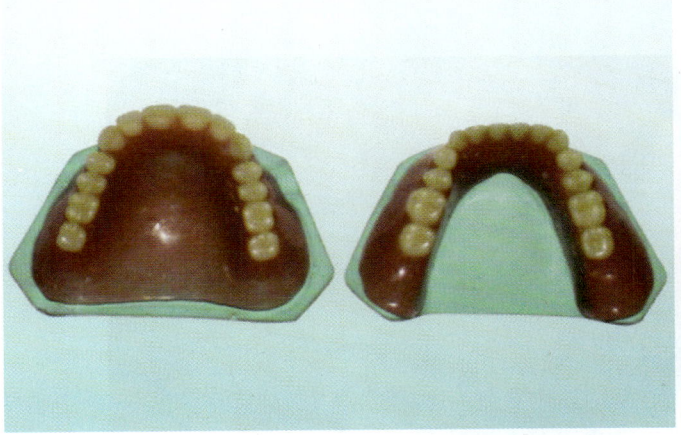

Fig. 6.12: Finished complete dentures

Injection moulding technique

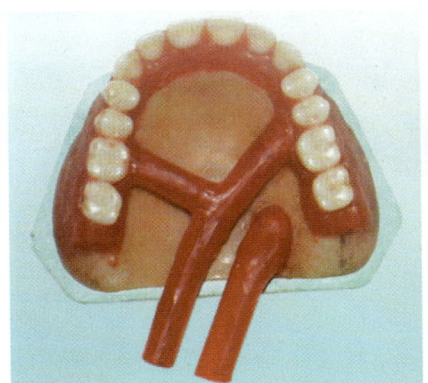

Fig. 6.13: Sprue fitting

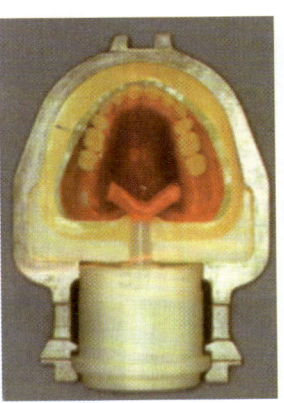

Fig. 6.14: Flasking

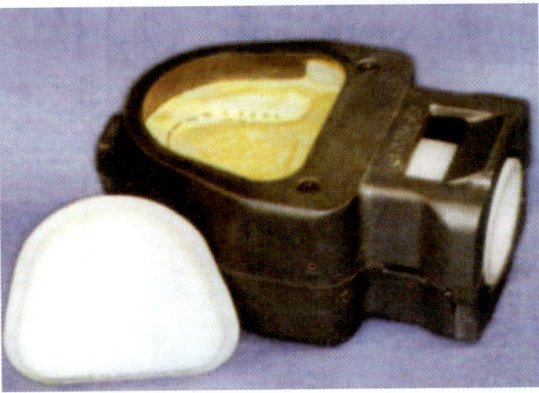

Fig. 6.15: Exposing teeth

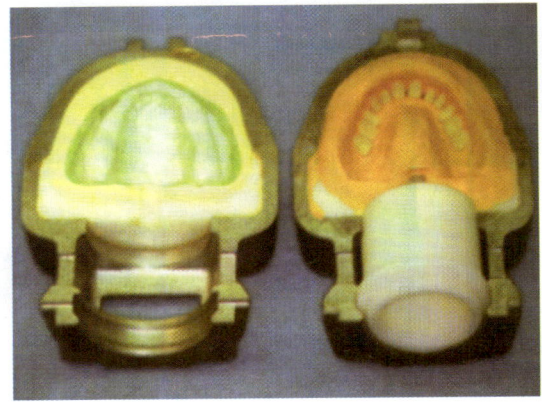

Fig. 6.16: Two halves after dewaxing

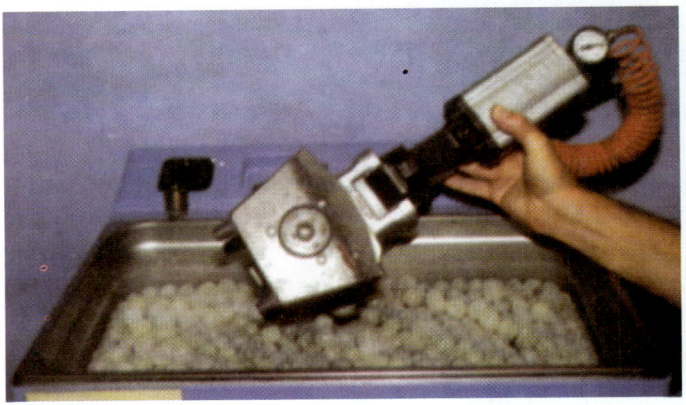

Fig. 6.17: Injecting resin dough and then curing

Figures 6.18a to j: Denture relining steps

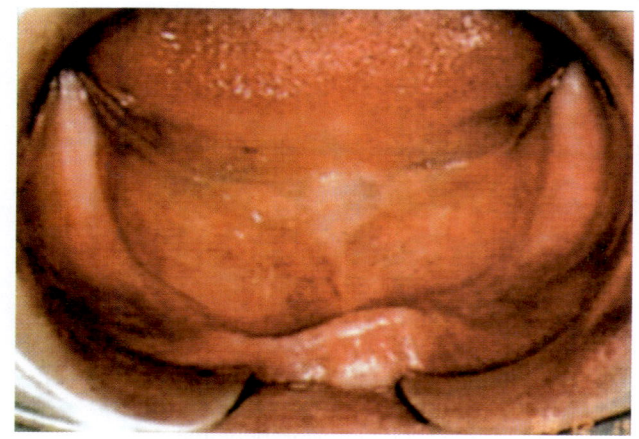

Fig. 6.18a: Resorption and clinical condition requiring soft reliner

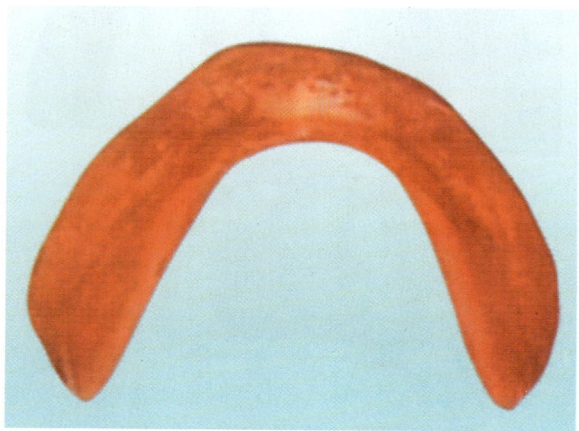

Fig. 6.18b: Denture surface before relining

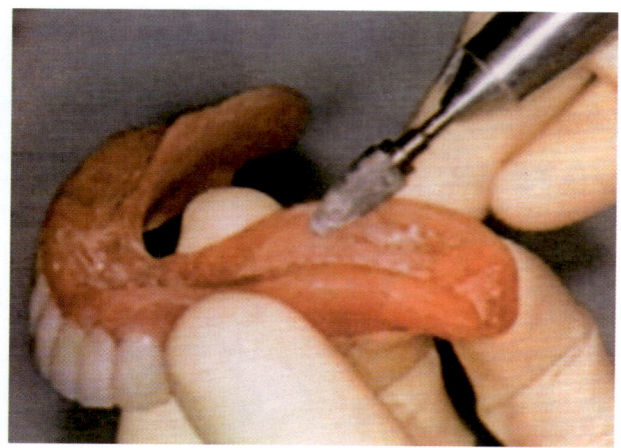

Fig. 6.18c: Relief area for relining

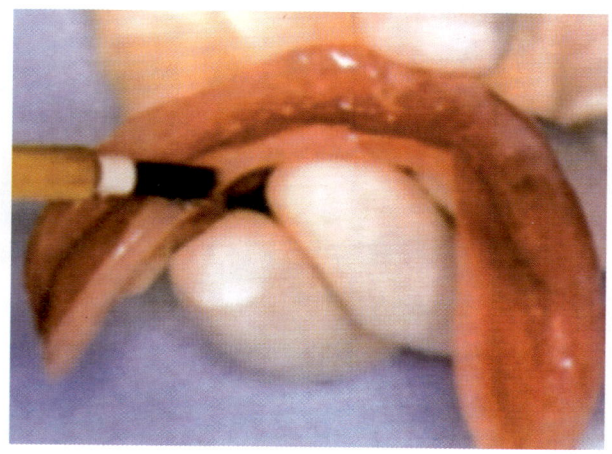

Fig. 6.18d: Application of reline primer

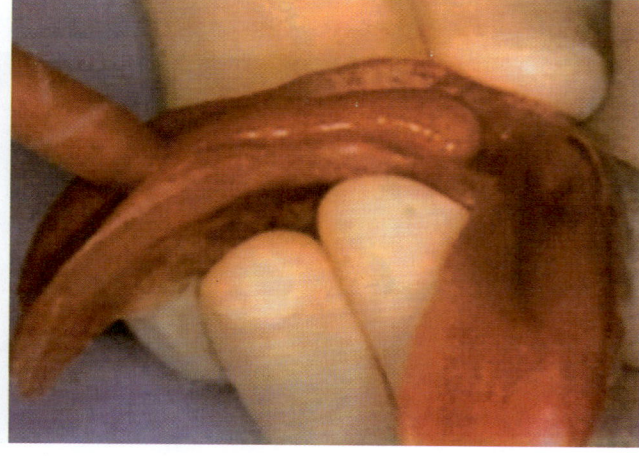

Fig. 6.18e: Applying reliner

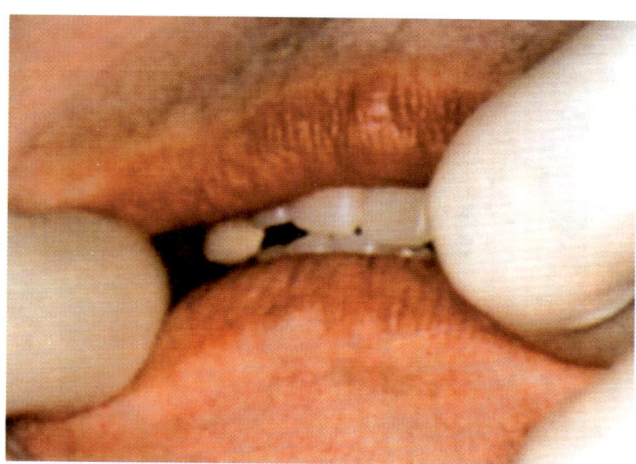

Fig. 6.18f: Seating in the mouth

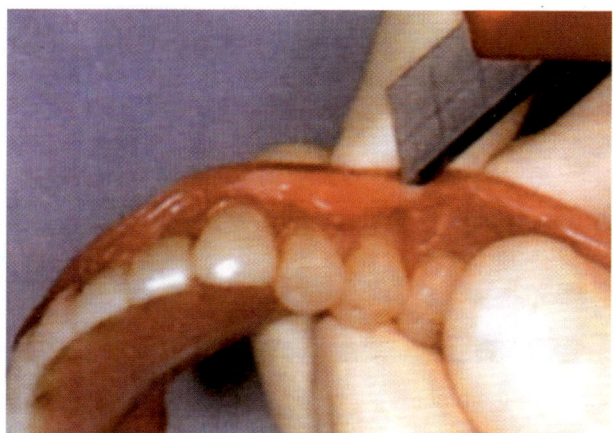

Fig. 6.18g: Trimming the excess

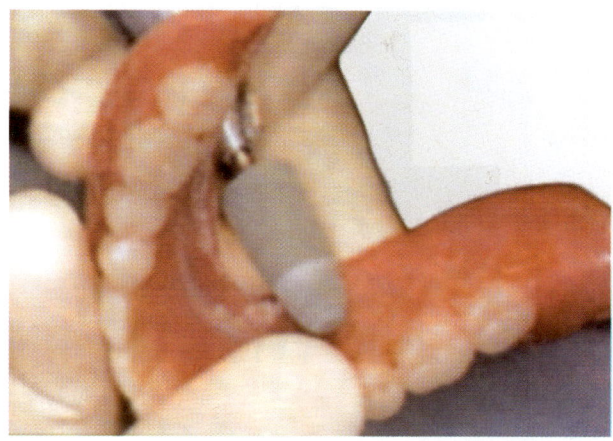

Fig. 6.18h: Finishing with silicone point (10,000 rpm)

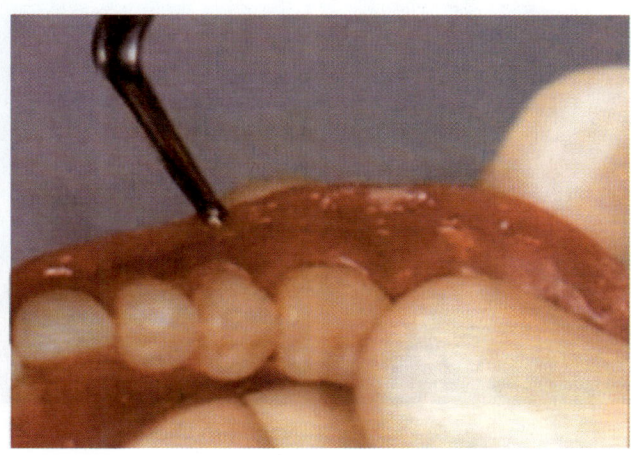

Fig. 6.18i: Final modification for smoothness

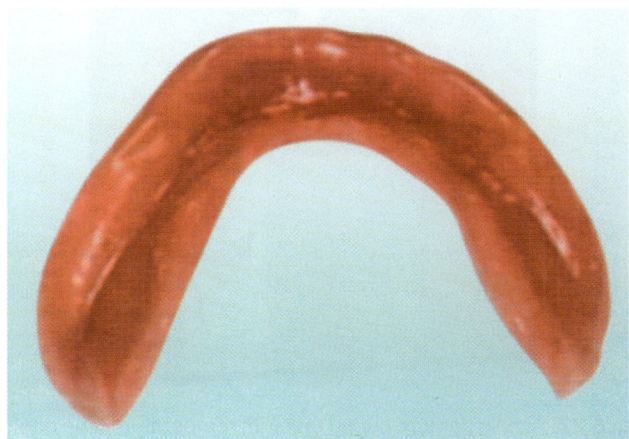

Fig. 6.18j: Finished relined denture

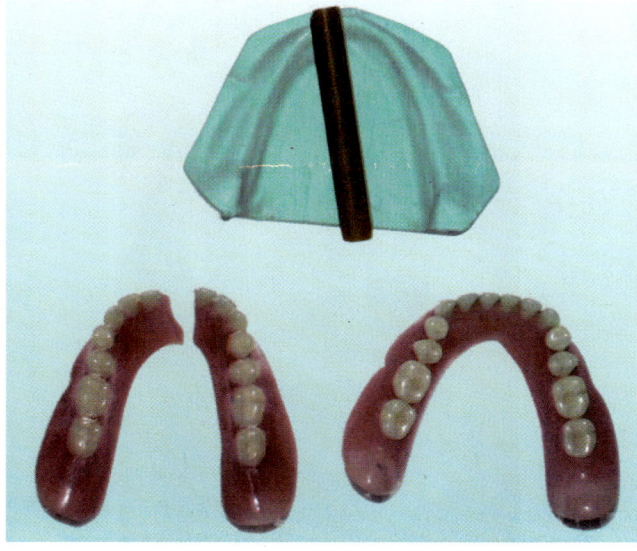

Fig. 6.19: Denture repair with sticky wax and cast

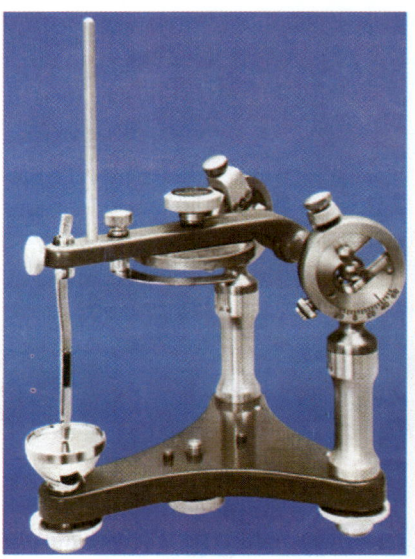

Fig. 6.20: Type ARH articulator

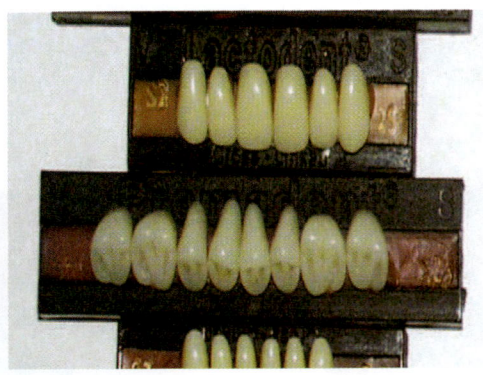
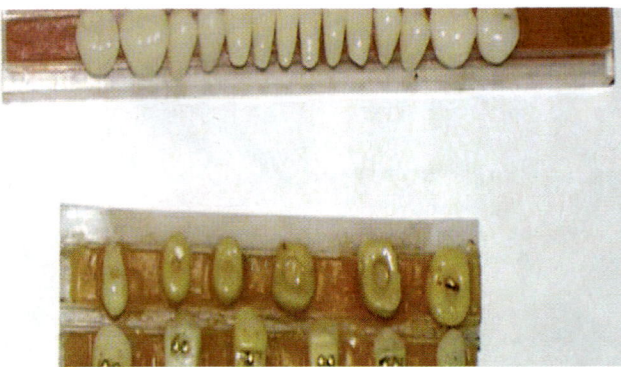

Fig. 6.21: Acrylic teeth and porcelain teeth sets

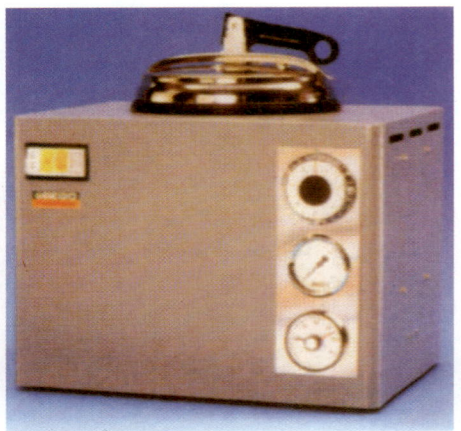

Fig. 6.22: Acrylic denture curing unit with temperature time controls

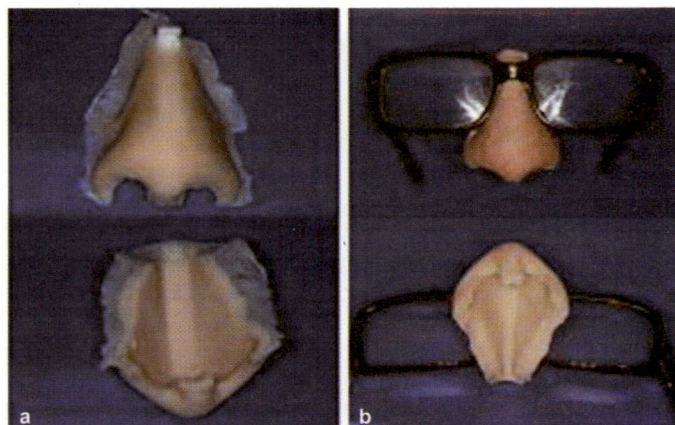

Figs 6.23a and b: Nose prosthesis

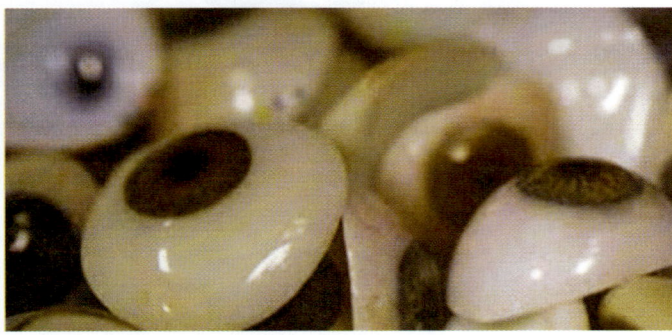

Fig. 6.24: Eye prosthesis

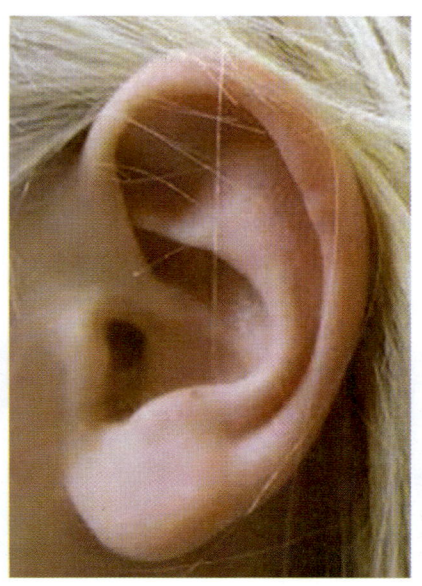

Fig. 6.25: Ear prosthesis

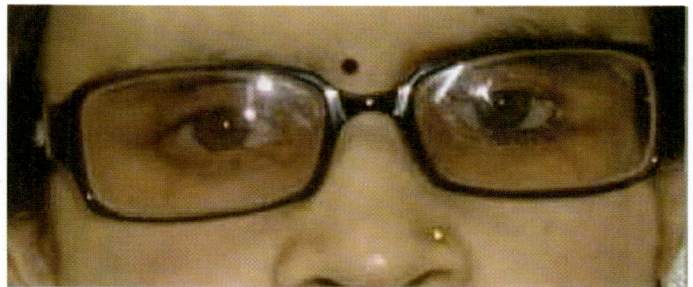

Fig. 6.26: Spectacle mounted prosthesis

CHAPTER 8: RESTORATIVE MATERIALS: DENTAL CEMENTS

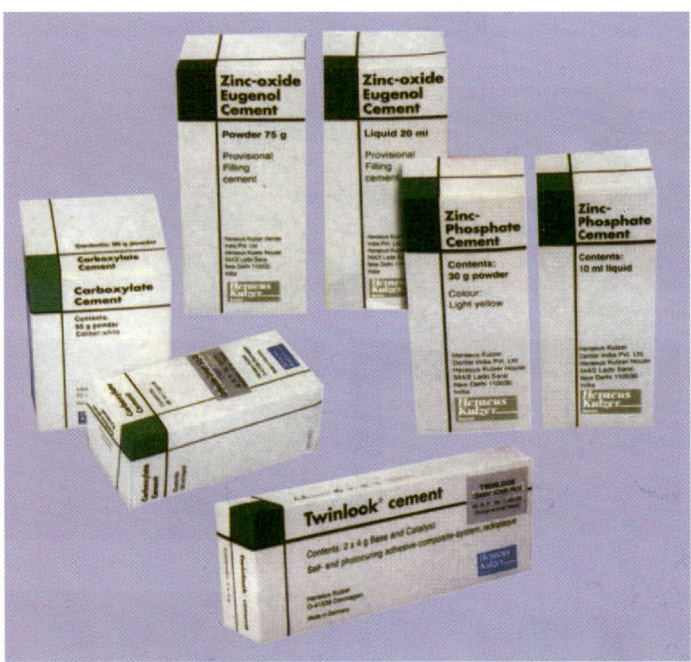

Fig. 8.1: ZnOE, ZnPO$_4$, zinc polycarboxylate cement

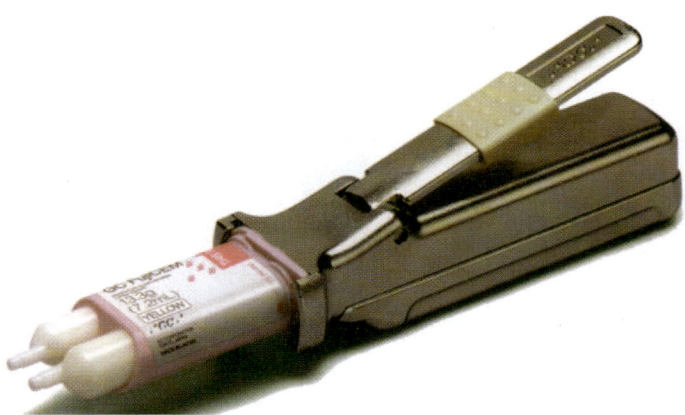

Fig. 8.2: GIC paste dispenser

Figure 8.3: Full range of glass ionomer cements

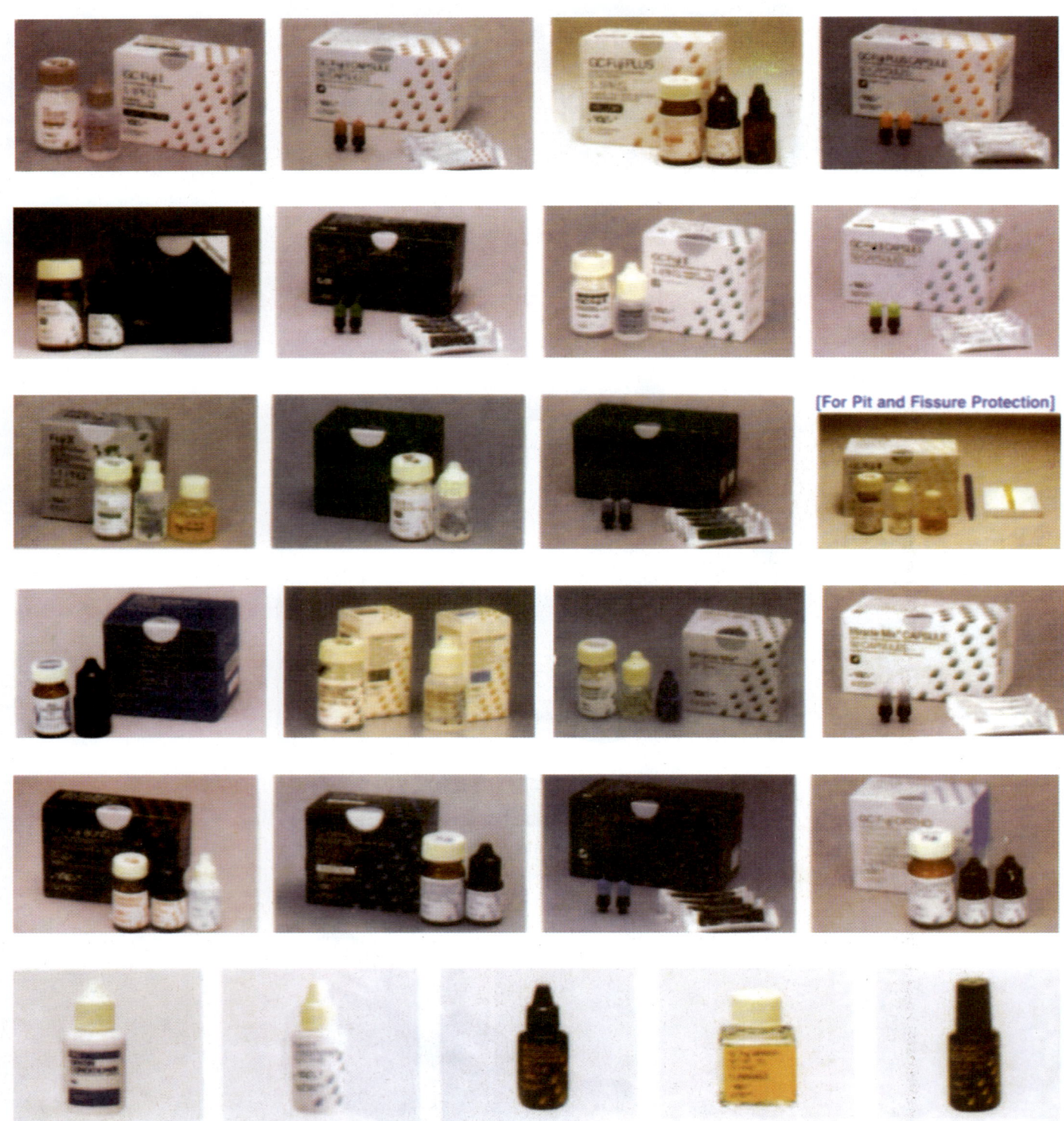

Fig. 8.3: Glass ionomer cement full range

CHAPTER 1

Orientation to Dental Science

CHAPTER SURVEY

- History of dentistry
- Introduction
- Special approaches
- Orientation to dentistry
- Oral environments
- Structure of tooth
- Properties of tooth
- Conservative dentistry

- Loss of tooth materials
- Stages of tooth decay
- Classification of cavities
- Conservative methods
- Specialities in dentistry
- Numerical values
- ADA specifications
- ADA acceptance programme
- Unique learning laboratory

HISTORY OF DENTISTRY

This is closely connected with the discoveries, innovations and applications of materials used in dentistry in fabrications of oral appliances as well as clinical treatments. Many dental materials with various desired wonderful properties have been formulated recently since the latter part of 19th century. This is due to the rapid advances in various basic sciences and technologies such as physics, chemistry, engineering, metallurgy (castings), resins, ceramics, information media, etc. during this period. The interactions of these areas with biological sciences lead to tremendous progress in dentistry.

PRE-HISTORIC PERIOD

Dental treatments or dentistry has the origin of toothache. All the cultures of the world believed that the toothaches were caused by tooth demons (tooth worms) or unbalanced body fluids. Due to lack of documentation, it is quite difficult to trace the growth of dentistry in the pre-historic period. However, a little information is available from the remnants of the human bodies, by determining their age by carbon dating, etc. procedures. In the earliest period, 4000–5000 years BC, few herbs, clay, etc. were used to relieve the pain. Later few instances of using gold and gold wires for restorations were noticed around 2500 years BC. Ancient Babylonians, Egyptians, Assyrians, etc. were familiar with few metals like gold, silver, copper, lead, tin, etc. and few of their alloys such as bronze. They also knew some metallurgy, alloying, drawing into wire, soldering, cutting, etc. They must have tried these for dental treatments.

MEDIEVAL PERIOD

Historians could not get more detailed information and perhaps there was no much progress in sciences up to the 15th and 16th centuries after Christianity. Dental treatments were conducted by skilled artisans, barbers, priests, painters, ceramists, metallurgists (goldsmiths), etc. Carious teeth were filled with ground mastic, alum and honey. Clove oil (eugenol) was discovered in India (1580). The discoveries, developments, and innovations were systematically documented since the 17th century onwards. However, the progress was very slow until the year 1840.

Pierre Fauchard (1678–1761) considered as the father of modern dentistry, had used lead cylinders, tin foil, etc. for a tooth filling. Agate, silver, gold, etc. were also used. He published in 1978, the first treatise describing many types of restoration, ivory artificial dentures, etc.

An interesting historical episode of denture is that of one worn by George Washington (1732–1799), the first president of United States of America. The denture base was carved by Dr John Greenwood (jr) from the hippopotamus tusk, and the teeth were from ivory and some of his mouth. This denture was very ill-fitting and gave terrible pain throughout his life.

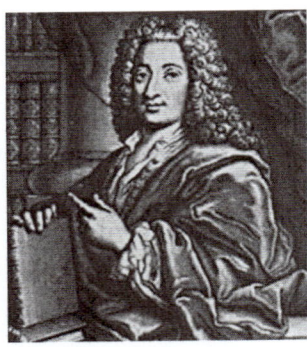

Pierre Fauchard, "Father of Modern Dentistry"

Silver coin triturated with mercury was tried by Taveau in 1816. However, dentists were scared of mercury health hazard, and there was an amalgam war from 1840 to 1850. Quality of silver alloys was slowly improved and finally it was GV Black in 1895 who formulated the standard present silver, tin copper amalgam alloys.

Gold foils were used by Pfaff in Germany to cap the pulp, and it was Arculanus (1848) who used direct filling gold restorations for the first time. The cohesive gold foils were developed by Arthur in 1855.

Pfaff in Germany (1756) described the method of recording the impression of edentulous arches with soft waxes and preparing the hard casts using plaster of Paris. Italian dentist Fronze in 1808 prepared porcelain denture base and porcelain artificial teeth of many shades. SS White dental manufacturing company started producing porcelain teeth and many dental materials like vulcanite denture base material, etc. around 1850s.

PROGRESS OF DENTISTRY SINCE 1840–1900

During the period 1840–1890 there was tremendous progress in many areas of basic sciences and technologies. Many of the present day major dental materials, fabrication technologies and clinical treatments were introduced during this time. For example, denture base material like vulcanite, rubber, bakelite, cellulose, restorative materials like zinc oxide eugenol, gutta-percha, zinc phosphate, silicate cement, ceramic teeth, standardized silver amalgam, etc. entered the field of dentistry. GV Black who formulated the silver amalgam alloys, knew almost all the phases of dentistry at that time.

Many dental journals were published and many dental associations were formed in United States and western countries. World's first dental college "Baltimore College of Dental Surgery" began in the year 1840 offering one year course leading to DDS (doctor of dental surgery). A group of dentists of United States, started American Dental Association (ADA) in 1859, but this began regular functioning only in 1992.

DEVELOPMENTS SINCE 20TH CENTURY

All the sophisticated restorative materials like elastic impression materials, elastomers, acrylic resins, composite resins, glass ionomer cement, etc. were developed and improved in 20th century. Also sophisticated technologies like a lost wax casting procedures, noble metal and predominantly base metal alloys, improvements in casting procedures, CAD-CAM techniques, abrasive and polishing methods, etc. were 20th century contributions. Similarly, clinical treatment techniques, various specialities of dentistry, implantology, etc. were developed in the later half of 20th century.

Selection of materials was done in the earlier periods according to their mechanical properties (resistance to fractures). Later more importance was given to aesthetic considerations. Since about 40–50 years, biological considerations were given the highest importance. Hence now we can consider dental materials as dental biomaterials.

Many dental associations like American Dental Association (ADA), British, Indian, Australian, French, Italian, as well the International Standard Organizations (ISO) are doing their best to prevent spurious materials entering into the market. Their research wings conduct all tests and biological aspects and finally recommend the materials for use in dental clinics.

The dental symbol adopted by ADA in 1965 as the official emblem, contains Greek letter Δ (delta) for dentistry, O (omicron) for odont (tooth) which forms the periphery of the design. Background design contains 32 leaves (permanent teeth) and 20 berries (deciduous teeth). In the middle, the staff entwined with a single serpent, God of dental health.

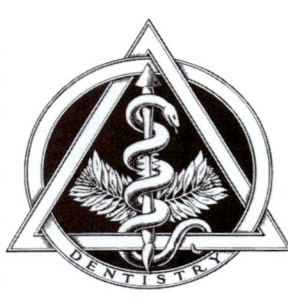

In India, the first dental college of surgery was formed in 1920 by Padma Bhushan Dr R Ahmed at Calcutta affiliated to Calcutta University offering one year BDS course. He is considered as the father of Indian dentistry. Due to his initiation, dental education spread out rapidly and now there are more than 270 dental colleges are offering BDS and MDS degrees courses.

• He founded India's first Dental College in Calcutta in 1928 from his own earnings and real hard work.

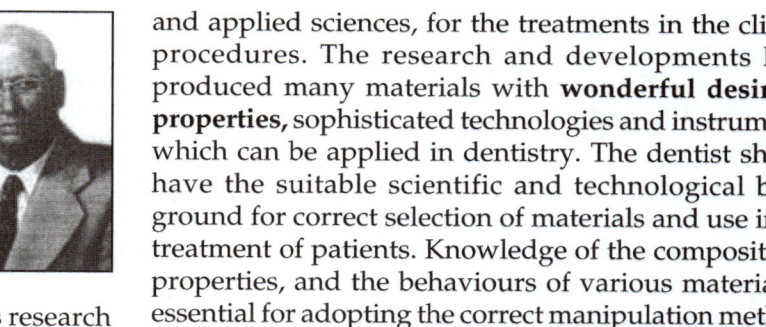

- The course in dentistry was for one year and changed to four years in 1935.
- He was the founder member of Indian Dental Association and was the president for three years from 1945 to 1948.
- He was awarded Padma Bhushan in 1964.

This history reveals the fact, the continuous research on the developments of materials, studies regarding their biocompatibilities and other properties. These resulted in producing newer materials, fabrication techniques and clinical applications. It is a must for dentists and technicians to be in touch with these progresses for selection of most suitable materials for clinical treatment and fabrication techniques.

Instead of barbers, artisans and priests dealing with dental problems in the pre-historic period, scientist-dental clinicians are now doing their jobs most efficiently. The importance of basic sciences and technologies in developing the dental biomaterials cannot be overemphasized. It is a known fact, that without using dental materials, no dental treatment in any specialities can be done.

ORIENTATION TO DENTISTRY

This orientation chapter is included specially for the new entrants to the courses in dental sciences, i.e. for the students who have been just admitted to the first year of the BDS degree course. The syllabus of the science of dental materials has been planned as **a bridge course** between the pure basic sciences, studied in the pre-university course level, and their various applications in dentistry. Different specialities of dentistry have been evolved by the interactions between the different basic sciences, technologies and clinical conditions.

Dentistry is said to be an art of science and skill applied in prevention, correction and treatments of dental problems. These are accomplished by
- **Educating the public, children and patients** regarding dental health awareness, maintenance of oral hygiene, and regular checking in the dental clinics. Fissure sealing is a preventive measure.
- **Correcting malocclusions,** abnormalities of the teeth, and facial deformities.
- **Restoring** the missing part of the teeth.
- **Fabricating** the desired appliances like dentures, crowns and bridges, orthodontic appliances, etc.
- **Treatment** of oral diseases by medicines, surgeries, etc.

The present trend in dentistry is to utilise the latest scientific innovations in the basic sciences, technologies and applied sciences, for the treatments in the clinical procedures. The research and developments have produced many materials with **wonderful desirable properties,** sophisticated technologies and instruments, which can be applied in dentistry. The dentist should have the suitable scientific and technological background for correct selection of materials and use in the treatment of patients. Knowledge of the compositions, properties, and the behaviours of various materials is essential for adopting the correct manipulation methods and precautions to avail their best properties.

MATERIALS USED IN DENTISTRY

These dental materials can be broadly classified according to their applications as
- Materials used for the prevention and intervention of oral diseases.
- Restorative materials used for direct filling and fabrication of indirect restorations.
- *Auxiliary materials* used in laboratory procedures.
- Clinical and laboratory equipment and facilities.

SPECIAL APPROACHES

This subject has become recently very complicated due to the **multiple interactions** between many highly advanced basic sciences (chemistry, physics, biology), engineering technologies and testing methods. Dentist should know all the requirements of materials suited for the clinical situations. Hence, one has to remember all the properties of the materials and adopt correct manipulative techniques to avail their best properties.

To help to remember all these properties the subject has been discussed in this book with the following special approaches (or order).
- The ideal requirements and properties of the materials are classified and presented in the following order:
  – Biocompatibility—chemical
  – Rheological—physical
  – Mechanical
  – Thermal
  – Optical (aesthetics)
  – Other minor items not included in the above.

(This systematic method has been very much appreciated as it helps recollection).
- Most of the side-headings correspond to the short or long essays or brief answer questions. These keywords are in bold prints for an easier **survey.**
- Periodic chart of elements and physical properties of the important elements used are given.
- American Dental Association specification numbers of techniques and material descriptions are given.

- Approximate numerical values of many useful properties are given in the tables.
- Simple line diagrams and graphical presentations are provided to make the explanations more clear and effective.
- Photographs of teaching models and some materials are printed with respect to chapters at the end. Most of these are from our **Museum of dental materials.**
- Approximate compositions of the materials are presented in tabular columns with the ingredients, weight percentages, and functions usually for the important reactive agents.
- Chemical structural formulae of important resins and chemicals and sometimes the reactions are also provided for reference.
- Model questions of different types, e.g. long essays (20 minutes), short essays (10 minutes) and brief answers (5 minutes) are given at the end of all chapters. The time durations, given in the brackets, should guide the students to limit their answers. The questions are prepared concerning to many question papers of different universities.

ORIENTATIONS TO DENTISTRY (SCOPE FOR STUDY)

Before commencing the study of materials and techniques used in dentistry, one should have a proper background of dentistry and suitable motivating orientations, regarding the necessity and methods of restorations. The following topics are specially dealt with certain details in this introductory chapter.

- Very hostile **oral environments** (chemical, mechanical, thermal, etc.) attacking the artificial restorations placed in the mouth.
- **Structure of the tooth and the surroundings** (enamel, dentin, pulp, cementum, periodontal attachment, etc.).
- **Properties of the teeth** (biological, physical, mechanical, aesthetics, etc.) with the tabulated numerical approximate values.
- **Conservative dentistry**
  - Causes for loss of tooth matter, dental caries, fractures, abrasions, erosions, periodontal reasons, etc.
  - Progressions of tooth decay (stages)
  - Brief classification of the prepared tooth cavities
  - Permanent restorations (inlays, onlays, crown and bridges, cast FPD, core build-up, etc.)
- **Stages of tooth decay and principles of restorations**
- **Specialities of dental sciences**
- **Importance of numerical values**
- **ADA specifications and acceptance programme**
- **Importance of Learning Laboratory or Museum.**

HOSTILE ORAL ENVIRONMENTS

Any dental treatment cannot be done without placing one or more artificial materials or appliances, temporarily or permanently in the oral cavity. The following are the important oral environments to be considered.

1. **Biological (chemical)**
   - Saliva and oral fluids are **slightly alkaline.** The pH of saliva varies between 7 and 9, but during the intake of food and fluids (citrus fruits, acidic drinks, etc.), the pH may vary between 3 and 11. These should be neutralised by the salivary buffers **within half an hour** otherwise, they **initiate tooth decay by dissolving the minerals of tooth enamel or dentin.**
   - Metallic appliances are containing Cu, Ag, Fe, etc. undergo tarnish and corrosion, whose products may be toxic and some may be cariogenic.
   - Some of the filling materials, may disintegrate or dissolve in oral fluids.
   - **Enzyme activities** converting food debris and carbohydrates, release certain by-products which attack the structure, dissolving the hydroxyapatite and initiate tooth decay in acidic environments.
   - **The formation of dentin** with the dentinal tubules effecting the tissue fluids, **challenge the bonding** of restorations.

2. **Physical and mechanical**
   - Large surface energies of enamel **(84 ergs/cm^2)**, and also of restorative materials cause adhesions of food debris is encouraging tooth decay.
   - However, the surface tension of saliva (54–56 dynes/cm) helps to retain the dentures.
   - Large dynamic forces of mastications acting several times **(~300,000 times per year)** can easily fracture most of the so-called strong restorative materials. The fatigue created, also decreases the life of the so-called permanent alloy-restorations. The static biting forces vary from 0–100 kg, maximum values (statistical average of the maximum value is about **77 kg,** Table 1.1).

Table 1.1	Average masticating forces (max)
Area (position)	*Force (newtons)*
Incisor regions	90–111
Cuspids region	133–334
Premolar region	220–445
Molar region	400–890
Average maximum	756 (77 kg)
Guinness record	4,337 (≃ 440 kg)

- Surface hardness and abrasive or attrition resistance of tooth enamel are very large, to serve the purpose. However, the tooth can abrade other softer restorative materials and also get abraded by harder restoratives, like porcelain.

3. **Thermal**
   - Normal oral temperature, 37°C can fluctuate during intake of cold or hot foods, between about 0–65°C and may cause pain to the patient by the thermal shock to the pulp if the restorations are conductors of heat. Materials used should not disintegrate, soften or undergo debonding by this thermal cyclings.
   - The coefficient of thermal expansion of tooth is about 11.4 ppm/°C. The restorative materials should have the same value to avoid microleakages.

4. **Aesthetics**
   Aesthetically tooth colour matching materials, selected and used are attacked by oral environments and undergo discolouration, i.e. change in **colour parameters (hue, value, and chroma).**
   The oral soft tissues are quite sensitive, allergic and toxic to some restorative materials. The delicate tooth pulp exposed due to caries or cavity preparations, should be well-protected from **chemical, electrical and thermal insults** and also from **trauma**. Hence, acidic, toxic, hazardous, carcinogenic, thermal and electrically conducting materials should be avoided. Pulp protecting agents (cement bases, cavity liners, etc.) are applied on the exposed pulp and dentinal tubules.

STRUCTURE OF TOOTH

A brief outline of the structure and the properties of the tooth is required as any conservative treatment is to replace the missing part of the tooth (or missing teeth), with artificial materials which ideally should have similar properties (Fig. 1.1).

1. **Crown and root:** Crown is the visible part of the tooth above gingiva, which is about 1/3 of the total length. The remaining 2/3 part (or more) is the root which is stably positioned, through the periodontal ligaments in the alveolar bone sockets.

2. **Enamel:** This outer part of the crown, is the **hardest** material of the body and has varying thicknesses 1–3 mm. It is a highly calcified, mineral phase apatite structure (96% by weight) with **hydroxyapatite, $Ca_{10}(PO_4)_6 (OH)_2$,** and a small amount of organic materials (2%) of soluble proteins, peptides insoluble proteins and citric acids. Rest 2% is water. The **hydroxyapatite has prismatic rod-shaped** structures

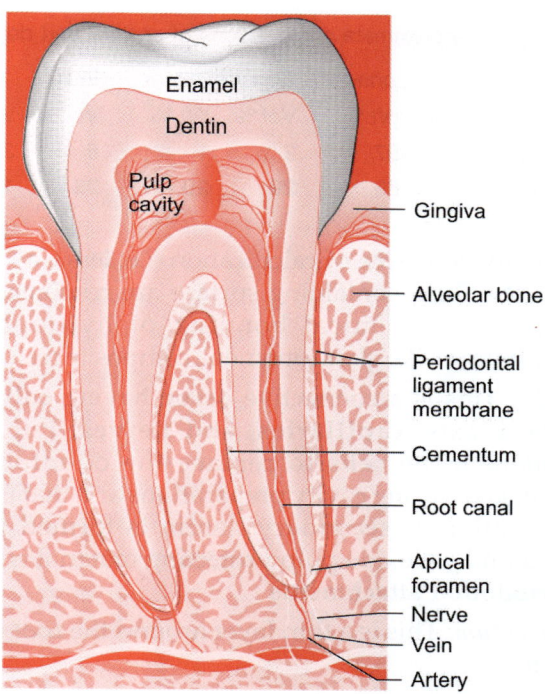

Fig. 1.1: Structure of the tooth

of diameters about 4–5 mm, extending from the dentino-enamel junction to the enamel surface (at right angles).

The organic material is mostly present on the enamel surface. The prismatic rod surfaces have **interlocking structures**, for high compressive strengths. As these rods have different refractive indices, dispersed at different densities, the structure is **optically anisotropic medium, which shows different colour parameters in different directions for different wavelengths. Hence, it is impossible to do perfect matching of colour parameters with artificial materials** (Table 1.2).

3. **Dentin:** This has a more complex structure. Degree of calcification is less. The inorganic hydroxyapatite phase is only about 65 to 70% by weight. The organic matter is about 20%, with collagen 18%, small amounts of citric acid, insoluble proteins, mucopolysaccharides and lipids. Prismatic structures are much smaller than those of enamel rods (Table 1.2).

The **dentinal tubules** of about 2.5 μm diameter extend from dentin–pulp interface with decreasing diameter of 0.5 μm to the dentin–enamel junction. Density of these tubules also decrease from about 50,000/mm^2 to 20,000/mm^2. Through these tubules, fluids flow out (as seen from the freshly cut dentin surface). Between the tubules, the intercellular substances as bundles of **fibrils of collagen** are embedded in calcified substances.

Table 1.2	Approximate compositions of enamel and dentin					
	Mineral phase		Organic phase		Water	
	Vol.%	Wt.%	Vol.%	Wt.%	Vol.%	Wt.%
Enamel	92	97	2	1	6	2
Dentin	48	69	29	20	23	11

The lower degree of calcification (i.e. less Ca^{++} ions) and the **fluid** containing surface are responsible to the lower chemical bonding of hydrophobic restoratives like glass ionomers, composite resins, etc.

4. **Pulp:** This is a connective tissue having **collagen, fibroblasts, capillaries, and nerves.** Pulp can replenish the cells to replace the odontoblasts damaged during cavity preparations and that is why reparative or secondary dentin is formed when calcium hydroxide pulp protecting material is used.

5. **Periodontal attachments**

   Cementum: This is a thin layer around the root of the teeth.

   Periodontal ligaments are the connective tissues between the cementum and alveolar bones.

   Gingival sulcus is a small V-shaped space, filled with fluid, above the cementum, between the extended free gingiva and enamel. This collects food debris, become a source of infections and periodontal diseases.

6. **Periapical area:** This is the junction or interface between the apex and alveolar bones. Through this, blood vessels and nerves enter into the root canal. If the pulp is infected, the endodontic, root canal treatment is done by **sealing the canal** perfectly, to prevent microleakages from restorations to the apex, which **cause more damages, inflammations** around periapical tissues, leading to periapical diseases.

PHYSICAL PROPERTIES OF TOOTH

The teeth are positioned and functioning under very hostile environments of chemical (oral fluids and foods) attacks, large dynamic masticating forces, abrasions, attritions, erosions, and thermal fluctuations. The **internal structure is a wonderful and astonishing one**, evolved for the **protection of delicate pulp, from chemical, electrical, thermal and mechanical insults.** The properties of teeth are of utmost importance to a clinician, for selection of materials for the replacements of missing parts of the tooth.

1. **Biological (chemical) properties:** These, in oral conditions are insoluble and almost impervious to bacteria and acidic materials. It becomes semi-permeable for small-sized molecules or ions like peroxides and fluorides. If the saliva or oral environments, **persist to be acidic, the enamel (hydroxyapatite) begins to dissolve causing tooth decay.**

2. **Physical and mechanical properties** (Table 1.3)

   The tooth enamel has
   - High proportional limit, 224 MPa and compressive strength (350–380 MPa)
   - High modulus of elasticity (~40,000–80,000 MPa)
   - High surface hardness (350 KHN) and abrasive resistance
   - Low tensile strength (10 MPa)
   - Low shear strength (90 MPa)
   - Low modulus of resilience (0.55 J/m^3).

These approximate values show that enamel is **brittle, rigid material** and can fracture by accidents/trauma easily. Surface hardness shows that it can abrade most of the restoratives, including alloys, but wear out by harder ceramic or chrome cobalt (base metal) appliances.

   - Large surface energy (84 ergs/cm^2) causes adhesion of food debris resulting in tooth decay, etc.

The dentin has
   - High proportional limit 148 MPa and compressive strength (300–350 MPa)
   - Higher tensile strength (than enamel) (50 MPa)
   - Higher shear strength (138 MPa)
   - Higher modulus of resilience (0.94 J/m^3)
   - Lower modulus of elasticity (14,000–18,000 MPa)
   - Lower surface hardness and abrasive resistance.

These properties show that dentin is **less brittle but tougher.** Its resilience makes it behave like a **cushion**

Table 1.3	Physical and mechanical properties		
Properties (approximate values)		Enamel	Dentin
Mechanical			
1. Density (gm/cm^3)		2.97	2.14
2. Proportional limit (MPa)		224	148
3. Modulus of elasticity (MPa)		84,100	18,300
4. Ultimate compressive strength (MPa)		380	300
5. Ultimate tensile strength (MPa)		10	51
6. Shear strength (MPa)		90	138
7. Modulus of resilience (joules/m^3)		0.55	0.94
8. Surface hardness KHN (kg/mm^2)		343	68
Thermal			
9. Specific heat (cal/ gm/°C)		0.18	0.28
10. Thermal conductivity cal/sec/cm^2/(°C/cm)		0.0022	0.0015
11. Thermal diffusivity (mm^2/sec)		0.469	0.183
12. Linear coefficient of thermal expansion ($\times 10^6$/°C) or ppm/°C		11.4	8.3

under enamel, by dispersing the large **dynamic energies** acting on the enamel and protect the delicate pulp, from mechanical trauma.

3. **Thermal properties:** Both enamel and dentin, luckily, are excellent insulators (low thermal conductivities 0.0022 and 0.0016 cgs units respectively, and low diffusivities). **This design** keeps the pulp well-protected from electrical and thermal shocks. The cement bases or pulp protecting agents, therefore, should be insulators of similar kind to protect the pulp from the thermal, chemical and electrical insults.

4. **Aesthetics:** The excellent aesthetics is due to transparency, translucency, and fluorescences. But due to the different, densities and orientations of enamel rods, the medium becomes *optically anisotropic. Different refractive indices, translucencies, etc. make the incident light radiation to reflect, refract, disperse, scatter, different amounts of light of different wavelengths in different directions in different areas of the teeth which makes it appear with different colour parameters.*

   It is not possible to produce any artificial, and so-called, tooth coloured anterior restorative materials which can exactly match with the colour parameters (HVC) of the tooth for different wavelengths at different directions.

CONSERVATIVE DENTISTRY

Conservative dentistry is a speciality of dental sciences dealing with diagnosis and treatments (prevention) of the diseases of the **calcified parts of the teeth, pulp and periapical regions**.

NEED OF CONSERVATIVE PROCEDURES

1. Loss of Tooth Materials

- **Dental caries (or tooth decay):** This is a bacterial disease of the teeth that results in **localised dissolution and destruction** of the calcified tissues like enamel, dentin, cementum, etc. Caries is first formed at the **pits and fissures** in the occlusal surfaces of the posterior teeth, or on the **proximal surfaces,** i.e. where adjacent teeth come into contact. When this extends to the pulp, it causes inflammation, infections, pain, etc. and cause pulp death and periapical infections.

  Plaque is a tenacious membrane, formed around the tooth. This contains salivary **mucin** and **microorganisms.** *Streptococcus mutans* and *Lactobacillus acidophilus* are found in caries. These *Streptococcus mutan* microorganisms found in the plaque produce **acids** by **fermentation of carbohydrates from the dietary source.** These acids decrease the pH due to which minerals in the enamel and the dentin dissolves and initiate caries. The cariogenic plaque provides the acidic environment for the progress of caries to the interior, finally resulting in periodontal diseases.

- **Periodontal diseases:** The plaque deposited on the tooth gets calcified to form hard calculus. Further, continued plaque deposition on the calculus makes it grow, causing gingival inflammations **(gingivitis)**. If this is not treated in time, it progresses further, destroying the tooth supporting (alveolar) bones and periodontal ligaments. **The tooth becomes mobile and finally lost**.

- **Fracture by mechanical trauma:** The tooth enamel is very brittle (having high compressive but low tensile and shear strengths). Dentin is slightly less brittle and more resilient. The dynamic impact forces by the trauma of accidents, can easily fracture the teeth, which then need the restorations.

- **Attrition:** This is the physiological wearing of incisal and occlusal surfaces of the teeth by chewing forces.

- **Abrasion:** This is also the loss of tooth matter by pathological (abnormal) wearing of the tooth due to frictional forces between the tooth and other harder materials.

- **Erosion:** This is the loss of the tooth material, by dissolution due to attack from the acidic materials, other than the caries process. (**Acid etching** with phosphoric acid is a kind of erosion.)

- **Resorption:** This also refers to the loss of tissues of the teeth due to special resorbing cells—**odontoclasts.**

- **Iatrogenic causes:** Excess removal of the healthy tissues, by the dentist during cavity preparation. This may be due to accidental chipping of the other healthy teeth or during shaping of the cavities for better fit or retention or strength of the restorations.

2. Few Other Situations

- **Hypoplasia:** Defective formation of the teeth due to disturbances of the developmental process by certain deficiencies (vitamins, calcium, etc.) or congenital disorders.

- **Malformed teeth:** Some of the teeth, may not have the correct size, shape or colour (aesthetic). These also require conservative treatments.

STAGES OF TOOTH DECAY AND PRINCIPLES OF RESTORATIONS

The accumulation of food debris in the pits, fissures and proximal areas, their conversions to carbohydrates, bacterial activities, acidic environments, etc. cause demineralization of the tooth structures and initiate caries or decay of the tooth. This usually commence from the pits and fissures or the proximal areas. The caries progress along the directions of enamel rods or dentin tubules and reach the pulp. **Pulp undergoes necrosis** (degeneration) and the apical areas are affected leading to abscess, periapical granuloma (reparative tissues) and cysts.

FIRST STAGE (Fig. 1.2a)

The **caries is initiated at the enamel portion**. The patient does not experience any symptoms of pain or sensitivity. Periodical dental check-up reveals this decay.

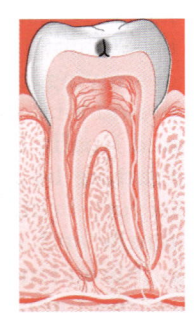

Restoration method is quite simple. Cavity preparation is followed by filling with a suitable restorative material like composite resin or glass ionomer cement, etc. or cementing inlay, onlay or crowns.

Fig.1.2a: First stage

SECOND STAGE (Fig. 1.2b)

Caries progress through the enamel rods and extend to **the dentin.** Fluids of dentin tubules conduct electric charges, (ions) and thermal energies under temperature changes between the pulp and the exposed dentin. Patient experiences sensitivity.

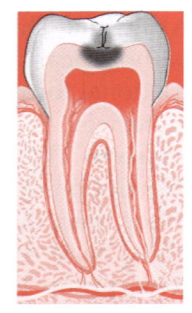

Restoration method is not very simple. Cavity preparation is followed by insulating cement bases, cavity liners, cavity varnishes and finally restorations or cementation of permanent restorations. Deep dentinal caries, very close to the pulp require pulp-protection with $Ca(OH)_2$ or ZnOE cements.

Fig.1.2b: Second stage

THIRD STAGE (Fig. 1.2c)

Pulp exposure may be caused by the progression of caries or sometimes during cavity preparations. This causes pulpitis. Patient experiences **lancinating (pricking)** pains, which is unbearable.

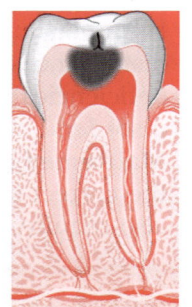

Restoration method is by root canal treatment (RCT) by removing all the pulp matter, draining the abscess, sealing with gutta-percha, etc. and finally placing a restoration.

Fig.1.2c: Third stage

FOURTH STAGE (Fig. 1.2d)

If not treated earlier, pulp undergoes **necrosis (degeneration)** and infection continues to the apical areas, leading to the formation of abscess, periapical granuloma (reparative tissues) or a cyst.

Treatment

The root canal preparation is followed by draining the abscess completely and conventional root canal treatment and **apicoectomy**.

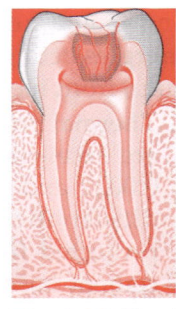

Fig. 1.2d: Fourth stage

CLASSIFICATION OF TOOTH CAVITIES

Conservative methods begin with carefully removing the carious legions by instrumentations and preparing required cavities, with suitable undercut designs, for silver amalgam and direct filling restorations, and no undercuts for cast metallic or ceramic restorations. The classification of cavities are given by GV Black, more than 100 years back, is continuing.

CLASS I CAVITY (Fig. 1.3a)

Cavities are formed in the pits and fissures of the occlusal surfaces of posterior (premolar, molar) teeth. These, lie in the very high stress acting areas and restorations used should be of materials of high strength to withstand large dynamic biting forces.

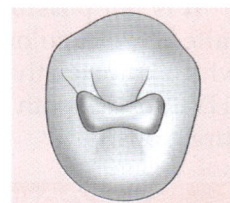

Fig. 1.3a: Class I cavity

CLASS II CAVITY (Fig. 1.3b)

Cavities are formed on the proximal surfaces of the posterior (premolar, molar) teeth, i.e. the areas of contact between the adjacent teeth. These are also high-stress acting areas, requiring the restorations of high strength.

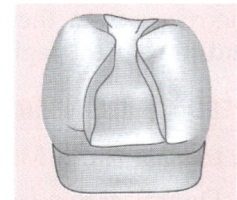

Fig. 1.3b: Class II cavity

CLASS III CAVITY (Fig. 1.3c)

Cavities are formed on the proximal surfaces, of the anterior teeth without involving the incisal edge. The restoratives should be **aesthetically pleasing** and exact colour matching with the adjacent teeth.

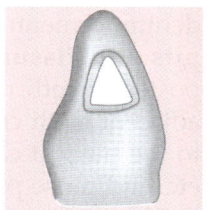

Fig. 1.3c: Class III cavity

CLASS IV CAVITY (Fig. 1.3d)

Cavities are formed on the proximal surfaces of anterior teeth involving incisal edge, require aesthetic restorations.

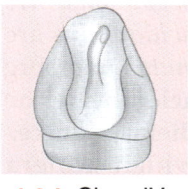

Fig. 1.3d: Class IV cavity

CLASS V CAVITY (Fig. 1.3e)

Cavities are formed at the **gingival third,** of the labial and lingual surfaces of all the teeth. Require aesthetic restorations.

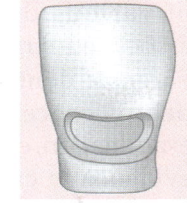

Fig. 1.3e: Class V cavity

CLASS VI CAVITY

All other cavity varieties, which are not included in the above classifications from class I to V.

These classifications are used for the sake of communication and selection of suitable restorative materials and procedures.

Conservative methods (Fig. 1.4) are mainly aimed at restoring the missing parts of the teeth, using temporary, semi-permanent (intermediate) and permanent materials. Some of the restorative fabrications (by casting or forming), are briefly introduced.

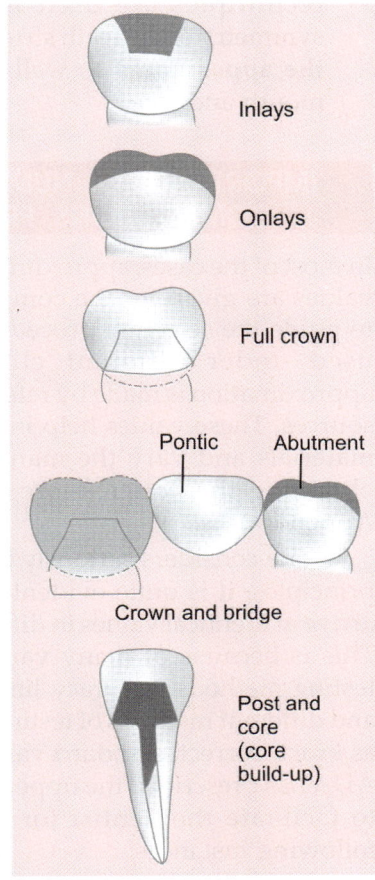

Fig. 1.4: Conservative methods

1. **Inlays:** These are intra-coronal restorations fabricated outside the mouth and restored. One or more (but not all) cusps may also be involved.
2. **Onlays:** Intracoronal restoration covering all the cusps, fabricated outside the mouth.
3. **Crowns:** Restorations covering all or most of the surface of the teeth. Temporary crowns are fabricated sometimes with acrylic and sometimes with readymade aluminum or stainless steel and permanent, by casting.
4. **Veneers:** These are thin tooth coloured (aesthetic) restorations on the labial side covering one or more metallic surfaces of crowns.
5. **Core build-up:** The lost tooth part is built up over the damaged tooth on which the crown is prepared. Post and cores are done by alloy castings. Ceramics and glass ionomers are also used for core build-ups.
6. **Fixed cast partial dentures** (crown and bridges) and removable cast **partial denture prosthesis and implants.**

SPECIALITIES IN DENTAL SCIENCES

Earlier, since about a century, dentistry was involved only with the conservation of missing parts of the teeth, extraction, if not possible to save, and providing artificial dentures of vulcanite, bakelite and later acrylic resins. All these were called as **operative dentistry** and teaching institutions of early 1950s were also named as **colleges of dental surgeries!** As the various basic sciences and medical specialities interacted, the **science of dentistry** also began to shoot up and grow in several branches and specialities. Later, teaching institutions were named as **college of dental sciences.** Now all these specialities are sustained due to the applications of various basic sciences and technologies. Hence, this subject is rightly named **Science of materials and technologies in dentistry.** Following are the main specialities:

1. **Conservative dentistry:** Formerly known as **operative dentistry** is one of the largest areas of specialities. This deals with diagnosis, treatments and prevention of the diseases of the **calcified parts of the teeth,** pulp and periapical regions, and also the conservations of the loss of teeth by trauma, abrasion, corrosions, etc. The two major divisions are:
   - *Conservative part* dealing with restorations of the coronal aspects and aesthetic treatments
   - *Endodontics* dealing with the study and treatment of pulpal and periapical pathologies.

   Materials used are many, such as restorative cements, metal, and alloy casting fabrications, metal-ceramics, endodontic materials, composite resins, silver amalgam, etc.

2. **Prosthodontia:** Perhaps the largest speciality area, deals with the restorations, maintenance of oral functions and aesthetics by replacement of the missing teeth and associated structures with artificial devices. These are required for comfort, appearance and health of the patients. The word **prosthesis** refers to the replacement of the absent (missing) parts of the human body by artificial parts like dentures, cranial replacements of the portion of the skull, post-surgical periodontal, etc. These are complete dentures, removable and fixed partial dentures, crowns, bridges, metal-ceramic appliances, implants, etc.

Materials used include, heat and chemically cured acrylic resins, high noble and base metal alloys, titanium and its alloys, metal ceramics, etc.

Auxiliary materials used in the laboratories for fabrications are, gypsum products (cast and die materials), waxes, impression materials, investment materials, etc. Denture fabrications, castings, metal ceramics, implants, etc. require sophisticated laboratories, technical skill, and training.

3. **Orthodontia:** This speciality deals with diagnosis, prevention, interception, and treatments of all malocclusions of teeth and associated alterations in their surrounding structures. Design, application and control of functional and corrective appliances to maintain, optimum occlusal relations with physiologic and aesthetic harmony among facial and cranial structures.

Materials used are wires of various compositions and properties like, 18–8 stainless steel, Elgiloy, β-Ti, Ni-Ti, PGP, metal alloy bands, fixtures, etc. Techniques involve fabrications of study models, various types of active and passive appliances (using acrylic resins), brazing and welding, etc.

4. **Pedodontia:** This is the dentistry for children, dealing with all the dental problems of infants or children **below the age of 14 years**. Pedodontists train the children, to accept dental treatments, apply preventive measures against dental caries and periodontal diseases, restore and maintain deciduous, mixed and permanent dentitions and also take measures **to prevent, intercept, and correct various occlusal problems**.

5. **Periodontia:** This branch of dentistry deals with examination, diagnosis and treatments of diseases affecting periodontium. **Periodontium includes all the tissues** which help to hold the teeth in the alveolar socket and support them during the function, e.g. gingiva, cementum of the teeth, periodontal ligament and alveolar socket.

6. **Oral and maxillofacial surgery:** This is concerning with the diagnosis, **surgical and adjunctive** treatments of diseases, injuries, and defects of the jaws and associated structures, including dental extractions and related procedures.

7. **Oral medicine and radiology:** This speciality is concerned with the diagnosis and treatment of oral diseases and oral manifestations of systematic diseases and also medically compromised patients.

8. **Community dentistry:** This speciality is concerned with the dental care and oral health of the **community as a whole** and its aggregates rather than that of individual patients.

9. **Oral pathology:** This branch of dentistry deals with the study of the characteristics, causes, and effects of various diseases of the oral cavity and its associated structures.

10. **Forensic dentistry (odontology):** This specialised field is concerned with the correct management, examination, evaluations, and presentation of dental evidence in criminal or civil legal proceedings in the interest of justice. Forensic dentists assist, legal authorities, by preparing dental evidence, to identify the persons in case death or murder, by recognising the signs and symptoms of human abuse.

11. **Aesthetic (cosmetic) dentistry:** A new branch of specialisation in dentistry deals with the improvement of aesthetics. In this field, **skills and techniques** are used to improve the art and symmetry of the teeth structure and face to **improve the appearances** as well as the function of teeth, mouth and face.

IMPORTANCE OF NUMERICAL VALUES OF COMPOSITIONS, PROPERTIES, ETC.

In most of the cases, approximate or ranges of numerical values are given for the compositions, properties, etc. to guide the selection procedure for various materials used under different clinical situations. This approximation is made by referring to various available sources. These values help in comparing the available materials and vary the manipulative techniques for obtaining the better, more suitable properties (*see* Appendix).

If one considers seriously by applying the scientific principles, it is quite evident that it is not possible to arrive at identical values in different experimental trials. This is because of many variable parameters, of the testing methods, accuracy limits of testing equipment and different methods of testing. Hence, there is nothing as exact, correct, standard values as such. That is why ADA has prescribed the upper or lower limiting values, to facilitate the dentist for selection. Consider the following instances:

1. **Compositions:** The exact compositions are not usually revealed by the manufacturers. There are always slight changes in the composition from batch to batch of productions. Also, different manufacturers use their own values. Approximate values can only be determined for research works, by chemical or spectroscopic analysis. These also give approximate values to the accuracy of some decimals. Different methods of chemical analysis also yield different values. Hence, it is better to express the compositions approximately. But these values help to control the manipulative variables suitably. These approximate

values are given in weight percentages or sometimes as some small ranges.

2. **Properties of materials:** Many of the properties like densities, melting temperatures, boiling points, coefficients of thermal expansions, surface tensions, viscosities, mechanical properties, hardness, etc. are also approximated as they depend upon many variable parameters of manipulations and determinations. For example, these are some of those variable parameters:
   - Preparation of the test samples.
   - Compositions
   - Sample dimensions
   - Surface textures (roughness, smoothness)
   - Temperatures
   - Types of testing equipment
   - The rate of loading (for viscoelastic materials)
   - Accuracy of measurements
   - Solvent actions, etc.

   For **metals and alloy castings or fabrications,** it is almost impossible to control the following parameters.
   - Rate of solidification, grain structure, lattice defects, porosities, coring, etc.
   - Precipitations of relative amounts of different phases, superlattices, etc.
   - Work hardening or annealing conditions
   - Dynamic forces resulting in fatigue conditions
   - Testing methods and equipment constants.

   With so many **uncontrollable variable parameters**, it is impossible to obtain consistent values for different trials.

3. **Compositions and properties of teeth:** Dentist should have a clear idea of the internal structures, compositions, behavior and various properties of the teeth. Accordingly, he has to decide the line of treatments and selection of materials for the restorations. That is why these are already given in tabular columns approximately. But the compositions and the properties (sometimes structures also) depend upon many of the following variable parameters:
   - From person to person
   - From tooth to tooth (incisors, canine, molars, etc.)
   - Samples collected from different parts of the same tooth or the different teeth
   - Age and sex of the person
   - Oral health and nature of food
   - Methods of testing, etc.

   That is why even the statistical average values obtained by different authors do not agree.

   All these examples reveal, **beyond doubt**, the fact that there are no exact or true values for compositions or properties, which agree with each other. This justifies the reasons for approximations done in this book. But the approximate values are definitely of much importance for comparison and selections. However, certain critical values, situations and ADA specifications are also to be remembered.

ADA SPECIFICATIONS

As the dentistry which is an art of scientific skill, progress, several major items of restorative materials and improved clinical and laboratory fabrication techniques were introduced. Due to the greater intensive interactions between the basic sciences and dental specialities, the qualities of the new materials also improved.

Around 1919, United States army requested the National Bureau of Standards (now National Institute of Standards and Technology—NIST), to set up standards for evaluation and selection of silver amalgam alloys. In 1928 American Dental Association (along with NIST) arranged to conduct research on evaluation of the various properties, compositions and selection criteria for dental materials to prevent the entry of substandard materials to the dental field so that patients can be protected from, the various **biohazardous** materials used, secure better quality treatments, and appliances.

ADA established research committees in 1966, which standardised the various methods of testing of the materials, the manufacturing techniques, and the instruments used. As the continuous improvements of the materials were taking place to satisfy the requirements of dentists and patients, **ADA had to revise**, from time to time the minimum standards prescribed by it, and the specifications to select the materials. These steps improved the quality of the products.

ADA ACCEPTANCE PROGRAMME

In 1966, ADA began to issue the manufacturers and their products acceptance certificates. For this the manufacturer should provide the following information to ADA as well as to the users:
- Serial or lot number of the products
- Detailed percentage compositions
- Physical and mechanical properties, as obtained by standard testing methods prescribed by ADA
- Corrosion and biocompatibility test reports
- Reports on clinical studies
- Data covering all the provisions of the official specifications.

ADA council may arrange at any time, testing of the various products, without informing the manufacturers. If any sample fails to give the standard specified properties the products name will be removed from the acceptance list. Extended clinical study reports also may be used for evaluation. The council also may revise the standards of specifications with adequate clinical study reports.

INTERNATIONAL STANDARDS

Federation Dentaire Internationale (FDI) and International Standard Organization (ISO) are the two international organisations for maintaining the quality standards of all the dental products, manufactured, throughout the world. Many countries like France, England, Australia, Italy have their own dental associations, doing similar responsible works of ADA. These also specify the standards for acceptance of the products.

Many FDI specifications are now accepted as ISO specifications. There are more than 80 countries which are members of ISO. The manufacturers can apply for ISO certificate. If these are accepted, then the material is considered to be of **International Standards.**

Many dental teaching institutions conduct mostly the clinical studies regarding the new products. Basic science and engineering technology departments (polymer science, composites, metallurgy, ceramics, etc.) of many Universities, have taken much interest in the research and development of new dental materials, technologies and instruments. Recently some private research organisations have also started taking an active part in this field. **These are, perhaps to avail the patient best clinical treatments, and fabricated appliances with recent non-biohazardous materials.**

The acceptance programmes of ADA and ISO are very invaluable for the dental profession throughout the world. Dentists are guided by the **criteria for the selection** of materials, clinical procedures and instruments, impartially. If the materials satisfy the ADA or ISO specifications, dentists, technicians, and patients need not have any doubts about reliability of materials and procedures.

IMPORTANCE OF LEARNING LABORATORY

One of the main problems for the Ist year BDS course students is to understand the clinical applications and significances of the knowledge of the science of dental materials. They do not have any knowledge of tooth morphology, histology, etc. in the first year. They also do not get the opportunity to attend to the patients in the dental clinics. Without adequate knowledge of dental materials even if the students are allowed to watch the patients for a few hours in the clinics, they will not get any benefit. In fact, in the first year, students

should be taught all the basic principles of the science of dental materials with a limited orientation.

To solve these problems, the students should be given free excess to all the materials used in dentistry and their manipulations.

A revolutionary step taken by the author is, establishing a **museum** of all materials and the various teaching models used in dentistry. The **first museum** was developed during 1976–1998 at College of Dental Sciences, Manipal. This first museum in India (or world) was very much appreciated by academicians, and students made the best use of it. The second museum was developed at CODS, KMC, Mangalore around the 1990s.

The third and perhaps the best museum of the dental materials and teaching models, has been developed at "Yenepoya University Dental College" with the excellent encouragement from the principal and support from the management. The special features of this museum has made it a **self-learning laboratory.** This is presented in a large hall of about 1000 square feet area, furnished with aesthetically fabricated glass showcases.

The following are the special features:

1. **Materials collections:** Almost every material used in dentistry, supplied by different manufacturers have been collected and presented in the aesthetically pleasing showcases, according to **important chapters**. These are again classified according to conventional methods, and arranged separately, with containers, manufacturers instructions, as well as clinical application models for reference.

2. **Teaching models:** Most of them are made with the available techniques in our own laboratory. These are specially prepared to assist teaching programmes, showing the step by step various clinical or laboratory fabrication procedures and theoretical scientific aspects. For example, we have the following:

   Lattice models, fracture models, cast pouring, different impression techniques, fabrication steps of acrylic dentures and miscellaneous techniques, prosthesis models of inlays, onlays, crowns, veneers, clear acrylic porosity models, dental burs, cross section of burs, cavity cuttings, casting steps for noble and base metal alloys, orthodontics active and passive appliances, interceptive appliances, etc. presented in proper order.

3. **Common instruments:** Gilmore needles, Vicat penetrometer, amalgamator, visible light curing units, soldering, welding unit, etc. to benefit the students.

4. **Literature:** Many pamphlets, brochures with attractive pictures, charts, manufacturer's instructions for

manipulations numerical values from books for reference and a small departmental library with technical books on basic sciences like polymer science, metallurgy, dental materials, etc. are arranged systematically.

5. **Antiques:** Good number of antiques in dentistry have been collected and preserved. There are old dental units, foot engines, pedaling buffing and grinding unit, vulcanite denture fabricating units, old ceramic furnace, etc. These are the rare collections which otherwise, will be forgotten by the future dentists.

6. An ambitious plan to collect ores of various materials used in dentistry, teeth, and skulls of animals for comparative anatomy is under progress.

This museum has not only helped our students but also in promoting dental health awareness, in public as well as school children.

This learning laboratory is an invaluable asset to the dental teaching institutions as expressed by the visiting dignitaries. It is hoped that the Dental Council of India will insist such self-learning laboratories for dental materials in every dental teaching institutions.

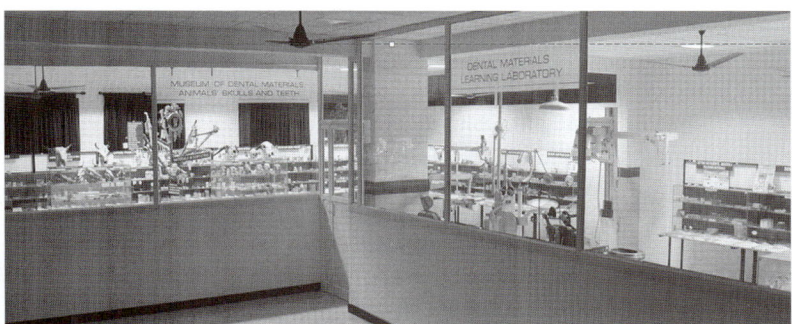
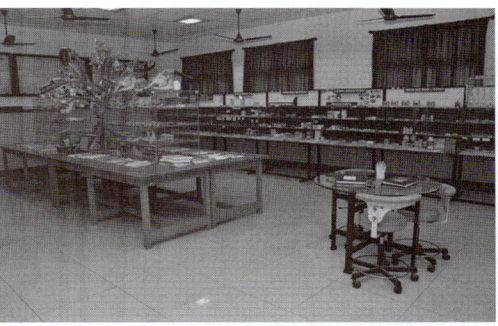
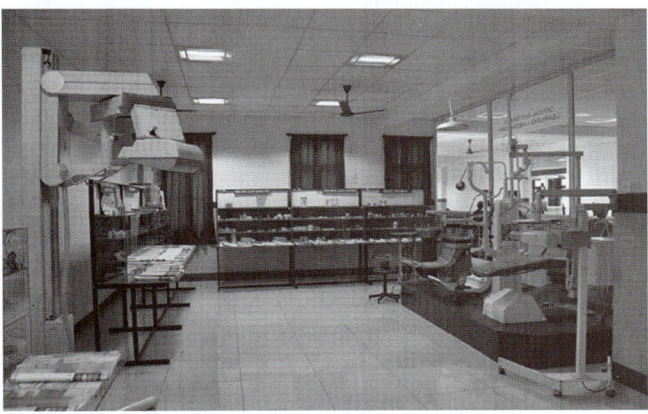
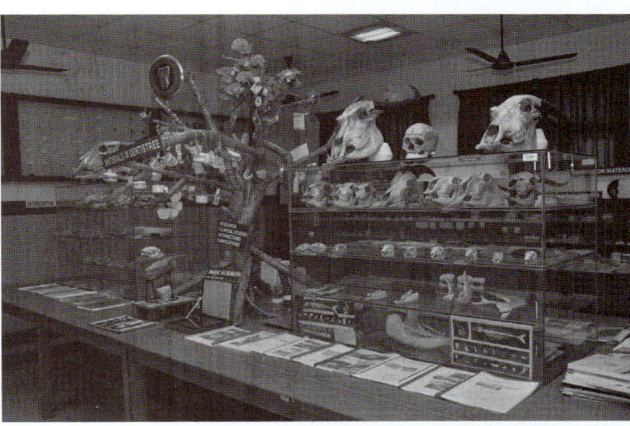
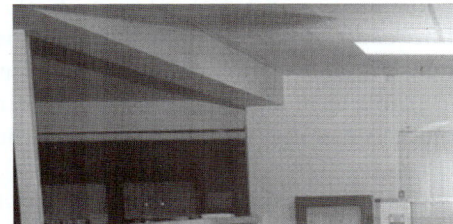
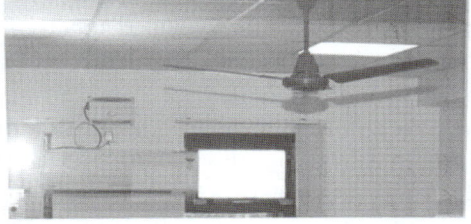
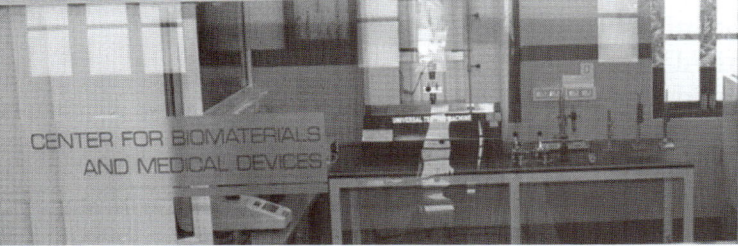
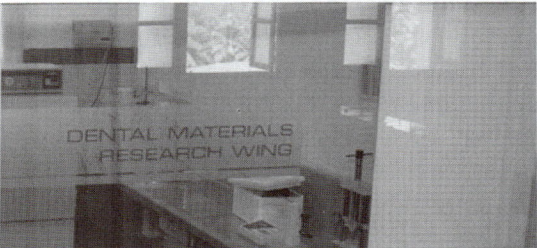

Unique Learning Laboratory: Museum of dental materials, teaching models, and a rare collection of skulls and teeth of domestic animals at Yenepoya Dental College.

CHAPTER 2

General Properties of Matter

CHAPTER SURVEY

- States of matter
- Interatomic bondings
- Crystal structure
- Deformations—stress, strain
- Stress–strain relations
- Elastic and non-elastic deformations
- Strengths, moduli of elasticities
- Testing of mechanical properties
- Complex stresses
- Dynamic forces
- Impact strengths

- Fatigue, failures, endurance limits
- Surface tension, contact angles
- Wetting, adhesion, and failures
- Surface hardness, testing methods
- Rheological—viscosity
- Viscoelasticity (creep)
- Thermal properties
- Conduction, expansion
- Colour—hue, value, chroma
- Colour matching

STATES OF MATTER

Matter is made up of a large number of electrically neutral atoms of the particular structure with definite number of neutrons and protons forming the nuclei and electrons in different shells (orbits) around them. The long range and short range electrostatic cohesive forces make them approach each other, forming crystalline (metals), semi-crystalline (polymers) and amorphous (vitreous—noncrystalline, ceramics, waxes), etc. solid structures at low temperatures, i.e. below their solidification temperatures. When the temperature of the solid is raised, the kinetic energy of vibrations of atoms increases, and at one stage, the atoms get debonded and solid is converted into a liquid. The **thermal energy** required to break completely or debond this solid structure, is the **latent heat of fusion.** This is also, the **heat energy required to convert one gram of a solid to liquid state** or liquid to solid state, by liberating heat at its normal melting temperature and at normal pressure. Similarly, heat required to debond atoms of liquid or convert one gram of a liquid into its vapour state at normal pressure and boiling point, is the **latent heat of vaporisation** (*refer* to Appendix, Table 9).

Applications

1. At higher pressures, the melting point decreases and boiling point increases. The boiling point of MMA monomer while curing the dentures in a flask under high pressure will be more than 100.8°C, which is its normal BP (*refer* to boiling monomer porosity in dentures).

2. The latent heats of fusion and vaporisation of water are 80 cal per gm at 0°C and 540 cal/gm at 100°C respectively. **Large latent heat of fusion is absorbed** from heat sources when the **alloy pellets are melted,** and an equal amount of heat is released during solidification in the casting, brazing, and welding procedures.

Depending on the internal energies or characteristic temperatures, matter exists mainly in three states, **solid, liquid and gas (or vapour)**

	Heat (Melt)		Heat (Vaporise)		Heat (above Tc)	
Solid	⇌	Liquid	⇌	Vapour	⇌	Gas
	Cool (Fuse)		Cool (Condense)		Cool (below Tc)	

When the vapour is heated above a critical temperature (triple point), Tc, it becomes a gas above which it cannot be liquefied only by pressure, e.g. CO_2 has its Tc = 31°C and below this temperature, it can be liquefied

14

only by pressure. At very high temperatures, the electrons escape from orbits and the **plasma state** is reached.

MATERIALS USED IN DENTISTRY

These can be broadly classified into

- *Metals and alloys* (solid solutions—ordered and disordered) used for fabrication of permanent appliances such as DFG, silver amalgam, noble and base metal alloys.
- *Ceramics:* Inorganic salts, like gypsum, cements, dental porcelains, etc.
- *Polymer resins:* PMMA and other resins, soft waxes and impression materials, hard denture base material resins, clinical instruments, etc.
- *Composites:* Ceramic–resin combinations like composite restorative resins.

These dental materials can also be broadly classified according to their applications as

- Materials used for the prevention and intervention of oral diseases.
- Restorative materials used for direct filling and fabrication of indirect restorations.
- Auxiliary materials used in laboratory procedures.
- Clinical and laboratory equipment and facilities.

GENERAL PROPERTIES

- *Metals:* These are characterised by metallic bonding, formation of positive ions in solutions, good conductors of heat and electricity, ductility, malleability, higher density, COTE, definite melting points, opacity, etc.
- *Alloys (disordered solid solution—ordinary alloys):* These have a certain range of melting temperatures lower ductility and malleability, higher strength, opacity, heat hardenability, etc., e.g. high noble, noble, predominantly base metal alloys.
- *Intermetallic compound (ordered solid solution):* These are more brittle than ordinary alloys, containing different phases in the microstructure, e.g. dental amalgam, ordered Au, Cu, etc.
- *Ceramics:* There are non-crystalline amorphous (vitreous) solid structures having high compressive strengths, brittleness, hardness, and fusion temperatures. These soften above their glass transition temperatures. These have low thermal conduction and thermal expansions.
- *Polymers:* Polymers are soft, flexible or rigid, fibrous properties, crystalline, semi-crystalline or amorphous structures, low density, less brittleness, lower glass transition temperature, higher COTE, thermal and electrical insulators, transparent inorganic glasses (PMMA).

- *Composites:* These have combined properties of ceramics and polymers.

These varied properties of different groups of materials are mainly due to their interatomic bonding energies, crystal lattice structures, compositions, etc.

1. INTERATOMIC BONDING

All the physical, chemical, mechanical and thermal properties of materials depend on their atomic structures, the interatomic cohesive binding energies, and the solid-state conditions. When two atoms are at a certain distance, like charges (+ve and +ve, or –ve and –ve) repel and unlike charges attract each other. The resultant force is attractive above, and repulsive below, a **certain minimum distance.** This represents the **interatomic distance,** at equilibrium. The energy required to bring these atoms from infinity or separate them completely is the **interatomic bonding energy.** If this **bonding energy is more,** the material has a higher melting temperature, lower thermal expansion, etc. The various properties depend on this, as well as the types of **atomic bondings,** namely **primary** and **secondary.**

1. **Primary bondings:** These are due to long-range electrostatic forces between the opposite charges.
   - **Ionic bonding** takes place between the +ve and –ve ions by strong electrostatic forces of attraction. In NaCl, the **sodium atom donates** its single electron of outermost shell, to **chlorine,** to completely fill its outermost shell. Sodium and chlorine atoms become +ve and –ve ions respectively and are held together firmly by electrostatic forces of attraction. **Such ionic bonded substances are chemically stable, insoluble in organic solvents and fusible,** e.g.

     $$Na^+ + Cl^- \rightarrow NaCl$$

   - **Covalent bonding is due to the sharing of one or more electrons** of the outermost orbit of the atoms. Hydrogen bonding takes place in this manner to form a stable hydrogen molecule. The organic molecules, such as CH_4, C_2H_4, etc. are formed in this manner. In polymers, the chain structure of polymers is formed by this strong covalent bonding with long-range attractive forces. These materials are generally,

E.g.:

Methane   Ethane   MMA

soluble in organic solvents and infusible (i.e. decompose on heating, without melting).

- **Metallic bonding:** The valence electrons of the outermost shell are rather loosely bound to the nuclei and hence get knocked out by thermal energies, even at low temperatures. These **free electrons** can move at random, in the space between the +ve ion lattices, as **electron gas cloud** and form a strong electrostatic field-bonding. The **free electron gas density** is responsible for the characteristic properties of metals, such as **conductivity, ductility, malleability, opacity, polishability**, etc. Gold, silver, platinum, palladium, etc. have high, free electron gas densities and therefore have excellent conductivity, malleability, ductility, etc. Organic compounds with hydrogen bondings, ceramics with oxygen bondings, do not have the free electrons, and hence, these have low thermal and electrical conductivities, ductilities, and high transparencies (Fig. 2.1).

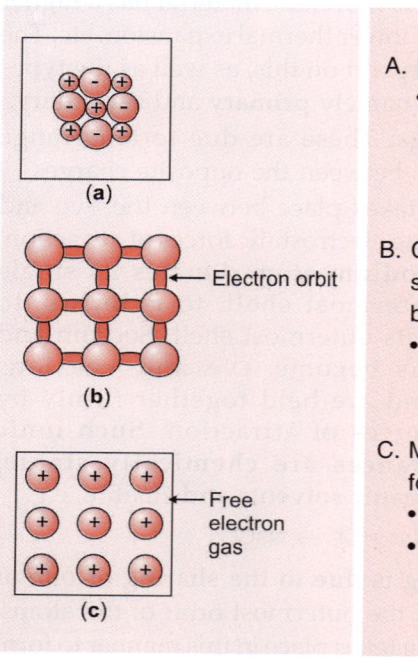

	A. Ionic bond formation
	• e⁻ transfer from one atom to another
(a)	
	B. Covalent bonding by sharing of electrons between two atoms.
	• e⁻ transfer from one element to another
(b) Electron orbit	
	C. Metallic bond formation
	• e⁻ sharing
(c) Free electron gas	• Formation of gas of e⁻ that bonds the atoms together in a lattice

Fig. 2.1: Primary atomic bondings

- **Secondary bondings:** These are **weak, short range, van der Waals** attractive forces due to **dipole moments** between the molecules having **temporarily asymmetric charge distributions.**

Examples

- The electric charge distribution in a **water molecule** is asymmetric. The proton (H^+) side is less −ve or more +ve (δ^+) than the oxygen side (δ^-), forming an electric dipole. The molecules rotate and become **loosely bonded** liquid structure by these short-range forces.
- In polymers, the mers join by long-range strong covalent bonding forces to form long chains. The

valency electrons can move to and fro between the ends of polymer chains inducing an opposite charges in the adjacent chains. This causes fluctuating dipoles and binds the **polymer chains with weak short range secondary bonding** (Fig. 2.2). When a polymer is heated above its characteristic glass transition temperature, **Tg**, the weak secondary bonds are broken, the polymer chains can easily slip one over the other, or it **becomes soft (thermoplastic). Tgs become higher if** the chains are **more cross-linked** by the strong covalent bonds.

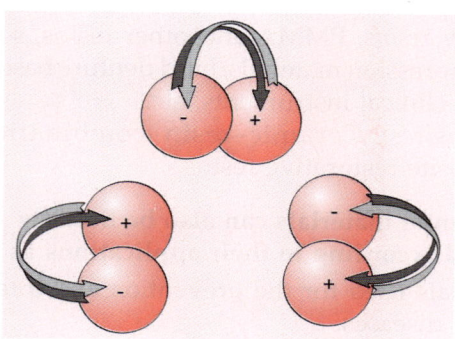

Fig. 2.2: "Secondary bonding fluctuating dipole bonds". Fluctuating positions of electrons relative to an atom's nucleus (the dipole is not fixed in direction)

- **Chemisorption** of gases by alloy liquids is followed by attraction due to van der Waals forces and get absorbed.
- **Adhesion** between two materials is by secondary bonding or by primary–chemical valency bondings.

2. CRYSTAL STRUCTURE

The attraction between the atoms, make them approach to the minimum equilibrium distance during solidification. They arrange themselves in crystalline ordered manner, so that **each atom is positioned, symmetrically with the neighbouring atoms, to have minimum energies.** Six different geometric arrangements have been recognized. These are cubic, tetragonal, orthorhombic, monoclinic, triclinic and hexagonal, depending on the spacing between the atoms, a, b, and c on the x, y and z axes and the angles α, β, γ formed between the faces.

Bravias has shown that there can be **14 varieties** of networks of lattice points so that each point has identical surroundings as shown in Fig. 2.3.

Most common varieties belong to cubic types.

Simple cubic crystal (SCC) has 8 atoms positioned at the corners of a cube (e.g. NaCl).

The **face-centered cubic (FCC)** structure has one atom at the center of each face in addition to those at the corners, e.g. Au, Ag, Cu, Pt, Pd, Al, Pb, Fe (γ), Co (β), Ni (β), etc.

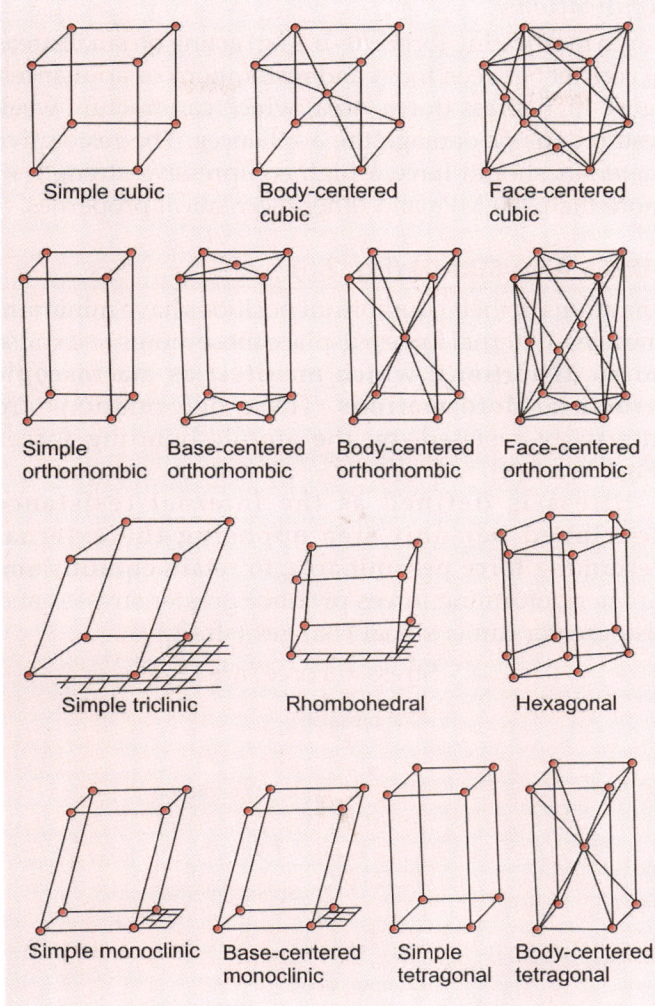

Fig. 2.3: Bravias unit cells of 14 space lattices

The **body-centered cubic (BCC) lattice** has one extra-atom at the center of the cube in addition to those at the corners, e.g.: Na, K , Ba, Li, Mo, Ta, Fe (α), Cr (α), W(α), β-Ti, etc.

Note

However, as the solidification process progresses, the diffusion of atoms is obstructed. **Perfect crystals are not formed**, during casting procedures. Lattice defects (point, line, dislocation and voids) make the as-cast structure soft, ductile and malleable. When work hardened, it becomes brittle and loses ductility.

Applications

- One of the conditions to form solid solutions, is that the metals should have same type of lattice structures. Au, Ag, Cu, Pt, Pd, etc. are the constituents of noble metal casting alloys, as all these have FCC structures.

- In the precipitation (order–disorder) heat treatment of gold alloy castings, the FCT Au-Cu phase precipitates causing lattice inhomogeneity and increase in strength.
- Changes in the allotropic forms, at certain temperatures cause different mechanical properties. Sudden cooling of Austenite (FCC) steel precipitates very **hard martensitic steel,** which has **distorted FCT** structure. Similarly the properties of **α-Ti (HCP)** change when heated above 885°C forming **β-Ti (BCC)**. This β-Ti has more suitable properties for active orthodontic appliances, and β **(BCC)** structure can be retained by alloying with **aluminum and vanadium**.
- **Superelasticity and elastic memories** of Ni-Ti alloys are due to changes in the lattice structures, by changes in temperatures or stresses and then recovering back, to earlier structure (*refer* to Ni-Ti alloys), by **twinning** recovery.

AMORPHOUS (NON-CRYSTALLINE) STRUCTURES

Many dental materials like waxes, resins, composite resins, glass-ceramics, etc. are non-crystalline. The atoms have only **short-range attractive forces,** by which atoms may tend to have crystallinity just in small sites. During solidification, there is no conduction of heat due to low thermal conductivity. They solidify, without any arrangements, like molecules in a liquid state. Hence, these are known as **supercooled liquids, or vitreous solids.**

Properties of amorphous materials

- No definite single melting point
- When heated, first softens above a certain temperature known as glass-transition temperature, the flow increases with temperature and finally becomes liquid.
- No **free-electron gas cloud:** Hence, these are poor conductors of heat and electricity.
- The coefficient of thermal expansion suddenly increases above Tg and varies with temperatures.

Examples

- Dental waxes, impression compounds
- Denture resins, composite resins
- Ceramics (glasses)

MECHANICAL PROPERTIES (DEFORMATIONS)

External forces or energies acting on the materials, cause elastic and non-elastic deformations, and fractures. Large dynamic masticating forces, frequently acting, many times, damage and fracture oral appliances and restorations in service. With the knowledge of stresses, strains, stress–strain relationships, the reasons for failures can be understood. Suitable remedial measures or selection of suitable materials and techniques can be adopted for the patients' benefit.

Units and measurements of force, work (energy), power and stress

1. **Force:** It is measured by the product, mass (m) × acceleration (a), $F = ma$

   Units: Dyne = gm·cm·sec^{-2}
   Poundal = pound·feet·sec^{-2}
   Newton (kg·m·sec^{-2}) = 10^5 dynes
   kg·m force = kg 9.8 m·sec^{-2} = 9.8 N
   1 Newton = 0.102 kgf

   When a force, F acts in a certain direction it has its rectangular components $F \cos \theta$ and $F \sin \theta$ (Fig. 2.4).

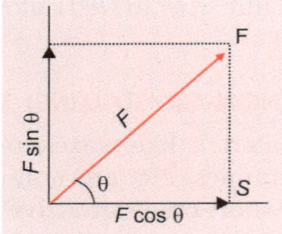

Fig. 2.4: Rectangular components of force

2. **Work = Energy** = Force × distance moved by the point of application of the force in its direction.
   $W = F. S \cos \theta$

   Units: Erg = dyne × cms
   Foot pound = poundal × foot
   Newton-metre = Joule = 10^7 ergs

3. **Power:** Rate of doing work = $\dfrac{\text{Work}}{\text{Time}}$

   Units: Ergs/sec, foot poundal/sec.
   Watt = Joules/sec = Newton-metre/sec
   = 10^7 ergs/sec.

   1 watt-hour = Energy consumed in one hour at the rate of 1 Joule/sec.

   1 kWh = 1000 watt hours

   1 Horse-power = 1 HP = 550 foot – poundal/sec = **746 watt**

4. **Stress:** Force per unit area
   Units: Dynes/cm^2 and psi (pounds per sq. inch)
   Pascal = Newton/metre^2 = 10 dynes/cm^2
   Mega Pascal = 1 MPa = 10^6 Pascals = 10^6
   N/m^2 = 10^7 dynes/cm^2

   1 MPa = 10.2 kgf·cm^{-2} = 145 psi
   or 1 kgf·cm^{-2} = 0.098 MPa

Applications

Large masticating forces (0–100 kg) acting on small areas of contact between tooth and restorations or appliances, cause high stress (force/area) which can fracture weak restorations or damage the appliances. The restorative materials should have a high compressive strength of more than 200 MPa and other mechanical properties.

STRESS AND STRAIN (Fig. 2.5)

The atoms in their equilibrium positions have minimum energies. External forces displace these atoms and cause **micro distortions, which manifest as macroscopic structural deformations.** These deformations are internally resisted, by the atomic bonding forces (Figs 2.6a to c).

Stress is defined as the internal resistance developed per unit area opposing the external deforming force per unit area, to retain equilibrium. Greater deforming forces produce greater stresses and also greater dimensional changes (strain)

Stress = Force/area.

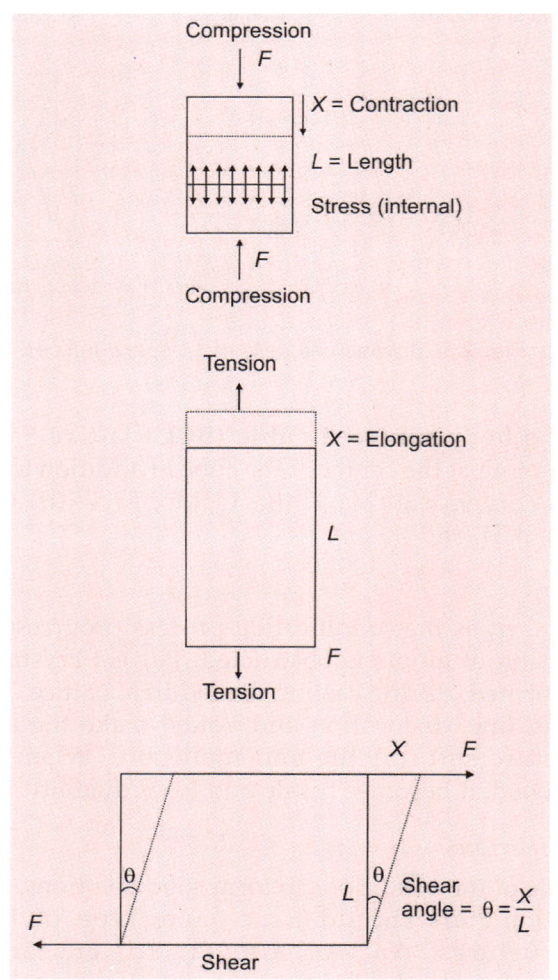

Fig. 2.5: Stresses and strains

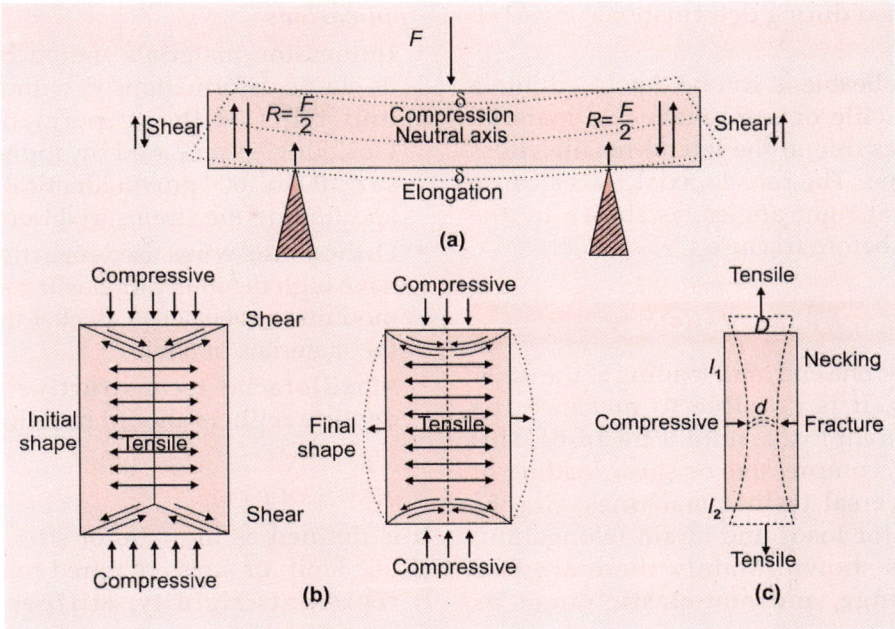

Figs 2.6a to c: Complex stresses: (a) Flexure, (b) compression, (c) tension

Types of Stresses

1. **Compressive stress** is developed **internally** to oppose the two external equal and opposite compressive forces acting along the same axis

$$= \frac{\text{Force}}{\text{Area}} = \frac{mg}{\text{Area}}$$

2. **Tensile stress** is developed **internally** to oppose two external equal and opposite tensile forces, acting along the same axis

$$= \frac{\text{Force}}{\text{Area}}$$

3. **Shearing stress** is developed **internally** to oppose the two external equal and opposite shearing forces acting along different axes

$$= \frac{\text{Force}}{\text{Area}}$$

Units of stress correspond to force/unit area, i.e. $\frac{\text{Dynes}}{\text{cm}^2}$

$\frac{\text{Newton}}{\text{m}^2}$ = (Pascal), $\frac{\textbf{Kgf}}{\textbf{cm}^2}$, psi, etc.

1 MPa = 145 psi

Strain is the deformation taking place per unit dimension. This has no units and is expressed as the ratio or percentage. **Strain is dimensionless quantity usually expressed in percentage.**

Types of Strains

1. Compressive strain $= \dfrac{\text{contraction}}{\text{original length}} = \dfrac{x}{L}$

2. Tensile strain $= \dfrac{\text{elongation}}{\text{original length}} = \dfrac{x}{L}$

3. Shear strain $= \text{shear angle} = \theta = \dfrac{x}{L}$

The strain causes the stress at the same instant, and both disappear simultaneously.

Complex Stresses and Strains

Pure tensile, compressive and shear stresses and their corresponding strains do not individually occur in practice. These combine and form complex stresses and strains.

1. Consider a rectangular bar, supported by two knife edges at distance '*l*' apart and a deforming force *F* act at the middle (refer, three-point bending test). The upper surface contracts producing compressive stress, lower surface elongates producing tensile stress and the layers at right angles, get sheared (Fig. 2.6a).

   The combined strains cause bending or flexure. In irregular crown and bridge structures or cast RPDs, the inhomogeneous stress distributions are studied, with models by optical methods. These complex stresses or strains are created due to the **resistance** between the lattices and cause slipping one over the other.

2. Distribution of stresses when a cylindrical sample is compressed and elongated shows the tensile and

shear strains formed during deformations (Figs 2.6b and c).

If the metal is malleable, it can be deformed into a thin sheet. Semi-ductile or semi-malleable material bulges at right angles due to the **lateral tensile stress** and gets drum-shape. The tensile axial forces cause compressive stress at right angles, as shown by the narrow neck region before fracture.

STRESS–STRAIN RELATIONS

By clamping a wire at one end, and loading at the other end in increments, it is possible to measure the elongations for different loads, until it fractures. This is done with tensile, compressive or shear loading of samples using **universal testing machines**. Graphs representing stress (or load) and strain (elongation) can be obtained as shown. Mainly there are two portions, **elastic range, and non-elastic range,** as shown in Fig. 2.7.

1. ELASTIC DEFORMATION

- **Proportional Limit (PL)**
  The first part of the graph OP is a straight line, showing that the stress is directly proportional to strain up to a certain limit, known as proportional limit.

  It is the **maximum stress up to which, the stress is directly proportional to strain** (up to this strain, the internal structure is not deformed permanently).

  For **tooth enamel, dentin, acrylics, stainless steel,** PL = **225, 147, 27.5, 1630 MPa respectively.**

- **Elastic Limit (EL)**

  According to Hooke's law, **within the elastic limit,** stress is directly proportional to strain

  $$\frac{\text{Stress}}{\text{Strain}} = \text{constant} = \text{modulus of elasticity} = \text{slope} = \frac{\text{LM}}{\text{KM}} = E$$

  The elastic limit is determined, in a similar manner. The incremental load is applied, or load is increased step by step **after removing each time, to check the complete elastic recovery.**

  The elastic limit can be defined as the **maximum stress up to which the elastic recovery is complete** or there is no permanent strain.

  The elastic and proportional limits have nearly same values, as they represent the same phenomena.

- **Flexibility or elastic range (F1)**
  It is the **maximum recoverable strain** or the strain at the proportional limit, **F1 = P/E.**

Applications

- **Impression materials** should have large flexibility or elastic deformations to withdraw through severe undercuts without permanent deformation. Flexibility is compared by applying a constant load, say, 100 to 1000 gm on identical cylindrical samples and finding the strains in different samples.
- **Orthodontic wires** used for active appliances should have high flexibility or elastic range (low stiffness or modulus of elasticity). Nickel-titanium and β-Ti are the materials of choice.
- **Maxillofacial reconstructive materials and soft denture reliners** should have high flexibility.

Modulus of Elasticity

It is defined as the ratio of stress and strain (within elastic limit) or stress required to produce unit strain. It represents **rigidity, stiffness or resistance to deformations**.

Young's Modulus of Elasticity (Y, E or Q)

It is the ratio of compressive or tensile stresses and corresponding strains. It is obtained from the slope of the straight line portion of the stress-strain graph, i.e. $\frac{\text{LM}}{\text{KM}}$ or the ratio

$$Y = Q = E = \frac{\text{Stress}}{\text{Strain}} = \frac{\text{Proportional limit}}{\text{Flexibility}} = \frac{P}{F1}$$

Units: dynes/cm^2, MPa, GPa (=1000 MPa), psi

Applications

- **Oral appliances** and restorative materials should have high proportional limit and high modulus of elasticity, E (as very large dynamic compressive masticating forces are acting on them frequently) to resist permanent deformations. E for acrylics (2,500), enamel (40,000), dentin (16,000), bones (18,000), $ZnPO_4$ cement (14,000), gold alloys (100,000) Cr-Co alloys (220,000), stainless steel (200,000) Ni-Ti (41,000), β-Ti (71,400), etc. in MPa.
- **Ideally, restorative materials** should have the same E as that of dentin (i.e. about 14,000 MPa). $ZnPO_4$ cement has nearly same value.
- **Orthodontic wires** for active appliances should have high flexibility or low E (i.e. Ni-Ti and β-Ti) and for reactive or passive appliances, high stiffness or E (like 18-8 stainless steel, elgilloy, Cr-Co or Cr-Ni alloys).
- **Alloys of metal-ceramic appliances** should have **high modulus of elasticity, to avoid sagging**, at high temperatures.

Modulus of rigidity or shear (η)

It is the ratio = η = Shear stress/shear angle or strain.

This is the resistance to shearing (torsion) forces. In liquids, the viscosity represents the ratio of **shear stress to the shear strain rate or resistance to flow.** Bond strengths of adhesive cements are measured by tensile or shear strengths.

Modulus of rupture or flexure strength **for brittle materials like ceramics is of importance. It is measured by the resistance to flexure and is related to complex stresses and strains**.

Dynamic Young's modulus

Dynamic Young's modulus of elasticity is more realistic than the static values. Dynamic Young's modulus E_D is obtained by measuring the **velocity of ultrasonic waves (v)** in the material of **density d. Dynamic modulus = v^2d.**

Modulus of Resilience (R)

It is the a**bility** of a material to absorb deforming **energies** without undergoing permanent deformation. In other words, it is the 'cushion-like' or 'springiness' property. It is measured by the work done on a material or energy stored, when stressed up to the proportional limit. Modulus of resilience, **R is the amount of energy** absorbed by a unit volume of material when stressed up to the proportional limit. It can be shown, **R = ½ stress × strain** or the **area of the triangular part of** the stress–strain graph up to the proportional limit (PL), i.e. Δ OAP.

$$R = \frac{1}{2} \text{ stress} \times \text{strain} = \frac{1}{2} P \times F = \frac{P}{2} \times \frac{P}{E} = \frac{P^2}{2E} \text{ J/m}^3$$

Applications

- **Tooth enamel and dentin have R = 0.5 and 0.93 J/m³** respectively. Higher R and lower E of dentin, show that **dentin is tough and acts like a cushion underneath, the hard, brittle enamel.**
- The **elastomers** have large R and permanent resilient properties. Highly plasticized PMMA have high flexibility and resilience. They are chosen for resilient-denture liners, tissue conditioners and maxillofacial reconstructive materials.
- Large modulus of resilience is a requirement for **orthodontic wires**, to store a large amount of potential energy of deformation and supply small constant forces for a long time.

Poison's ratio

When a tensile force is applied along one axis to produce elongation, compressive strain is produced at right angles, proportionately. If D and d are initial and final diameters, l_1 and l_2 are initial and final lengths (Fig. 2.6c).

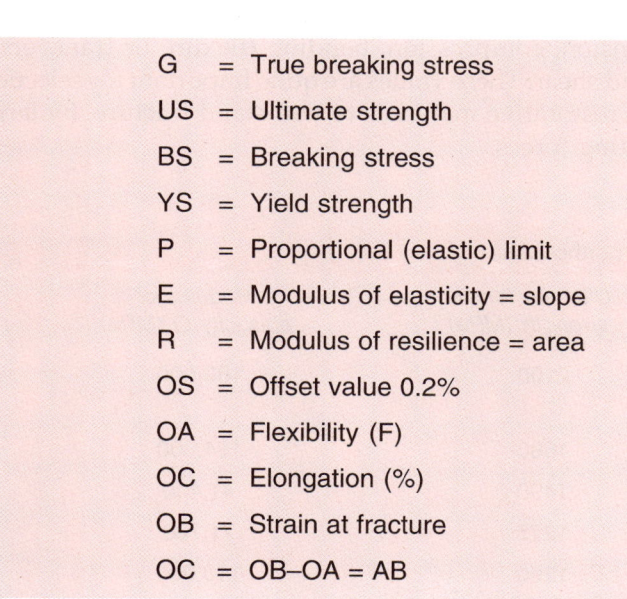

G	=	True breaking stress
US	=	Ultimate strength
BS	=	Breaking stress
YS	=	Yield strength
P	=	Proportional (elastic) limit
E	=	Modulus of elasticity = slope
R	=	Modulus of resilience = area
OS	=	Offset value 0.2%
OA	=	Flexibility (F)
OC	=	Elongation (%)
OB	=	Strain at fracture
OC	=	OB–OA = AB

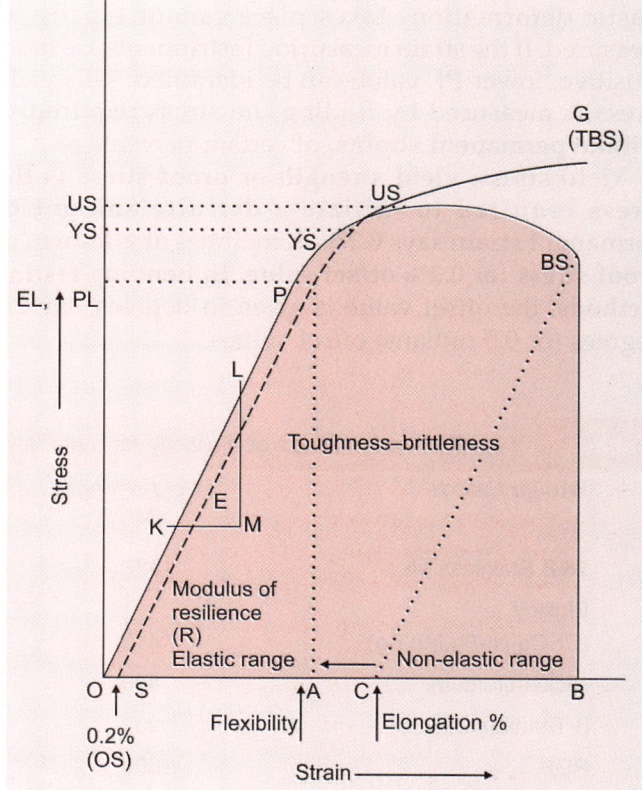

Fig. 2.7: Stress–strain relationship

Table 2.1	ADA specification 1997 or ISO Draft 2002 for yield strengths of casting alloys			
	ADA specification 1997 (minimum)		ISO Draft 2002 (minimum)	
Casting alloys	Yield strength (MPa)	Elongation (%)	Yield strength (MPa)	Elongation %
Type I—soft	80	18	80	18
Type II—medium	180	12	180	10
Type III—hard	240	12	270	5
Type IV—extra hard	300	10	360	3

Poison's ratio $\sigma = \dfrac{\text{Lateral contractional strain}}{\text{Longitudinal, elongational strain}}$

$$= \frac{D-d}{D} / \frac{l_2 - l_1}{l_1}$$

For most of the dental materials $\sigma = 0.3$

For ideal isotropic medium $\sigma = 0.5$ and can be found by ultrasonic testing methods.

The shear modulus η and Young's modulus E are related by:

$$\eta = \frac{E}{2(1+\sigma)} = 0.38\,E$$

2. NON-ELASTIC DEFORMATION

The stress at which the change from elastic to non-elastic deformations takes place cannot exactly be measured. If the strain measuring instruments are more sensitive, lower PL value can be identified. This yield stress is measured by finding the stress required to **initiate permanent strains**, of certain percentages.

Yield stress, yield strength or proof stress is the stress required to initiate a definite amount of permanent strain says 0.2%. Sometimes, it is known as **proof stress for 0.2% offset value. In bending testing methods,** the offset value is given in degrees, say 2.9 degrees (or 0.5 radians) offset values.

Yield strength is slightly more than the proportional limit. **It indicates the possibility of permanent deformation when higher stress is produced.**

Yield strength value can be measured accurately and hence is often referred for selection. **The dental casting alloys are classified** according to their minimum yield strengths at 0.2% offset value and percentage elongations (ability to undergo plastic deformation) in the quenched conditions, as per ADA specification No. 5, (1997) or ISO Draft (2002) (Table 2.1).

The orthodontic wires of the following alloys have their yield strengths at 0.2% offset values, ultimate tensile strengths, modulus of elasticities (Table 2.2).

These values, vary according to the compositions, diameters, work hardened, annealed and tempered conditions of the wires.

Ultimate Strength

This is the maximum stress up to which the material resists fractures and is represented by the peak value in the graph. Ultimate strengths are different under tension, compression, bending (flexure or transverse) and shear. These values are quite important for selection of restorative materials to withstand fracture, by large biting forces.

Table 2.2	YS, UTS, and modulus of elasticity for materials used in orthodontia		
Wrought alloys	Yield strength (MPa)	Ultimate tensile strength (MPa)	Modulus of elasticity Q (MPa)
18-8 Stainless steel	1580	2100	180,000
Elgilloy (Cr-Co-Ni-Fe,Mo,Be)	1410	1680	184,000
Nickel-titanium	430	1490	41,400
β-Titanium	930	1275	71,700
PGP	1000	1200	110,000
PSC	750	1000	120,000

The ultimate tensile strengths of alloys are given in Table 2.2. For some restoratives, the UTS values in MPa are; tooth enamel = 10, dentin = 51, human bone = 140, GIC-type I = 5.5, GIC type II = 6–15, composite resins = 40–60, amalgam = 30–50, porcelain = 25–35 MPa, etc.

Breaking Stress

When the stress slightly exceeds the ultimate strength value, the atoms begin to tear out or separate at the **V-shaped micro notches, surface defects, and lattice defects** and finally fracture.

The **actual stress** beyond the proportional limit is more than that measured. Due to plastic deformations, the area of cross sections decreases and the true stress is not calculated. That is why the breaking stress appears less than the ultimate strength value.

True Breaking Stress

By substituting actual area of cross-section at different loads, **true stress** can be calculated. Graph OPG represents the true stress–strain relation and G gives true breaking stress (TBS).

Toughness and Brittleness

The total area under the entire stress-strain graph with the strain-axis refers to the work done to fracture the material of unit volume or **the energy absorbed before fracture, which is a measure of toughness.**

A material is said to be tough if the **plastic deformation or this area is more,** i.e. the ductility and malleabilities are higher, e.g. metals and alloys.

A material is said to be **brittle if the area is small** that is negligible plastic deformations, e.g. gypsum products, ceramics, glass, etc. These have low tensile, shear and flexure strengths, but higher compressive strengths (Fig. 2.8).

Fracture Toughness

It is defined as the amount of energy or the stress intensity required to fracture, or the ability of the material to get plastically deformed without fracture.

Brittle materials get easily fractured by deforming forces or trauma. The surface flaws such as V-shaped cracks, notches, and internal cracks produced during solidification of insulators like porcelain, become the **centers of stress concentrations,** specially, at the tip of the cracks, imperfections, and voids. The large stress concentrations **tear the lattices** or separate the atoms causing **crack propagations.** Fracture toughness is also defined as the energy required to produce a fine crack of unit length (MPa $\sqrt{m}$ or Newton/meter$^{3/2}$. It is measured by Charpy and Izod impact testing, punch out shear testing; three-point flexure-bending method,

Stress–Strain Relationship–Mechanical Properties of Materials: Comparison

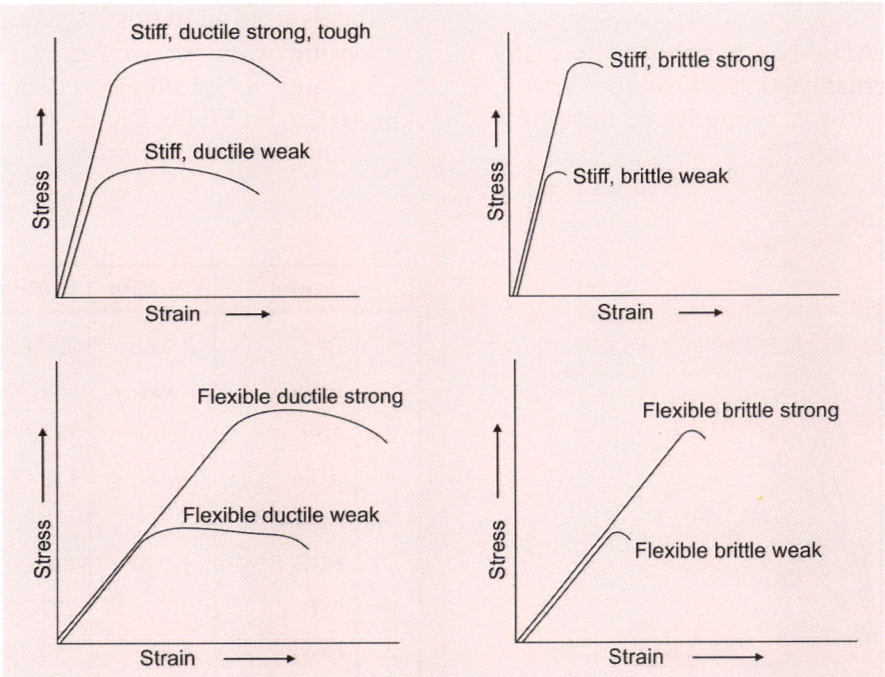

Fig. 2.8: Significance of stress–strain graphs

Vicker's hardness indentation methods. Types: Ductile, brittle, shear, tensile, flexure, impact, etc.

The fracture toughness depends on the size of the cracks inside, or notches and flaws on the surface. The values are expressed in **MPa·m½**, where m is in meters.

Examples
- The fracture toughness of **composite resins, porcelain, ceramics, tooth enamel and dentin are 0.75–2.2, 2.2, 1.5–2.1, 0.61–1.8, 3.08 units respectively.**
- **High copper silver amalgam** restorations fracture more easily than low copper variety, as the latter has higher fracture toughness.
- **Dispersion toughening of porcelain:** Addition of hard (tough) materials like zirconia (ZrO_2), alumina (Al_2O_3), leucite, lithia disilicate crystals, etc. to porcelain, can resist crack propagation and increase fracture toughness, **up to about 3.3. MPa·m½** (*refer to ceramics*).

Percentage Elongation (Plastic Strain)

When a wire is stretched to fracture, initial elastic deformation is completely recoverable up to elastic limit OA in Fig. 2.9. After the fracture of the wire, the parts are joined and the increase in the distance between any two points marked on the wire earlier can be measured. The percentage of this increase in length (per original length) gives the percentage of **non-elastic, permanent elongation** (OC = OB–OA = AB, if, elongation is plotted), otherwise, strain (AB) × 100%.

Applications
- According to the ADA No. 5, specification (1997), classification of dental casting alloys, the types 1, 2, 3, and 4, a minimum % elongation, in annealed condition, should be 18%, 12%, 12% 10% or minimum 18%, 10%, 5%, 3% respectively (ISO Draft 2002). Type iv alloys, after hardening, percentage elongation should have a minimum value of 3%. Base metal alloys. Cr-Co-Ni, etc. have very low values of % elongation 1.5–8% (Table 2.1).
- **The percentage elongation depends upon the alloy components, work hardened and annealed conditions, as well as the method of heat treatments. Large values are useful** for burnishing, bending or deforming, clasp adjustments of appliances, etc.

Ductility and Malleability

Metals and alloys have a large number of free-electrons in the lattice space due to metallic bonding. These are responsible for their ability to undergo **non-elastic permanent deformations** when stressed above the elastic or proportional limits.

Ductility is defined as the ability to undergo permanent deformations, by **tensile loading** (or stress), or it is the ability to be **drawn into a wire**. The ductilities can be compared by their percentage strain (elongation), percentage decrease of areas of cross-sections, or the number of cold bends, **at fracture**.

Malleability is the ability to undergo plastic deformations by **compressive loading** (stresses), or it is the ability to be beaten into a **thin sheet**. These can be compared by measuring the percentage increase in the areas at fracture.

Metals used in dentistry, having their ductilities in decreasing order are Au, Ag, Pt, Pd, Fe, Ni, Cu, Al, Zn, Sn, Pb. and malleabilities in decreasing order are, Au, Ag, Al, Cu, Sn Pt, Pb, Zn, Fe, Ni.

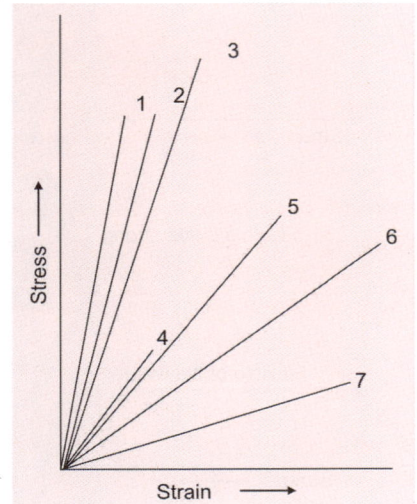

	Wires	Y.S. MPa	E. MPa
1.	Cr-Co	1300	200,000
2.	Elgiloy	1400	184,000
3.	18-8	1600	180,000
4.	α-Ti	450	112,000
5.	Au alloy		
	PGP, PSC	1,000	110,000
6.	β-Ti	930	71,700
7.	Ni-Ti	430	41,400

Fig. 2.9: Stress–strain relationships representing properties of different orthodontic wires

Ductilities and malleabilities decrease, by increasing slip resistance, i.e. by
- Alloying, solution hardening
- Work hardening
- Age hardening heat treatment
- Precipitation heat treatments.

Applications

- High ductility and malleabilities are useful in adapting metallic restorations, to the margins by burnishing direct filling gold foil, type I and II, casting gold alloys, silver amalgam restorations, etc.
- Gold and silver have highest ductility and malleabilities. Very thin, pure direct filling gold foils of submicron thickness (no. 3, 4, 5, 6, etc.) are available for restorations.
- Very thin platinum foils are used in the procedure of fabrication of porcelain jacket crowns.
- Very thin tin foils were used earlier as separating medium in the denture-fabrication procedures.
- Orthodontic wires are drawn from cast ingots into very thin wires.

DETERMINATION OF MECHANICAL PROPERTIES

Many varieties of sophisticated instruments involving different principles are used for testing the different properties of dental materials.

ADA has specified the methods of preparing the test samples and the methods of measurements for various dental materials. Even then, it is very difficult to control many variable parameters such as voids, lattice imperfections in cast alloys, work hardened or heat-treated conditions, etc. That is why, very rarely consistent values, but often—different values are obtained for different trials. **The values of the properties of various dental materials, obtained by different authors, are not concurrent or exact, but only representative figures,** helping the dentist to compare and select the suitable materials and techniques. (The values given in this book are also, therefore, some average representative values.)

STRENGTHS OF MATERIALS

The ultimate strength can be defined as the maximum stress the material can withstand by compressive, tensile, shear, flexure loading, before it fractures.

The ultimate, compressive, tensile, torsion and shear strengths are measured by using **universal testing machines**, tensiometers, etc. In all these cases, proper sized samples are to be prepared (Figs 2.10a and b).

The instruments also show the stress–strain relations, proportional limits, modulus of elasticity, etc. and the values can be easily computed, at **different rates of loadings**.

For **viscoelastic** materials, the properties depend on the **rate of loading.** For example, modulus of elasticity of silver amalgam can vary from about 40,000 to 80,000 MPa, at a higher rate of loading.

1. Tensile Strength

For ductile materials, the ultimate tensile strength can be measured directly using a tensiometer. A dumbbell-shaped cylindrical specimen is clamped rigidly at the ends and pulled apart to fracture. UTS is the maximum force per unit area required to fracture. Brittle materials may fracture at clamping points due to stress concentrations. **Diametral compression test for tension, Brazilian** or **indirect tensile** testing method is used for brittle materials. In this, a circular disc of diameter D, thickness t, is loaded (P) diametrically until it fractures.

This method does not give reliable values for strain-rate sensitive (viscoelastic) materials. Many dental restorative materials—cements, ceramics, composite resins, silver amalgam, etc. can be tested by this method. This UTS value is important, as brittle materials, have low UTS and fracture easily. For 18-8 stainless steel wire, UTS = 2100 MPa, tooth enamel = 10 MPa, dentin = 51 MPa.

2. Compressive Strength

Many dental materials are brittle, have high compressive strengths and low tensile strengths. When a compressive force is applied, complex stresses, created inside (cylindrical sample diagram, Figs 2.6a to d) give

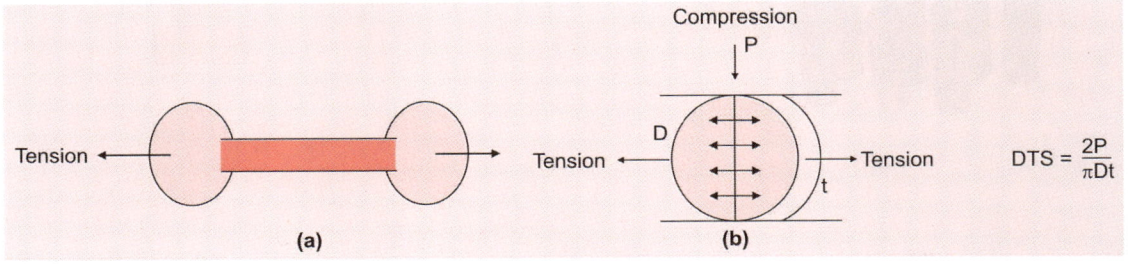

Figs 2.10a and b: Tensile strength testing. (a) Uniaxial tension, (b) diametral compressive test for tension

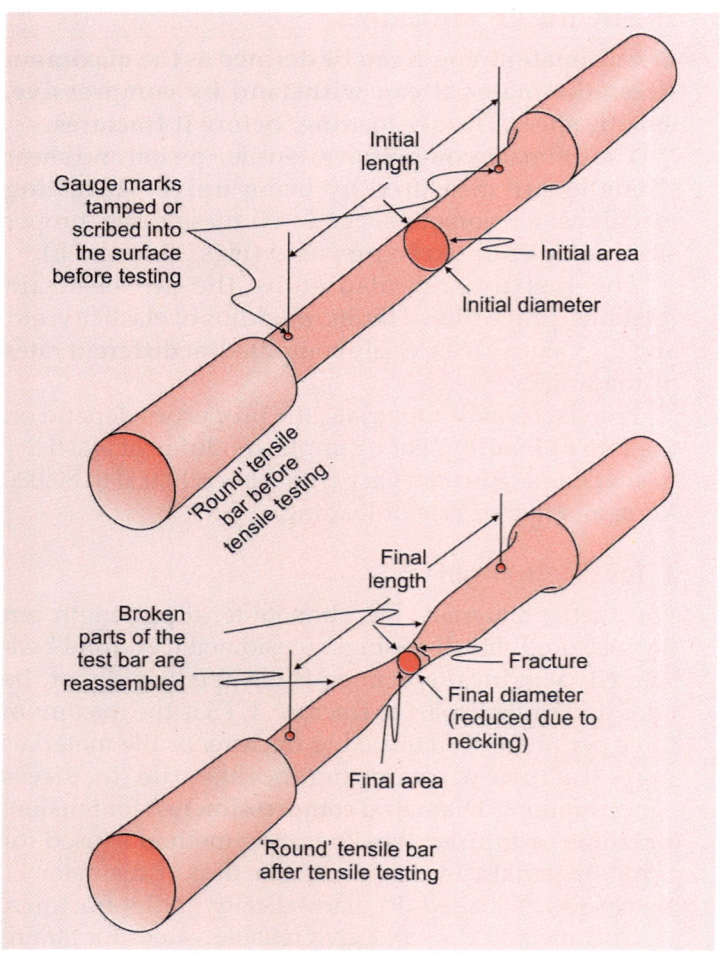

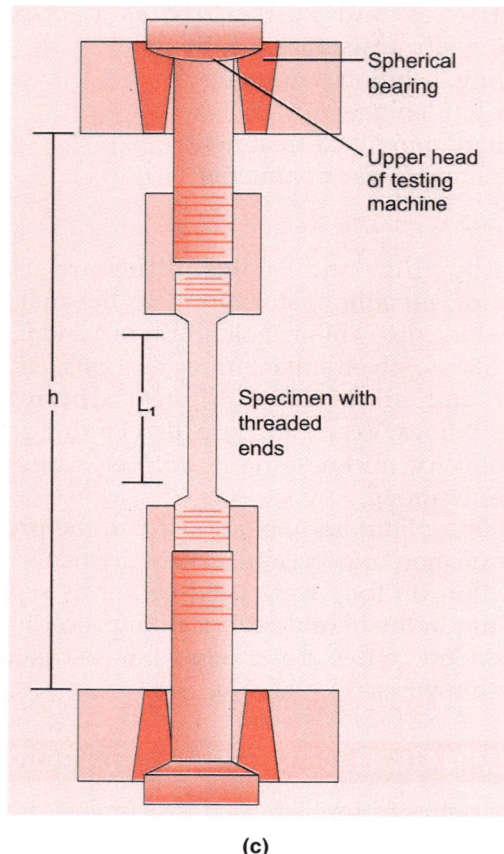

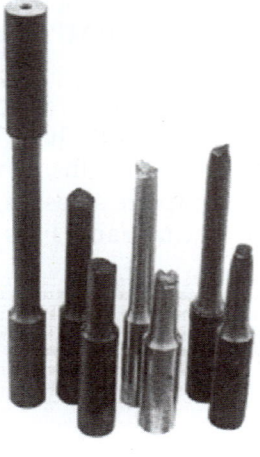

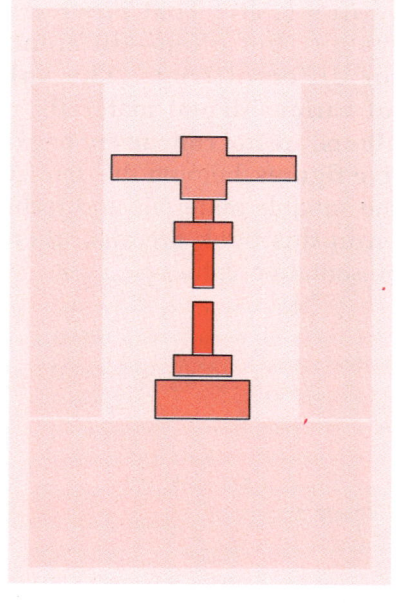

Figs 2.11a to d: UTM fractured testing samples

unreliable values. If the too long cylinder is used, the **buckling** in the middle takes place. Usually a cylindrical sample of a **length twice its diameter** is used for testing. The universal testing machines give stress–strain graphs (Fig. 2.11e). From this modulus of elasticity, resilience, PL, EL, and yield strengths can be found. The Young's modulus (E) is nearly same for compressive and tensile methods. The restorative materials should have higher compressive and tensile strengths comparable to tooth enamel and dentin (380 and 10 MPa, 350 and 51 MPa, respectively).

Examples: Compressive strengths in MPa: Heat cure acrylics = 75, $ZnPO_4$ cement = 80–100, $ZnPO_4$ base = 110–130, zinc polycarboxylate cement = 60–70, GIC = 60–150, porcelain = 150, amalgam = 300–500, composite resins = 300–450, etc. (pages 355–357).

3. Shear Strength

It is the maximum shearing stress at shear failure. **Push-out or punch test** method (i.e. applying an axial load to push out a sample, through the other side), is used.

- For cylindrical punch of diameter (d),

$$\text{Shear strength} = \frac{\text{Load}}{\pi \times \text{Diameter} \times \text{Thickness}} = \frac{P}{\pi dt} \text{ MPa}$$

- For rectangular punch of cross-section l and b, shear

$$\text{strength} = \frac{P}{2(l+b)t} \text{ MPa}$$

- For the punch of square cross-section of side(s) shear

$$\text{strength} = \frac{P}{4st} \text{ MPa}.$$

Applications

The interfacial force of retention, under shear, is quite important for bonding metal-ceramics, composite-resin restorations, etc. The shear strengths for amalgam, dentin, acrylics, porcelain, enamel, $ZnPO_4$ cement are 188, **138**, 122, 111, **90** and 13 MPa, respectively (Fig. 2.11f).

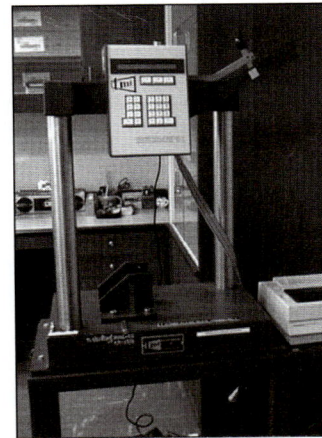

Fig. 2.11e: Universal testing machine

Bond strengths are measured by shear or sometimes by tensile testing. The samples sometimes are subjected to thermal cycling between 5°C and 50°C, several times, to study the bond strengths. Zinc phosphate cement easily gets debonded compared to zinc polycarboxylate cement which is chemically bonding with enamel.

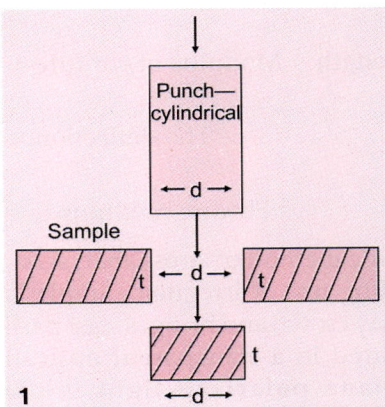

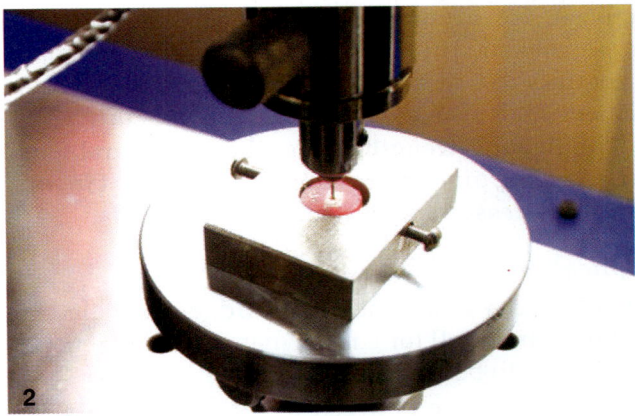

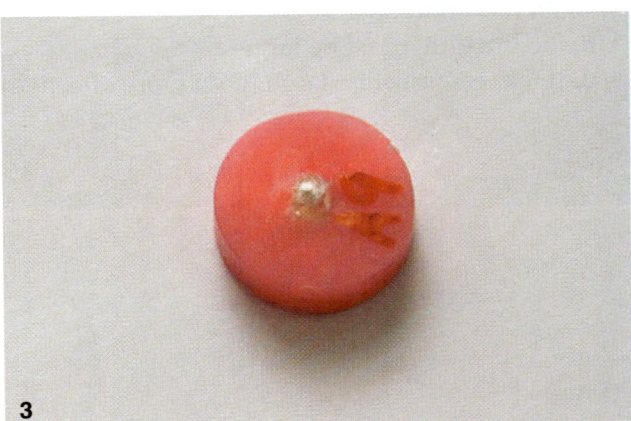

Fig. 2.11f: (1) Punch-pushout test for shear strength, (2) shows measurement of pushout bond strength of MTA cement with root dentin. The dentin of thickness 3 mm and with a hole (apical foramen) 1 mm diameter embedded in the acrylic and filled with MTA. The specimen is placed in a special jig and load is applied with a plunger of 1 mm diameter. The load required to shear is recorded, (3) shows the sheared specimen during testing

4. Complex Stresses: Testing

Flexure (Transverse) Strength, Modulus of Rupture

This is a bending test. The load, P is applied at the middle of a rectangular bar of breadth (b), depth (thickness) (d), supported by two knife edges at a distance—l apart, and the depressions (δ) are measured **(3 point-bending test)**. If P is the fracture load (Fig. 2.12).

$$\text{Flexure strength} = \text{Modulus of rupture} = \frac{3Pl}{2bd^2}$$

$$\text{The deflection} = \delta = \frac{Pl^3}{4Ebd^3}$$

$$\text{Flexure modulus } E = \frac{Pl^3}{4bd^3\delta}$$

Photoelastic method of stress analysis is used for the 3-point bending test of irregular samples. A model of the sample (say crown and bridges, cast partial dentures, etc.) is prepared in a **transparent optically isotropic material. Plane polarized light** is passed while (stressing) loading and viewed through a **Nicol Prism analyzer. Isochromatic fringes** representing constant stresses, obtained in different concentrations are analysed to get the stress distributions and properties. The **finite element analysis** method is used for this study.

The flexure strength, rather than diametral tensile stress testing, gives more realistic values, as it involves complex stresses and real clinical situations.

Applications

1. **For stability of a** (cantilever) **bridge,** the deflection δ **should be small** for large dynamic loads. Hence, the bridge is to be designed, such that:
   - l, the distance between the abutments should be small (i.e. short span bridges)
   - b, the breadth, must be large
   - d, thickness, must be large (d³ is more effective).

2. **Bending:** Many instruments used in clinical practices are bent frequently. (For example, **files** and **reamers, during root canal preparations.**) If the applied stress is more than a critical value (yield strength), it is permanently bent and damaged. The bending moment increases with the angular deflections as shown. Thicker reamers can have higher angular deflections. The initial straight line portion indicates the elastic deflections for safe use without causing permanent bending, or damage. Elastic memory—Ni-Ti alloys are used nowadays (Figs 2.13a and b).

3. **Permanent bending** is to be done in many cases, such as **clasp adjustments** for cast partial dentures, fabrication of orthodontic appliances, etc. In these cases also complex stresses, compressive on the inner part and tensile on the outer part, are introduced.

4. **Torsion or twisting** is another type of loading, producing complex stresses. The endodontic files are twisted through a handle. The angle of twist θ is directly proportional to the torsional moment. Graphs of torsional moments against the angle of rotation, for files of different numbers, are represented as shown. Twisting, above the corresponding elastic limit angle, should not be done to prevent permanent damage (Fig. 2.14).

5. **Tear strength:** It is the **minimum force required to initiate tearing** of a crescent or trouser shaped specimen of unit thickness, with a right-**angled V-notch.**

   High tear strength is required for impression materials to use in **thin sections** (thick impressions get distorted while setting or cooling, by **relaxation of internal stresses**). Agar-agar and alginates have low tear strengths about 900 gm/cm and 700 gm/cm, respectively. Elastomers have higher tear strengths about 2000–7000 gm/cm and hence can be used in thinner sections.

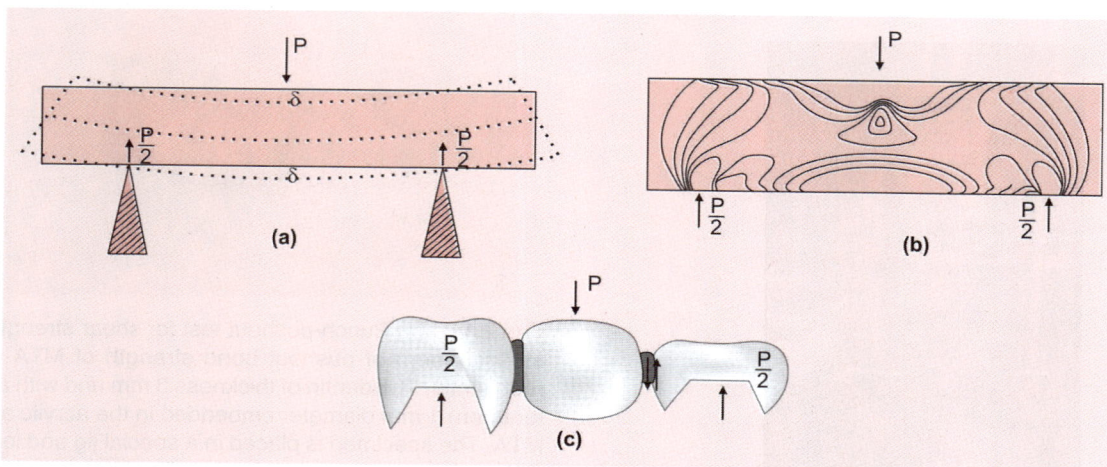

Figs 2.12a to c: (a) Three-point bending test, (b) stress distribution by photoelastic method, (c) example: Crown and bridge

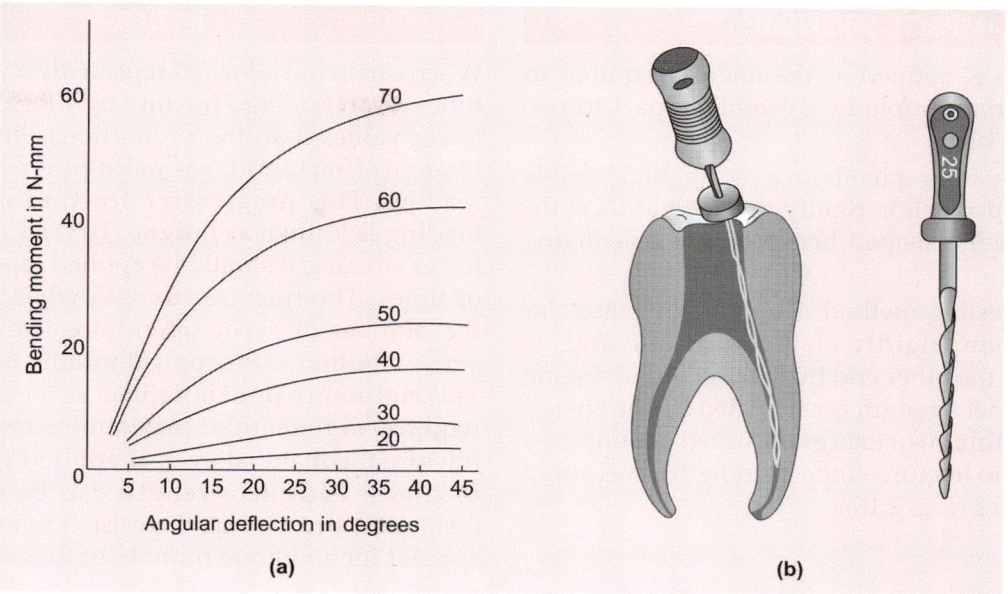

Figs 2.13a and b: (a) Bending moment and angular deflection for endodontic reamers, (b) Ni-Ti flexible file

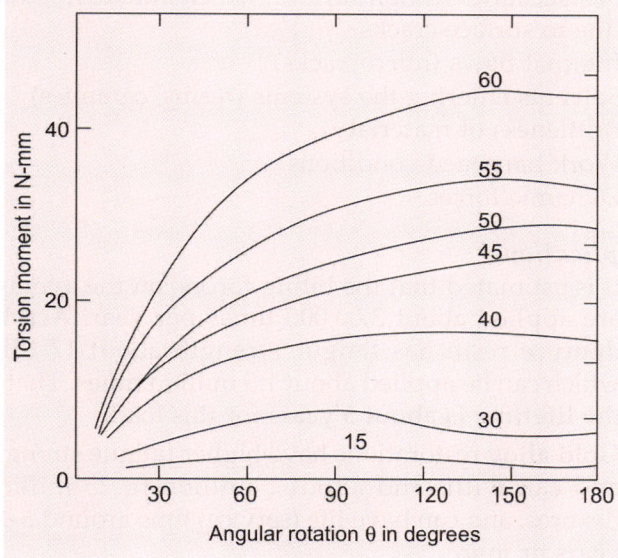

Fig. 2.14: Torsion moment and angular rotation graph for endodontic files, sizes 15 to 60

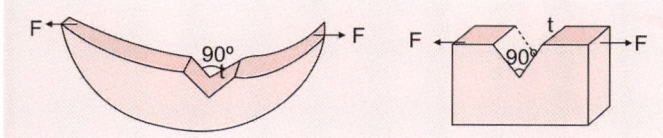

Fig. 2.15: Tear strength testing samples of thickness t cm. Tear strength is expressed as T = F/t gm/cm

Polysulphides have higher tear strengths but greater softness or flexibility (strain in compression). Polyethers have lower tear strengths 1800–4800 gm/cm and lower flexibility (or high stiffness) (Table 3.17).

DYNAMIC FORCES

Dental restorations and many oral appliances, like dentures, crowns, bridges, cast partial dentures, cements, etc. are subjected to large **dynamic impact forces,** which are more damaging, than the applied static forces.

Dynamic mechanical properties, even though depending on the static properties, sometimes are measured by different methods. Properties measured are the dynamic modulus of elasticity, resilience, Poison's ratio, etc., by different techniques for brittle and resilient materials.

Dynamic modulus of elasticity is defined as $E_D = \dfrac{Stress}{Strain}$ for small cyclic deformations by a given stress at a certain frequency.

This is measured by forced oscillations technique, using a vibrating yoke of definite mass striking on a sample at a certain frequency. The ultrasonic method involves measuring its velocity (v) in a sample of density d, using **piezoelectric transducers, $(E_D = v^2 d)$**. This method is very suitable for viscoelastic materials like acrylics, silver amalgam, dentin, athletic mouth protectors, etc. The testing also can be done, after thermal cycling between (5°C and 50°C) to find the variations. Elastomeric materials also can be tested by this non-destructive method.

The cyclic stretching method can be used to find the dynamic modulus of resilience (R_D) of elastomers which is the ratio of, **R_D = energy lost/energy applied.**

IMPACT STRENGTHS

Impact strength is defined as the energy required to fracture a material sample by dynamic impact forces, i.e. by a sudden blow.

In the **Charpy** testing method, a rectangular sample with a **V-shaped notch** is rigidly clamped at its ends, and hit by a wedge shaped heavy bob of a swinging pendulum.

In the Izod testing method, **U-notched** rectangular shaped specimen, rigidly clamped at one end, is suddenly hit, at the other end by the bob of a swinging pendulum. Impact strength is calculated by the energy lost (by the pendulum) or energy absorbed per unit area of the specimen to fracture. Impact strength is measured in kg cm or joules (Fig. 2.16).

Applications

1. **Denture base materials** should have high impact strengths to protect it from fractures by dynamic masticating forces, accidental falls or trauma. The PMMA denture base resin has **low impact strengths** of about 0.25 Joules, which is its main **drawback.** When it is modified by **butadiene rubber,** the impact strength becomes more than double, about 0.6 Joules.

2. **Silver amalgam cavity design:** The energy required to fracture a material by impact forces is directly proportional to the modulus of resilience (R) and volume of the restoration V.

   Hence, resistance to fracture is directly proportional to V × R, i.e. = KVR where K is a constant of geometric configuration or cavity design factor.

   This shows that the cavity designed, should have a large volume and no thin sections (ledges) on the occlusal surface. However, at present, cavity preparation is minimized as silver amalgam posterior composite resins gradually replace.

FATIGUE

When a material is loaded repeatedly (cyclically) several times it can undergo fracture by stresses even at much lower values than the proportional limits. Separation of atoms (fracture) takes palce progressively in cyclic loading. This **progressive fracture under repeated loading is known as fatigue.** To fracture a material by lower stresses, it should be applied repeatedly number of times. The fracture strength when plotted against the number of cyclic operations shows a minimum stress required to be applied infinite number of times. This **endurance limit** is defined as the **minimum stress** required to fracture or maximum stress which cannot fracture the material **even if applied infinite number** of times. **Fatigue strength** can be defined as the maximum stress which is resisted when it is cyclically applied for a definite number of times (Fig. 2.17).

Factors which decrease the fatigue strengths or endurance limits and life of restorations are:
1. Surface flaws (rough surface) which initiate fracture, due to surface cracks
2. Internal flaws (microcracks)
3. Solvents entering the systems (resins, ceramics)
4. Brittleness of materials
5. Work hardened conditions
6. Dynamic forces.

Applications

- It is estimated that the biting forces, on the average are applied about 3,00,000 times per year. **Acrylic denture** resin has fatigue strength about 17 MPa which can be applied about 1.5 million times. That is the **lifetime is about 5 years** for this load.
- **Gold alloy** restorations have higher fatigue strength and can withstand about 1 million to 25 million flexures, and can have life (service) time around **5–50 years or more.**

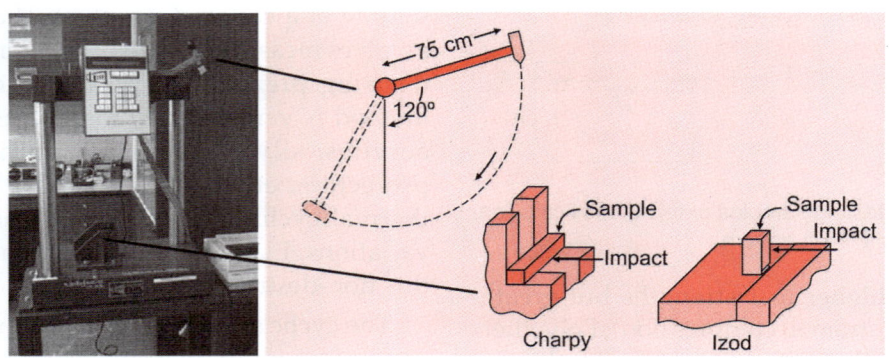

Fig. 2.16: Impact strength testing, samples

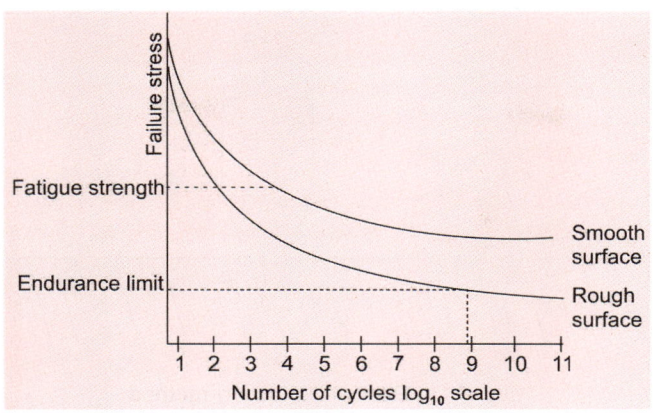

Fig. 2.17: Fatigue and failure stress—number of cycles

- **Dental instruments** sometimes undergo fracture, suddenly, due to fatigue.

SURFACE HARDNESS

It can be defined as **the resistance offered by the surface of a material to scratching, abrasion, indentation or penetrations**. Theoretically, any method of measurement should involve only the surface layer of atomic thickness, which of course is not practicable. In micro-hardness testing methods, attempts have been made to reduce the depth or area of indentations to minimum values and also to get the hardness of localised small sites of particular phases of alloys.

For higher abrasive resistance, materials should have higher surface hardnesses and surface integrities. As diamond has the highest surface hardness (>7000 KHN) **diamond instruments** are used for cutting, abrading or finishing of all other materials **without any attrition.**

The surface hardness of a material depends upon
1. Atomic binding forces
2. The composition of phases of cast alloys
3. Work hardened and annealed conditions
4. Heat treatments
5. Proportional limits and ultimate strengths
6. Modulus of elasticity and resilience
7. Ductility and malleabilities.

But there are no exact relationships (or proportionalities) between the mechanical properties and surface hardnesses. Certain relationships established between surface hardness and ultimate tensile strengths for semi ductile materials, are also not reliable.

METHODS OF MEASUREMENTS OF SURFACE HARDNESS

These involve the principles of scratching (abrasion), indentation, penetration and elastic rebounds
1. Moh's scratch test and Bierbaum's modifications

2. Indentation methods
   - Brinnel's, Rockwell's and Brale methods
   - Micro Vicker's and Knoop's hardness—diamond point hardness.
3. *Penetration methods:* Shore-A and Barcol's durometers.

1. Moh's Scratch Tests (*Refer* to page 349)

Scratching one ore by another ore: Moh could compare the hardnesses of various mineral ores available and arranged them according to numbers 1 for softest talc and 10 for hardest diamond. Hardness of tooth enamel lies in between 5 and 6. As the method was inaccurate and could not be used for many materials, Beirbaum modified the method by scratching a sample by a sharp hard indentor with definite loads and measuring the depths and width's of scratches. This method is now obsolete.

2. Indentation Methods

Brinnel's Hardness Test (BHN)

A hardened steel or tungsten carbide ball of diameter D mm is pressed on the flat surface of a sample with a definite load, P, for 30 sec. The diameter of the indentation, 'd' mm is measured with the help of calibrated eye piece of a traveling microscope. Brinnel hardness number is computed by formula (force/unit area)

$$\text{BHN} = \frac{2P}{\pi D \left[D - (D^2 - d^2)^{\frac{1}{2}}\right]}$$

The applied load can be varied according to the hardness of the materials (Fig. 2.18).

For measuring the hardness of materials used in dentistry, small **Baby-Brinnel** testing instrument having **D = 1.6 mm and P = 123 kg** is used.

Advantage

This method is quite simple and certain relationships between BHN and proportional limit or ultimate tensile strengths of gold alloys have been found.

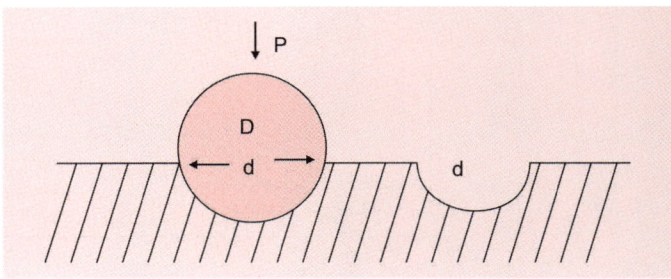

Fig. 2.18: Brinnel's testing method

Disadvantages

This method cannot be used for:

- Brittle materials like ceramics, gypsum products, dental cements, etc.
- Elastically recovering materials, as 'd' decreases on removal of indentor
- Small sites of different phases of alloys
- Getting accurate real values of the hardness of surfaces, as the depth or area of indentation is quite large
- Rubber-like materials like elastomers, hydrocolloids.

Some BHN values (approximate)

Direct filling gold foil = 24 BHN and after condensation = 68 BHN, Gold alloys type I (45), Type II (95), Type III-H (120), Type IV-H (220), Cr-Co alloys. 265, etc. in BHN (kg/mm²) (*refer* to page 350).

Rockwell's Hardness Test

A hardened steel ball of 12.7 mm diameter or a conical diamond point indentor is held on the surface under a **minor load of 3 kg. Then the major load of 30 kg is applied for 10 min and the depth 'a' of indentation can be directly** measured with a micrometer dial gauge. RHN is calculated by a certain formula or read on the calibrated scales. (For different applied loads P = 60, 90, 120, 150 kg, different scales are referred.)

If b is the depth of indentation left after 10 minutes of removal of the major load, the **percentage elastic** (Fig. 2.19) **recovery** $= \dfrac{a-b}{a} \times 100$.

Advantages

- Rockwell's method is also quite simple and RHN is directly obtained from different scales (for different loads), i.e. R_A, R_B, R_C, R_D, R_E, R_F, R_G, etc.
- Can be used for hard and brittle materials
- Can also be used for ductile materials
- Can be used for comparing hardness of elastomers, rubbers, etc.
- Percentage elastic recovery can be found

Disadvantages: Cannot be used for:

- Very hard base metal alloys

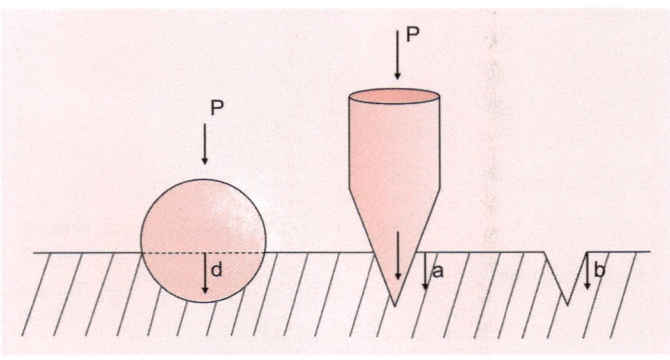

Fig. 2.19: Rockwell's testing method

- Small sites of different phases of alloys
- Getting accurate real hardness of surface, as depth of indentation is quite large.

Some RHN values (approximate)

Gypsum products: Type III stone = 60 RHN
Type IV die stone = 80 RHN
Type V HE, HS die stone = 90 RHN

Microsurface Hardness: Vicker's Diamond Pyramid Test

The earlier explained methods do not give the real surface hardness. As the depths of indentations are more, the resistance offered has the influence of internal lattice structures and properties. To get more **realistic values, the depths of indentation must be reduced to a minimum**. This is done by using, diamond pyramids of large angles and measuring the diagonals of indentation.

Vicker used a square-based diamond pyramid of a large angle **136°**. The metal work surface has to be **well polished**. Indentor is held for 10 seconds on this surface with definite loads, P (5 to 120 kg) and the average diagonal d = $d_1 + d_2$ is measured in mm and k is a constant second.

If the angle of indentor is α (Fig. 2.20a).

$$DPH = VHN = \frac{2P \sin \dfrac{\alpha}{2}}{d^2} = \frac{P}{Kd^2} \ kg/mm^2$$

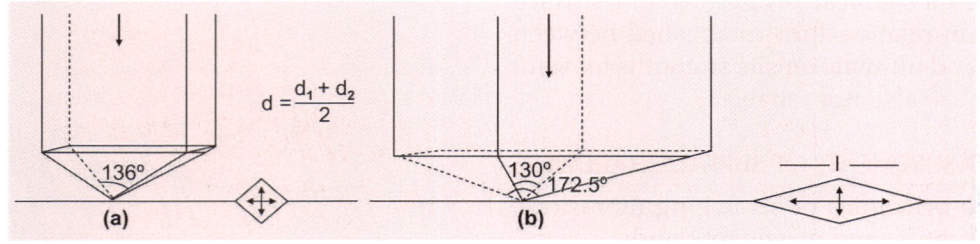

Figs 2.20a and b: (a) Vicker's diamond point indentor, (b) Knoop's diamond point indentor

Advantages
- VHN can be directly found from tables for different diagonals 'd' and for different loads.
- As the depth of indentation is negligible, **more realistic values** are obtained.
- Can be used for very hard (base-metal alloys) and very brittle (ceramic) materials.
- Can be used for small sites of metallurgical **phases of alloys**.

Disadvantages
- Elaborate methods to obtain polished alloy surfaces
- During polishing, work hardening taking place is to be taken care off by annealing
- Cannot be used for elastically recovering materials and elastomers (*refer* to pages 350 and 351).

Some VHN values (approximate)
Tooth enamel = 300 VHN
Tooth dentin = 60 VHN
Titanium alloys = 125–350 VHN
Noble metal alloys (N) = 175–400 VHN
Nickel-Chromium alloys = 210–380 VHN
Cobalt-Chromium alloys = 300–465 VHN
Porcelain = 400–700 VHN
Alumina (Al_2O_3-recrystallised) = 1800 VHN

Microsurface hardness; Knoop's method—KHN:
A rhombic based diamond point indentor with opposite sides at **130° and 172° 30'** is used under different loads (P = 10 kg, ... 100 kg). Indentor is held under the load for 10 min. time, on the **highly polished** surface of the material. These form a rhombic indentation of **negligible depth**. The major diagonal 'l' is measured, under scattered light, after the indentor is removed (Fig. 2.20b).

$$KHN = \frac{P}{Kl^2} \frac{kg}{mm^2}, \text{ where K is a constant}$$

Advantages
- KHN values can readily be found from reference tables
- Can be used for very hard and brittle materials
- Due to negligible depth **more realistic** values are obtained
- Alloys having elastic recoveries can be tested. This is because, when the indentor is removed, the elastic recovery, contraction takes place, along the minor diagonal only, leaving the **major diagonal unaffected**.
- Can be used for small sites of alloy phases.

Disadvantages
- Very high polishing needed, may cause work hardening which requires annealing.
- Rubber-like elastomers cannot be tested.

Some KHN values (approximate)
Tooth enamel = 340 KHN, dentin = 68 KHN, cementum = 40 KHN and hard calculus = 80 KHN, heat cure acrylics = 18–20 KHN, diamond = 7,000–10,000 KHN, silica/quartz = 800 to 820 KHN.

Note (i): This is the most common method, for testing almost all materials used in dentistry, approximate values are given in separate tables (*refer* to Appendix, page 349).

Note (ii): Comparison of surface hardnesses of different materials should be done only with reference to particular testing method and the load-scales.

3. Penetration Method: Barcol Shore-A Durometer

The instrument consists of a blunt pointed stainless-steel indenter of 0.8 mm tip diameter, tapering to a cylinder of 1.6 mm. This is connected through a lever to an adjustable loading spring and a pointer, moving on a scale. The scale is graduated from 100 to 0. The spring load can be adjusted so that when the depth of penetration is maximum (softest material) pointer reads 0 and when there is no penetration (hardest material) it reads 100 (Fig. 2.21).

A sample of definite thickness say, 5 cm, is prepared and allowed to **harden completely**. The durometer indenter is placed on it, for some time until the viscoelastic material shows maximum recovery and hardness number is noted in Table 2.3 where (l = light, m = medium, h = high, p = putty consistencies).

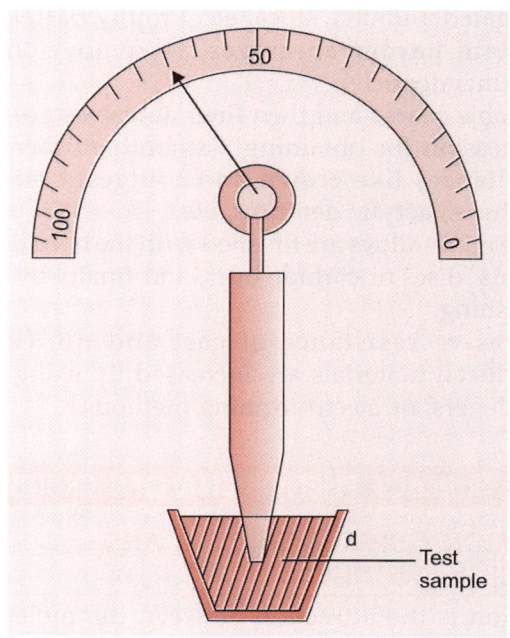

Fig. 2.21: Barcol Shore-A Durometer

Table 2.3	Consistencies and hardness of elastomers	
Material	*Consistencies*	*Shore-A hardness no.*
1. Elastomer	Polysulphides (l, m, h)	20, 30, 35 respectively
2. Elastomer	Add. polysilicones (l, m, h, p)	35, 50, 60, 70 respectively
3. Elastomer	Polyethers, (l, m, m + thinner, h)	38, 48, 43, 55 respectively
4. Resilient liners	....	45–85
5. Maxillofacial polysilicones	....	25
6. Polyethylene, polyvinyl acetate	....	65

l = light, m = medium, h = heavy, p = putty consistencies

Applications in dentistry

Abrasive resistance of the surfaces, mostly depend upon the surface integrity and hardness. **Cutting, abrasion, polishing, finishing, etc.** are the various procedures, involved in the finishing of fabricated oral appliances, preparation of tooth cavities, restorative procedures, maintenance of oral hygiene, etc. Even though tooth enamel is the hardest part of the body, with a surface hardness around 340 KHN, it undergoes attrition by harder foods, opposing metallic, and ceramic appliances, and chemical attacks.

1. Suitable restorative materials of same SH as enamel, should be chosen, to avoid abrasion of tooth or material.
2. Diamond points and carbide burs are used for cutting tooth enamel and hardened steel burs for dentin preparations (SH = 68 KHN).
3. Dentifrices should have **mild abrasives** and not hard levigated alumina, silica, etc. **Prophy pastes** should contain **harder abrasives,** to remove the hard calculus deposits.
4. Suitable coarse and then finer abrasives are used in succession for obtaining a smooth surface of oral appliances like crown and bridges, cast partial dentures, acrylic dentures, etc.
5. Base metal alloys are finished with the hard diamond points, discs or carbide burs, and finally by electro-polishing.
6. Abrasive resistance of cast and die (gypsum products) materials are increased by using surface hardeners, or electroforming methods.

SURFACE PHENOMENA OF LIQUIDS

COHESION (SURFACE TENSION) AND ADHESION (WETTING)

Cohesion is the attraction between the molecules of **same substance** (e.g. molecules of water) and adhesion is the attraction between the molecules of **different** materials (e.g. water molecules and glass surface molecules, adhesives). Due to cohesion, the molecules well inside a liquid, are attracted equally by nearby molecules from all directions. The resultant force becomes zero (energy becomes minimum) and the molecules are 'free' to move, within the liquid.

However, the molecules on the free surface, are acted by **unbalanced cohesive forces** towards the interior, tending to retain a minimum number of molecules on the surface or **minimum surface area**. This surface tension causes the liquid surface to act like a **stretched elastic membrane,** e.g. horizontal liquid surfaces, spherical—small liquid drops, raindrops, mercury drops, etc. have a minimum area of surface.

Surface tension is defined as the unbalanced force acting on the free surface of a liquid, tending to reduce the surface area to a minimum. It is measured **by force acting on unit length of a straight-line imagined on the free surface of a liquid, stretching the molecules apart.** It is measured in **dynes/cm or Newton/meter.**

Factors affecting surface tension
- Nature of the liquid molecules, i.e. the cohesion between the molecules.
  For example: Water at 20°C = 72.8 dynes/cm, Benzene = 29 dynes/cm, Mercury = 465 dynes/cm, at 20°C, Saliva = 40–45 dynes/cm at 37°C, Blood = 50–54 dynes/cm at 37°C
- **Temperature:** ST decreases as temperature rises. Water has surface tensions 76, 72, 68, 59, dynes/cm, at 0°C, 20°C, 50°C and 100°C, respectively.
- **Chemical impurities:** Which decrease surface tension are known as **surfactants, detergents, wetting agents or debubblizers,** e.g. soap solutions or detergents like sodium lauryl sulphate, sodium stearate, sodium laureates, etc. having –COONa hydrophilic groups. **These deplete the number of water molecules on the free surface and reduce surface tension and angle of contacts. One in 5,000 parts, i.e. 0.02% of sodium laureate in water decreases surface tension from 72 to 35 dynes/cm (1 N/m = 1000 dynes/cm).**

SURFACE ENERGY

The surface molecules have higher energies due to **unbalanced forces**. Surface energy is defined as the **work required** to bring the molecules from inside, to form a new surface of unit area or **the energy of molecules in unit area of the free surface.** It is expressed in **erg/cm^2** which has the same magnitude (since ergs/cm^2 = dynes/cm) of surface tension. SE for water at 20°C = 72.8 ergs/cm^2.

Surface energy of tooth enamel = 84 ergs/cm^2 (0.084 J/m^2)

ANGLE OF CONTACT AND WETTING

When a liquid is placed on a solid surface, it spreads out and wets the surface. The surface energies of solid, induce secondary bonding between the solid and liquid molecules. The surface tension of liquid, oppose the spreading, an area of the liquid surface should be minimum (i.e. it tries to retain spherical shape). These reduce the wetting and form contact angle of more than 0°.

 The angle of contact (θ) is the angle made by the tangent, drawn to the liquid surface at the point of contact with the solid surface, the angle being measured within the liquid (Fig. 2.22).

 Smaller θ, shows greater wetting, due to the higher surface energy of solid and lower ST of liquid, and a clean surface.

Wetting of solid surface by the liquid is more, when
- The contact angle is small
- The surface energy of solid is more
- The surface tension of the liquid is less
- Surface is clean without oxide layer or contaminations.

Applications

- **Waxes are hydrophobic** and do not wet when wax patterns of dentures, inlays, crowns, etc. are invested, causing collection of air-bubbles on their surfaces.

The **wax patterns are coated with surfactants** or washed with detergents, leaving a thin film of **wetting agent on** the surface.

- **Some elastomeric** impression materials are hydrophobic, and air bubbles get collected, when the stone cast is poured. Hence, hydrophilic elastomers are preferred (page 342).
- **Fluxes** are applied on base-metals soldering surface to remove the oxide layers (fluoride fluxes for stainless steel) by reducing or dissolving the oxides and help to wet the surface with the solder liquid.
- **Fluoride** applications on tooth enamel reduce the surface energy, wetting, and collection of debris.
- **Surfactants** are included in type V die stones for better wetting and decrease W/P to improve strength.

ADHESION

The attraction between molecules of different materials causes adhesion. The secondary bonding causes weaker adhesion. The primary bonding causes stronger adhesion. When the molecules of a gas or liquid approach the surfaces, they are attracted by secondary bonding and get **adsorbed** on the surface. If these atoms then chemically combine with the surface molecules, it is known as **chemisorption.** Oxygen, hydrogen, etc. gases get adsorbed in molten gold alloy liquid during casting procedures. **Passivation of base metals by Cr, Al, Ti are by chemisorption.**

 The weak secondary bonding, cannot hold two solid surfaces together since very few molecules come close to each other (less than 0.0007 microns). If a drop of water/liquid is placed in between the two glass slides, the wetting causes strong adhesion.

Conditions for strong adhesions are
- Greater wetting, i.e. smaller contact angle
- The higher surface energy of adherend

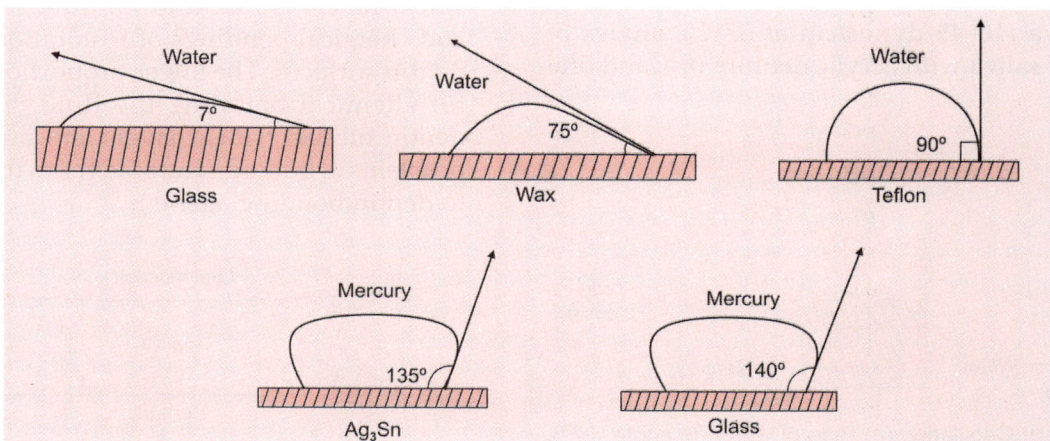

Fig. 2.22: Angle of contacts of water and mercury with different solid surfaces

- The lower surface tension of adhesive
- Clean surfaces, without oxide layers
- The larger area of surfaces (by acid etching)
- Chemisorption of adhesive (dentin bonding poly-carboxylate cements).

Applications

1. **Capillarity:** Penetration of liquids through capillaries is due to the creation of **negative pressure** when the angle of contact is obtuse ($\theta < 90°$). For example when a capillary glass tube of radius r, is held vertically, in water or a liquid of surface tension T, the rise of liquid level, approximately is given by, $h = \dfrac{2T \cos \theta}{rdg}$, where d = density of liquid and θ = contact angle. If θ is acute, $> 90°$, there is capillary depression (like mercury in glass capillary tube held in mercury) (Figs 2.23a and b).

2. **Penetration coefficient:** Due to setting contraction, poor bonding, and dissimilar coefficients of thermal expansions, many restorative materials, and cements leave a marginal gap with the tooth cavity walls. Through these oral fluids can **percolate** or cause **microleakage.** These attack and deteriorate the cavity walls. The **penetration coefficient** is given by

$$PC = \frac{T \cos \theta}{2\eta} \text{ where } \begin{array}{l} T = \text{surface tension} \\ \eta = \text{coefficient of viscosity} \\ \theta = \text{angle of contact} \end{array}$$

   In case of pit and fissure **sealants,** the restorative materials should be thin and flow into the fissures, i.e. high T, low η and small θ. (Examples: Thin or unfilled composite resin, type III GIC.)
   In the interproximal spaces and occlusal fissures, the negative pressure caused by the trapping of saliva can cause penetration and collection of food debris, which deteriorates the surface.

3. **Retention of dentures:** The force of surface tension, **T, of saliva (40–45 dynes/cm** at 37°C), angles of contacts of saliva with acrylic denture (θ_1), and oral mucosa (θ_2) cause adhesion and **retention of the denture** to the oral tissues with force,

$$F = \frac{AT}{t} (\cos \theta_1 + \cos \theta_2) \text{ dynes}$$

Where A = area of the surface of the denture, t = the thickness of saliva film. For better retention, area A must be large, better close fitting (i.e. small thickness of film) and θ_1 and θ_2 must be small. Angle of contact of saliva with acrylic, initially is quite large (75°), but gradually decrease due to adsorption of saliva components. The viscosity of saliva also is a factor to be considered for **retention, and dislodging of dentures** (Fig. 2.24).

4. **Trituration of silver alloy and mercury amalgamation:** When the alloy powder is added to mercury, it does not react by itself. **Large surface tension (465 dynes/cm), high angle of contact (~135°)** of **mercury and a thin oxide film** on the alloy particles, prevent wetting. Trituration removes the oxide layer by friction and forces mercury to come into contact with the surface of alloy particles to react.

5. **Adhesion of food debris to tooth:** The large surface energy of enamel **(~84 ergs/cm²)** cause adhesion and retention of food debris, specially, in the interproximal and occlusal areas. These cause tooth decay. This adhesion is decreased, by reducing the wettability or surface energy of enamel. Application **of fluorides** reduces this surface energy, and hence this method has been used to **reduce the caries incidence** specially in school children.

6. **Adhesion of tooth restoratives:** Mechanical retention can be increased, by preparing the tooth cavities with undercuts, or by acid etching, and then applying thin bonding agents. Chemical bonding is achieved by using polycarboxylate cements and suitable bonding agents. **Removal of smear layers** is found to improve the mechanical and chemical bondings of restorations to exposed dentin surfaces. The lower proportion of Ca^{++} ions for chemical bonding, the fluid circulations in dentin tubules, smear layers, etc. are some of the problems of bonding restoratives to the dentin (*refer to dentin bonding agents*).

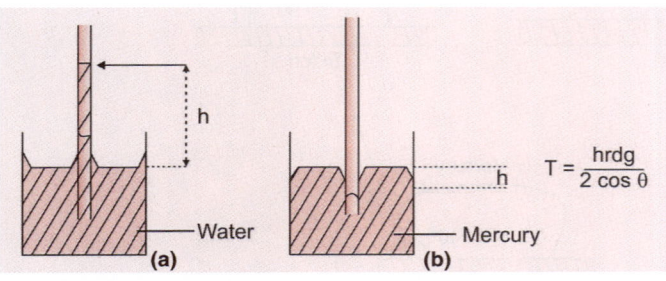

Figs 2.23a and b: Capillarity. (a) Rise of water (θ, acute = 7°), (b) depression of Hg (θ = obtuse, 140°)

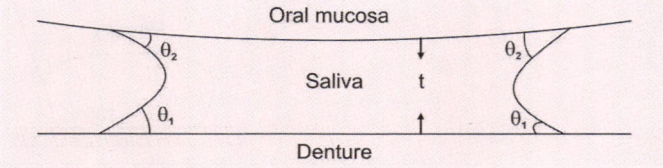

Fig. 2.24: Retention of denture by surface tension of saliva

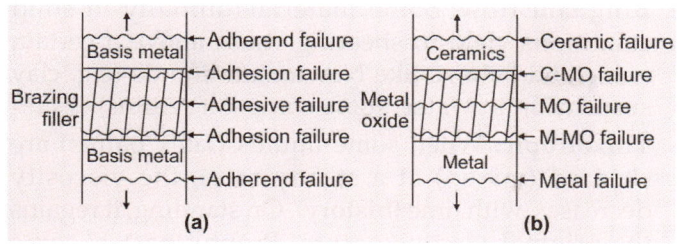

Figs 2.25a and b: (a) Brazing bond failures, (b) metal-ceramic bond failures (*refer* to page 271)

7. **Soldering (brazing):** The **oxide layer** (passivating effect) in the chrome-cobalt, stainless steel and titanium alloys, prevent the wetting and adhesion of the brazing materials. **The fluoride fluxes are specially useful to reduce the oxide layers and dissolve them. The adhesion and flow** of molten solder to unwanted areas is **prevented by applying antifluxes.**

8. **Metal ceramics:** The mechanical bonding is achieved by preparing rough surface and mismatching of coefficients of thermal expansions. Chemical bonding is achieved by forming a metal oxide layer in between them.

9. **Surfactants, wetting agents or detergents** are applied for wetting wax patterns.

10. **Bond failures:** These result from failures in mechanical interlocking, chemical bonding and internal structure of materials used.
   - In soldered materials, the failures can take place at the represented sites (Fig. 2.25a).
   - In a metal-ceramic bonded appliance, the failures are represented as shown
     (M = metal, MO = metal oxide, C = ceramic)
     (Fig. 2.25b).

Suitable techniques of bonding are to be employed for the different materials which are to be carefully selected to prevent failure.

RHEOLOGICAL PROPERTIES—VISCOSITY

Rheology is the study of flow and deformation properties of materials under external forces. Many dental materials are used in the fluid and paste forms which gradually set or harden. Gypsum products—investments, impression materials, restorative materials, waxes, casting alloy liquids, etc. are first manipulated and used in the fluid or paste conditions, within their working times and allowed to set or attain certain rigidity (setting time). The deformations taking place may be elastic, viscous or viscoelastic.

VISCOSITY

The **fluid resistance against flow is viscosity.** In a steady (streamlined) flow condition, different adjacent layers of liquid (or gases) move with different velocities, varying from zero to a maximum value having,

$$\text{Velocity gradient} = \frac{dv}{dh}$$

This is because of the attractive intermolecular forces resist the slipping of the adjacent layers. If A = area of layers, the resisting force, $F = \eta . A . \frac{dv}{dh}$, $dv = dx/dt$

The constant η is coefficient of viscosity,

$$\eta = \frac{F}{A}\frac{dh}{dx}.dt, \quad \frac{F/A}{\frac{dx}{dh}}\bigg/t \quad \text{or} \quad \eta = \frac{\text{Shear stress}}{\text{Shear strain rate}}$$

This has a certain similarity (except time dependence), with the modulus of rigidity, i.e. $\frac{\text{Shear stress}}{\text{Shear strain}}$ of solids

Definition

The coefficient of viscosity is defined as the shearing force or resistance acting between the two adjacent layers of unit area, of a fluid, to maintain unit velocity gradient for streamlined flow.

Units of coefficient of viscosity

$$\eta = \text{dynes}-\text{cm}^{-2}\sec = \text{Poise}$$

$$= \text{Newton}-\text{m}^{-2}-\sec = \text{Pas} = 10 \text{ Poise}$$

Viscosity of dental materials is expressed as **centipoise (CP).**

$$1 \text{ CP} = 10^{-2} \text{ Poise or 1 Poise} = 100 \text{ CP}$$

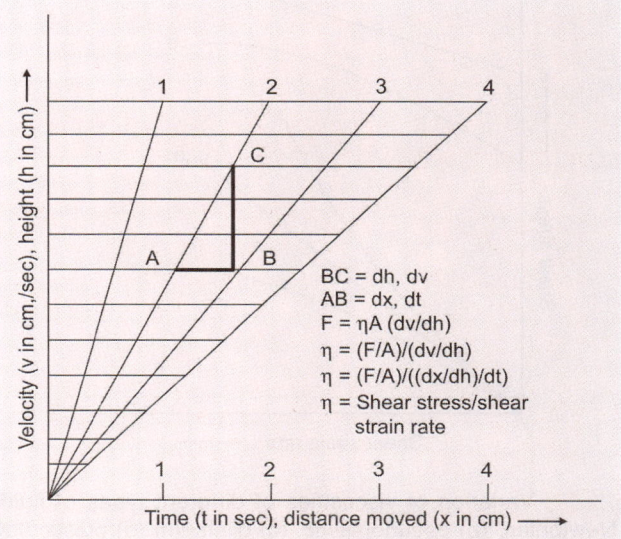

BC = dh, dv
AB = dx, dt
F = ηA (dv/dh)
η = (F/A)/(dv/dh)
η = (F/A)/((dx/dh)/dt)
η = Shear stress/shear strain rate

Fig. 2.26: Viscous fluid flow

For water at 20°C, viscosity = 1 CP = 0.01 Poise
For elastomers at 20°C, viscosity = 60,000 to 4,50,000 CP.

Methods of measuring, η, viscosity
- Capillary flow (Poiseuille's method, Ostwald's method)
- Rotational viscometers (Searle's cylinders, cone-plate)
- Parallel plate, reciprocating rheometers
- Stoke's falling body method, etc.

Factors affecting viscosity η
- Decreases as the temperature rises, for non-setting liquids (water)
- Increases with time and temperatures for chemically setting materials (impressions pastes, cements)
- Composition, fillers, plasticizers, diluents, impurities, etc.
- The shear rates (shear thinning—pseudoplastic)

Dependence of η on shear rate (Fig. 2.27)
a. **Newtonian liquid:** η is constant, i.e. independent of shear rate (e.g. water, oils, etc.).
b. **Pseudoplastic:** The **viscosity** (slope of stress–strain rate graph) **decreases** at higher shearing stresses, i.e. liquids become thinner on vibration, stirring or vigorous mixing (e.g. blood, saliva, dental plaster mix, some impression pastes, cements, fluoride gels, etc.).
c. **Dilatant:** The **viscosities increase** with a shear rate; i.e. these become thicker and show higher resistance to deformation at higher shear rates (e.g. some fluid resins, agar, alginates).
d. **Plastic flow:** Some materials initially in solid condition, yield above certain shear stress and behave like non-Newtonian liquids.

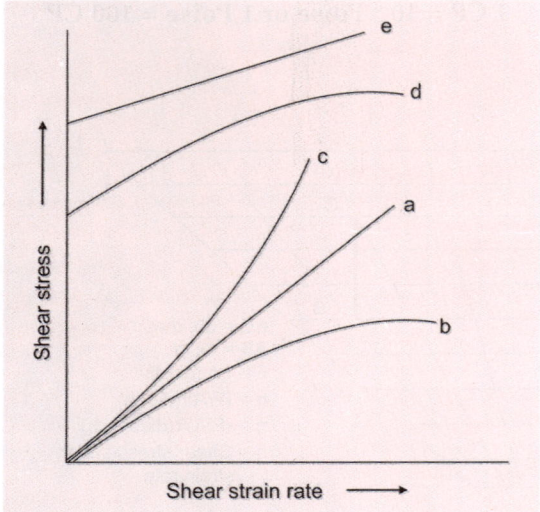

Fig. 2.27: Variation of viscosities of different types of fluids. (a) Newtonian, (b) pseudoplastic, (c) dilatantm (d) plastic flow, (e) Bingham flow

e. **Bingham flow:** Some materials initially in solid conditions yield to shearing stress above a certain value and behave like Newtonian liquids (e.g. clay suspension in water, some composite resins).
f. **Thixotropic:** When some liquids (latex paints) are sheared (mixed) at a steady rate), the viscosity decreases, with time **(history)**. On standing, it regains the original viscous nature. Prophy pastes, some impression pastes and resin cements, dental plaster, etc. have thixotropic properties which are beneficial in clinical practices.

Applications in dentistry
- **Elastomeric impression materials:** These are supplied in two paste forms which on mixing have different viscosities, low (light body), medium (regular body), high (heavy body), and very high (putty) consistencies. These are adjusted with fillers and plasticizers. According to different clinical situations and impression techniques (single mix, double mix, syringe, etc.), suitable materials are chosen, to get an accurate reproduction of finer details. In case of **pseudoplastic** impression pastes, a part of the mix is loaded on the tray, another part is **syringed out**, (when it **becomes very thin** and can flow better) on the prepared teeth surface. The two are brought into contact and allowed to set (*refer* to monophase add. polysilicones).
- **Gypsum products,** when mixed with water, the pseudoplastic mix is obtained. Vibrations or shaking of the mix while pouring the cast makes it thinner and flow better on the impression.
- **Cement consistencies:** Can be adjusted with P/L ratios, for use as a base, restoration or cementation (luting). The consistency increases with time as well as the temperature of the mixing pad. More powder can be added to get higher strength, by cooling the mixing pad or glass slab, powder and liquids. Pseudoplastic (zinc phosphate, ZOE) luting cements have an additional advantage. While cementing the crown or bridge, it is pressed hard against tooth when the luting cement in between becomes thinner and excess flows out leaving the thin layer, as required.
- **Casting alloy liquids** can be made thinner by adding certain trace elements like iridium, which increases the flow or castability so that incomplete castings can be avoided.
- **Cold cure–pour and cure fluid resin,** as well as the agar-agar investments, are dilatants. This helps packing with higher pressure, in pour and cure denture technique.

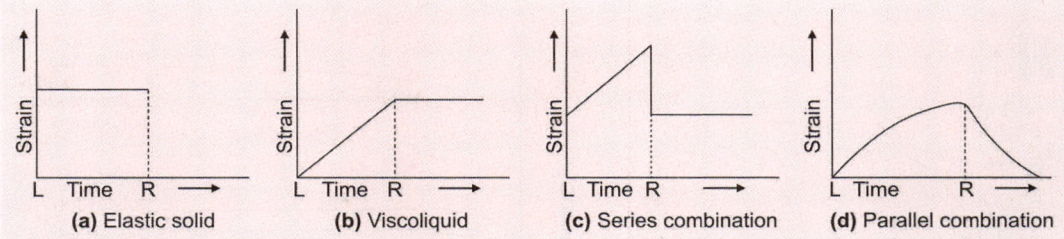

Figs 2.28a to d: Deformation with respect to time, L: Instant of loading, R: Instant of unloading

VISCOELASTICITY (CREEP)

The **mechanical properties of** many dental materials depend on **the rate of loading, i.e. strain rate.** This shows, that their behavior is **intermediate to that of a rigid solid and viscous liquids.** For example, when the rate of loading is increased about 10 times the modulus of elasticity of silver amalgam increased from about 25 GPa to about 62 GPa. Such materials, also **show time-dependent deformations, creep or flow,** like viscous liquids. **This is because both phenomena (deformation and flow) have the same principles of resistance to slip.** The modulus of elasticity of rigid solids is the constant of proportionality of stress and strain (E = stress/strain), whereas the coefficient of viscosity is the constant of proportionality between shearing stress and shear strain rates (η = stress/strain rate).

Viscoelastic behavior of many dental materials in clinical procedures are of much importance. Elastomeric and hydrocolloid impression techniques, amalgam restorations, orthodontic elastics, etc. involved distortions due to **time-dependent stress and strain relaxations.**

THEORETICAL EXPLANATION FOR VISCOELASTIC DEFORMATION (OPTION)

1. For an ideal solid, stress is directly proportional to strain. Strain remains constant until stress is removed and vanish immediately (Fig. 2.28a).
2. For an ideal liquid, a shearing stress is directly proportional to strain rate. Strain increases with respect to time and remains constant when the stress is removed (Fig. 2.28b).
3. When these properties act in **series**, the changes in strain can be represented as shown in Fig. 2.28c.
4. When these properties act in **parallel**, the changes in the stress and strain of materials can be represented as shown in Fig. 2.28d.
5. In actual viscoelastic materials, the interactions of these properties take place in a complex manner, partly in series and partly in parallel. These will result in an instantaneously recoverable elastic strain (BC), time-dependent recovering anelastic strain (CD), and residual viscous strain (DE), as shown in Fig. 2.29.

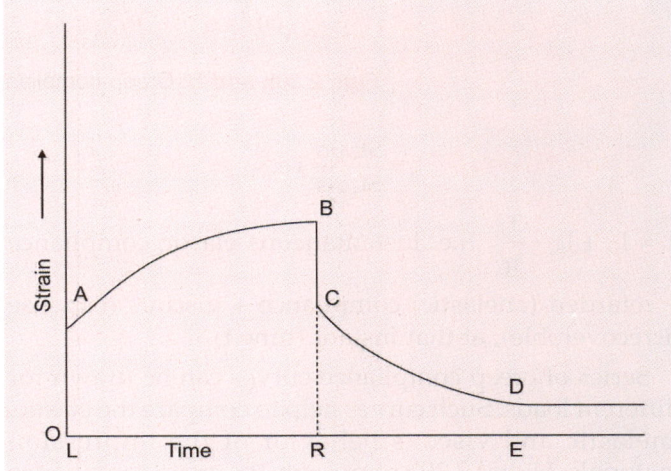

Fig. 2.29: Viscoelastic strains of elastomeric impressions, series plus parallel combinations

Application

Elastomeric impressions: After complete setting, shearing load or stress is applied parallel to the tissue surface to dislodge the impression. The deforming strain produced is partly elastic OA and partly time-dependent AB. Applied load immediately vanishes but stress and strain persist and recovery begins to take place, from B.

The elastic recovery **BC is instantaneous.** The time dependent, **creep or anelastic recovery CD** takes place initially quickly, but later quite slowly, until a permanent **irrecoverable viscous strain DE** is left behind. To achieve maximum dimensional accuracy or minimum distortion, dental stone cast **pouring is to be delayed for about 30 minutes (OE).**

Creep compliance (optional)

As the external load vanishes the internal stress produced causes the recovery of strain (BCD) first faster, then slowly (Figs 2.30a and b). The magnitudes of this residual strains can be more easily understood by creep-compliance curves (Figs 2.30a and b).

Creep compliance J_t is the ratio of strain to stress at the given instant.

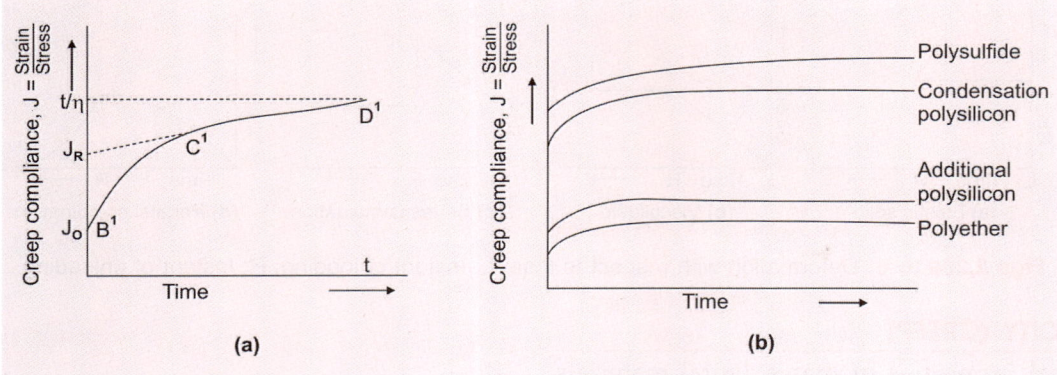

Figs 2.30a and b: Creep compliance curves. (a) General, (b) elastomers

$$J_t = \frac{Strain}{Stress} \text{ i.e.,}$$

$J_t = J_O + J_R + \dfrac{t}{\eta}$, i.e. instantaneous elastic compliance + retarded (anelastic) compliance + viscous response (irrecoverable), at that instant (time t).

Series of creep compliance curves can be drawn for different loads. Such curves help to compare the elastic, anelastic and viscous behavior of the impression materials. Figure 2.30b represents the creep compliance of the common elastomeric impression materials. These show, that **polyether has least flexibility, least permanent deformation, and highest elastic recovery properties, followed by addition polysilicones, condensation polysilicones and polysulphides. Polysulfides have high flexibility** and **viscous behavior.** It requires a **longer time** to recover and more delay in pouring the cast.

- **Hydrocolloid impressions:** Exhibit viscoelastic properties after gelation. The strength properties are better at **higher rate of loading**. The impressions are dislodged with a **single sudden jerk to improve tear strength** (or minimise the chance of tearing) and to get the highest elastic recovery. But as the dimensional change due to syneresis, is very predominant compared to the anelastic recovery, the stone cast is to be poured **immediately.**
- **Creep and flow:** Creep and flow are the **time-dependent deformations** (increase in strains) **taking place in viscoelastic materials by constant static load** or repeated **dynamic loads.** Usually, creep and flow refer to the crystalline and amorphous materials respectively but sometimes the terms are used for both. The posterior restorations of silver amalgam are subjected to large dynamic impact forces repeatedly several times. The restoration gets gradually deformed and flows or creeps on the occlusal surface as thin ledges. This easily fractures,

creating crevices at margins, which collect food debris and enhances caries. Proper selection of alloy and manipulation methods are used for minimising creep (refer to silver amalgam). Microstructure, having more γ_1 and γ_2 phases, increase creep, and η phase rods decrease creep, as these interconnect growing γ_1 crystals.

- Impression compounds have higher creep and flow at higher temperatures, and also is controlled by their compositions.
- **Stress relaxation (elastics in orthodontia):** This refers to the decrease in stress with respect to time for viscoelastic materials, kept under constant strains. For example in orthodontia, small constant forces are applied, to bring the tooth nearer and to align them by using stretched elastic bands (Fig. 2.31).

  The initial stress gradually decreases (relax) and become constant after about 2 or 3 weeks. The low residual stress is not adequate, and hence the elastics are to **be changed frequently** by the patient. For the **elastic bands** of the same dimensions, the **plastic** band shows large stress, whereas, the **latex** band shows more constant but smaller stresses, for a long time. The **stress relaxation is high in plastic bands.**
- **Acrylic dentures** have viscoelastic properties, due to which, distortion of denture takes place in long service.

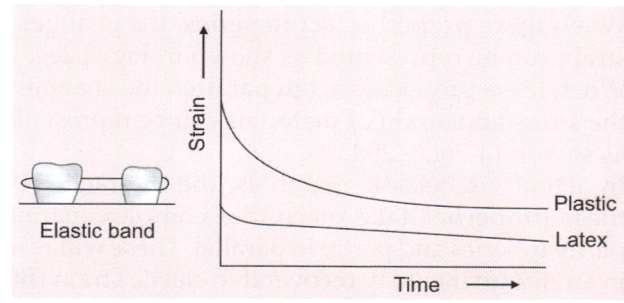

Fig. 2.31: Viscoelastic stress relaxation for plastic and latex stretched elastic bands

- **Viscoelastic palatal mucosa easily gets displaced** while taking impressions, according to the load applied. The viscoelastic property causes a delay in recovery.

To get an accurate impression, of mucosal tissues in their resting position, the patient should not wear the old denture for several hours before taking the impression.

- **Casting alloys in metal ceramics:** Creep of alloys, depends on its composition and is **more at higher temperature**. Metal ceramics, fixed or removable partial dentures can undergo a higher creep rate (or sag) during the laboratory procedures, resulting in deformation of the appliances.

THERMAL PROPERTIES

Heat is a form of energy corresponding to the kinetic energies of vibrations and movements of the atoms and molecules of the substances in solid, liquid or gaseous states. These energies increase with temperatures.

Temperature is the measure (or degree) of hotness of a material. It is measured (by thermometers) by the heat-induced changes in certain physical properties like expansions, electrical resistances, wavelengths of electromagnetic radiations, etc. Different scales of measurements are, Kelvin (absolute), Celsius (French) Fahrenheit (British), Reumer (German).

For example, melting point of ice

$0°C = 32°F = 0°R = 273° K$ at 1 atm. pressure

Boiling point of water

$100°C = 212°F = 80°R = 373°K$ at 1 atm. pressure

Conversion to centigrade.......

$x°C = \dfrac{5}{9}(F°-32) = \dfrac{5°R}{4} = (K°-273)$ in centigrades

Heat is measured (calorimetry) by the changes in the temperatures of the material in calories, joules or BTU. **One calory is the amount of heat required to raise the temperature of 1 gram of pure water by, 1°C (i.e. from 14.5 to 15.5°C). 1 cal = 4.18 Joules**.

Specific heat is the thermal capacity of 1 gm of a substance. It is the amount of heat required to raise the temperature of 1 gm of a substance by 1°C. For water sp. ht = 1 cal/gm = 4.18 joules/gm.

Thermal capacity is the amount of heat required to raise the temperature of the **entire mass** by 1°C, = M × S. Lower the specific heat, less heat is required to raise the temperature.

The quantity of heat is measured by the product of mass, specific heat and change in temperature

$$Q = MS\ (\theta_2-\theta_1)\ cals.$$

Heat flows by conduction, convection, and radiation from the region of higher temperature to that of lower temperature. When heat is absorbed, the temperature of the object rises, and it expands proportionately.

The principle of heat exchanges

When two materials at different temperatures are intimately mixed.

Heat lost by hot body = Heat gained by the cold body
= Mass × sp. ht × change in temperature.

HEAT OF FUSION (LATENT HEAT)

When a solid is heated, the kinetic energies of vibration of atoms increase, and finally they get detached from each other, at its characteristic temperature and converted to a liquid state.

Latent heat of fusion is the amount of heat required to convert one gram of a substance from its solid to a liquid state at its normal melting temperature. This is the thermal energy required to break the solidbonds of the atoms and make them move at random, with varying velocities in the restricted space occupied by the liquid. Similarly, when a liquid is converted into solid, this amount of heat is to be lost or taken out of the substance (Appendix, Table 9) (for ice., L = 80 cal/gm).

For example, latent heat of fusion is supplied to the alloy pellet to melt into liquid, which during solidification get released to investment material in casting procedure or during brazing procedures.

Latent heat of vapourisation is the heat required to convert 1 gm of a liquid into its vapour at its normal boiling point. For water L = 540 cal/gm at 100°C and normal one-atmosphere pressure.

THERMAL CONDUCTION

Conduction of heat from a hot region to cold region takes place through the free electrons present in metals and vibrations of atoms depending on interatomic distances.

Thermal conductivity or coefficient of thermal conduction (K) is the **amount of heat** conducted per second through one cm^2 area of the surface of a material of 1 cm thickness, when the opposite surfaces are maintained at a steady temperature difference of 1°C. **The units are cal/sec/cm²/unit temp. gradient,** i.e. cal/sec/cm²/(°C/cm). All metals are good conductors of heat as well as electricity, whereas, most non-metals, polymers, ceramics, etc. are good insulators, due to the absence of free electrons.

Applications in dentistry

1. **Tooth structure: Enamel and dentin have very low K, i.e. 0.0022 and 0.0016** cgs units respectively. These help to protect the sensitive pulp from **thermal and electrical insults.**

2. **Tooth restorative materials should be good insulators to protect the pulp**. But the permanent restorations of direct filling gold, metal alloy inlays, crowns, bridges, and silver amalgam are not good insulators. Hence, the **pulp should be protected by insulating bases**, and pulp capping agents.

3. **Ideally, impression materials should be good conductors** of heat so that thermoplastic materials can be softened uniformly and all impression materials should harden or set uniformly (or simultaneously) to **minimise the distortion due to relaxation of internal stresses**. Unfortunately, all impression materials are **not good conductors** and suitable precautions are to be taken for precision impressions.

4. **Denture base materials:** The common PMMA denture base material is a very poor conductor of heat. The patient cannot feel the real hotness or coldness (taste) of the food.

THERMAL DIFFUSIVITY

This is the rate at which a body with a nonuniform temperature distribution approaches equilibrium by conduction of heat from higher temperature to lower temperature regions of the body.

This is expressed as the ratio

$$D = \frac{\text{Thermal conductivity}}{\text{Specific heat} \times \text{density}}, \text{i.e.}$$

$$D = \frac{K}{Sd} \ cm^2/sec, \ mm^2/sec, \ m^2/sec$$

Applications

1. **In deep cavities** the exposed pulp or dentin is protected from thermal insult when the oral temperature fluctuates due to hot or cold foods. Hence, the restorative materials should have **low thermal conductivities as well as low thermal diffusivities, that is high specific heat.**

2. **Direct filling gold,** silver amalgam, and the metallic restorations have high thermal conductivities and diffusivities. The patient may experience thermal shocks when the oral temperature fluctuates. Tooth enamel, dentin, and most non-metallic restorations, like $ZnPO_4$, GIC, composite resins have low K and low D. These are desired properties, i.e. to protect the pulp from thermal insults or shocks. The **thickness** of such restorations or cement bases should be adequate for **effective pulp protection.**

THERMAL EXPANSION

When the thermal energy is given to a material (i.e. heated), the amplitude of atomic vibrations and hence the inter-atomic spacing increases. The cumulative effect of this is thermal expansion (or contraction when cooled). The coefficient of linear thermal expansion is the increase in length per unit original length per degree centigrade (Kelvin) rise in temperature. If l_1 and l_2 are the lengths of a specimen at $t_1°C$ and $t_2°C$ temperatures,

$$COTE = \alpha = \frac{l_2 - l_1}{l_1(t_2 - t_1)}/°C$$

Units of $COTE = \dfrac{m}{m}/°C$ or $\dfrac{cm}{cm}/°C$ or $\dfrac{mm}{mm}/°C$, i.e. $/°C$

Since the values are very small $COTE = \alpha$ is given in $10^{-6}/°C$ or parts per million$/°C$, i.e. ppm$/°C$, by multiplying α with 10^6.

The coefficient of volume expansion can be shown as,

$$\gamma = \frac{V_2 - V_1}{V_1(t_2 - t_1)} = 3\alpha$$

Applications in dentistry

1. **Impression materials** ideally should have COTE = 0, to reduce dimensional changes of impressions due to thermal contraction from 37°C to room temperature and also distortions due to relaxation of internal stresses-induced during manipulation as well as due to nonuniform thickness of impression, $(x = \alpha (t_2 - t_1) \times \text{thickness})$.

   Since all impression materials have high α, (impression compound ~300–350 ppm$/°C$, elastomers 150–225 ppm$/°C$), suitable precautions and modifications of impression techniques (using a spacer of uniform thickness, wash impression, secondary impression, etc.) are used.

2. **Restorative materials** should have the value, **same** as that of enamel crown, i.e. $\alpha = 11.4$ ppm$/°C$. (Dentin has $\alpha = 8.3$ ppm$/°C$.) Almost all restorative materials have α differing from 11.4 ppm$/°C$.

   This large difference in COTE causes dissimilar thermal contractions and expansions of restorations and tooth structure **when cold and hot foods or drinks are used**. This causes **marginal or microleakages** which induce further decay of cavity walls. Larger the deviation COTE of the cement from 11.4 ppm$/°C$, greater is this **percolation,** e.g. acrylics $\simeq$ 80–120 ppm$/°C$, composite resins = 20–60 ppm$/°C$, silver amalgam = 25ppm$/°C$, GIC = 10–11 ppm$/°C$ (least microleakage), ceramics, silicate cements 7–8.5 ppm$/°C$).

3. The **brazing** (soldering) material should have **COTE same** as that of the substrate, to avoid distortion and detachment when heated or cooled.

4. **Metal ceramics:** Thermal bonding of metal and ceramics can be obtained by making their COTEs slightly different, i.e. **mismatching.** The α of alloys used is lowered by adding metals of low COTE like Pt, Pd, etc. to about 13–13.5 ppm/°C, whereas α of **ceramics is** raised, by using more leucite or devitrifiers such as Na or K ions to about 12.5–13.0 ppm/°C.

5. In the casting procedure, the metal alloy liquids after solidifying in the moulds at approximately 930°C for noble metals and 1300°C for base metal alloys, cool down to room temperature (or 37°C) undergoing **large thermal contractions, approximately 1.3 or 2.0%.** This is to be **compensated** by large setting expansion and thermal expansions of the investment materials. Cristobalite, a polymorphic form of quartz, used as a refractory material, is selected due to its large thermal expansion at lower temperatures.

COLOUR PARAMETERS AND COLOUR MATCHING

Aesthetic considerations in prosthodontics, and conservative (cosmetic) dentistries have received greater importance in recent years. Many advances in ceramics and its fabrication, spectrum of different colours (red to violet) on a screen, techniques, availability of anterior restoratives like glass ionomers, composite resins, compomers, etc. have created many problems, demanding challenging artistic abilities and skill, from dentists and technicians. This requires applications of basic scientific knowledge of certain areas in optics, such as:

- Laws of reflection, refraction, dispersion, diffraction, transmission, scattering, fluorescence, etc.
- Spectral distributions of visible lights emitted from various illuminating sources reflected and scattered from the surfaces.
- Colour parameter measurements
- Physiological and psychological factors of vision
- Optical anisotropy of tooth structure
- Problems involved in colour matching
- Variations of colour parameters in service, etc.

Visible light is a small part of the electromagnetic energy spectrum, with the wavelength (λ) extending from 400 nm (violet) to 800 nm (red), i.e. lying in between ultraviolet and infrared regions. The energy of such radiations depend on the wavelength (λ) or the frequency (ν) as

$$\varepsilon = h\nu = \frac{hc}{\lambda} \text{ ergs}$$

where Planck's constant, h = 6.62×10^{-27} ergs and velocity of light, c = 3×10^{10} cm/sec. Depending on this **photon energies,** different physiological responses are produced in the nerve cones and rods in the retina, which are interpreted as colours by the brain. The physical responses of substances, to various energy ranges, are utilized in industries, as well as in health sciences. The electromagnetic energy spectrum can be represented as in Table 2.4.

The photons of different energies (of ν or λ) ranges are emitted, during energy transitions/changes taking place mainly in the nucleus (γ-rays), innermost orbits of atoms (X-rays), outer orbits (UV, visible, infrared rays), atomic vibrations (thermal, microwaves or radio waves), etc. Analysis of these photon radiations has given deep insight into the atomic and molecular

Table 2.4	Electromagnetic radiation spectra		
	Frequencies (ν Hertz)	Wavelength (λ m)	Main uses
γ-rays	$3 \times 10^{19} - 3 \times 10^{22}$	$10^{-11} - 10^{-14}$	Industries, medicine
X-rays	$3 \times 10^{16} - 3 \times 10^{19}$	$10^{-8} - 10^{-11}$	Industries, medicine **Dentistry radiography**
Ultraviolet	$3 \times 10^{14} - 3 \times 10^{16}$	$10^{-6} - 10^{-8}$	Industries, medicine **Polymerizing resins** visible
Red to violet	$5.75 \times 10^{14} - 7.5 \times 10^{14}$	$8 \times 10^{-7} - 4 \times 10^{-7}$	**All visual fields**
Infrared	$3 \times 10^{12} - 3 \times 10^{14}$	$10^{-4} - 10^{-6}$	**Thermal energy (curing, etc.)**
Microwaves	$3 \times 10^{8} - 3 \times 10^{12}$	$1 - 10^{-4}$	Thermal **(curing)** Communications
Radiowaves	$< 3 \times 10^{8}$	>1 meter	Communications

structures, methods of analysing the compositions, and reactions of chemical compounds and in many other fields. Spectrophotometers, colorimeters, electron microscopes (SEM), etc. involved in this basic science knowledge.

DISPERSION OF LIGHT

When white light is passed through a glass prism, it is dispersed according to their wavelengths and form a spectrum of different colours (red or violet) on a screen. The lights of different energies or wavelengths (colours), reflected or scattered from an object, enter or get focused on the retina. **These physical excitation energies, incident on the optical nerve endings as rods or cones, produce physiological nerve impulses,** which are conveyed through the optic nerves to the brain for interpretation as colours. Nerve rods show responses to white light and the **cones** show responses mainly to three colours, **blue, green, and red—tristimuli.** These three **primary colours** have approximate wavelengths, blue (430–460 nm), green (510–570 nm) and red (610–780 nm).

COLOUR TRIANGLE: PRIMARY, SECONDARY AND COMPLEMENTARY COLOURS

When the primary colours B, R, G, are mixed with correct proportions, white colour is obtained. The **secondary colours** are obtained by mixing of any two primary colours in the correct proportions (Fig. 2.32).

B + G → cyan, G + R → yellow, R + B → magenta

If these are mixed in any proportions, an infinite number of colours is formed. Our eyes are not so much sensitive, but are capable of distinguishing seven (VIBGYOR) or ten colours, and their combinations.

(P-PB-B-BG-G-GY-Y-YR-R-RP-P, purple), cyan (B+ G), yellow (G+R), magenta (R+B) are complementary to red, blue, and green, since on mixing they give white colour.

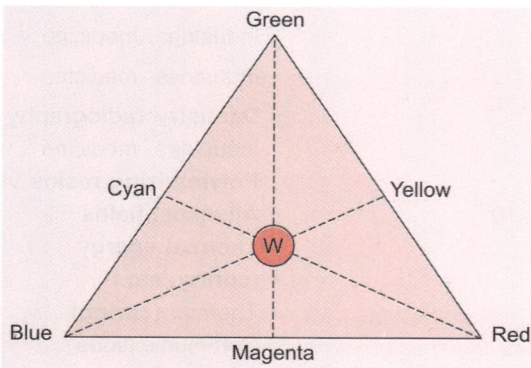

Fig. 2.32: Colour triangle

COLOUR PIGMENTS

When white light is passed through a red glass filter, it allows only red light and absorbing all the other colours. Similarly, if a colour pigment, like HgS is added, it absorbs all other colours except its own red, and the material appears red by reflection of light. As inorganic substances are more stable, these are used as colour pigments, e.g. green (CdS), pink (Fe_2O_3).

COLOUR PARAMETERS

Perception of colour is by the **physiological responses of optic nerve ends (cones) due to the physical excitation (tristimuli). Colour sensation is the subjective experience due to objective tristimuli.** According to **Grassmann's laws, the eye can distinguish differences in colours only by three dimensions or parameters, i.e. hue, value, chroma.**

1. **Hue:** It is the **colour** corresponding to the **dominant wavelength** of light, or it is the **subjective interpretation** of the (monochromatic) dominant wavelengths of light, incident on the nerve-cones of retina. This forms a continuous spectrum of colours, purple to red end. In visual techniques these are considered as purple, P, PB, B, BG, G, GY, Y, YR, R, RP, purple, i.e. ten colours, which are further measured in segments of 0, 2.5, 5, 7.5, 10, (i.e. say Y 10 or YR 0, YR 2.5, YR 5, YR 7.5, YR 10 or R 0, R 2.5 .... etc.)

2. **Value:** It is the **luminous reflectance** of a colour of a surface, and is **independent of hue. It is the brightness or lightness (value = 10) or darkness (value = 0)** of a colour of the surface. The shades of teeth and restorative materials are grouped as of higher (brighter) or lower (darker) values. In the visual technique, values of perfect black to perfect white surfaces are sometimes represented from 0 to 10 (or 0–100).

3. **Chroma: It is the colour saturation or excitation purity:** The chroma is represented by purity or by the excitation with increasing saturation 0–1 or grey (0), 2, 4, 6..... 18 (highly saturated).

MEASUREMENT OF COLOUR PARAMETERS

Methods used mainly are:
1. **A visual technique using Munsell's colour system**
2. **Instrumental techniques:** Colorimeters, spectrophotometer, chromaticity diagrams, etc.

Munsell's Colour System

The three colour parameters **hue, value, and chroma** are presented in a three-dimensional system. **The hue** of 10 colours, P, PB, B, BG, G, GY, Y, YR, R and RP are

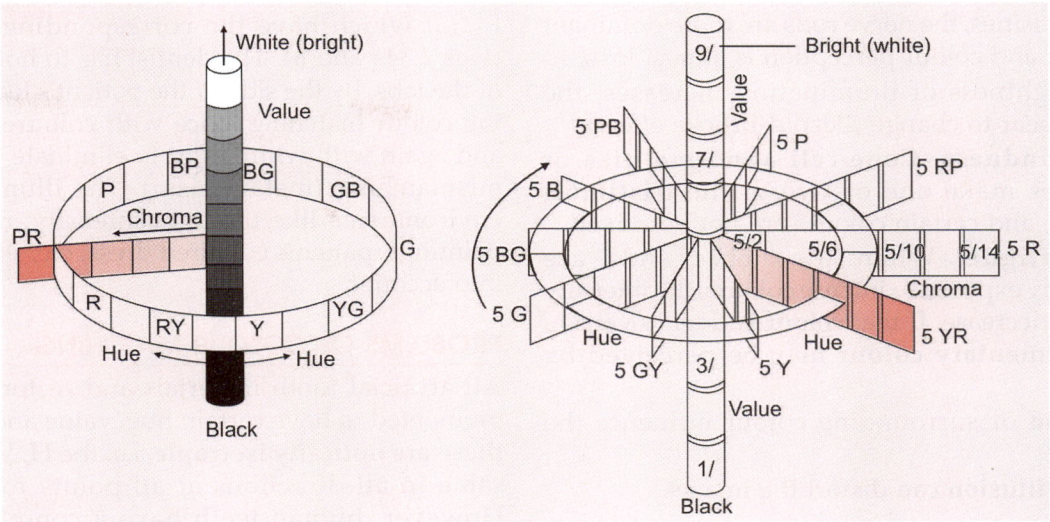

Fig. 2.33: Munsell's colour system—hue, chroma, value, scales

painted with **continuous change** on a circular strip, with 0, 2.5, 5, 7.5 gradations as shown for each colour (Fig. 2.33).

The value of brightness or whiteness is presented by **10 tabs** with varying brightness, or whiteness from the lowest lightness or darkness, along with the vertical axial cylinder.

The chroma colour saturation (excitation purity) is represented along the radial tabs with increasing saturation 0–1 or grey (0), 2, 4, 6.....18 (highly saturated) for every hue and values as shown.

The measurement of colour parameters is done by:
- Moving the sample along the hue strip and matching it, say H = 5 YR
- Along the vertical cylindrical tabs and matching it say V = 6
- Along the chroma tabs, say C/8. Then the colour parameters of the sample are:

$$HVC = 5YR\frac{6}{8}$$

Colour difference from the standard value can be calculated using Nickerson's formula

$$I = \frac{C}{5} \Delta H + 6 \Delta V + 3 \Delta C$$

Where C = average chroma. Trained observer can identify the difference of more than a factor 5.

Instrumental techniques are more complicated as it involves the systematic matching of the tristimuli values (R, G, B) of the light reflected from the surface, and comparing them with those of the standard gas-filled light source of Commission Internationale de Ecllairage (CIE) and then with average daylight. Chromaticity diagrams also are used to find luminous reflectances.

FACTORS AFFECTING COLOUR MATCHING

Sources of Illumination
- Incandescent, fluorescent, and white light have different spectral distributions. These vary with the brightness (voltage of power supply) of emitted light.
- Surrounding reflectors, wall paints of the clinics, colour of the patient's dress (even lipsticks), etc.

Nature of the Object
- **Transmission,** scattering and absorption of colours.
- **Reflections:** White surface reflects all colours, black surface absorbs all colours, coloured surfaces absorb all other colours, and reflects their own colours.
- **Translucent materials:** Cause greater lightness.
- Surface gloss or roughness: Glossy surface reflects more.
- Fluorescent materials emit light of higher wavelengths.
- Careless addition of pigments, change HVC.
- **Metamerism:** Certain colours match properly in one source and **mismatch in other.**
- **Isomerism: Exact matching of any 2 shades at all sources or colours.**

Observer's Physiological Aspects
- The human eye is almost equally sensitive to all the colours, but has a **higher response to green.**

- At low intensities, the nerve rods are more dominant than cones, and colour perception is almost lost.
- As the brightness of illumination increases, the colours appear to change (Bezold-Brucke effect).
- **Colour blindness:** Cone-cell abnormalities or deficiencies make one or two of the **tristimuli ineffective,** and certain colours are not perceived.
- **Colour fatigue:** When the nerve ends are continuously exposed to intense colours, the intensity appears to decrease. If that colour suddenly vanish, its **complementary colour** may be perceived by fatigue.
- **Background** or surrounding colour influence the perception.
- **An optical illusion** can distort the images.

COLOUR MATCHING OF RESTORATIONS WITH TOOTH

Very careful selection of materials for restorations, artificial teeth, fabrication of ceramic crowns, veneers, metal ceramics, etc. is to be done to achieve the goal of **perfect colour matching.** The hue, value, and chroma of patients, teeth should exactly match with those of selected materials and fabrications (Table 2.5). Manufacturers supply visible light cured composites, compomers, enamel and dentin ceramics, etc. of various shades (HVC values) for selection and use. They also provide the corresponding **shade-guides,** to assist the colour matching. These shade-guides have many shade tabs, marked A_1, A_2, A_3, A_4, B_1......, C_1......, D_1......, E_1........which have the corresponding HVC values (Figs 2.34a and b). The dentist has to hold closely, one of the tabs, by the side of the patient's teeth, and verify the colour matching, once with **coloured light (blue)** and again with **white light** to eliminate the chances of mismatching (metamerism). The illuminations and environments like the light intensity, reflecting wall paintings, patients coloured dress, etc. should be taken into account.

PROBLEMS OF COLOUR MATCHING

All artificial tooth materials and restorations can be pigmented to have certain hue, value and chroma. **But these are optically isotropic,** i.e. the H, V, C values are same in all directions at all points for all colours. However, human teeth have a complex structure, comprising, **optically internal anisotropic structures of enamel and dentin** having different thicknesses at different regions. **The orientations, and density distributions of the enamel rods, of different refractive indices are different in different directions,** which make the anisotropy still worse.

The hue, value and chroma of teeth depend on
1. Patients
2. Oral health conditions, i.e. discolouration of the teeth
3. Placement and position of the teeth
4. Patients' age, sex, etc.
5. Nature of light intensity, wavelength, etc.

Due to this extreme optical anisotropy, it is perhaps impossible to select a perfectly colour matching material.

Table 2.5	Colour parameters of few materials		
Material surface	*Hue dominant λ nm*	*Value, luminous reflectance, 0–100*	*Chroma; excitation purity 0–1*
Human teeth	566–586	36–45	0.35–0.4
Glass ionomer	577–579	55–68	0.2–0.27
Composite resin	576–580	52–79 (brighter)	0.15–0.30
Veneer resin	577–580	56–64	0.26–0.31
Denture resin	601–623 (reddish)	22.5–28.6	0.30–0.38

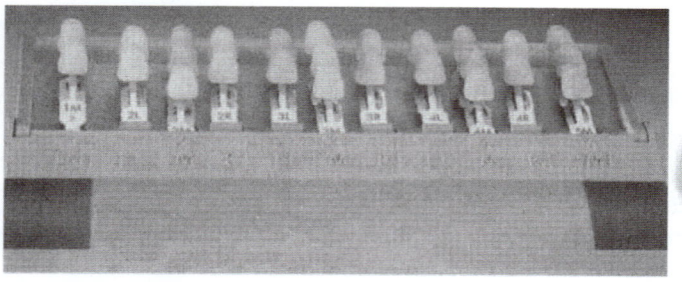

(a)

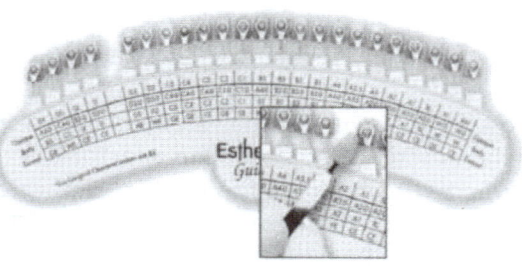

(b)

Figs 2.34a and b: Shade-guides: (a) Vitapan 3D shade-guide, (b) Esthet-x composite shade-guide

MODEL QUESTIONS

I. Long Essays (20 minutes each)

1. Explain the different types of stresses and strains. Describe the stress–strain relationship and give the significances of elastic and nonelastic deformations.
2. Explain the term surface hardness. Describe the indentation methods of determination and add a note on abrasive and polishing agents (also *refer* to Chapter 26).
3. Explain the term strengths of materials. Briefly outline the methods of determination of strengths and give their significances in dentistry.

II. Short Essays (10 minutes each)

1. Atomic bonding
2. Crystal lattices (also *refer* to alloys)
3. Stress and strains
4. Modulus of elasticity
5. Modulus of resilience
6. Yield strength
7. Flexure strength
8. Strengths of materials, and testing methods
9. Ductility and malleability
10. Impact strength
11. Surface hardness
12. Microhardness tests
13. Surface tension
14. Adhesion
15. Viscosity
16. Viscoelasticity
17. Creep (also *refer* to silver amalgam)
18. Thermal expansion
19. Thermal conductivity
20. Colour parameters
21. Colour matching
22. Fracture toughness

III. Brief Answers (5 minutes each)

1. Covalent bond
2. van der Waals forces
3. Metallic bonds
4. Amorphous solids
5. Stress and strains
6. Complex stresses
7. Proportional limit
8. Yield stress
9. Flexibilities
10. Ductility
11. Malleability
12. Percentage elongation
13. Ultimate strength
14. Tensile strength
15. Compressive strength
16. Torsion
17. Bending
18. Moh's scratch test
19. Brinnel's hardness test
20. Rockwell's hardness test
21. Vicker's diamond point hardness
22. Knoop's hardness number
23. Shore-A Penetrometer (durometer)
24. Microcrystalline layer (*refer* to polishing)
25. Contact angle
26. Capillarity
27. Surfactants
28. Retention of denture
29. Penetration coefficient
30. Adhesion of food debris to tooth
31. Adhesion failures
32. Pseudoplasticity
33. Creep
34. Creep compliances
35. Thermal expansion
36. Thermal diffusivity
37. Primary and secondary colours
38. Hue, chroma, value
39. Optical isomerism and metamerism
40. Shade guides

Impression Materials (Auxiliary Materials)

These are very important auxiliary materials used in clinical laboratories to obtain the **exact negative replica of the oral structures**. From these, positive hard replica cast can be prepared for construction procedure of oral appliances or study models for diagnostic purposes. As the procedures for **fabrications** of **prosthesis** like acrylic dentures, metal, and ceramic appliances are complicated and involve high temperatures, sophisticated equipment and laboratories, such positive duplicates are used by the technicians or dentists in the absence of the patients.

DEFINITION

"**An impression can be defined as an exact negative replica of the teeth and its associated oral tissues with accurate reproduction of all finer details, maintaining correct spatial dimensions**".

Cast is an exact positive hard replica of dentulous or edentulous arches of oral tissues used in fabricating procedures of oral appliances.

Model or study casts are the exact positive hard duplicates of dentulous or edentulous arches used for diagnostic and fabrication purposes in orthodontia, prosthodontia, pedodontia, etc. specialities.

Die is also an exact positive hard duplicate of single or sometimes few teeth used in fabrication procedures of inlay, onlays, crowns and bridges, etc.

IMPRESSION MATERIALS

Impression materials are used to register and reproduce the forms and relationships of teeth and associated oral tissues.

Impressions of a **portion of a tooth, a single tooth, several teeth, entire dentulous or edentulous arches or even perioral and extraoral structures may be recorded.**

Impression materials are generally carried to the patient's mouth by an **impression tray.** The trays support the impression materials and not allow it to flow down since most materials are in semisolid conditions during impression recording. After the material sets in a patient's mouth, the impression is pulled out with the help of the tray. This gives the negative replica of the patient's mouth which is poured with a gypsum product to get a positive replica on which the oral appliances are fabricated. Therefore, the impression stage is the first stage and a very important stage involving the fabrication of dental appliances.

IDEAL REQUIREMENTS OF IMPRESSION MATERIALS

1. Biocompatibility and Chemical Properties

- Nonpoisonous, nonirritant, nonallergic to oral tissues (e.g. ZnOE impression pastes is allergic, irritant for few patients)

- Acceptable taste and odour for patients
- Chemically inert in oral conditions
- Should not absorb or dissolve in oral fluids which may cause dimensional changes
- Hydrophilic, to avoid incomplete wetting or collection of air bubbles causing voids while taking impression or pouring casts
- Compatible with die or cast materials and pattern waxes.

2. Rheological (Fluidity Flow) Properties

- **Low viscosity** or good flow property while inserting, to get an accurate reproduction of finer details.
- **Viscosity should increase quickly** while setting to avoid distortion due to inadvertent shaking by the patient and during tray removal.
- **Pseudoplastic nature** helps to increase flow by stressing to get better details, e.g. monophase additional polysilicones.
- Suitable mixing and working times by controlling the rate of chemical reactions, and should have short setting times, i.e. dentists command setting properties short setting time, i.e. **command set** properties.

3. Mechanical Properties

Good ability to **reproduce the finer details** within a tolerance of ± 20 microns. For this, it should have **finer particles** and no dimensional changes during setting and before pouring the casts or dies.

- **High elasticity and complete elastic recovery**, so that it can be withdrawn through severe undercuts without distortions or dimensional changes. The elastic recovery should be complete in a short time to get dimensional accuracy, e.g. addition polysilicones have highest elastic recovery: 99.93%.
- **Adequate compressive strength** to avoid dimensional changes while pouring the cast or die materials, e.g. silver amalgam—dies cannot be condensed in elastomeric impressions.
- **High tear strength** to withstand tearing or shearing stresses during withdrawal of impression, e.g. due to low tear strengths of hydrocolloids, i.e. 750 gm/cm to 800 gm/cm, a thicker section of impression is required, but this will cause distortions. Elastomers have better tear strengths, 2,000 gm/cm–4,000 gm/cm and can be used in thin sections.
- **High flexibility or strain in compression** is needed to permit withdrawal through severe undercuts.

4. Thermal Properties

- Thermoplastic materials should have **low softening temperatures** (45–55°C) and set or harden at 37°C.
- **Very low or zero coefficient of thermal expansions (COTE)** to minimise contraction while taking out of the mouth. But most of the impression materials have very high COTE, due to which, large contraction takes place with distortion **if the thickness is not uniform.**
- **High thermal conductivity** to soften or harden or set the impression simultaneously, to avoid internal stresses cause distorts by stress relaxations.
- Properties should not change while kneading at high temperatures in case of thermoplastic materials.

5. Aesthetic Properties

- **Good colour contrast** is required to identify the margins. Two-paste systems have one paste coloured to check uniform mixing with all the coloured streaks eliminated. Different colours are added to identify the elastomers according to their consistencies as well as preliminary and secondary impressions.
- **Fairly good colour stability.**

6. Other Minor Requirements

- **Good dimensional stability** during setting and also in-between the interval of cast pouring. Hydrocolloids undergo dimensional changes by syneresis and imbibition, quickly and hence **cast pouring should be done immediately**. Elastomers have elastic recovery close to 100%.
- Adhesion to tray or retention should be good to reduce distortion during removal and before pouring cast. Should not adhere to oral tissues.
- Long shelf-life, readily available and inexpensive.
- Able to sterilize and reuse.
- Able to be used repeatedly to obtain many copies of dies without dimensional changes.

Note: **None of the materials satisfy all the ideal requirements**, specially thermal properties which cause distortions. Many do not have adequate flow to obtain mucostatic impressions. The ability to reproduce very fine details accurately, elastic recoveries, flexibilities, etc. are to be compromised, and impression techniques should be modified such as multiple mix techniques, laminate techniques, etc. to avail fairly good satisfactory impressions.

CLASSIFICATION OF IMPRESSION MATERIALS

This is done according to the various properties, **to help the dentists to select the proper materials, apply suitable precautions during manipulations and use the correct impression techniques according to the requirements of clinical situations to obtain the best results.**

1. Chemical Compositions

- Impression compounds
- Impression waxes
- Impression plaster
- Zinc oxide eugenol impression pastes
- Hydrocolloids: Agar-agar, alginates
- Elastomers: Polysulphides, polysilicones (condensation and addition types), polyethers.

2. Mechanical Properties

- *Elastic impression materials:* These, when deformed, should recover elastically, e.g. hydrocolloids (agar-agar and alginates), elastomers (polysilicones, polysulphides and polyethers).
- *Nonelastic impression materials:* Impression compound, impression waxes, impression plaster, zinc oxide eugenol impression pastes.

3. Force Exerted on Soft Tissues

- *Mucostatic* impression materials—theoretically should not exert any force which distorts the soft tissues during the recording of impression. Clinically impression plaster, agar-agar, light body elastomers, zinc oxide eugenol impression pastes can be considered as mucostatic impression materials.
- *Mucocompressive:* These exert considerable force on soft tissues causing distortion. (Theoretically all are mucocompressive), impression compound, viscous alginates, R, H, P, consistencies of elastomers are usually considered as mucocompressive, clinically.

4. Nature of Setting

- Materials which set by physical (thermal) changes.

  For example: Impression compound, agar-agar, impression waxes.
- Materials which set by chemical change or chemical reactions, e.g. zinc oxide eugenol impression pastes, impression plaster, elastomers, alginates.

5. Oral Conditions

- **Edentulous condition:** All impression materials (impression compound, impression waxes, impression plaster, ZnOE impression pastes, hydrocolloids, elastomers)
- **Dentulous condition:** Hydrocolloids and elastomers are only to be used.

6. Dispensing System

- Powder: Impression plaster, alginates
- Two-paste systems: ZnOE impression pastes, polysulphides and polysilicones
- Three-paste systems: Chemically activated polyether (base, reactor, thinner)
- Single paste systems: Light-activated polyether
- Gels: Agar-agar
- Supplied in the form of cakes, cylinders, sticks, sheets and cones—impression compound, impression waxes.

7. Clinical Applications

- Primary/preliminary impressions, e.g. impression compound, impression waxes, alginates, elastomers (heavy and regular bodies)
- Secondary/corrective wash impressions, e.g. impression plaster, ZnOE impression pastes, elastomers, polysulfides, polyethers, polysilicones (light bodies), agar-agar
- Border moulding impression, e.g. green stick compound
- Cavity impressions for inlays and onlays, e.g. elastomers
- Crown and bridge impression, e.g. hydrocolloids—agar-agar, alginates elastomers—polysilicones, polysulphides, polyethers
- Partial denture impressions, e.g. hydrocolloids—agar-agar, alginates, elastomers—polysilicones, polysulphides, polyethers.

8. Special Uses

- Syringe materials, e.g. light body elastomers, agar-agar
- Tray materials, e.g. heavy body elastomers, tray compound, putty like elastomers
- Border moulding impression material—green stick compound (impression compound)
- Cast duplicating materials: Hydrocolloids, elastomers, PVC.

Note

- The impression plaster is explained in detail under **gypsum products chapter**
- The impression waxes are explained in detail under **waxes chapter.**

IMPRESSION TRAYS

Impression trays are rigid metallic (stainless steel) or plastic (acrylic) devices, used for supporting the unset impression materials for carrying to the mouth, recording the impression, allowing to set or harden, removal of impression without distortion, and pouring the cast or model materials. Trays of different sizes, shapes, and materials are used according to situations and techniques (Fig. 3.1).

Classification

It can be according to:

1. *Availability*
   - Stock trays of standard sizes (stainless steel)
   - Special custom-made, individualised secondary impression trays (acrylics)
   - Special rim-lock trays (metal)
   - Reusable and disposable trays (plastics).
2. *Methods of retention*
   - Perforated trays
   - Nonperforated trays
   - Rim-lock trays
3. *Impression materials/techniques*
   - Perforated for alginates
   - Nonperforated for impression compound
   - Special trays for ZnOE and elastomers
   - Rim-lock trays for agar-agar
4. *Arch size of patients*
   - Maxillary (upper) arch—U_1, U2, U3, U4 sizes
   - Mandibular (lower) arch—L_1, L_2, L_3, L_4 sizes
5. *Type of impressions*
   - Trays for full length (complete) impressions
   - Trays (perforated, reusable, disposable) for sectional impressions
6. *Oral conditions*
   - Dentulous impression trays—perforated for hydrocolloids, adhesive coated for elastomers
   - Edentulous impressions—nonperforated trays

STOCK TRAYS AND CUSTOM-MADE SPECIAL TRAYS

1. **Stock trays** are available in standard sizes. There are two varieties:
   a. Reusable stock trays are supplied with or without perforations and usually made out of stainless steel
   b. Disposable stock trays are usually perforated and made up of polymer resins such as nylon or polystyrene.

Advantages
- Eliminates time and expense of fabricating trays
- Metal stock trays are rigid.
- They can be sterilized and reused.

Disadvantages
- The nonuniform thickness of impression
- Must be sterilized before using for other patients
- Requires more material
- Inaccurate impression due to the improper tray extensions.

2. **Special trays are fabricated** from a preliminary or primary cast of the patients mouth. These are disposable trays, usually made out of shellac or similar thermoplastic materials and also by acrylic resins—heat cure acrylic resins or cold cure acrylic resins.

Advantages
- Less to moderate impression material is required and less wastage
- Uniform thickness of impression is achieved, using spacers
- Since trays are disposable no sterilization is required
- A more accurate impression is obtained.

Disadvantage
Trays are fabricated in the laboratory. So, it is a time-consuming process.

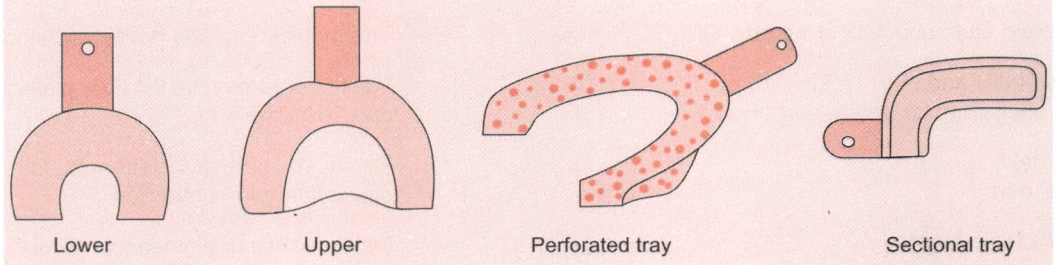

| Lower | Upper | Perforated tray | Sectional tray |

Fig. 3.1: Metal/plastic stock trays

Selection of Trays

1. Based on relative need of retention of impression materials—perforated trays are used for hydrocolloids which produce mechanical interlocking, when the material flows through the holes and gelates.
2. Based on the type of impression materials to be used—nonperforated trays for impression compound, perforated trays for hydrocolloids, special trays—zinc oxide eugenol impression paste and elastomers.
3. Based on patients arch size
   U_1, U_2, U_3, U_4—for upper or maxillary arches
   L_1, L_2, L_3, L_4—for lower or mandibular arches
4. Based on the arch length
   • Full arch length trays
   • Sectional trays

Properties Required for Impression Trays

• Trays should not be too rigid, as they can distort or displace the soft tissues.
• Trays should not be too flexible, the flexible trays are likely to deform during impression recording and relax after removal of impression, producing a distorted impression.
• Impression materials should adhere to the tray. Retention can be improved by coating the surface of special trays with tray adhesives supplied by the manufacturer in the case of elastomers or by using perforated trays in case of hydrocolloids. Partial detachment may cause gross distortion of impression recorded.

NON-ELASTIC IMPRESSION MATERIALS: IMPRESSION COMPOUND

It is a mucocompressive, thermoplastic, nonelastic impression material used to record the preliminary impressions of edentulous arches in the preparation of complete dentures (and is also used as a special tray material).

Note: **Thermoplastic materials,** get softened by heating and hardened by cooling without any chemical change.

Alternative names
• Impression compound
• Dental compound
• Model compound
• Modeling compound
• Impression composition

ADA specification No. 3

Types of impression compounds available are (Table 3.1)

1. Type I impression compound (low fusing) (fusion temperature approximately above 45°C), e.g. impression compound, green stick compound.
2. Type II Impression compound (high fusing) (fusion temperature almost above 70°C), e.g. tray compound.

Dispensing: Available in the form of sheets, cakes, cones, sticks, etc.

Composition: Refer to Table 3.1

Properties

1. **Setting action:** Setting action is by physical change. It can softened by warming above its Tg (45–50°C) and hardened by cooling, which is reversible.
2. **Biological property:** It is nontoxic, nonirritant, nonpoisonous to the oral tissues.
3. **Rheological property:** Impression compound is highly viscous and mucocompressive impression material.

Flow is the ability of amorphous material to undergo plastic deformation under the influence of external forces or by its weight.

Table 3.1 The composition of impression compound

Ingredients	Percentage	Functions
1. Natural or synthetic resins		
a. Copal resin	20%	Thermoplasticity and gives flow and cohesions
b. Rosin	20%	
2. Waxes (beeswax, carnauba wax or paraffin wax)	7%	Thermoplasticity and produce a smooth surface
3. Various types of oils and fats (stearic acid, shellac, gutta-percha)	3%	Plasticizer to improve the flow, plasticity, workability and flexibility
4. French chalk, talc, diatomaceous earth	50%	Fillers: To improve the strength, to reduce thermal expansion and contraction
5. Rouge (Fe_2O_3) ferric oxide	Trace	Mainly as colour pigments of reddish-brown colour to the compound

Measurement of the Flow of Impression Compound

A cylindrical sample of 10 mm diameter, and 6 mm height is prepared and maintained at 37°C or 45°C for some time and a load of 2 kg is applied for 10 minutes. The decrease in the height x mm is measured. The flow $= \frac{x}{6} \times 100\%$. The ADA specification No. 3, for the flow, is given in Table 3.2.

Factors Affecting Flow

- **Temperature:** Higher the temperature, greater is the flow. But if the temperature is quite high the **leaching of plasticizers cause grainy and sticky surface.**
- **Wet kneading** causes trapping of air or water which act as plasticizers and increase the flow, which can record the finer details better. But at the same time, it distorts while removing the impression (flow should not be >6%).
- Prolonged kneading also increases flow.

4. **Thermal properties**
   - *Fusion temperature:* Fusion temperature can be defined as the temperature at which an amorphous material begins to soften. The fusion temperature of the impression compound is about 43.5°C.
   - *Thermal conductivity:* Impression compound is a poor conductor of heat. So, this property should be taken into consideration during cooling and heating of the material. When the compound is heated, the outside part always softens first and the **inside part softens last.** Since it is important that the compound must be uniformly softened when it is placed in the tray, adequate time must be allowed for the material to be heated uniformly throughout its mass. Similarly, adequate time must also be allowed for uniform hardening. Premature removal of the impression before complete hardening may result in severe distortion of impression.
   - *Coefficient of thermal expansion (COTE):* They have high thermal expansion **and contraction** coefficients. The COTE value is 200–500 ppm/°C (as it contains waxes and resins). Contraction, while cooling from mouth temperature to room temperature may be as great as about 1.4% to 2.31%. Lower the temperature of the compound at the time of taking impression, less will be the error due to its thermal contraction.

5. **Dimensional stability**
   Residual mechanical stresses are commonly incorporated in the impression compound during heating and manipulation as well as during the actual process of recording the impression. As a result, **warpage (distortion) may occur during storage period** due to relaxation of these internal stresses.
   For most accurate results, the model should be poured as soon as possible after recording the impression.

Manipulation of Impression Compound

Requirements: Temperature controlled water bath (thermostat) or air bath or open flame (open flame is not recommended because uneven heating may burn off some of the ingredients).

Main techniques of softening the impression compound are:
1. Wet kneading (more common)
2. Dry kneading

Procedure to Record the Impression

1. **Wet kneading technique** for softening consists of submerging the compound in a water bath maintained at about 60°C, warm water taken in a small plastic bowl. Usually the process takes several minutes because of the low thermal conductivity of the material.
   - After the material becomes sufficiently soft, it is customarily kneaded with fingers to produce a uniform state of plasticity.

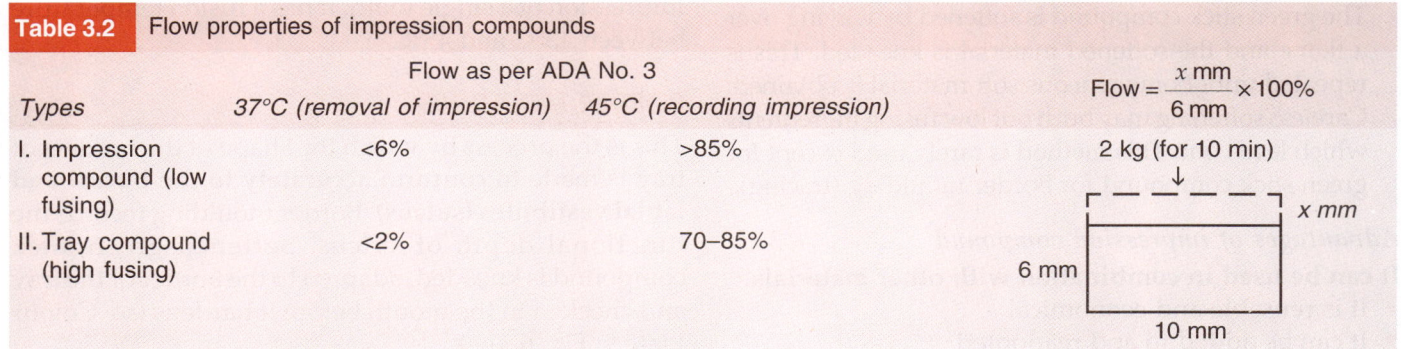

Table 3.2	Flow properties of impression compounds		
	Flow as per ADA No. 3		
Types	37°C (removal of impression)	45°C (recording impression)	
I. Impression compound (low fusing)	<6%	>85%	
II. Tray compound (high fusing)	<2%	70–85%	

$$\text{Flow} = \frac{x \text{ mm}}{6 \text{ mm}} \times 100\%$$

2 kg (for 10 min)

- At this point, the impression compound is placed in a non-perforated stock tray.
- After the compound is moulded to the shape of the impression tray, it is inserted into the mouth.
- The impression is **retained until** it cools to the body temperature of 37°C, with adequate pressure.
- Since it has a low conductivity, it **hardens** initially on the outer surface, then on the tissue side, and the inner portion may be considerably hotter and softer.
- Premature removal from the mouth results in warpage or distortion.
- After the impression compound completely hardens, the impression is removed from the mouth washed, dried, trimmed and the cast is poured (*see* Colour Plate 4, Fig. 3.1).

Precautions

- When the direct flame is used the **compound** should not be allowed to ignite or boil, so that the essential constituents are not volatilised.
- Prolonged immersing or heating in a water bath, makes it brittle and grainy and some of the low molecular weight ingredients may leach out causing **stickiness and grainy surface** (temperature also should not exceed (60–65°C).
- Undue kneading of the compound to produce plasticity can incorporate water into the material and the flow after hardening will be increased. So, it should be avoided.
- Water bath should be lined with a napkin to prevent the compound from sticking to the sides of the bowl.
- Adequate time must be given for uniform softening and hardening due to low thermal conductivity.
- Premature removal from the mouth should be avoided as it may result in distortion of the impression.
- Cast should be poured as soon as possible. Delay causes relaxation of internal stresses and distortion.

2. **Dry kneading technique**

The green stick compound is softened by waving over a flame and the softened material is kneaded. This is repeated until homogeneous soft material is obtained: Careless softening may burn out low fusing ingredients which leach out. This method is rarely used except for green stick compound for border moulding (tracing).

Advantages of impression compound

It can be used in combination with other materials.

- It is reusable and economical
- It can be added to and readopted

- It has a long shelf-life of about 5 years.
- Nontoxic, well-tolerated by the tissue of the mouth.

Disadvantages of impression compound

- **It is nonelastic** and cannot be used when undercut exists, or dentulous cases.
- Does not reproduce all the fine surface details required, as it is mucocompressive.
- As it cannot be sterilized, it tends to become unhygienic and should not be reused ideally.
- Its thermal properties are not ideal, it has large COTE, and it is a very poor conductor of heat, which leads to distortion.

A certain amount of pressure is required to record the impression and this causes compression or **displacement of soft tissues,** resulting in a poor quality of the impression.

Uses

- Type I impression compound is used to record the **preliminary impressions of edentulous arches** in preparation of complete dentures.
- Green stick compound (type I) is used to take tube impression (copper band impression) for inlays and crowns. It is also used for border moulding technique for the peripheral extension of the special tray.
- Type II impression compound (tray compound) is used to prepare special trays for recording secondary impressions or corrective wash impressions.

GREEN STICK COMPOUND

TRACING COMPOUND OR BORDER MOULDING COMPOUND

It is a low fusing impression compound, supplied as cylindrical rods of about 10 cm in length, 6 mm in diameter and green in colour. It is softened by warming over a gas flame and then kneaded **(dry kneading technique)**. It is used for border extension of special trays in border moulding technique. It is also used for copper tube impression for recording the preliminary impression of a single tooth. It has a fusion temperature between 43°C and 45°C.

BORDER MOULDING

This is the process by which the shape of the borders of tray is made to **conform accurately to the buccal and labial vestibules (sulcus).** Border moulding records the functional depth of sulcus. Softened green stick compound is kneaded, adapted to the border of the tray and checked in the mouth before it hardens (*see* Colour Plate 9, Fig. 6.3).

COPPER TUBE IMPRESSION TECHNIQUE OR COPPER RING TECHNIQUE

A cylindrical copper tube or band is filled with softened green stick compound. The filled tube is then pressed over the prepared teeth, when the compound flows on the prepared teeth. After the compound has been cooled the impression is withdrawn. The contour of the entire tooth may not be reproduced accurately because of the fracture of compound during withdrawing from the mouth. However, the form of the prepared cavity is accurately recorded. After this procedure, secondary or corrective wash impression is recorded with **light body elastomers** (Fig. 3.2).

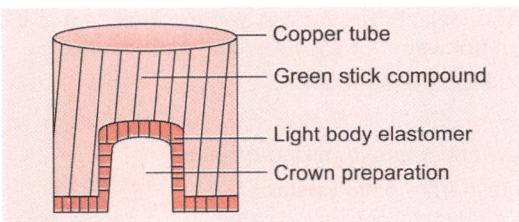

Copper tube
Green stick compound
Light body elastomer
Crown preparation

Fig. 3.2: Copper tube impression

The function of the **green stick compound is to strengthen the thin copper tube** while obtaining a tube impression of a single tooth with a rubber base impression material. Otherwise, the impression will be squeezed with fingers when it is removed from the tooth and distortion will occur.

TYPE II TRAY COMPOUND/ IMPRESSION COMPOUND

The tray compound is more viscous when it is softened and more rigid when hardened. Since reproduction of finer details is not essential for tray compound, it is generally stiffer and has less flow than the regular impression compound. It has a higher fusion temperature of more than 70°C. It is usually supplied in the shape of a tray which may be black or white in colour. It is made up of thermoplastic resins, waxes, fillers and colour pigments. It has a flow value of less than 2% at 37°C and 70–85% at 45°C. This is mainly used to prepare special trays which will later hold the secondary impression material to record the final impression commonly referred to as corrective wash impression.

Tray compound lacks in strength and is dimensionally unstable. Hence it is not widely used in recent days. It has been replaced with stronger materials like **cold cure-acrylic resins.**

ZINC OXIDE EUGENOL IMPRESSION PASTES

It is **mucostatic, inelastic, chemically setting** impression material, used for recording secondary or corrective wash impressions of edentulous arches in the preparation of complete dentures.

Alternate names
- Metallic oxide pastes
- ZnOE impression pastes (Table 3.3).

TYPES OF ZnOE IMPRESSION PASTES

According to ADA specification No. 16, there are 2 varieties
- Type I: Hard set, fast set, thinner consistency
- Type II: Soft set, slow set, thicker consistency.

The difference between these 2 types are related to their consistences, setting times and hardness after setting.

Dispensing

It is usually supplied as two pastes systems in collapsible tubes, i.e. base ZnO paste and reactor-eugenol pastes. It is also available in powder and liquid system (powder—ZnO and liquid—eugenol) (Table 3.3).

Setting Reaction

When equal lengths of the two-paste are mixed in presence of moisture.
- An **acid–base** reaction takes place in which ZnO combines with water to give zinc hydroxide. Zinc hydroxide reacts with eugenol to give zinc eugenolate salt (chelate product) and water as the by-product (Fig. 3.3).
- The water formed is utilized in the further reaction and hence is termed **autocatalytic reaction.**
- The setting reaction is anionic and ionic medium is increased by adding certain ionizable salts (which acts as accelerating—$CaCl_2$, $MgCl_2$, acetic acid, sodium acetate, etc.) and water.

PROPERTIES OF ZnOE IMPRESSION MATERIALS

1. **Biological property**
   These materials are nontoxic, but those containing eugenol can be irritant giving a tingling or burning sensation to the patients and leaving a persistent taste, which some patients may regard as unpleasant. Occasionally, eugenol may produce allergic responses in some patients. For this type of patients, eugenol free zinc oxide impression pastes are available (the alternate organic acids replace eugenol such as *ortho*-ethoxybenzoic acid).

Table 3.3	The composition of ZnOE		
Ingredients		wt%	Functions
Base paste			
1. Zinc oxide		87%	Reactive ingredient
2. Fixed vegetable oil or mineral oil (linseed or olive oil)		13%	Paste former plasticizer, retarder, masks the irritation of eugenol
3. $CaCl_2$ (sometimes)		2%	Accelerator
The composition of ZnOE reactor paste			
1. Oil of clove or eugenol		12%	Reactive ingredient
2. $CaCl_2$ or $MgCl_2$		5%	Accelerators
3. Gum or polymerized rosin		50%	1. Facilitates the speed of the reaction and produces a smoother, homogeneous mix
			2. Gives body and coherence to the mixed material
			3. Imparts thermoplastic property to set material so that it can be softened in hot water for easy removal from the cast
4. Fillers (silica, kaolin, talc)		20%	Paste former, increase strength
5. Lanolin		3%	Plasticizer
6. Resinous balsam (Canada or Peru balsam)		10%	Increases flow and improve mixing qualities
7. Colour pigments		Trace	1. To distinguish from other pastes
			2. Enables thorough mixing as indicated by a homogeneous colour

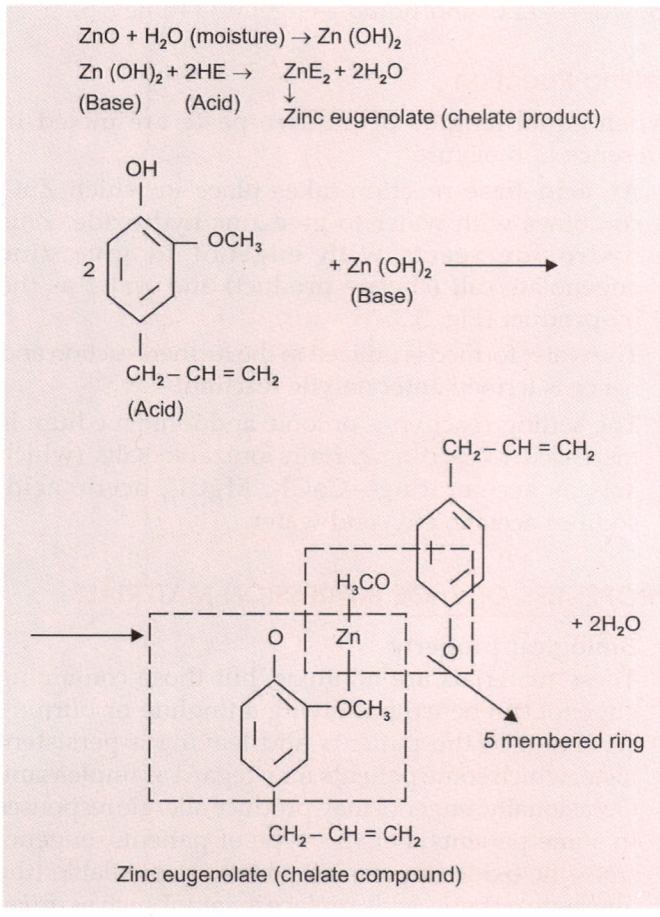

Fig. 3.3: The setting reaction of ZnO and eugenol

2. **Rheological properties**
   - **Setting times:** Should not be too long as it causes inconvenience to the patients and should not be too short as the material cannot be manipulated properly (Table 3.4).
     According to ADA specification No. 16:
   - **Initial setting time:** It is defined as the time from the beginning of mixing until the material ceases to pull away or string out when its surface is touched with a metal rod of the specified dimension. The initial setting times for both the types of pastes (soft and hard) are **3–6 minutes**.
   - **Final setting time:** It is defined as the time from the beginning of mixing until the material gets maximum hardness so that the impression can be withdrawn from the mouth with a minimum distortion or final setting time is the time elapsed from the start of mixing to the instant when penetration falls below 0.2 mm as measured with penetrometer or similar instruments.
     Final setting time for **type I material is <10 minutes**
     Final setting time for **type II material is <15 minutes**
   - **Hardness is measured by Krebs penetrometer:** It is used to find the hardness of set material. Hardness is measured by noting the extent to which a loaded needle will penetrate on a small specimen of a set material (minimum depth of penetration). The hardness is expressed in **mm** within a given time. The penetrometer is equipped

Table 3.4 Factors affecting setting time

Factors	To decrease ST	To increase ST
1. Temperature	Higher the temperature Shorter ST (by warming glass slab and spatula)	Lower the temperature longer ST (by cooling, glass slab and spatula but not below the dew point)
2. Humidity	Higher	Lower
3. The ratio of ZnO paste to eugenol paste	More eugenol paste	More ZnO paste
4. Mixing time	Longer and faster (should be <1/2 minutes)	Slower and shorter
5. Chemical modifiers	Accelerators glacial acetic acid, primary alcohols, moisture, heat, etc. ($CaCl_2$, $MgCl_2$ or a drop of water)	Retarders (boroglycerin, inert oils, and waxes) by cooling

with a needle of **50.8 mm** in length and **1.02 mm** in diameter and the total weight of the needle is **100 gm. 30 minutes** after the start of the mix, the loaded needle is applied to the specimen surface for **10 sec** and penetration is recorded to the nearest **0.1 mm**. The values of penetration is reported as the minimum constant value of the depth of penetration, reached in three successive readings when measured at an interval of 30 seconds.

- Penetration hardness for type I material (hard set) is **<0.5 mm**
- Penetration hardness for type II materials (soft set) is between **0.8 mm and 1.5 mm** (Table 3.5)
- Hard set (type I) material has more fluid consistency before setting, greater hardness, and brittleness after setting. Soft set Type II material is tougher and not brittle. It has a buttery consistency and longer final setting time.

3. **Consistency (fluidity):** An accurate impression will be recorded or obtained only in case of a mixed material having a thinner consistency and good flow properties.

Consistency can be measured by spreading the material under a specified load when placed between the two glass plates immediately after mixing (Fig. 3.4).

- **Consistency measurement:** **0.5 ml** of the mixed paste to be tested, is taken on a thin plastic sheet and placed over a glass plate, **90 seconds** after the start of mixing, a second plastic sheet, and glass slab of **500 gm** weight are carefully placed on the top of the soft paste. **10 minutes** from the start of mixing the weight is removed and major and minor diameters of the slumped mass (disc) are measured to the nearest millimeter. The average value of three trials is reported to the nearest mm value.

4. This is **mucostatic** and gives accurate finer details.
5. **Dimensional stability: Has very low dimensional** changes during setting **(<0.1%)** and **there is no dimensional change after setting or hardening.**
6. **Elasticity:** It is **inelastic** impression material and cannot be used for recording **undercuts.** The set material may distort or fracture when removed over undercuts.
7. **Strength:** The strength of hardened ZnOE impression paste is about **7 MPa, after 2 hours** from the start of the mixing.
8. **Compatibility with stone and die materials is quite satisfactory:** The paste can be removed from the stone by softening in hot water at 60°C.
9. **Shelf-life:** The materials can be stored in the dental office up to 1 year (follow manufacturer's instructions).

Table 3.5 Properties of type I and type II zinc oxide eugenol materials

Types	Consistencies (under 500 gm wt)	Setting times Initial	Final	Hardness (penetration depth)
1. Thinner, harder fast setting	30 mm–50 mm	3–6 min	<10 min	<0.5 mm (harder)
2. Thicker, softer and slow setting	20 mm–45 mm	3–6 min	<15 min	0.8–1.5 mm (softer)

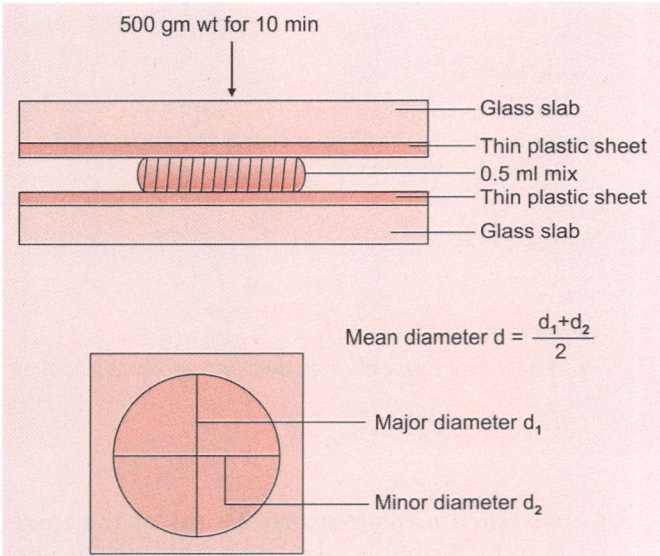

Fig. 3.4: Determination of consistency of ZnOE paste

Manipulation Techniques

Instruments

Glass slab or oil impervious paper pad (the paper pad is preferred to avoid cleaning of glass slab to which the material adheres firmly, and the used paper is thrown out after use). Stainless steel spatula is used for mixing.

Procedure

The proper proportioning of two pastes is generally obtained by squeezing out ropes of pastes of the **same lengths** (1:1) on the glass slab. The diameters of the strips of pastes (thickness) should not vary from the opening of the tube. A flexible stainless steel spatula is to be used for mixing. The reactor paste is first collected and applied over the base paste and mixed with broad strokes in a sweeping motion until a uniform homogeneous colour mix is obtained, mixing time is approximately one minute.

The mix is now collected and spread over the dry tissue bearing surface of the special tray and placed in the mouth. It is held firmly in position until the material has uniformly hardened. After the material has set, the impression is removed from the mouth. If the impression is not properly obtained, **another increment of a fresh mix can be placed** on the distorted area, and better impression can be obtained or scrap out the old material from the special tray and record a new impression.

The impression obtained is well rinsed under running cold water for removal of saliva/debris, disinfected, dried and cast is poured with dental stone. The cast can be separated from impression by immersing in hot water at 45°C to 60°C for 5–10 minutes. Separating medium is not required when making the cast. ZnOE impression material sticks well to dried skin and instruments, so it is advisable to coat the lips of the patients with petroleum jelly which allows the extra material to be wiped out (*see* Colour Plate 9, Fig. 6.4).

Advantages

- *Mucostatic therefore gives an accurate reproduction of finer details*.
- Dimensionally stable.
- The fresh mix can be added to and readapted if the impression is found faulty.
- Adheres well to dried surfaces of compound, resin and shellac bases (no tray adhesives are required).
- It has sufficient resistance so that borders can be built up if the tray is slightly deficient in any area.
- Allows adequate working time for unhurried border moulding in the mouth.
- No separating medium is required before pouring the cast
- Easy to manipulate, not very expensive and has reasonable shelf-life.

Disadvantages

- Cannot be used when undercut exists as it is **nonelastic**.
- Some patients find eugenol content unpleasant, and it may cause a burning sensation and irritate the oral tissues.
- Requires special trays which involves time-consuming process.
- Instruments are difficult to clean.

Uses

- For recording corrective wash or secondary impressions of edentulous arches in the preparation of complete dentures.
- For corrective lining in preliminary impressions. Modified ZnOE pastes can be used as:
  - **Surgical paste** is used for intraoral bandage after some surgical procedures in the mouth.
  - **Bite registration paste** is used to record the occlusal relationship between maxillary and mandibular arches.
  - **Noneugenol paste:** It is used to record secondary impressions in patients who find eugenol an irritant.

Modifications of ZnOE Impression Pastes

1. Surgical Paste

A modified ZnOE paste with **longer setting time** can be used as surgical paste after some dental surgical procedures such as **gingivectomy** (surgical removal of gingiva) as an **intraoral bandage** to protect cut surfaces and to prevent infection of tissues. These materials are used to cover and protect wound surface after surgery, by shielding the incised tissues from infections which may be caused by irritations from food, air, tongue or cheek movements.

These materials are available as two pastes or powder–liquid systems.

Two-paste systems

This is similar to the conventional ZnOE impression pastes with the following modifications:

- More amount of fillers to prevent dislocation or fracture of the material during mastication
- More amount of eugenol: Eugenol is weak antiseptic and has a slight sedative effect.
- More amount of plasticizer: To increase its softness
- It also contains antibiotics such as tetracyclines.

Powder and liquid system

Powder
- ZnO: 63%—reactive ingredient
- Rosin: 30%—plasticizer
- Asbestos fibres: 5%—to improve the setting of dressing material
- Zn acetate: 2%—accelerator

Liquid
- Eugenol: 80%—reactive ingredient
- Vegetable oil: 20%—plasticizer, retarder.

Manipulation

Once the bleeding from the operated area has stopped, mix the two pastes and apply over the wound and smoothen the surface. The dressing should cover the wound but should not interfere with occlusion.

Drawbacks

- This may cause chronic gastric disturbances if kept for a longer time
- This may produce irritation and burning sensation.

2. Bite Registration Paste

ZnOE impression paste with slight modifications can be used as bite registration paste to record the occlusal relationship of maxillary and mandibular teeth or arches during the preparation of a wide variety of dental appliances such as complete dentures, partial dentures, crowns, bridges, etc.

The interocclusal record is necessary to produce the required occlusal relationship in the restorations and it is required at several stages in the construction of oral appliances.

Compositions

The composition is similar to the conventional zinc oxide eugenol impression pastes with slightly more **plasticizer added (petroleum jelly)** to reduce the tendency of the paste sticking to the mouth tissues (also refer elastomers—addition polysilicones).

Advantages

- This offers almost **no resistance** for the closing of mandible thus allowing a more accurate inter-occlusal relationship.
- **This is more stable** than the one made in wax.

Disadvantage

Eugenol may be irritant to some patients.

3. Non-eugenol Pastes

Eugenol present in ZnOE impression paste may be irritant to some patients. To cater for this type of patients eugenol-free impression pastes are developed.

Drawbacks of eugenol

- This causes a burning sensation when contacts soft tissues.
- Some patients find the taste and odour of eugenol extremely disagreeable.
- Causes allergic response in some patients.
- Leaching of eugenol from surgical paste may cause the patients a **chronic gastric disturbance.**

It has been found that a material similar to ZnOE product can be formed by a **saponification reaction** to produce an insoluble soap, if the ZnO reacted with carboxylic acid.

$$ZnO + 2\ RCOOH \rightarrow (RCOO)_2\ Zn + H_2O$$

Number of chemicals will produce a reaction with metallic ZnO in a manner comparable to eugenol. Eugenol is replaced by an organic acid such as *ortho-ethoxybenzoic acid (EBA)* in these non-eugenol pastes. Bactericides and other medicaments can be incorporated without interfering the reaction.

ELASTIC IMPRESSION MATERIALS

HYDROCOLLOIDS

The term hydrocolloid is used to describe the state of matter in which matter is divided into particles of size between 10^{-4} and 10^{-7} cm and dispersed in another medium.

A colloid consists of **large molecules** or agglomerates of molecules, which are dissolved or dispersed in a dispersing medium such as water.

Definitions

- **True solutions:** If the size of the dispersed particles are small **($<10^{-7}$cm)** and cannot be seen by a naked eye or through a microscope the system is termed as **true solution.**
- **Suspension or emulsion:** If the size of the dispersed particles are larger **($>10^{-4}$ cm)** and can be seen by a naked eye or through a microscope, the system is termed as suspension or emulsion.
  - Solids distributed in liquids is called suspension, e.g. fine saw-dust in water
  - Liquid distributed in liquids is called as an emulsion, e.g. oil and water
- The **colloidal state** is an **intermediate state** between true solution and suspension.

Colloids have two phases

1. *Dispersed phase* (dispersed particle): It is a **substance** which is distributed in the form of colloidal particles is dispersed in a suitable dispersion medium.
2. *Dispersion phase* (dispersion medium): It is a **medium** in which colloidal particles are dispersed.

Types of Colloids

- Solids and liquids in air—**aerosol**
- Solids, liquids or gases in liquids—**lyosol**
- Liquids in solids—**gel**
- Solids in liquids—**sol**
- Gases in solids—**solid foam**

Hydrocolloids can be defined as colloids with water as the dispersion medium.

- **Sol** is a colloidal system, in which the dispersed phase is a solid and dispersion medium is a liquid.
- **A gel is a heterogeneous biphasic system in which liquid is dispersed in a solid dispersion medium.**
- **Gelation:** It is a process of conversion of viscous liquid sol, into a **semifluid jelly-like substance**. It is a gelation (solidification) process and is brought by either a physical change or a chemical change. The temperature at which, sol gets converted to a gel in case of (reversible hydrocolloids) is known **gelation temperature.**

Mechanism of Gelation (Fig. 3.5)

When aggregates of molecules are dispersed in a liquid or water, the material is in the sol form. By a reduction in temperature or by a chemical reaction, the aggregates of molecules in a colloid can be made to join or agglomerate together to form a network of chains, **fibrils or micelles.** This fibril network encloses the dispersion medium (i.e. water is held in the interstices

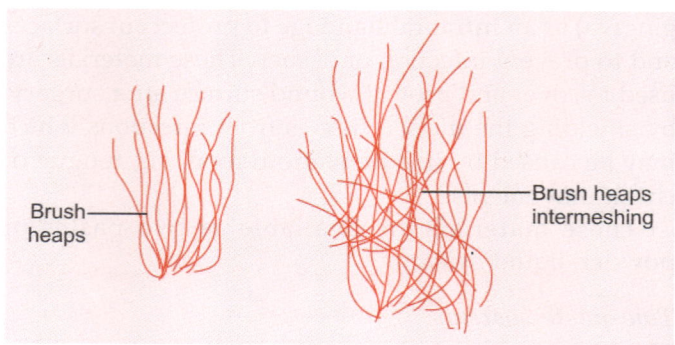

Fig. 3.5: Gelation: Intermeshing of brush heaps

between the fibrils by capillary action). These growing fibrils may **branch and intermesh** to form a **brush heap structure**. As the molecules are joined together to form fibrils, the consistency of the colloid becomes that of jelly, and it is in the gel form. Therefore, the higher the concentration of the brush heaps or fibrils, the stronger will be the gel structure. In case of agar-agar, the fibrils are held together by **secondary forces, i.e. van der Waals forces** and in alginates fibrils are held together by **primary valency bonds, i.e. covalent bonds.**

Sol → fibrils (micelles) → brush heaps → gel (intermeshing of brush heaps)

Reversible hydrocolloids: If hydrocolloid can be easily changed by cooling into **gel form** and back into the **sol form by heating,** the material is known as reversible hydrocolloid. This process (sol ⇌ gel) can be repeated several times by temperature changes.

Gel to sol: On heating, the gel converts to sol form. As the temperature rises, the kinetic energy of the molecules in the fibrils increases and the fibrils separate from each other to form a sol.

Sol to gel: When the temperature is reduced by cooling, the secondary intermolecular forces once again come into play and molecules join together to form fibrils and gel.

Reversible hydrocolloids do not return to the gel state at the same temperature at which they change to sol. The gel must be heated to a higher temperature known as liquefaction temperature to attain sol condition. **The temperature lag** or the difference between the gelation temperature and liquefaction temperature of a gel is known as **hysteresis,**

i.e. agar-agar, $\text{gel} \underset{37°C}{\overset{80°C}{\rightleftarrows}} \text{sol}$

Irreversible hydrocolloids: If a hydrocolloid changes from colloidal solution (sol) to an elastic gel by a **chemical reaction,** the resultant gel cannot be converted back to its original sol state. Such a hydrocolloid material is described as an irreversible hydrocolloid.

The molecules in the irreversible hydrocolloid are joined together by primary valency bonds. These bonds are very strong and cannot be affected by temperature changes except at which decomposition takes place.

For example, *alginate* impression material: Sodium alginate sol in water reacts with calcium sulphate, as

Sodium alginate + calcium sulphate →
calcium alginate (gel) + sodium sulphate

General Properties of Hydrocolloids

Dimensional Stability

Hydrocolloids are dimensionally unstable because of **syneresis and imbibition**. A large amount of water, dispersion medium in the sol and dispersed phase in the gel is enclosed loosely within the gel fibrils. If the water content of the gel is reduced, the gel will shrink and if the gel then takes up water the gel will swell or expand. If these materials are used for obtaining impressions, any change in dimensions of the impressions after it has been removed from the mouth is a source of error.

Syneresis

Hydrocolloids loose water content on standing in **a dry atmosphere**. The gel may lose water by **evaporation** from its surface or **by exudation of fluid** onto the surface of the gel. The gel may also lose some of the more soluble constituents. Syneresis results in the formation of small droplets of exudates on the surface of the hydrocolloids, which is not pure water. It may be either **alkaline or acidic, slightly,** depending on the composition of gel. The loss of water or fluid will lead to the **shrinkage of the gel.** This effect is known as syneresis.

Imbibition

If a hydrocolloid gel is placed in water, it will absorb water and swells and this phenomenon is known as imbibition, which alters the original dimension of the gel.

The reversible hydrocolloids will imbibe only as much water needed to replace the amount of water, which they have lost by syneresis. The hydrocolloids appear to exhibit, **gel-memory** in this respect.

Irreversible hydrocolloids will continue to undergo imbibition if they are placed under water. They imbibe until their water content is much higher than that of the original gel.

Remedy

To ensure optimum accuracy, the model or cast should be poured immediately after recording the impression. If it cannot be poured immediately, **store the impression in 100% relative humidity chamber** for not more than one hour. For shorter periods the surface of the impression can be **covered with a damp napkin or wet cotton**.

Gel Strength

Hydrocolloid gels are relatively **weak viscoelastic materials**, and easily undergo tensile fracture, i.e. tearing and flow. However, such a gel can support greater stresses when the stress is applied rapidly.

Factors to Increase the Gel Strength

- **Greater the density** or concentration of dispersed phase in the sol, greater will be the fibrils formed on gelation and greater will be the strength.
- **Lower the temperature,** stronger will be the gel for reversible hydrocolloids. As the temperature rises, more fibrils may revert to the sol phase and strength decreases.
- **Fillers:** Strength of the gel can be controlled by the manufacturer by adding an appropriate amount of fillers (modifiers).
- **The rate of loading: Faster loading** causes greater resistance to deformation, i.e. it maximizes elastic recovery and minimizes permanent deformation. The impression should be removed from the mouth **with a single, sudden jerk. These behave as viscoelastic materials**.

AGAR-AGAR IMPRESSION MATERIAL
(REVERSIBLE HYDROCOLLOIDS)

Agar is chemically an organic, hydrophilic hydrocolloid (polysaccharide) extracted from certain **seaweeds,** and is **a sulfuric ester of a linear polymer of galactose**.

Agar-agar (in Dentistry)

It is a mucostatic, elastic, reversible hydrocolloid impression material, earlier used mainly to record impressions of dentulous arches in the preparation of crowns, bridges, partial dentures, etc. In recent days these are most widely used as duplicating materials to duplicate the casts.

ADA Specification No. 11

These materials are supplied in two forms:
1. *Tray material:* It is supplied in plastic or metallic disposable tubes.

Table 3.6	The composition of agar-agar impression materials (gel)	
Ingredients	%	Functions
1. Agar	13–17%	To provide the dispersed phase of sol and the continuous fibril structure of the gel
2. Borax	0.2–0.5%	To improve the viscosity of the sol and strength of the gel
3. Potassium sulfate	1–2%	Gypsum hardener—to counteract the inhibiting effect of borax and agar on the setting of gypsum model material
4. Alkyl benzoate	0.1%	Preservative—to prevent the growth of mould in the impression material during storage
5. Diatomaceous earth	0.3–0.5%	Filler—to control the viscosity, rigidity, and strength
6. Water	85.5%	To provide the continuous phase in the sol and second continuous phase of the gel
7. Thymol	Trace	Bactericide
8. Glycerin	Trace	Plasticizer
9. Colour and flavouring agents	Trace	To improve the appearance and taste

2. *Syringe material:* It is supplied in small cylinders of correct size to fit the syringe.

The only difference between the two types is the difference in colour and greater fluidity in the syringe material, composition of agar-agar impressions material (Table 3.6).

Gelation Mechanism

When the gel is heated, the kinetic energy of the fibrils will increase, so that the interfibrillar distance increases and the gel is converted to sol because cohesion is less. When the temperature of the sol decreases the kinetic energy of sol particles decrease forming fibrils and these fibrils adhere to form a brush heap structures. The fibrils are joined by weak **van der Waals forces**. The water is enclosed loosely in the interstices between fibrils. When the gel is heated to 70°C weak van der Waal's forces disappear due to the increase of their kinetic energy.

Liquefaction temperature of the gel, i.e. the temperature at which the gel is converted to sol and gelation temperature, i.e. temperature at which the sol is converted to gel are different. **This temperature lag** or difference is known as **hysteresis**, which makes hydrocolloid suitable to use in dentistry.

Properties of Reversible Agar-agar Hydrocolloids (Agar-agar)

1. **Biological properties:** It is nontoxic and nonirritant to the oral tissues.
2. **Rheological properties**
   - **Viscosity:** After liquefaction, it is sufficiently fluid to record all the finer details. It is available in two viscosities—tray and syringe. Its low viscosity classifies it as a **mucostatic** impression materials.
   - **Gelation time:** It is a function of both temperature and composition. It is approximately **5 minutes** and is shorter at lower temperatures.
   - **Gelation temperature:** It should not be too high as it may burn the soft tissues or too low as it may not flow properly and distorted impression will result. According to ADA specification No. 11, it should not be less than 37°C and should not be more than 45°C.
3. **Physical properties**
   - **Gel strength:** According to ADA specification No. 11, the compressive strength should be **more than 0.245 MPa. It is about 0.4–0.7 MPa.**

   Strength is higher for
   - Higher concentration of dispersed phase-brush heaps
   - Lower temperature
   - Higher filler content
   - Higher rate of loading
   - **Tear strength:** It is about **715 gm/cm,** which is very low. So, the thickness of the impression should have a minimum of 3–5 mm. Tear strength also depends on the rate of loading, i.e. rapid removal with a single sudden jerk is recommended to **maximize tear strength, elastic recovery and to minimize permanent deformation.**
   - **Flexibility:** According to ADA specification No. 11 agar-agar should have **4–15% flexibility**. It is measured as the amount of strain produced when a sample is stressed by **100–1000 gm/cm^2**. The material should be flexible enough for easy removal over undercuts.

• **Permanent deformation and elasticity**

These materials are classified as elastic but they are not perfectly so. They undergo a small percentage of deformation known as a **permanent set** due to **viscoelastic nature** of the material.

When agar-agar impression material is held between the tray and the tissues, it is important to know the extent of any deformation of the material during removal of impression from the mouth.

The permanent deformation of the material after stressing is measured as **percentage deformation of set** (percent set) that occurs in a cylindrical specimen after the specimen has been **compressed to 10% strain for 30 sec**. According to the current ADA specification No. 11, the permanent deformation value should not exceed 1.5% (Fig. 3.6).

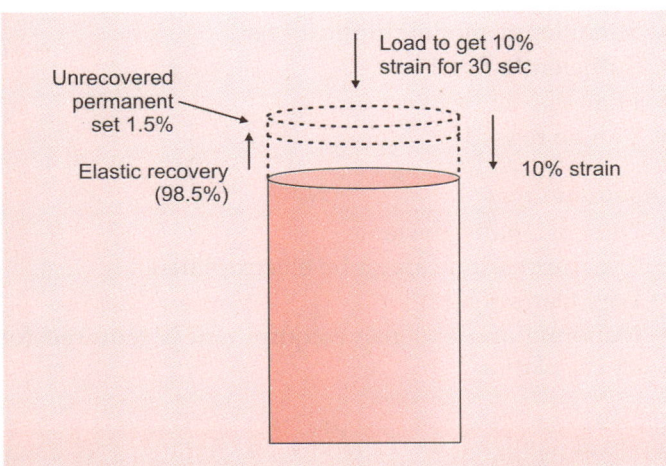

Fig. 3.6: Testing sample for finding elastic recovery

Elastic recovery = 100 – permanent deformation
(ER) = 100 – 1.5 = 98.5%

Most of the commercially available agar-agar impression materials have permanent deformations of 1% and recovery of 99%.

Permanent deformation is more for

• Greater percentage compression or strain
• Longer time of compression
• The greater thickness of the sample
• The lower rate of loading
• Repeated cyclic loading

To minimise deformation, **the impression is removed with a single sudden jerk.**

• **Dimensional stability:** Reversible hydrocolloids are dimensionally unstable because of syneresis and imbibition (*refer* to properties of hydrocolloids). So, the cast should be poured immediately within 15 minutes after recording the impression.

4. **Minor properties**

Compatible with gypsum products with cast and die materials.

5. **Electroplating:** Cannot be done

6. **Disinfection:** The impression can be **disinfected** by using *iodophor, bleach* or **2%** *glutaraldehyde.*

Manipulation Procedure

Apparatus required is hydrocolloid conditioner

Reversible hydrocolloids usually are conditioned before use by using a specially designed hydrocolloid conditioner. This consists of three temperature controlled compartments containing water (Fig. 3.7).

• Liquefaction compartment at 100°C boiling water temperature.
• Storage compartment at 65°C.
• Conditioning or tempering compartment at 45°C.

1. **Liquefaction of the gel (gel ⇌ sol)**

The filled syringes and tubes are placed in one of the water baths of a hydrocolloid conditioner at about 100°C for 10–15 minutes. This rapidly converts gel to sol. Insufficient boiling will lead to a stiff granular mass that will not reproduce the finer details. If the material is to be reliquefied after a previous use, approximately three minutes should be added to the boiling time, each time the material is reliquefied. At higher altitudes, the temperature of boiling water will not reach 100°C. In such cases a pressure cooker can be used, or an agent such as **propylene glycol** can be added to the water until a temperature of 100°C is attained.

2. **Storage of the sol**

After the agar gel has been converted to sol, the tubes and syringes are placed in storage bath which is maintained at **63–65°C**. It can be stored at this temperature for several hours. A lower temperature may result in some gelation and inaccurate reproduction of fine details. The material in the syringe is never allowed to drop below this temperature. Otherwise, it will undergo gelation, and it is then difficult to squeeze.

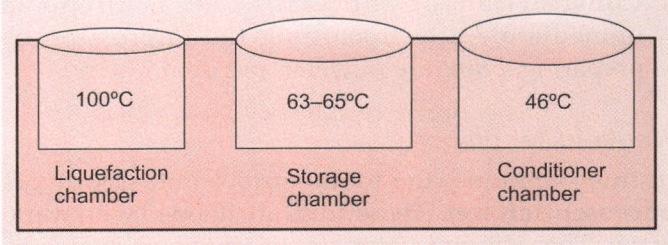

Fig. 3.7: Hydrocolloid conditioner

3. **Conditioning or tempering**
The material that is used to fill the tray must be cooled or tempered before the impression is taken. The stored agar sol is squeezed on to a perforated water cooled tray, a gauge pad or glass is placed over the top of the tray and the tray is placed in conditioning bath at 43°C or 45°C for 10–15 minutes. The purpose is to:

- Increase the viscosity of the sol, so that it will not flow out of the tray, and becomes homogeneously viscous.
- Reduce the temperature of the sol, which also decreases gelation time so that the material will not be uncomfortable to the patient.

The temperature at which the hydrocolloid is held, influences the rate of gelation. The lower the temperature the shorter should be the time in the conditioning.

4. **Impression recording**
In order to secure maximum detail the prepared cavity (or tooth) is first filled by injecting the syringe material taken directly from the storage bath. Before placing the tray material in the mouth the water soaked outer layer of tray material is blotted with a dry gauge. Failure to do so may prevent firm union between the tray and syringe material. The tray is immediately brought into position and seated with passive pressure.

5. **Gelation:** Gelation is accomplished by circulating cold water at about 18–23°C, through the tray for not less than 5 minutes. The coolest areas of the sol are converted to gel rapidly. Circulation of the ice water will induce rapid gelation and more concentration of stress in hydrocolloid which is nearer the tray, and distorted impression may result.

6. **Removal:** After gelation, the impression is removed rapidly from the mouth with **a single sudden jerk** in a direction parallel to the long axis of the tooth.

7. **Washing:** The impression is rinsed thoroughly with water, and excess water is removed by shaking the impression. The impression is disinfected using suitable disinfection procedure.

8. **Construction of the cast:** Cast is prepared immediately after recording the impression by preparing a mixture of water and dental stone.

Wet-field Technique

In this technique, the tooth surface and tissues are **purposely left wet**. These areas are flooded with **warm water.** Then syringe material is injected quickly in bulk to cover the occlusal and the incisal areas. Immediately,

tray material is seated over the syringe material. The hydraulic pressure of the viscous tray material, forces the fluid syringe material into the areas to be recorded. Theoretically, there is less chance that these materials will tear when the impression is removed from the mouth. Wet and warm conditions improve the flow of the material in the mouth.

Uses of agar-agar impression materials

- It was used to take impressions of dentulous arches in preparations of crowns, bridges and partial dentures.
- It is mainly used now as a duplicating material to duplicate casts and models

Advantages

- Reproduces finer details
- Suitable for model duplications
- Sufficiently flexible
- High elastic recovery
- Can be reused

Disadvantages

- Dimensionally unstable
- The impression cannot be electroplated
- Low tear strength
- Elaborate and expensive equipment is required for manipulation.

ALGINATE IMPRESSION MATERIALS (IRREVERSIBLE HYDROCOLLOIDS)

Alginate is one of the most widely used dental impression materials. It is irreversible hydrocolloid elastic impression material which sets by chemical reaction. It is used to record the impressions of **dentulous arches** in the preparation of crowns and bridges and the preliminary impressions of edentulous arches in the preparation of complete dentures.

Dental alginate impression materials change from the **sol phase to the gel** phase by **chemical reaction**. Once the gelation is completed, the material cannot be converted to a sol. Hence, these type of hydrocolloids are called as **irreversible hydrocolloids**.

Alginate is based on **alginic acid** which is prepared from a brown seaweed, algae, a marine plant. Chemically, it is **a linear polymer of anhydro β-d-mannuronic acid of high molecular weight.** Alginic acid is insoluble in water but the salts obtained with sodium and ammonium are soluble. Sodium potassium or triethanol amine alginates are used in dental impression materials (Fig. 3.8).

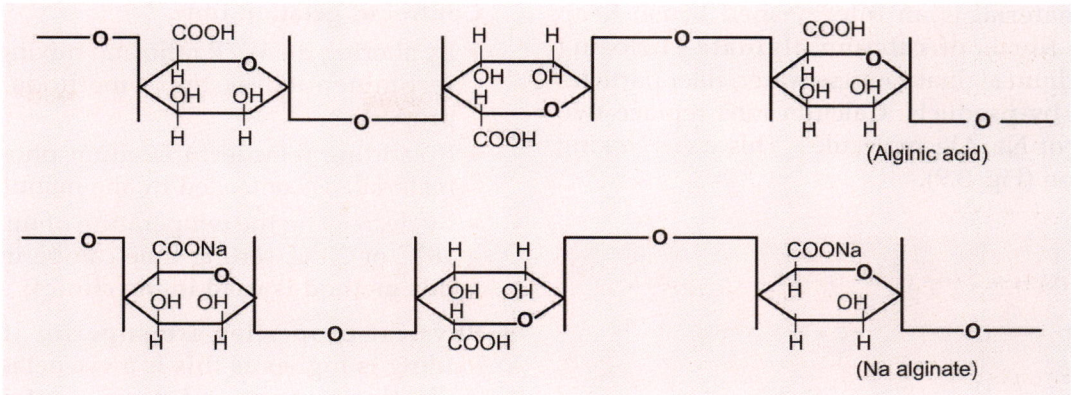

Fig. 3.8: Structure of alginic acid and sodium alginates

Dispensing

The material is supplied as a powder in sealed bulk containers or in weighed small packets or sachets of plastic or metal foils for longer storage time.

As per ADA No. 18, there are two types

- Type I—fast set, with setting time, 1–2 min
- Type II—normal set with setting time 2–4 min.

Gelation Reaction

On mixing the powder with water, a sol is formed, and the alginate, calcium salt, and trisodium phosphate begin to dissolve. Calcium sulphate rapidly reacts with soluble alginate to produce an insoluble calcium alginate gel. The production of calcium alginate gel is so rapid that it does not allow sufficient working time.

Trisodium phosphate reacts with calcium sulphate in **preference to the soluble alginate** to give a precipitate of calcium phosphate. This **reaction delays** the supply of calcium ions required for the gelation reaction and thereby **increases the working time** (Table 3.7).

$$2Na_3PO_4 + 3CaSO_4 \rightarrow Ca_3(PO_4)_2 + 3Na_2SO_4$$

When **all the sodium phosphate has reacted**, the calcium ions begin to react with soluble alginate quickly to produce **calcium alginate as a gel**. As the reaction proceeds, the degree of cross-linking increases and gel develops elastic properties.

$$Na_nAlg + \frac{n}{2}CaSO_4 \longrightarrow Ca\frac{n}{2}Alg\ (gel) + \frac{n}{2}Na_2SO_4$$

Table 3.7	Composition of alginate impression powder	
Ingredients	%	Functions
1. Soluble salts of alginates of (Na, K, ammonium or triethanolamine alginate)	15%	– Main reactive ingredient – Forms sol with water – Reacts with calcium to form a gel of calcium alginate
2. Calcium sulphate dihydrate	16%	Reactor—releases calcium ions to react with soluble alginate to form insoluble calcium alginate gel (accelerator).
3. Trisodium phosphate	2%	Retarder—to react preferentially with calcium ions, delay gelation and increase working time.
4. Diatomaceous earth	60%	Filler—to increase the strength and stiffness of the gel structure (that is not tacky) and controls the viscosity of the mix.
5. Zinc oxide	4%	Filler—has some influence on physical properties and setting time of the gel.
6. Potassium titanium fluoride	3%	Gypsum hardener—to counteract inhibiting effect of alginate on the setting of die materials and improves the surface of the stone model.
7. Flavouring agent	Trace	To provide pleasant taste (wintergreen or peppermint) to make of more acceptable to the patients
8. Colour pigments	Trace	To provide characteristic colour, sometimes changing.

The set material is an intermeshed brush heap structure of fibrils of **calcium alginate** enclosing unreacted sodium alginate, excess water, filler particles and reaction by-products. Calcium ions replace two sodium ions of Na_nAlg molecules. This cross-linking causes gelation (Fig. 3.9).

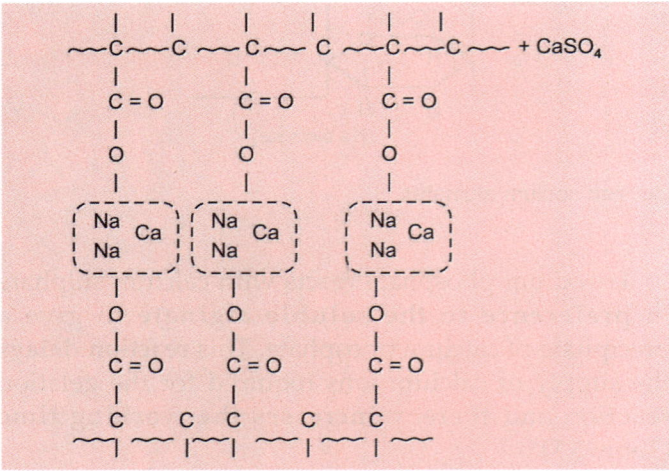

Fig. 3.9: Cross-linking of sodium alginate by Ca^{++} ions, replacing two Na^+ ions

Properties

1. Biological

- They are nontoxic and nonirritant to the oral tissues (alginate has diatomaceous earth as filler has finely divided silica particles). Some of these particles are present in the alginate dust which rises from the container **while tumbling, fluffing or shaking. These** silica particles are found to be a source of health hazard, **silicosis if inhaled.**

Remedy: The container is allowed to settle for a while after tumbling. Then it is held away from the face while opening to avoid breathing the dust (or **use dust-free alginates).**

- It has pleasant taste, odour, and good compatibility.

2. Rheological

- **Gelation time**

It is the time from the beginning of mixing until the gelation occurs. It is measured as the time from the beginning of mixing until the material is no longer tacky or sticky when it is touched with clean, dry fingers. Based on the gelation time, there are two types of alginates.

Type I—fast set (1–2 minutes)

Type II—normal set (2–4 minutes)

Control of gelation time

- By altering the W/P ratio and mixing time are not recommended as these methods affect other properties.
- By adding retarder, trisodium phosphate to the material, as controlled by the manufacturer.
- By decreasing the temperature of mixing water to 18°C or 20°C, setting time can be increased, and **this method is used in the clinics.**

3. **Physical properties are superior if the rate of loading is higher as this is a viscoelastic material.**
   - **Elastic recovery and permanent deformation:** These materials are classified as elastic but they are not entirely so. They undergo a small amount of deformation known as a permanent set due to their **viscoelastic** behavior. It is measured as the percentage of deformation that occurs in a cylindrical sample after it is compressed by 10% strain for 30 seconds. According to ADA No. 18, it should be **less than 3%** (Fig. 3.6).

Elastic recovery (ER) is about 100–300 or 97%

It is a time dependent property and is a function of
- Percentage compression
- Time under compression
- Time after removal of the compressive load
- Severity of undercuts

Permanent deformation decreases when
- Percentage compression is less
- Impression is under compression for a shorter time *(remove the impression with a single sudden jerk)*
- When recovery time is longer (remove the impression from the mouth after 8 minutes).

- **Gel strength**
According to ADA specification No. 18, it should be **more than 0.343 MPa** (about 0.5–0.8 MPa).

- **Factors affecting strength**
  - The decrease in W/P ratio within limits, increases strength
  - Both under- and over-spatulation decrease strength
  - **The higher rate of loading increases strength**

- **Tear strength**
Varies from 300 to 700 gm/cm, which is quite low. Hence, the **thickness should be between 3 and 5 mm.**

- **Flexibility**
According to ADA specification No. 18, it should be between **5 and 20%.** It is measured as the amount of strain produced when a sample is stressed between 100–1000 gm/cm². Most alginates have values of 12–14%.

- **Dimensional stability**

  These are dimensionally unstable due to **syneresis and imbibition,** so cast should be poured **immediately** after recording the impression (refer: properties of hydrocolloids).

4. **Minor properties**
   - **Compatible with gypsum die materials**
   - **Electroplating cannot be done**
   - **Trays used** should be perforated for mechanical retention
   - **Shelf-life is quite short**

     They deteriorate rapidly at higher temperatures. Therefore, it is better not to stock the material more than one year, and it should be stored in cool dry environment.

Manipulation Techniques

Instruments

Plastic mixing bowl, alginate mixing spatula with curved end and a perforated tray of suitable size.

Proportioning

The container of the powder should be shaken before use, to get uniform distribution of components. The powder dispensing cup is slightly overfilled tapped gently with a spatula to fill the voids in the dispensing cup and to ensure a reproducible volume of the powder is used in each mix. The blade of the spatula is used to scrape off the excess from the top of the cup. Water/powder ratio is taken 3:1 by volume as per manufacturer's instruction using the measures supplied for examples,

For maxillary impressions—2 scoops of powder (15 g) + 2 measure of water (48 ml)

For mandibular impressions—1 scoop of powder (7.5 g) + 1 measure of water (24 ml).

Hand mixing

The measured powder is shifted into a clean rubber bowl and the measured quantity of water is added. The powder is incorporated into the water by careful spatulation. Once the powder has been wetted, the material is mixed with a vigorous **figure 8 motion or stropped** between the blade of the spatula and sides of the mixing bowl, with intermittent rotation of the bowl in the opposite (anticlockwise) direction. The mix is collected and again stropped repeatedly to form homogeneous conistency. Mixing time is quite short, (only about 45 sec).

Manufacturers supply mechanical mixing instruments have control of speed and time of mixing. This gives a reproducible mix.

Under spatulation results

- Inadequate wetting and lack of homogeneity
- The mix will be a grainy and poor recording of details and mechanical properties.

Over-spatulation results

- Reduction in working time
- Decrease in strength due to the destruction of gel fibrils as they form and intermesh.

The final mix should be smooth and creamy that does not drip off the spatula when it is raised from the bowl.

Loading the tray

The mixed alginate is quickly transferred to a perforated tray by using mixing spatula and is generally added to the posterior portion of the tray and pushed towards anterior portion.

Impression recording

The loaded tray is carried to the patient's mouth to record the impression. The posterior portion of the tray is usually seated first and then the anterior portion. The tray should be held gently until the alginate sets.

Removal of impressions

After the seal between impression and peripheral tissue is **broken,** the tray and the impression should be removed with a **single sudden jerk** to minimize the permanent deformation and maximize recovery.

Washing

It should be **washed** under running tap water, and excess water should be shaken off. The impression can be disinfected by immersing it in a **sodium hypochlorite** or **glutaraldehyde solution or iodophor** for 10 minutes. The disinfectants can also be sprayed on the impression.

Construction of cast

The cast should be poured **immediately** with a mix of dental stone and water, as they are not dimensionally stable, due to syneresis and imbibition.

Precautions

- The instruments must be clean. Small amounts of gypsum impurities left in the bowl, earlier will accelerate the reaction.
- After tumbling, the powder container, the dust coming out should not be inhaled which may lead to a **health hazard**.
- Correct water/powder ratio, as specified by the manufacturer is to be followed. Variation in W/P ratio effects is setting time, permanent deformation, flexibility, and strength.

- Air should not be incorporated during mixing.
- Both under- and over-spatulation should be avoided.
- The temperature of water used for mixing should be in between 18 and 23°C.
- The thickness of the impression should be **3–5 mm** to avoid tearing of the material.
- The tray should not be disturbed during gelation.
- The impression should be held in the mouth for at least 2–3 minutes after the material has gelled, because strength and elasticity of the gel increase with time thus permitting superior reproduction of undercuts.
- Dislodge the impression with a **single sudden jerk.**
- The cast should be poured immediately. For shorter periods it can be stored in 100% humidity or its surface can be covered with a **damp napkin or wet cotton**.

Advantages
- Reproduces excellent surface details
- High elastic recovery
- Records undercut fairly accurately
- Comfortable with the patient
- Hygienic since fresh material is used each time
- Not very expensive
- Easy manipulation procedure.

Disadvantages
- Dimensionally unstable
- Low tear strength
- Cannot be electroplated
- No proper storage medium
- Cannot be added in increments, if faulty.

Uses
- It is used to record the impressions of dentulous arches in preparation of crowns and bridges, partial dentures to a limited extent.
- To record preliminary impression in preparation of complete dentures.
- To record the impression in orthodontia to prepare study models
- To record the impression to construct athletic mouth protectors
- For duplicating cast and models.

Modified Alginates

1. Dust-free alginates (DFAs)

The alginate powder is finely divided, and considerable amount of dust may be involved while dispensing the powder. Some of the silica particles in the dust are of such a size and shape which may lead to a possible health hazard if inhaled. The dimensions of 10–15% siliceous dust particles present in the powder are similar to asbestos fibres that produce **fibrogenesis and carcinogenesis**. Therefore dust should be avoided.

In an effort to reduce the dusting encountered after tumbling, few manufacturers have incorporated a **de-dusting agent (glycerin or glycol)** into the alginate powder to agglomerate the particles. This causes the powder to become denser than in the uncoated state. No detectable levels of dust have been measured at the operators level. This type of alginate powders are **dust free or dustless alginates** (*see* Colour Plate 5, Fig. 3.6).

Some varieties are
- Rapid—setting elastic DFA (2 min 10 sec)
- Normal—setting high precision DFA
- Rapid—setting chromatic DFA (3'30")
- Extra—rapid setting orthodontic DFA (2'35") and (1'50").

2. Siliconized alginates
Silicon polymers have been incorporated into alginates and have been modified and developed into a much stronger material. These materials are supplied in two consistencies (tray and syringe viscosities). These materials have superior resistance to tearing when compared to unmodified alginates. These materials are considered as hybrids of alginates and silicone elastomers, but their properties closely match to those of alginates.

3. Alginates in the form of sol
Alginates can also be supplied in the form of a sol containing water but without the source of Ca^{2+} ions. A reactor of $CaSO_4$ can be added to the sol in this case.

Alginate sol in water + $CaSO_4 \rightarrow$ Calcium alginate gel

4. Chromatic or colour indicator alginates (modified by the addition of chemical indicators).

The primary purpose of adding indicators is to show the different stages during manipulation and help the operator while recording the impression. Chemical reaction take place by a change of colour in each stage of manipulation. The indicator incorporated show the different stages of the reaction which has been reached.

For example: Violet colour—during spatulation
Pink colour—during loading
Light yellow (peach)—when material sets.

5. Hard and soft set alginates
These alginates are produced by adjusting the **percentage of fillers to control** the flexibility of set

impression material, e.g. hard set alginate has a flexibility range of 5–8%.

6. **Alginates containing disinfectants**

   These type of alginates are recently developed which contain disinfectants in the original material itself which *destroys the microorganisms*. These materials need not to be disinfected after recording the impression, but ideally all the impression have to be disinfected to avoid transmission of deadly diseases, e.g. quaternary ammonium salts or chlorohexamine are added to alginate powder.

   Note: The patients have to be strictly informed **not to swallow** the impression materials.

Laminate technique (agar-alginate combination)

In this technique, the agar syringe material is injected into the prepared cavity or surfaces in the mouth and the *chilled alginate* material mix is taken in a perforated tray, held over the injected agar sol and allowed to set or gelate. Alginate gels by chemical reaction, whereas agar gels by precisely contact with cool alginates.

Advantages

- Cost of equipment is lower because only the syringe material needs to be heated.
- Less preparation time required.
- Eliminates water cooled impression trays
- Records all surface details very clearly because of agar
- Cost effective technique to produce adequate details.

Disadvantages

- Poor dimensional stability due to syneresis and imbibition.
- The bond between the agar and alginate is not always strong.
- High viscosity alginate displaces the agar during seating (Table 3.8).

Table 3.8	Common causes for failures and remedies of hydrocolloid impressions	
Failures	**Causes (and remedies are suggestive)**	
	Agar-agar	*Alginate*
1. Grainy material surface	• Inadequate boiling • Too low storage temperature • Too long storage time	• Inhomogeneous mixing • Prolonged mixing • Excessive gelation (delay in using) • Too low $\frac{W}{P}$
2. Separation of tray and syringe material	• Water left on the surface of tray material • Premature gelation of either material	• Not applicable due to chemical bonding
3. Tearing	• Inadequate thickness • Premature removal • Delay in seating tray material	• Prolonged mixing • Inadequate thickness • Moisture contaminations • Premature removal
4. External bubbles	• Gelation of syringe material	• Pregelation before seating • Air trapped while mixing
5. Irregular voids	• Too cold material	• Water and debris on the tissues
6. Distortion	• Movement of the tray during gelation • Removal before completion of gelation • Improper removal from the mouth • Delay in pouring the cast	• Movement of the tray during gelation • Removal before completion of gelation • Improper removal from the mouth • Delay in pouring the cast
7. Rough and chalky stone model surface	• Inadequate cleaning • Excess water or surface hardener left • Incomplete gelation • Improper mixing or high $\frac{W}{P}$ of the cast or die stone • Too cold water circulation	• Inadequate cleaning of the impression • Excess water or surface hardener left in impression • Incomplete gelation (early removal) • Inadequate mixing or high $\frac{W}{P}$ of stone die and cast material.

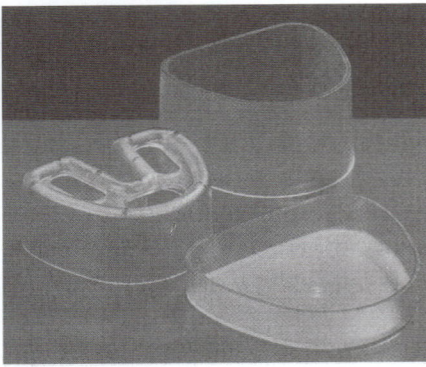

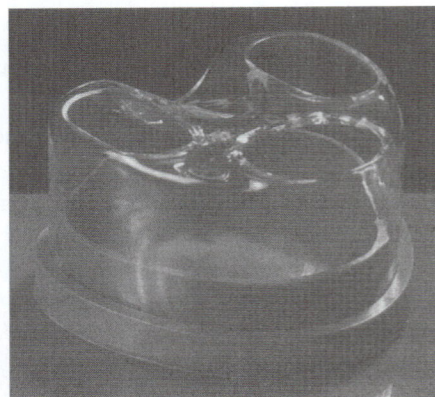

Fig. 3.10: Plastic and glass duplicating flasks

Duplicating Materials

These are the materials used to make an accurate replica of models or casts. Duplicate refractory casts are used in the construction of prosthetic appliances, partial dentures, and orthodontic models. It is required for two reasons:

- The cast on which the wax pattern of metal framework is to be formed must be made from a refractory investment since it must withstand the high casting temperatures.
- The original cast is required for checking the accuracy of the metal framework and for processing the acrylic portion of the denture (*see* Colour Plate 5, Fig. 3.5).

Materials

According to ADA specification **No. 20**, there are two types

- **Type I:** Thermoreversible—agar-agar and PVC gel
- **Type II:** Non-reversible—alginates and elastomers

Further, these are known as

- Class I: Aqueous—agar-agar, alginates
- Class II: Nonaqueous—PVC gel, elastomers.

Requirements as per ADA specification No. 20

- Maximum permanent deformation = 3% (for all)
- Strain in compression = 4–25% (for all)

- Minimum compressive strength
  Type I = 2,200 gm/cm^2 = 0.215 MPa
  Type II = 2,600 gm/cm^2 = 0.255 MPa
- Minimum tear strength = 900 gm/cm (for all).

Properties

Type I aqueous—agar-agar

- Excellent reproduction of finer details
- Sufficient strength, flexibility and tear strength to duplicate undercuts
- Dimensionally unstable
- Reusable
- More number of duplicates becomes less accurate.

Type I nonaqueous—PVC gel

Sufficient strength, flexibility, and chemical stability which permits large numbers of duplications.

Type II aqueous—alginate

- A simpler method (no heating equipment)
- Dimensionally unstable
- Not reusable

Type II nonaqueous elastomers (polysilicones and polyether)

- Excellent reproduction of finer details
- Good dimensional stability
- Can be used to get **many duplicates**
- Compatible with duplicating die materials
- But expensive and cannot be reused.

Duplicating procedure

Purpose of duplicating: To prepare multiple casts for fabrication of cast partial denture (CPD).

Agar duplicating material is the most common type used in the dental laboratory. Technique for duplication in the involves placing the cast in the duplicating flask. Agar gel is heated to 100°C to convert the gel to sol and then allowed to cool to 50°C before use (Fig. 3.10) (*see* colour plate 4, Figs 3.3a and b).

The fluid material is then poured through a hole in the top of the flask until it **overflows through another hole**. When gelation is completed the master cast is removed with a single sudden jerk to minimize permanent deformation. The duplicating cast should be poured immediately with a die or refractory material (gypsum or phosphate bonded) to avoid dimensional changes due to syneresis and imbibition.

ELASTOMERS
(ELASTOMERIC IMPRESSION MATERIALS)

Elastomers are rubber-like materials with long chained polymers, slightly cross-linked and coiled structures having glass-transition temperatures (T$_g$) much lower than the room temperatures. These exhibit large elastic *deformations and elastic recovery properties even under small stresses.*

Elastomeric Impression Materials

These are the materials which deform elastically while removing from undercut areas and spring back to their original form.

Elastomeric impression materials can be used to record the impressions of dentulous arches in the preparation of crown and bridge work, partial dentures, onlays, and inlays. They are also be used to record the edentulous arches impressions in the preparation of complete dentures.

Different elastomeric impression materials are

1. *Polysulphides*
2. *Polysilicones*
   - Addition polysilicones
   - Condensation polysilicones
3. *Polyether*
   - Light-activated poly ether
   - Chemically activated polyether.

ADA Specification No. 19 for Elastomers

Classification of elastomers according to various properties

This is required to select quickly, the most suitable material for the clinical condition.

1. **According to chemical nature/chemical name**
   - *Polysulphides*
   - *Polysilicones*
     - Addition polysilicones
     - Condensation polysilicones
   - *Polyethers*
     - Light-activated polyethers
     - Chemically activated polyethers
2. **According to viscosity** (viscosity is controlled by the amount of fillers):
   - Very high viscosity material—**putty**-like elastomers.

- High viscosity material—**heavy** body elastomers.
- Medium viscosity material—**regular** body elastomer.
- Low viscosity material—**light** body elastomer—syringe consistency.

3. **According to method of polymerization**
   - Addition polymerization materials, e.g. polyether, addition polysilicones
   - Condensation polymerization materials, e.g. condensation polysilicones and polysulphides.

4. **According to method of dispensing**
   - Single paste system: Light-activated polyether
   - Two paste system (base + reactor paste) polysulphides, addition, and condensation polysilicones.
   - Two-paste system having pseudoplastic property—supplied in a single consistency which can be used as a tray and syringe **monophase** material, e.g. addition polysilicones.
   - Single paste (base paste) with reactor liquid, e.g. condensation polysilicones.
   - Three paste system—base + reactor + body modifier (thinner)
     For example chemically activated polyether.

5. **According to dimensional stability, flow and permanent deformations** (Table 3.9).

Table 3.9	Classification according to dimensional stability—ADA No.19		
Types	Max. permanent deformation%	Max. flow in compression%	Maximum dimensional change in 24 hours%
I	2.5	0.5	0.5
II	2.5	0.5	1.0
III	2.5	2.0	0.5

6. **According to their clinical impression techniques** (Table 3.10).

Table 3.10	Classification according to impression techniques		
Kind of impression	The object of impression	Combinations
1. Double mix, single impression	Cavity impressions for inlays and onlays	Light + heavy body
2. Double mix, double impression (reline technique)	Cavity impressions for inlays, onlays, etc. impressions of a crown and impressions of a partial denture	Putty + light body or putty + regular body
3. Individual tray method (tube impression)	Impression for a crown (single tooth)	Regular body or light body
4. Single mix, single impression	Cavity impressions for inlays and onlays. Impressions for partial dentures	Regular or heavy having **pseudoplastic** property or light or regular body

POLYSULPHIDE IMPRESSION MATERIALS

This impression material was mainly used in recording dentulous impressions in the preparation of crowns and bridges, inlays, and onlays, where more working time is required.

Vulcanization

The process of heating the rubber with sulphur to produce cross-linking.

Dispensing methods

These are supplied as a 2 paste system in collapsible tubes, and are available in all 4 viscosities, **light, regular, heavy body and putty-like consistencies**.

> **Note:** L → Light body, R → Regular body, H → Heavy body, P → Putty consistency

Alternate names

- **Thiokol** corporation material: By the name of the first manufacturer.
- **Mercaptan** impression material: Due to mercaptan –SH groups.
- **Vulcanizing** impression material: By processing terminology.

The composition of polysulphide base and reactor pastes (Tables 3.11 and 3.12).

Chemistry of Polysulphides

On mixing the 2 pastes, terminal and pendant SH groups of polysulphide prepolymer get oxidized by PbO_2 and produce **chain extension and cross-linking.** The reaction results in the rapid **increase in mol. wt.** and mixed paste is converted to rubber. It is a condensation process, chain lengthening is brought about by terminal –SH group and cross-linking is brought about by **pendant SH groups. The chain lengthening increases the viscosity of the rubber, and cross-linking gives three-dimensional network and elastic properties to the material. Higher cross-linking makes the material more rigid or less flexible.**

Table 3.11	The composition of base paste		
	Ingredients	Base paste%	Functions
1.	Moderately—low molecular wt. polysulphides (pre-mol wt. 2000–4000) with **terminal SH groups**	74–80%	This is a reactive ingredient which further polymerizes and cross-links with the pendant SH groups to form rubber
2.	Moderately low molecular wt polysulphide prepolymer with **pendant SH groups**	2%	Undergoes cross-linking which reduces permanent deformation under compression or tension during, removal from the mouth
3.	Reinforcing fillers (e.g. titanium dioxide, lithophone, zinc sulphide, zinc oxide, silica, as fine particles of 0.3 µm size	16–56% L–16% R–26% H–36% P–56%	Paste former improves strength, gives body and control viscosity
4.	Dibutyl phthalate (plasticizer)	0.5%	To control the viscosity of the mix

Table 3.12	The composition of reactor (accelerator or catalyst) paste		
	Ingredients	%	Functions
1.	PbO_2 (lead dioxide) (or, $-Cu(OH)_2$) (cumene hydroxide)	78%	Oxidizing agent causes polymerization and cross-linking by SH groups, gives a characteristic dark brown colour to the paste and has a bad smell
2.	Sulphur	0.5–3%	To facilitate the reaction or as a promoter
3.	Dibutyl phthalate (plasticizer)	17%	To form a paste with PbO_2 and sulphur
4.	Inert oil (oleic acid, stearic acid, Mg stearate)	Trace	Paste former
5.	Deodorants	Trace	Reduces unpleasant smell

It is an exothermic reaction with 3°C–4°C rise in temperature. It is a condensation reaction in which water is formed as a by-product (Figs 3.11a to d). The viscosity increases and PbO also can enter into the system. **This is step-growth condensation polymerization with H_2O as a by-product.**

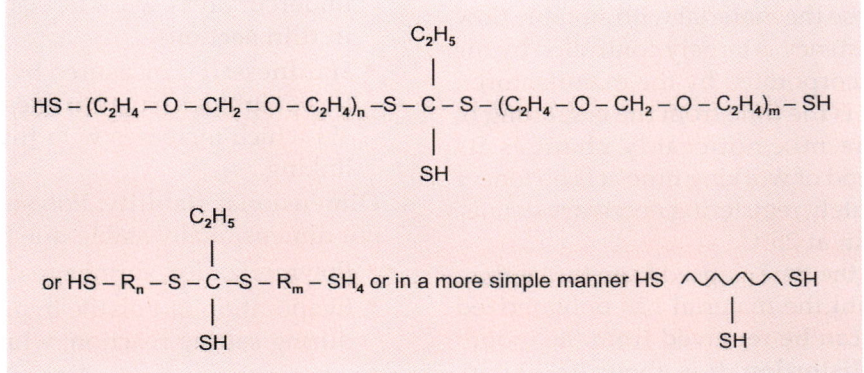

HS - (C_2H_4 - O - CH_2 - O - C_2H_4)$_n$ - SH,

represented as

HS - R_n - SH or simply HS ⌇⌇⌇⌇ SH

Fig. 3.11a: Moderately low molecular weight polysulphide with terminal—mercaptan –SH group

HS – (C_2H_4 – O – CH_2 – O – C_2H_4)$_n$ –S – C – S – (C_2H_4 – O – CH_2 – O – C_2H_4)$_m$ – SH

with C_2H_5 above C and SH below C

or HS – R_n – S – C –S – R_m – SH_4 or in a more simple manner HS ⌇⌇⌇⌇ SH

Fig. 3.11b: The polysulphide with pendant mercaptan

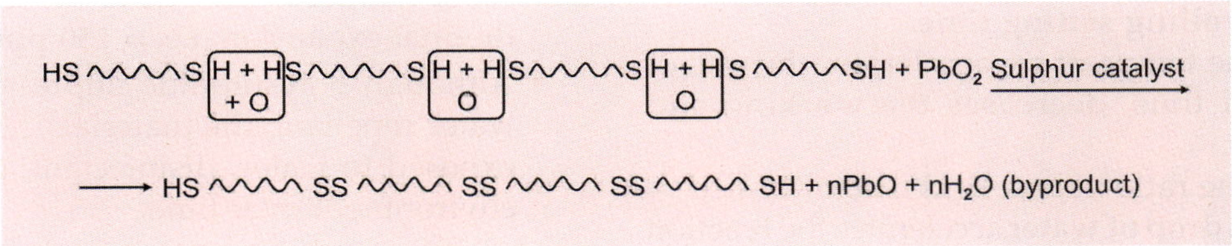

HS ⌇⌇⌇S H + H S ⌇⌇⌇ S H + H S ⌇⌇⌇ S H + H S ⌇⌇⌇SH + PbO_2 Sulphur catalyst ⟶
+ O   O   O

⟶ HS ⌇⌇⌇ SS ⌇⌇⌇ SS ⌇⌇⌇ SS ⌇⌇⌇ SH + nPbO + nH_2O (byproduct)

Fig. 3.11c: Polymerization—setting, and propagation of polysulphide by step-growth

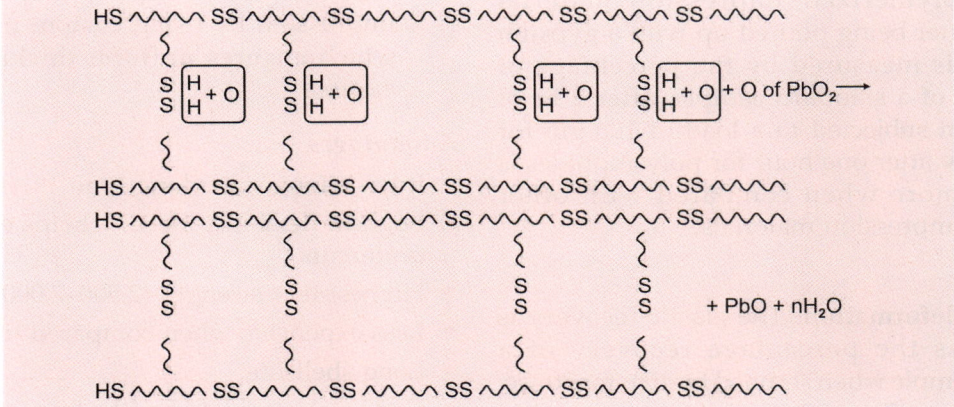

HS ⌇⌇⌇ SS ⌇⌇⌇ SS ⌇⌇⌇ SS ⌇⌇⌇ SS ⌇⌇⌇ SS ⌇⌇⌇

S H + O   S H + O   S H + O   S H + O + O of PbO_2 ⟶
S H   S H   S H   S H

HS ⌇⌇⌇ SS ⌇⌇⌇ SS ⌇⌇⌇ SS ⌇⌇⌇ SS ⌇⌇⌇ SS ⌇⌇⌇
HS ⌇⌇⌇ SS ⌇⌇⌇ SS ⌇⌇⌇ SS ⌇⌇⌇ SS ⌇⌇⌇ SS ⌇⌇⌇

S   S   S   S
S   S   S   S   + PbO + nH_2O

HS ⌇⌇⌇ SS ⌇⌇⌇ SS ⌇⌇⌇ SS ⌇⌇⌇ SS ⌇⌇⌇ SS ⌇⌇⌇

Fig. 3.11d: Cross-linking reactions

Properties of Polysulphides

1. Biological

- Non-toxic, non-poisonous and non-irritant to the oral tissues.
- It has got **bad odour** due to the presence of PbO_2 and mercaptan groups
- This can be easily disinfected by standard disinfectants like glutaraldehyde.

2. Rheological

Polysulphides are available in varieties of viscosities, light, regular, heavy, putty-like consistencies. It helps the operator to choose the material with suitable flow property. The consistency is largely controlled by the amount of fillers incorporated by the manufacturer.

- **Working time:** It is the time from the beginning of mixing until the mix noticeably changes its viscosity. At the end of working time, it is no longer capable of adequately registering necessary details. It is about 3–6 min at 25°C.
- **Setting time:** It is the time elapsed from the beginning of mixing until the material has polymerized sufficiently, and **can be removed from** the mouth with **minimum distortion**. It is about 10–20 min. The **mixing time is about one minute**.
  The working time and setting time can be measured by **Vicat** penetrometer or **reciprocating rheometer**.
- **Factors controlling setting time.**
- Increasing the temperature accelerates the rate of reaction and thus, decreases the working and setting times.
- By altering the ratio of base and reactor pastes
- Addition of a **drop of water** accelerates the reaction and setting time is decreased.
- Oleic acid can be used as an effective retarder.
- **Flow after one hour:** This property is important because it relates to the amount of deformation that the polymerized impression material undergoes after being poured up with a gypsum product. It is measured by the percentage of deformation of a standard sample, **after 1 hr** of setting, when subjected to a load of 100 gm for 15 min. Flow after one hour for polysulphides is 1.5%. It is more when compared with other elastomeric impression materials.

3. Mechanical

- **Permanent deformation:** The elastic recovery is measured as the percentage recovery of a cylindrical sample when strained by 10% for 30 sec. This is about 97 to 98%. The percentage of permanent deformation becomes 2–3%.

Elastic recovery properties improve with time due to viscoelasticity. The longer the impression remains in the mouth, higher is the accuracy.

- **Flexibility:** Polysulphide is one of the **least stiff** or **highly flexible of elastomeric materials.** This flexibility allows the set material to release from undercut areas and be removed from the mouth with minimum, stress. It is measured as the strain produced when a sample is stressed at 1000 gm/cm². Flexibility value of polysulphide is 14–17%.
- **Tear strength:** It has a high tear strength of 2500–7000 gm/cm. So it can be easily removed from the undercut areas without tearing, or it **can be used in thin sections.**
- **Hardness:** It is measured by **Shore-A-Durometer**. Polysulphides have hardness (L = 20, M = 30, H = 45) which increases with filler amount and cross-linking.

4. Dimensional stability: Polysulphide elastomers are not dimensionally stable due to following reasons.

- Polymerization shrinkage during cross-linking
- Evaporation of volatile byproducts such as water during setting reaction, which causes shrinkage.
- After setting, incomplete elastic recovery due to its time-dependent viscoelastic property.
- Large thermal contraction which causes deformation by a change in temperature from mouth to room temperature, due to the large coefficient of thermal expansion, i.e. **= 150 ppm/°C.**
- Although polysulphide impression materials are water repellant, the materials can absorb fluids if exposed to water, disinfectant, or high humidity environment over time.

For accurate polysulphide impressions

- The cast should be poured immediately after taking the impression.
- Minimize the amount of materials used to take impression by using custom made acrylic trays which **ensures uniform thickness** of impression material.

Advantages

- It has a longer working time
- Highest flexibility 14–17% helps easy removal over undercuts
- Highest tear strength (2,500–7,000 gm/cm)
- Less expensive when compared to other elastomers
- Long shelf-life.
- Can be electroplated with silver.
- It is compatible with die stones.

Disadvantages

- **Disagreeable odour** and taste due to the presence of PbO_2
- Long setting time
- Dimensional change due to evaporation of byproducts, i.e. water (3–6%)
- It will stain clothes
- Second or multiple die pouring is less accurate.

Uses

- To record dentulous impressions for preparation of crowns, bridges, inlays, onlays, partial dentures, etc.
- To record impressions of edentulous arches in the preparation of complete dentures.

CONDENSATION POLYSILICONES

It is also called as room temperature vulcanizing (RTV) silicones.

Dispensing

It is supplied in 2 forms
- Two-paste form in collapsible tubes, i.e. base + reactor or
- The base paste and reactor liquid.

Materials are available in all 4 viscosities or consistencies (L, R, H, P) in different indicating colours). Composition of condensation polysilicones (Table 3.13).

Setting Reaction

Moderately low molecular wt. silicone prepolymer with OH terminal group + ethyl silicate → ortho-silicate rubber (Fig. 3.12)

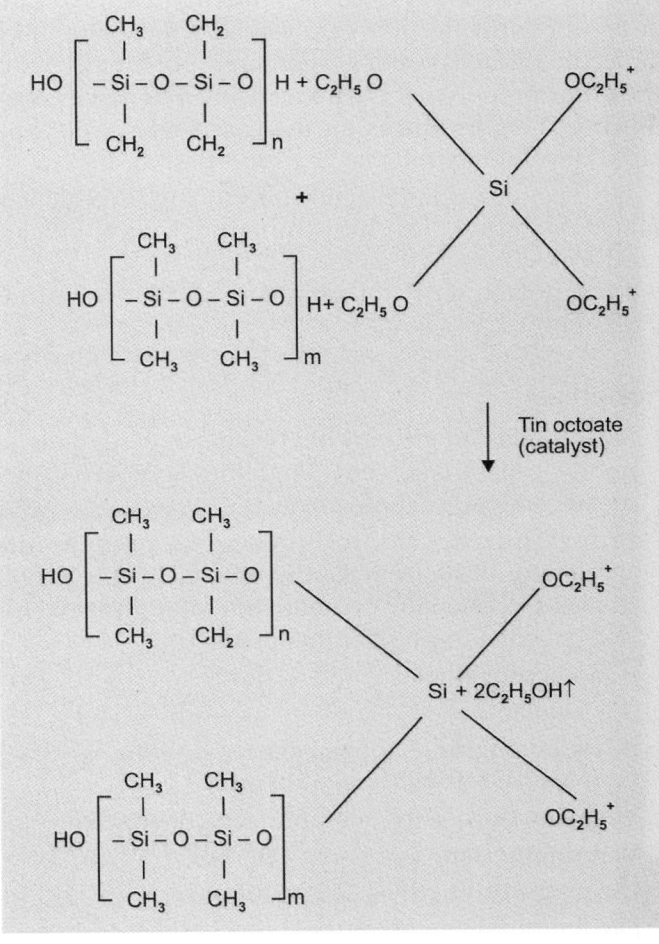

Fig. 3.12: Cross-linked condensation polysilicone rubber

On mixing the two components like base and reactor pastes, the reaction begins immediately in which the terminal hydroxyl groups of prepolymer chains react

Table 3.13	Composition of condensation polysilicones
Base paste: Ingredients	**Functions**
1. **Moderately low molecular wt. silicone** prepolymer with hydroxyl terminated groups	It undergoes polymerization and cross-linking to form rubber
2. Reinforcing fillers (copper carbonate, colloidal silica of particle size ranging from 2–10 microns) 35–75% (L, R, H, Putty consistencies)	1. Acts as paste former 2. Increases the strength of rubber 3. Gives body and controls consistency and modifies physical properties.
Reactor paste: Ingredients	**Functions**
1. Tri or tetra-functional **ethyl silicate**	As a cross-linking agent
2. Organometallic compound, **tin octoate**	As a reaction **catalyst** or activator
3. Reinforcing fillers or thickening agents	To form a paste and control viscosity
4. Colour pigments (organic dies)	To indicate the complete uniform mix To distinguish from the base paste

with the cross-linking agent, tetraethyl orthosilicate, under the influence of a catalyst, i.e. **tin octoate**. Each molecule of cross-linking agent can potentially react with four prepolymer chains, causing **extensive cross-linking**. This produces an increase in viscosity and rapid development in elastic properties.

It is a condensation reaction producing ethyl alcohol as a by-product. The multifunctional ethyl silicate produces a network or cross-linked structures that reduce permanent deformation and flow values (Fig. 3.6b).

Properties

- Silicone elastomers may be considered essentially as nontoxic materials even though they contain a heavy metal catalyst, i.e. tin octoate.
- Proper mixing has to be done to prevent the accelerator paste from coming into contact with soft tissues. Occasionally patients show allergic reactions with silicone impression materials.
- It has acceptable taste and odour.
- It is available in all 4 consistencies—L, R, H, P.
- It has mixing time approximately—**1 min**, working time **3 min**, setting time **6–10 min.**
- Very low flow after one-hour setting—0.09%
- Very high elastic recovery—99.5%
- Large tear strength—2300–3500 gm/cm
- Flexibility—4–9% (less than polysulphides)
- Hardness is measured by Shore-A-durometer, hardness No. is **43** (regular body)
- *Dimensional stability:* These materials are dimensionally **not very good** due to:
  - Polymerization shrinkage during cross-linking, about 0.6–1%.
  - Condensation reaction and liberation of byproduct, i.e. ethyl alcohol, there will be a measurable weight loss of 0.9%, and shrinkage.
  - Incomplete clastic recovery due to **viscoelastic nature.**
  - **Large thermal contraction** when the material is removed from mouth to room temperature. COTE, i.e. $\alpha = 190$ ppm/°C.
  - These materials are **nonaqueous and hydrophobic** in nature but if placed in a moist environment or water, these can absorb water and can change the dimension.

Advantages

- It has adequate working time and setting times
- Clean, pleasant odour and there is no staining

- Adequate tear strength
- Better elastic recovery properties on removal
- Available in a complete range of viscosities, thus allowing flexibility in choosing an impression material.
- Can be electroplated with silver or copper.

Disadvantages

- Lower flexibility than polysulphides
- Poor dimensional stability due to the release of by-products, ethyl alcohol
- Less accuracy if poured immediately, cast pouring is **delayed by 20–30 min** for maximum elastic recovery.
- Requires a very **dry field**. Since condensation silicones are hydrophobic, air bubbles are likely to occur in the impressions, as the material is readily repelled by water or saliva.
- Poor to adequate shelf life (1–2 years)
- Slightly more expensive
- Putty-wash method is technique sensitive
- The liquid component of the reactor paste material may be hazardous if not handled properly.

Uses

- Used for recording dentulous impressions in preparation of crowns, bridges, inlays, onlays and to some extent for partial dentures.
- Used to record the edentulous impressions in the preparation of complete dentures.

ADDITION POLYSILICONES

Alternate Names
- Polyvinyl siloxane
- Vinyl polysiloxane

Dispensing Methods
- Supplied as two paste systems and available in all four viscosities.
- Also available in a **single consistency called single phase or monophase** material. It can be used both as a tray and a syringe material due to **pseudoplastic property**.

Addition polysilicones set by addition polymerization reaction which are mainly used to record the dentulous impressions in the preparation of crowns, bridges, inlays, and onlays, partial dentures, etc. The composition of addition polysilicones (Table 3.14).

Table 3.14	The composition of addition polysilicones
Base paste: Ingredients	**Functions**
1. Polymethyl hydrogen siloxane or moderately low molecular weight silicone pre-polymer with silane terminal groups	Takes part in the polymerization reaction
2. Reinforcing fillers (powdered silica)	Controls the viscosity of the set material and modifies physical properties.
Reactor paste: Ingredients	**Functions**
1. Polydimethyl vinyl siloxane or moderately low molecular weight silicone prepolymer with a vinyl terminal group	Take part in a chemical reaction and main reactive ingredient
2. Reinforcing fillers (powdered silica)	Paste former increases strength gives body and controls viscosity, modifies physical properties
3. Chloroplatinic acid (H_2PtCl_6)	As a catalyst
4. Low molecular weight liquid polymer (polydimethyl hydrogen siloxane)	As a retarder and provide working and setting times
5. Finely divided platinum or palladium (powder)	To absorb the gas evolved or as a scavenger for the H_2 gas
6. Colour pigment (different for L, R, H, P)	To distinguish it from base paste for evaluating complete mixing and identification

Setting Reaction

Silane terminal siloxane + vinyl terminal siloxane $\xrightarrow{H_2PtCl_6}$ Silicone rubber without by-product

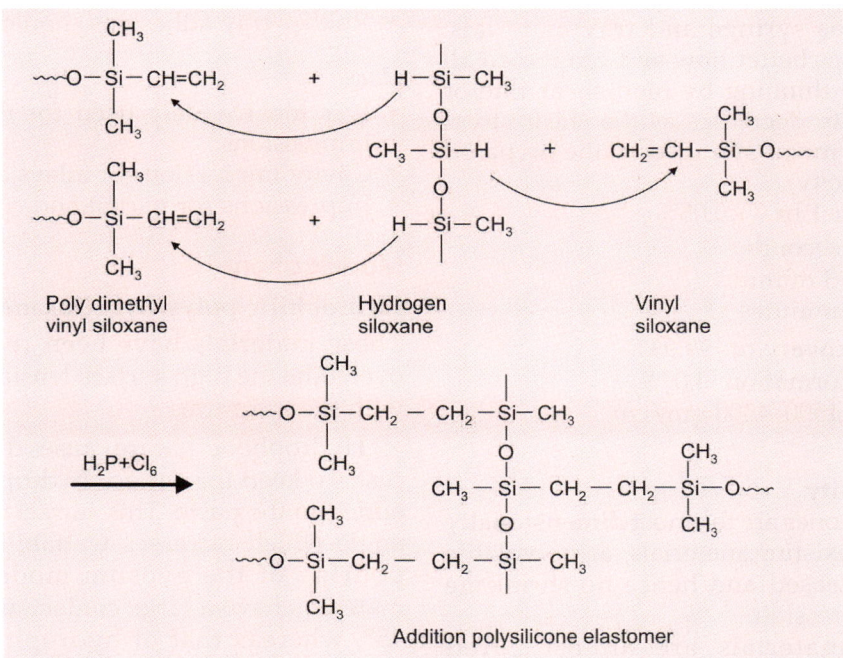

Fig. 3.13: Simplified setting reaction of addition polysilicone, chloroplatinic acid (H_2PtCl_6) as catalyst

On mixing the two pastes, a platinum catalyzed addition reaction occurs causing cross-linking between the two types of siloxane prepolymers to form silicone rubber. The reaction does not have by-products which result in a **minimum dimensional change** during polymerization reaction (Fig. 3.13). There are no by-products as long as the correct proportions of vinyl siloxane and the hydrogen siloxane are maintained and no impurities are present. Side reactions will produce hydrogen gas. The hydrogen gas could also be formed if moisture or residual silane groups are present. It could also be due to the decomposition of the catalyst producing hydrogen gas. The present-day silicones contain a noble metal such as platinum or palladium to act as a **scavenger for the hydrogen gas evolved.** The hydrogen gas evolved can result in **pinhole voids** in the impression which might affect the master cast. The remedy is to pour the impression **one hour after** recording the impression or elimination of impurities if present or subjecting the impression to vacuum before pouring the stone cast (*see* Fig. 3.6).

Properties

- Highly biocompatible with oral tissues and have acceptable taste and odour.
- They are available in all four consistencies and various consistencies serve different purposes, i.e. putty and heavy bodies are used for primary impressions, whereas light and regular body are used for recording secondary impressions.
- **Consistencies** are measured by standard methods (Table 3.15), and depend on the amount of fillers.

Table 3.15	Addition polysilicone—consistencies and viscosities	
Varieties	Consistencies (mm)	Viscosities $\frac{N}{m^2}$. sec
1. Light body (L)	36–55	10–70
2. Regular body (R)	30–40	40–150
3. Heavy body (H)	30–32	200–300
4. Putty body (P)	13–30	400–700

- **Psuedoplasticity:** Addition polysilicones exhibit pseudoplastic properties (monophase material). This can be used both as syringe and tray materials. Syringed material has better flow and can record all finer details due to thinning by high shear rate or shear force. Viscosity decreases as the shear stress increases, when the mix is syringed on the prepared tooth (pseudoplasticity).
- Very low flows after 1 hr – <0.05%
- Mixing time: 35–45 seconds
  Working time: 2–3 minutes
  Setting time: 6–8 minutes
- **Excellent elastic recovery of 99.93%**
- Low permanent deformation: 0.07%,
- High tear strength: 1500–4300 gm/cm
- Low flexibility: 3%
- **Dimensional stability**
  – Addition polysilicones are the **most dimensionally stable** of all the existing materials, as no volatile by-product is released and hence no shrinkage occurs in the impression.
  – Clinically set materials are almost cured completely and there is very low polymerization shrinkage (<0.4%, which is negligible).
  – The only cause for dimensional change is thermal contraction as the material cools from, mouth temperature to room temperature, due to large
    COTE = 190×10^{-6}/°C or 190 ppm/°C
- Hardness: Measured by Shore-A-Durometer for the regular body is 50 which varies from 35 to 75 for the light body and putty consistencies.
- **Compatibility with die-stones:** Difficult to wet the surface of impressions and hence it is very difficult to get water-air bubble free stone cast/die. Hence,

surfactants should be added to the surface of the impression to reduce the surface tension and get bubble free cast/die.

Advantages

- Produce highly accurate impressions
- Pleasant to handle and no disagreeable taste
- Excellent elastic recovery–**99.93%**
- Shorter setting time
- Dimensionally more stable as there is no elimination of byproducts
- Can be electroplated with silver or copper
- Multiple die-pour is possible

Disadvantages

- More expensive with automatic mixing devices
- Shorter working time
- It may release hydrogen gas on setting and produce pinpoint voids in the impression if absorbent is not present in the material.
- Hydrophobic material causes difficulty in obtaining cast/die, without air bubbles.
- Rubber-tray adhesives should be applied.

Uses

- It is most widely used for the crown and bridge impressions
- Cavity impressions of inlays and onlays
- Impressions for partial and complete dentures.

Modifications

Hydrophilic polyvinyl siloxane

These materials have been recently introduced to overcome the high surface tension and incompatibility with the moisture.

Hydrophobic nature causes difficulty in pouring the cast. To keep the surface hydrophilic, the surfactant is added to the paste. This surfactant reduces the contact angle which increases wettability and simplifies the pouring of the gypsum model. The hydrophobic materials have a large contact angle of approximately 95°, whereas that of hydrophilic materials have a smaller contact angle of 30°–35° and have better wetting.

POLYETHERS

This material was introduced in Germany in 1960. The commercial names are **Impregum, Remitec, Polyjel, Permadyne,** etc.

Dispensing

It is dispensed as 3 pastes system, base, reactor and body modifier (thinner). It is available in 3 viscosities, i.e. light, regular and heavy bodies.

Table 3.16	Composition of chemically active polyether impressions pastes
Base paste ingredients	**Functions**
1. Imine terminated polyether of moderately low molecular weight	Undergoes cross-linking to form rubber
2. Colloidal silica	Fillers
3. Glycol ether phthalate	Plasticizer
Reactor paste	
1. Ester derivative of aromatic sulphonic acid	Releases free cations, opens ring and cause cross-linking
2. Colloidal silica	
3. Glycol ether phthalate	Plasticizer filler
Body modifier	
Octyl phthalate (thinner)	It reduces the stiffness/viscosity of the unset
+ 5% methylcellulose	material and gives more working time (retarder)

Setting Reactions

When the base paste is mixed with catalyst paste, **the cation ring-opening addition polymerization** occurs, the ionized form of sulphonic acid provides the initial source of cations and in each stage of the reaction involves the **opening of an aziridine ring** and production of a fresh cation. The reaction is an addition polymerization reaction without the formation of by-products. Since each polyether molecules have 2 imine terminal groups, individual propagation reaction also may produce simple chain lengthening reaction and cross-linking. As the reaction proceeds, the viscosity increases and eventually relatively rigid cross-linked rubber is produced (Fig. 3.14).

Properties

- **Biological properties**

  This material is nontoxic, non-poisonous to the oral tissues but it can be an irritant. It can cause irritation due to the presence of an aromatic sulphonic acid catalyst in the reactor paste. Therefore, the direct contact with skin or soft tissues to the reactor paste should be avoided. Thorough mixing of the reactor with base should be accomplished to prevent any **irritation** to the oral tissues.

  It can also cause **hypersensitivity** in some patients who are allergic to this material (due to the presence of ethylene imine rings in the base paste).

It can also cause contact dermatitis in some patients
- **Consistency**

  Available in 3 consistencies, i.e. L, R, and heavy bodies.
- **Mixing time:** 45 seconds to 1 minute
  - Working time: 2 minutes
  - Setting time: 3–5 minutes
- Flow after 1-hour setting is <0.03%, is **quite low**
- Permanent deformation: 1.1%

Imine terminated polyether

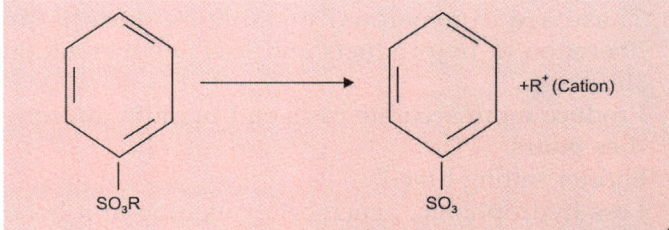

Imine ring or aziridine ring

Structure of the aromatic sulphonic easter acting an initiator by releasing a cation, R^+

Setting Reaction

Base imine terminated polyether + reactor sulphonic acid $\longrightarrow$ polyether rubber

Fig. 3.14: Cross-linking occurs by cationic polymerization via the imine end groups

- Lower elastic recovery: 98.9%
- Lower tear strength: 2700 gm/cm—**least,** compared to other elastomers
- Lower flexibility about **2%** (more stiffer)
- Higher hardness **62** measured by Shore-A-Durometer for a regular body (highest)
- **Dimensional stability:** They have high dimensional stability due to:
  - Addition polymerization reaction without by-products
  - Low polymerization shrinkage, volumetric contraction is only 0.4% (negligible)
  - Weight loss after 24 hours is just 0.2%
  - But larger COTE, $\alpha = 300$ ppm/°C, causes greater thermal contraction and shrinkage
  - Polyether absorbs water and swells under most clinical conditions. But this is not a problem unless the impression is exposed to the water after removal from the mouth. So, **electroplating is not possible** since the electroplating bath consists of water.

Advantages

- Have **pseudoplastic properties**, that is, the same mix can be used as a tray and syringe material. Addition of **thinner to the base and reactor pastes** increases flow properties.
- These are dimensionally stable as there is no liberation of by-products and less polymerization shrinkage.
- Produce more accurate casts and **permits multiple dies pours**.
- Shorter setting time.
- Less hydrophobic, hence better wetting and good casts are obtained.
- Long shelf-life, and no objectional odour distortion on removal from the mouth.
- Lower stiffness
- Cast pouring can be **delayed for a few hours and even for a week.**

Disadvantages

- Expensive when compared with other elastomers
- High stiffness
- Lower tear strength
- Electroplating is not easy
- Not available in complete ranges of viscosities
- The catalyst can be sensitive to the patients.

Uses

For recording impressions:
- In the preparation of crowns and bridges
- In cavity preparations for inlays and onlays
- In fabrication steps of partial and complete dentures.

Light Activated Polyether (Introduced in 1988)

Dispensing

Available in 2 viscosities, light body supplied in disposable syringes and **heavy body,** packed in collapsible tubes.

Composition

- Visible light curing polyether—**urethane dimethacrylate elastomer resin**
- Visible light cure photoinitiators—**camphoroquinone and photoaccelerators—dimethyl aminoethyl methacrylate**.
- Silicon dioxide as fillers. (It has a refractive index close to that of the resin to provide them translucency necessary for depth of cure.)

Properties

Most of the properties are similar to the chemically cured polyethers with the following advantages:
- Excellent elasticity
- Command setting, infinite working time and short setting times.
- Very low volume shrinkage on setting
- The impression can be stored up to two weeks.

Properties of Elastomeric Impression Materials (Table 3.17)

Manipulation of VLC Polyethers

Mixing is not required. Light body material is syringed into cavity preparation. The **special transparent tray** is loaded with heavy body material and placed in the patients mouth. After the tray is seated in the mouth, both materials are **cured simultaneously** using a visible light curing unit. The curing time is approximately 3 minutes. **The light source is a tungsten-halogen bulb with a** filter, $\lambda = 460–480$ nm.

Advantages

- **Command setting,** property, i.e. infinite working time and short setting time
- Excellent mechanical and clinical properties
- No mixing is required, hence no trapping of air or voids and less wastage.

Disadvantage

Requires a special **tray that is transparent** to the visible light, to cure the material.

Manipulation of elastomers

(see color plate 6, Figs 3.9a to f)

The steps to be followed while manipulating the elastomeric impression materials are:
- Selection of materials

Table 3.17 Comparative properties of elastomer impression materials for reference

Materials	Consistencies	Viscosities 45 sec After mixing in cP Water=1 cP	Shore-A hardness numbers	Tear strength gm/cm	Flow %	Strain in compression %	Permanent deformation %	Dimensional change in 24 hours %
Polysulphides	L	60,000	20	2500–7000	0.5–2	14–17	3–4	0.4
Regular	R	110,000	30	3000–7000	0.5–1	11–15	3–5	0.45
Heavy	H	4,50,000	35	-	0.5–1	9–12	3–6	0.44
Putty	P	-	-	-	-	-	-	-
Condensation polysilicones	L	70,000	15–30	2300–2600	0.05–0.1	4–9	1–2	0.6
Very high	P	-	50–65	-	0.02–0.05	2–5	2–3	0.38
Addition polysilicones	L		35	1500–3000	0.01–0.03	3–6	0.05–0.4	0.15
Reg	R	150,000	50	2200–3500	0.01–0.03	2–5	0.05–0.3	0.17
Heavy	H		60	2500–4300	0.01–0.03	2–3	0.1–0.3	0.15
Putty	P		50–75	-	0.01–0.1	1–2	0.2–0.5	0.14
Polyethers	L		35–40	1800	0.03	3	1.5	0.23
Thinner + Reg	R+T		30–50	2500	0.04	6	2	0.23
Reg	R	130,000	35–60	2800–4800	0.02	2–3	1–2	0.24
High	H		40–50	3000	0.02	3	2	0.19

- Preparation of custom/special trays
- Proportioning and mixing
- Impression techniques
- Application of wetting agents (surface tension reducing agents) on the impression (as it is hydrophobic)
- Pouring of stone dies.

1. **Selection of materials**
   The selection of the rubber impression material should be based on the clinical use of the material and the properties required.

2. **Preparation of custom/special trays**
   A special tray with spacer has to be prepared with acrylic resins by using the primary/preliminary cast of the patients mouth. For putty elastomers perforated stock trays or disposable trays can be used.

3. **Adhesion to the tray** (*see* Colour Plate 6, Fig. 3.9a)
   Elastomers are not adhesive to the trays. Adhesion can be obtained by application of adhesives to the trays. For **polysulphides, butyl rubber** or **styrene dissolved in chloroform or ketone** can be used.
   For polysilicones—**polydimethylsiloxane and ethyl silicate** can be used to create a physical bond with the impression trays.

4. **Proportioning and mixing**
   - **Two pastes system:** Equal lengths of 2 pastes are squeezed on a glass slab or a paper pad provided by the manufacturer. The reactor paste is collected on a stainless steel spatula and distributed over the base paste and mixed in a **sweeping** motion. The mixing is continued until the mixed paste is of **uniform colour. The** mixing should be finished within 45 secs. If mixture is not uniform, curing will not be homogeneous and distorted impression will result.
   - **Base paste and reactor liquid system:** Certain length of the base paste is dispensed on to a mixing pad, and the liquid is placed inside the rope of the paste with a stated number **of drops per unit length of paste.** Paste and liquid are mixed using the stainless steel spatula until uniform colour is obtained.
   - **Two pastes putty system:** The putty is so stiff that it must be dispensed with a scoop and may be mixed with the heavy spatula or kneaded in the hands until a mix free from streaks or uniform colour, is formed.
   - **Base putty + reactor liquid:** Base putty is dispensed with a scoop, depressions are made on the surface of the putty base, and the appropriate number of drops of liquid are added. A stiff spatula

is used to mix the putty base and reactor liquid. Once the reactor is well incorporated, mixing may be continued by hands for 30 secs, until a uniform coloured mix free from streaks is obtained.
Initially mixing by hands is avoided since a high concentration of reactor liquid in contact with the skin may cause allergic reactions.

Automatic mixing using automixer (*see* Colour Plate 5, Fig. 3.7d)

It is used for light and medium viscosity materials specially for addition polysilicones and polyether. There is greater uniformity in proportioning and mixing. Mixing time is reduced, and possibilities for contamination of materials is much less. Few air bubbles may get incorporated.

Impression Techniques

Following important impression techniques are used to obtain the best clinical performances.

1. **Multiple mix technique: (Double mix single impression technique or syringe-tray method)** (Fig. 3.15).
   Tray used is a special tray and consistencies used are **a heavy body as a tray material and light body as a syringe material**. This technique can be used with polysulphides, polysilicones, polyethers. This method is referred to as multiple mix techniques because two separate mixes are made on two separate mixing pads and spatula (*see* Colour Plate 5, Figs 3.7c and 3.8).

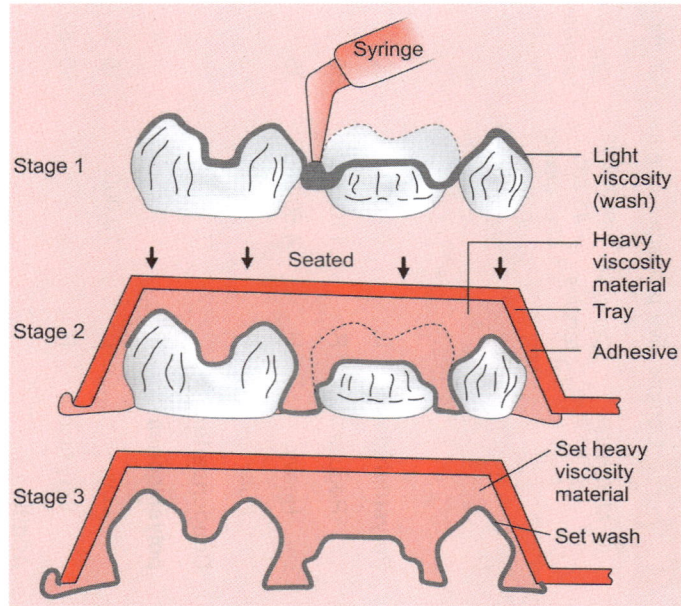

Fig. 3.15: Single stage–double mix–single impression technique for heavy and light body elastomers

Steps

- The light body material is first mixed and injected into the impression area.
- Meanwhile, the heavy body material is mixed and loaded on the tray and seated over the light body material.
- The light and heavy body materials **set together** to give a single impression in which light body material recording all the finer details and supported by the heavy body material.
- When both the materials set together, the impression is removed with a steady force to minimize permanent deformation and to maximize tear strength.
- The impression is cleaned with running tap water, disinfected, the excess water is shaken off, and a gentle stream of air is blown to remove the residual moisture.
- Cast/die is prepared by pouring type IV die stone material or type V die stones.

Advantages

- Less impression material is needed than for the stock trays.
- Trays are used for a single patient, so sterilization is not needed.
- Uniform thickness of impression material minimizes distortion resulting from thermal and curing shrinkages.
- Produce dimensionally accurate and stable impression.

Disadvantages

- Construction of special trays is time-consuming
- The monomer may be sensitive to some patients. These techniques are mainly used for tooth cavity impression for inlays, onlays, crowns, bridges, etc.

2. **Reline technique: Double mix double impression technique,** or **putty wash technique**
   - Tray used is an adhesive treated perforated stock tray
   - Consistencies required are:
     a. Putty material for the primary impression
     b. Light body for secondary impression or corrective wash impression.

   This technique is widely used with condensation and addition polysilicones. It is a two-stage method in which the primary impression is taken with putty material and the secondary impression is recorded with light body materials (Fig. 3.16).

Steps

Primary impression

Putty material is placed in a perforated stock tray and the impression is taken before (cavity preparation or

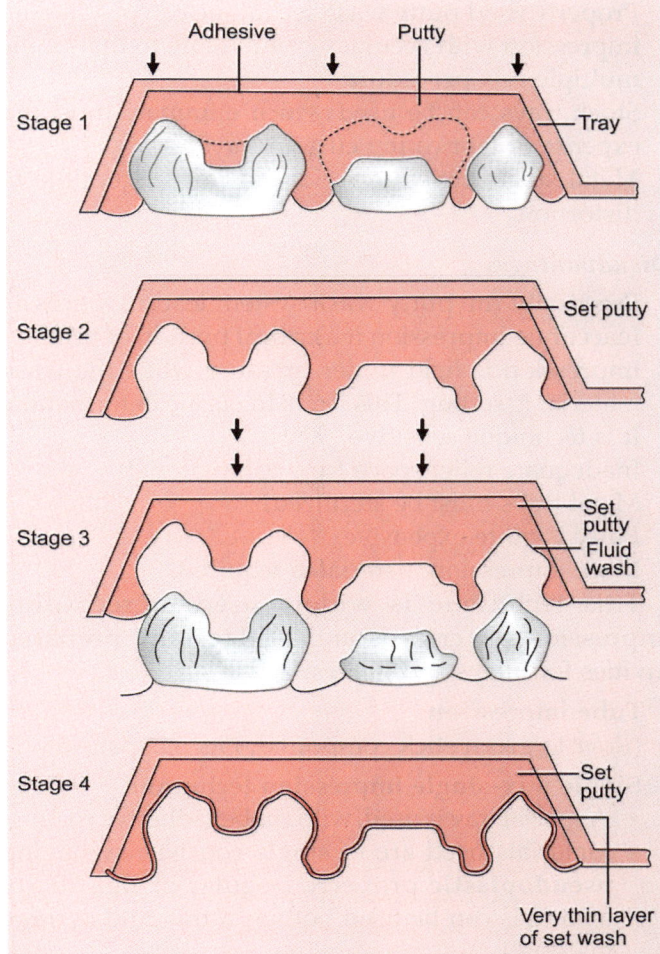

Fig. 3.16: Two-stage impression reline technique for putty and light body elastomers (preferred for condensation polysilicones)

crown cutting). **Space for the wash material** is provided by either cutting away some of the putty material from the original impression or by using a **spacer** between the putty and the teeth when recording the primary impression. When the putty material has set, the impression is removed and washed.

Secondary/corrective wash impression

After the cavity preparation, the light body material is mixed and injected into the cavity preparation. The tray is reinserted (to act as a custom tray for the light body with primary impression) and held gently until the wash material sets. The impression is removed with a steady force, washed, disinfected, dried and die is poured.

Advantages

- Rapid curing of putty elastomer, that is, the primary impression need be held in the mouth only for few minutes.

- Properly used putty wash technique can produce an impression with accuracy comparable to that of the multiple mix procedure.
- Stock trays can be used which eliminate time and expense of fabricating custom trays.
- Metal stock trays are rigid and not susceptible to distortion.

Disadvantages

- Practically the putty wash system lead to a grossly inaccurate impression if a critical portion of primary impression is held under pressure while the wash material is setting. This leads to elastic deformation. It is technique sensitive.
- Inadequate relief space for wash material.
- Metal trays must be sterilized.
- Putty is quite expensive.
- More impression material is required.

This technique is widely used in recording impression for crowns and bridges and prepared cavities for inlays and onlays.

3. **Tube impression**

   (*Refer* to green stick compound, Fig. 3.2, page 55)

4. **Single mix–single impression technique**
   - A special tray is used, with rubber adhesive coating.
   - Materials used are of single consistency having **pseudoplastic** property (regular or light body materials can be used both as a tray and **syringe** material).
   - This technique is used with addition polysilicones and polyethers as they have pesudoplastic properties **(monophase materials).**

   As these materials are subjected to low shear stress during spatulation to maintain its high viscosity. They can also be used as a syringe material because at the higher shear rates the viscosity decreases, as much as ten folds. **A pseudoplastic mix becomes thinner when stressed more. One part of the mix is loaded on a tray, and another part is taken in a syringe.** The syringe mix is injected on the prepared teeth, and these are held in contact until both set together. This thinner mix has a better flow and records all the finer details, whereas the thicker tray mix gives the support for the syringe materials (*see* Colour Plate 5, Fig. 3.7c).

Common Causes for Failures of Elastomeric Impression Materials

1. **The rough or uneven surface**
   - Incomplete polymerization due to premature removal, and improper mixing

- Too high accelerator/base paste ratio
- Too rapid polymerization, by high temperature or humidity.

2. **Bubbles**
   - Rapid polymerization preventing flow
   - Incorporation of air during mixing
   - Inadequate flow.

3. **Irregular voids**
   - Presence of moisture, water or debris on the tooth.

4. **Distortion**
   - Poor adhesion to the tray and detachment of impression.
   - Special tray, gets distorted if the resin has not completely polymerized
   - Delay in the seating of tray causes the mix to start polymerizing before seating.
   - Too thick and non-uniform impression material.
   - Too much pressure applied continuously even after setting commence.
   - Movement of the tray during polymerization.
   - Premature and improper removal of the tray from the mouth.
   - Delay in pouring the cast for polysulphide or condensation polysilicones.
   - Too early pouring the cast (before 20–30 min after taking impressions) in case of additional polysilicones and polyethers.

5. **Rough and chalky surface**
   - Inadequate cleaning of impression
   - Excess water or wetting agent left over the impression
   - Too high W/P ratio and improper mixing of the dental stone mix.
   - Premature removal of the stone cast.

Measurements of Properties of Elastomers

1. **Consistency**

   It is measured by the diameter of the disc formed when **0.5 ml** of the mixed material is placed under a fixed load, of **575 gm wt. for 15 minutes** after mixing. The larger the **diameter of the disc** formed, the more fluid is the material. The consistency is controlled by the molecular weight of the polymer and amount of fillers. **Consistency values for:**

   Light body: 36–55 mm
   Regular body: 30–40 mm
   Heavy body: 20–32 mm
   Putty body: 13–30 mm

2. **Working and setting times**
   - *Vicat penetrometer method:* The elastomer standard mix is filled in a small container of certain

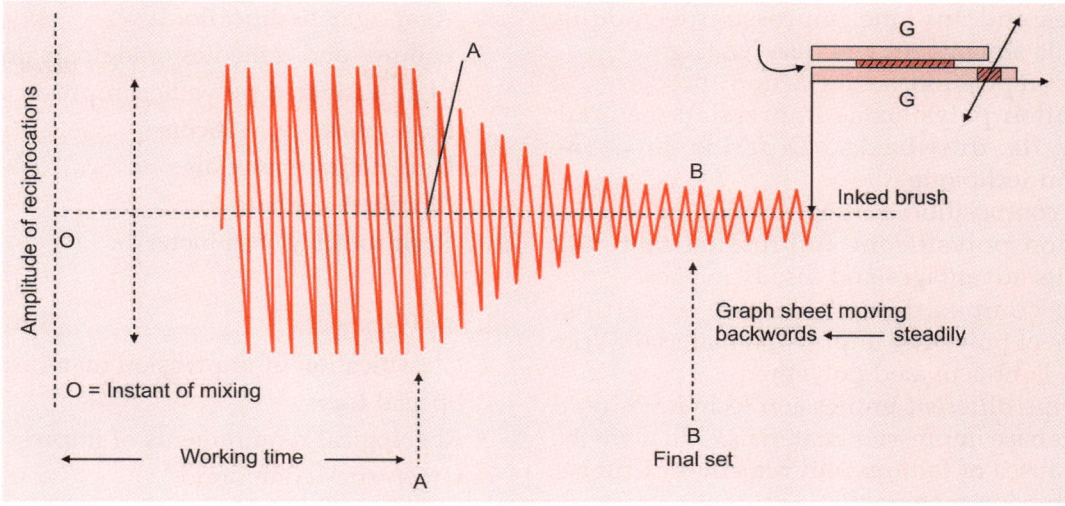

Fig. 3.17: Reciprocating rheometer—trace

depth and the needle (cylinder), loaded with a definite weight, is lowered on it at definite (10 or 20 seconds) time intervals until it can reach the bottom (for detail refer to the setting time measurement in gypsum products). This refers to working time. Procedure is continued until the indenlations of penetrometer completely recovers. This refers to the final setting time.

- *Reciprocating rheometer*
- *The reciprocating rheometer method:* The standard mix is placed between temperature controlled two glass plates G and G. One of the glass plates (say lower one) is vibrated by an electric motor at a constant rate of 10 cycles per second. The amplitudes of vibrations are recorded continuously with the help of an inked brush or stylus on a graph sheet, moved steadily.

As the material begins to set, viscosity begins to increase, and amplitude begins to decrease due to the increase in resistance as shown by point A. This time **OA** refers to the working time (Fig. 3.17).

As the viscosity increases to a maximum value correspondingly, the amplitude decreases to minimum value at the instant B. This time OB, interval refers to the final setting time.

Modified digital and automatic recording system displays this graph on a screen, and such instruments are used for measurements of working times of composite resins, cements, rubbers, etc.

Note: Bite registration elastomers

Addition polysilicones and polyethers are used for bite registration for checking the occlusal relationships in the fabrication procedures of dentures (*refer* to bite waxes and ZnOE pastes). Addition polysilicones having similar compositions of light bodies are supplied in automixing cartridges.

This has the advantages of adequate flow, negligible resistance, short, suitable setting time, stiffness, good elastic recovery, and dimensional stabilities. These are the requirements of bite registration materials.

MODEL QUESTIONS

I. Long Essays   (20 minutes each)

1. Explain the term oral impression and purpose. Mention the different impression materials used. Classify them according to their physical properties and methods of setting. Add a note on impression trays.
2. Describe in detail, the ideal requirements of the impression materials and give any three classifications of impression materials.
3. Describe the composition, properties, and manipulation of impression compound. Explain the precautions to be followed.
4. Explain the composition, setting action and properties of zinc oxide eugenol impression pastes. Give their advantages and disadvantages.
5. Give the composition, gelation-mechanism, properties, and manipulation of agar-agar hydrocolloids.
6. Give the composition, setting action, properties of alginate impression material. Add a note on the manipulation technique.
7. Give the causes for failures and remedies of hydrocolloid impressions (agar-agar and alginate)
8. Give the composition and chemistry of setting of polysulphide impression material. Describe its

properties and any one impression technique. Mention its advantages and disadvantages.

9. Give the composition, setting action, properties of condensation polysilicone impression material. Mention its drawbacks. Describe any one impression technique.

10. Give the composition, setting reaction, properties of addition polysilicone impression material. Mention its advantages and disadvantages.

11. Give the composition, chemistry of setting, properties of polyether impression material. Write a note on light-activated polyether.

12. Describe the different impression techniques used for rubber base impression materials. What are the various causes of failures and remedies of rubber base impression materials?

13. Explain the structure of elastomeric impression materials and classify the available impression materials. Add a note on pseudoplastic elastomers.

14. Classify elastomeric impression materials. Define working time and setting times of elastomers and explain how they are measured. Add a note on consistency of elastomers.

II. Short Essays   (10 minutes each)

1. Impression trays
2. Impression compound
3. Composition and properties of zinc oxide-eugenol impression materials

4. Agar-agar hydrocolloid
5. Failures and remedies of alginate impression
6. Light-activated polyether impression material
7. Monophase polysilicones
8. Duplicating materials
9. Modified alginates
10. Reciprocating rheometer

III. Brief Answers   (5 minutes each)

1. Classification of impression materials
2. Special trays
3. Rheological requirements of impression materials
4. Green stick compound
5. Wet field technique
6. Bite registration pastes
7. Surgical pastes
8. Non-eugenol pastes
9. Dimensional changes of elastomer impressions
10. Tray adhesives
11. Syneresis and imbibition
12. Elastic recovery of impression materials
13. Wash impressions
14. Primary impressions
15. Gelation
16. Thermal properties of impression compound.

CHAPTER 4

Gypsum Products: Cast and Die Materials (Auxiliary Materials)

Introduction

Most of the oral appliances like dentures, crowns, bridges, etc. are prepared by skilled technicians outside the mouth, in specially equipped laboratories. The fabrication techniques involve high temperatures and complicated lengthy procedures. For this, an exact positive, hard replica of the oral structure of the patient is obtained by the dentist. These casts or dies are prepared by pouring their thin mix into the accurate impressions of the oral structure and sent to the technicians. The technician prepares the wax patterns and converts into the oral appliances like acrylic dentures, orthodontic appliances or alloy castings by wax elimination methods.

Definitions

The model or cast is a hard exact positive replica of the entire oral structure including soft tissues with accurate reproduction of finer details and spatial dimensions. Die refers only to the positive hard replica of one or few teeth prepared for receiving the appliances. Most common and suitable materials used for these casts and dies are the various gypsum products.

GYPSUM

It is calcium sulphate dihydrate $CaSO_4.2H_2O$ a mineral available in many parts of the world. This is purified by washing, powdering and then heating (or calcination). It loses some water of hydration and is converted into the calcium sulphate hemihydrate, i.e. $CaSO_4.\frac{1}{2} H_2O$. This is again reacted with water and used, perhaps first time at Paris, and hence known as plaster of Paris.

GYPSUM PRODUCTS

Different manufacturing methods of calcination, produced different types of gypsum products, like type I (impression plaster), type II (model plaster), type III (hard model or cast, dental stone), type IV (die stone) and type V (high strength–high expansion die stones). These varieties are used in dentistry frequently.

Calcination

On heating the gypsum powder, the following changes take place at different temperatures (Key Box 4.1).

Key Box 4.1

$$CaSO_4.2H_2O \xrightarrow{110°C-130°C} CaSO_4.\frac{1}{2}H_2O \xrightarrow{130°C-200°C} CaSO_4 \xrightarrow{200°C-1000°C} CaSO_4$$

Dihydrate orthorhombic Hemihydrate (monoclinic) Hexagonal anhydrite Orthorhombic anhydrite

Manufacturing Methods

1. **Dry-calcination** method is used to manufacture types I and II, β-calcium sulphate hemihydrates:
    Gypsum ore is purified by washing, drying and powdering. This is heated in a pan or kettle, open to atmosphere for some time to a temperature of about 110°–130°C to convert most of the gypsum into its hemihydrate. **This β-calcium sulphate hemihydrate has monoclinic lattice, spongy, irregular large crystal particles.** The remaining some amounts of uncalcined gypsum, as well as the calcium sulphate anhydrides formed by overheating, are impurities. However, they help to accelerate the setting reaction by acting as nuclei (embryo) of crystallization. This β-hemihydrate is slightly modified to obtain suitable properties, by some additions, for use as impression materials, and model plaster.

TYPE I: RIGID IMPRESSION PLASTER

Compositions of Powder

- Dry calcined, β-hemihydrate $CaSO_4.\frac{1}{2}H_2O$
- Impurities present (uncalcined dihydrate, + small amounts of anhydrides)—accelerator
- Chemical accelerators (K_2SO_4,......) decrease setting time, and also setting expansions
- Chemical retarders (borax,.......) increase setting time but decrease setting expansions.
- Balancing agents = 4% K_2SO_4 + 0.4% borax—decrease setting expansion only
- Sometimes sugar or potato starch is added to get *soluble-plaster* for dissolving and separation of cast from impression.
- Colouring material (alizarin S).

TYPE II: DENTAL (MODEL) PLASTER COMMONLY KNOWN AS PLASTER OF PARIS

Composition of Powder

- Dry calcined β-calcium sulphate hemihydrate
- Uncalcined gypsum + anhydrites or increase setting times and decrease setting expansions
- *Chemical accelerators and chemical retarders* to increase working time, to decrease setting times and both decrease setting expansions.
    (This is supplied in plastic lined large container—bags, to protect from moisture.)

2. **Wet calcination:** α-calcium sulphate hemihydrates—*type III—hydrocal, dental stone, or class I stone*
    Purified gypsum is heated under steam pressure to about 110°–130°C in a **closed kettle, rotary-kiln or autoclave**. The calcium sulphate hemihydrate formed has **prismatic, monoclinic, regular small crystals.** This is called as dental stone, hydrocal or autoclaved calcium sulphate hemihydrate.

COMPOSITION OF TYPE III: DENTAL STONE, CLASS I STONE

- Wet calcined α-calcium sulphate hemihydrate
- Uuncalcined gypsum + anhydrites
- *Chemical accelerators and chemical retarders in combination increases working time and decreases setting times as required and also both decrease setting expansions.*
- Balancing chemicals (4% K_2SO_4 + 0.4% borax)—decrease setting expansions to a minimum.
- Colours (green, yellow, pink, etc.)—to identify margins of casts.

TYPE IV: DIE STONE, IMPROVED STONE, CLASS II STONE, DENSITE

This α-hemihydrate is prepared by boiling gypsum in 30% calcium chloride or 0.5% sodium succinate solution, washing in boiling water, drying and powdering. This has a fine *monoclinic prismatic crystal structure*. This is then added with small amounts of uncalcined gypsum impurities (if required), chemical accelerators, retarders, balancing chemicals, and colour (as in type III stone) (*see* Colour Plate 7, Fig. 4.1).

TYPE V: HIGH STRENGTH, HIGH EXPANSION: DIE STONE

This α-hemihydrate manufactured like type IV stone is added with (1) small amounts of surfactants like lignin sulphonate (to wet, with mixing water thereby lower W/P and increase strength), and (2) minimum amounts of chemical accelerators and retarders, and not balanced, i.e. not to decrease setting expansion, (3) colour.

Note I: Gypsum products (α or β) can also be prepared synthetically, i.e. obtained as a by-product in phosphoric acid manufacturing industries. These are more expensive, but have consistent slightly better properties (Fig. 4.1).

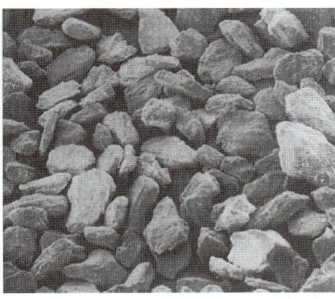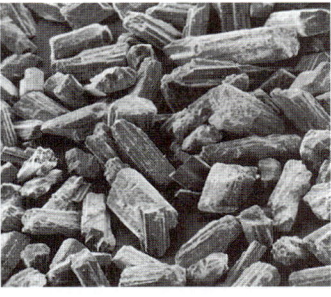

Fig. 4.1: Forms of hemihydrate. (a) β-hemihydrate (plaster of Paris)—spongy, porous, irregular, (b) α-hemihydrate (dental stone)—well-formed crystals, regular, denser

CLASSIFICATION OF GYPSUM PRODUCTS

Classifications are done to select the most suitable materials, according to

1. Manufacturing Method

- Dry calcination: Types I and II
- Wet calcination: Types III, IV, and V
- Dehydration by boiling with chemicals: Types IV and V (sometimes)
- Synthetic: By-product in phosphoric acid industries

2. Crystal Structure

- Spongy irregular particles monoclinic = Type I, II—β hemihydrates
- Prismatic regular particles monoclinic = Type III, IV, V—α-hemihydrates

3. Applications

Type I: Impression plaster (rigid, non-elastic)
Type II: Model plaster for edentulous casts, articulation, the base for the stone cast.
Type III: Model stone for dentulous casts, for denture-flasking and binder in alloy casting (GBI) investments.
Type IV: Die stone—hard dies, master casts
Type V: High strength, high expansion die stone—for enlarged dies (gypsum-bonded investments and divestments).

4. Balanced

Types I, III, IV—minimum setting expansions, divestments
Unbalanced: Types II, V—large setting expansions.

Setting Action

When gypsum products are mixed with water, they react and again form calcium sulphate dihydrate, according to as:

$2CaSO_4 \frac{1}{2} H_2O + 3H_2O \rightarrow 2\ CaSO_4.2H_2O + heat$ (3,900 cal/gm mol).

Water–powder (W/P) ratio: It is the amount of water added (in ml) to 100 gm of powder. Calculations show that the minimum W/P required is 18.61%.

Different W/P ratios are required for chemical reaction for different types and are an important factor in controlling the properties (*refer* to Tables 4.1a to c).

A decrease of W/P : Increases strength
Increases setting expansion
Decreases setting time

Approximate W/P for:

Type I : 55–75%
Type II : 45–55%
Type III : 28–35%
Type IV : 22–24%
Type V : 19–20%

Theoretical minimum value = 18.61%

Crystalline (dissolution-precipitation) theory of setting: When the $CaSO_4.\frac{1}{2} H_2O$ is added to water it dissolves partly (solubility is about 0.8% at room temperature) and reacts to form $CaSO_4.2H_2O$ whose solubility is only about one fourth, i.e. 0.2%. The solution becomes **supersaturated with the dihydrate**, which precipitates on the already present $CaSO_4.2H_2O$–impurities as nuclei (or embryo) and crystallize. Further, continuous precipitation causes crystal growth as star-like spherulite structures. The spherulites begin to intermesh, increasing the viscosity of the mix. This thick mix is in the mouldable state. After some time, it becomes friable, soft solid, and then the excess of water is suddenly drawn inside by capillary action, with the loss of gloss and gradually becomes hard (Fig. 4.2). Strength (or rigidity) increases with time.

Gloss disappearance time is the time elapsed from the instant of the addition of powder until the surface-gloss just disappears.

The set mass is porous due to the trapping of excess water (added to facilitate mixing) and form voids between the spherulites or individual (monoclinic) crystals of about 5–20 microns in length.

Setting Time

It can be defined as the time interval from the instant of addition of powder to water (or mixing) until the set material attains **certain rigidity or strength**.

Methods of measuring setting times

1. **Gloss-disappearance method:** This may be sometimes close to the initial setting time, slightly more or less, as measured using a smaller Gilmore needle.

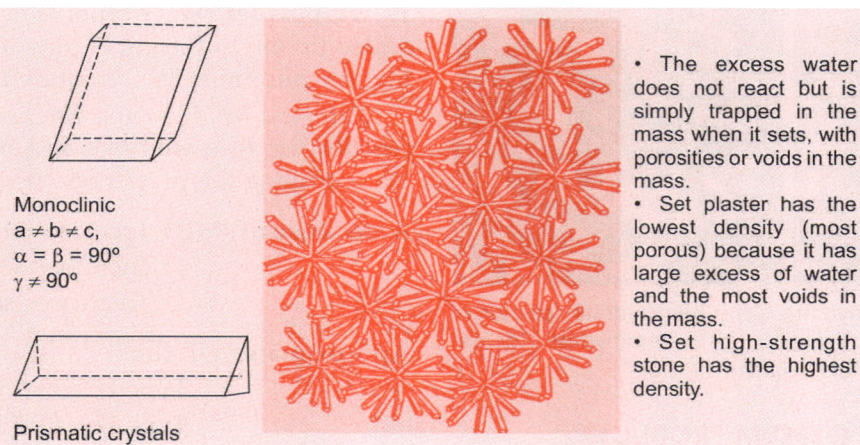

Monoclinic
a ≠ b ≠ c,
α = β = 90°
γ ≠ 90°

Prismatic crystals

- The excess water does not react but is simply trapped in the mass when it sets, with porosities or voids in the mass.
- Set plaster has the lowest density (most porous) because it has large excess of water and the most voids in the mass.
- Set high-strength stone has the highest density.

Fig. 4.2: Setting action of gypsum products

2. **Indentation, Gilmore needles method**
   - **Initial setting time:** It is the time interval from the instant of, the addition of powder to water (or mixing) until the smaller Gilmore needle of weight **1/4 lb** and tip diameter **1/12"** just fails to produce indentation.
   - **Final setting time:** It is the time interval from the instant of the addition of powder to water (or mixing), until the bigger Gilmore needle of weight **one pound** and tip diameter **1/24"** just fails to produce indentation (Fig. 4.3).

   Procedure: A weighed amount of powder is **sifted** to a measured volume of water in a clean plastic bowl, starting a stopwatch. It is thoroughly mixed for 45 or 60 seconds **with constant speed** and spread on a glazed tile. The smaller Gilmore needle is vertically placed, at every half-minute interval, until

it fails to indent. Then the bigger Gilmore needle is used similarly. These can be repeated for different W/P ratios, accelerators, retarders, mixing times, etc.

3. **Vicat penetrometer method**
   According to this, setting time is the interval from the instant of the addition of powder to water (or mixing), until the Vicat needle of **300 gm** weight and **1 mm** diameter, fails to penetrate a depth of 5 cm thick plaster mix (Fig. 4.4).

   The mix prepared as above is carefully filled in a container of 5 cm height. The Vicat needle is lowered on it, at every half-minute interval, until the needle **fails to reach the bottom** (floor) of the vessel, or penetrate 5 cm thickness. Values are close to initial

Weight 1/4 lb

Weight 1 lb

1"/12

1"/24

Fig. 4.3: Gilmore needles

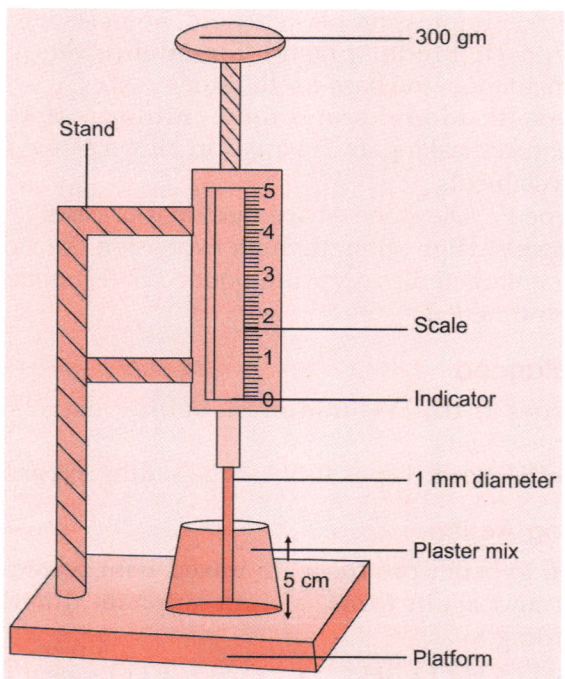

300 gm

Stand

Scale

Indicator

1 mm diameter

Plaster mix

5 cm

Platform

Fig. 4.4: Vicat penetrometer

setting times found by smaller Gilmore needle. This is a standard method prescribed by ADA specifications. Accordingly, setting times for type I = 4 ± 1 min and for all other types are 12 ± 4 minutes.

4. **Ready for use time**

   It is the **subjective judgment** of the experienced technician, depending upon the use of the cast or the die. This may be about 30 minutes or more when the cast attains about 80% of its wet (1 hour) strength. The relative mixing, working and setting time intervals for a certain W/P ratio are graphically represented (Fig. 4.5).

   Setting times should be suitable for the particular manipulative situations. Hence, the technician must be able to modify the working and setting times, which have already been adjusted by the manufacturer.

Controlling the Setting Time of Gypsum Products

1. Setting times are controlled by the manufacturer by varying the compositions. Setting times are decreased by increasing:
   - The solubilities of hemihydrate or the difference in solubilities, (i.e. to get higher supersaturation), with finer particles or certain chemicals, K_2SO_4, NaCl <2.0%, accelerators, etc.
   - The number of nuclei of crystallization/unit volume, by adding impurities like uncalcined dihydrate or calcium sulphate anhydrite (hexagonal $CaSO_4$).
   - The rate of crystallization, with the addition of chemical accelerators.

2. Setting times can be controlled by the technician, by changing:

   - Number of nuclei of crystallization per unit volume
   - Rate of crystal growth

Factors Affecting the Setting and Working Times

- **Water/powder ratio:** Smaller the W/P ratio, shorter is the setting time as more number of nuclei of crystallization are formed per unit volume.
- **Mixing time or speed:** Longer time of mixing or faster mixing, fractures the growing spherulites, producing more nuclei of crystallization, which decrease setting time.
- **Impurities added:** Uncalcined gypsum or gypsum powder—'terra alba' slurry, to increase the number of nuclei of crystallization and decrease setting time. Hexagonal anhydrite decreases working time and orthogonal anhydrite increases the working times.
- **Chemical accelerators:** Some chemicals like NaCl <2.1%, Na_2SO_4 <3.4%, K_2SO_4 at all concentrations, act as accelerators of crystallization. These increase the solubility of the hemihydrate and increase supersaturation, due to which setting is faster.
- **Chemical retarders:** Some other chemicals like **borates**, **citrates**, **acetates**, NaCl >2.0%, Na_2SO_4 >3.4%, etc. prevent the growth of spherulites by their complexes enveloping the spherulites **(poisoning of the nucleus)** and increase working and setting times. Careful addition of **accelerators and retarders gives suitable large working and short setting times.**
- **Finer particles** of the hemihydrate powder dissolve more quickly, help the reaction to take place faster, and also increase the number of nuclei of crystallization. Due to these, setting times decrease.
- **Temperature of water:** At higher temperatures the solubility of hemihydrate decreases faster than

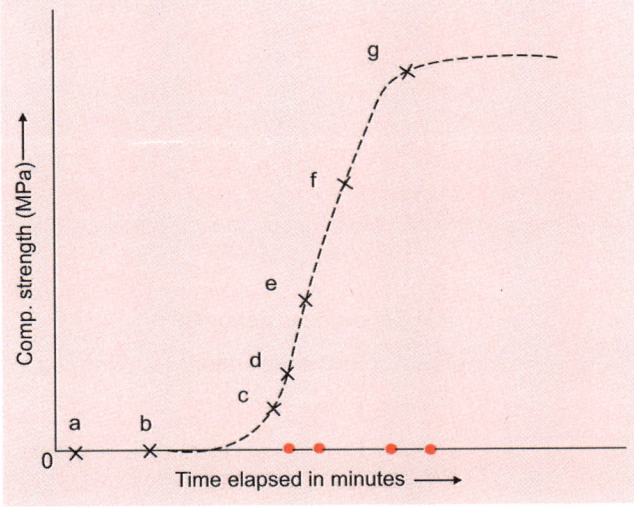

a = Mixing time
b = Working time
c = Setting time (GDT)
d = Initial setting time (GN)
e = Setting time (Vicat's)
f = Final setting time (GN)
g = Ready for use (20–30 min)

Fig. 4.5: Stages of setting (hardening) of gypsum products

dihydrate, i.e. supersaturation decreases which increase setting time. However, at the same time, setting reaction becomes faster at higher temperatures, which may nullify the previous. In addition, at temperatures above 80°C the reverse, i.e. calcination also takes place. Due to all these factors the setting time

- Increases very slightly from 0 to 50°C
- Increases rapidly from 50° to 80°C
- Does not set at all above 80°C

- **Old stock:** The $CaSO_4 \frac{1}{2} H_2O$ is hygroscopic and may absorb moisture causing less soluble dihydrate envelope on the hemihydrate particles. Hence, the setting time is **longer for** older and moisture exposed gypsum products. (Therefore purchase only small amounts at a time and store in dry condition.)

Accelerators and Retarders

Manufacturer, as well as the technicians, control the working and setting times, as required for the particular situations. The setting time can either be decreased or increased.

The best method for the technician to control these without seriously affecting the mechanical properties is by using chemicals.

1. **Accelerators:** K_2SO_4 at all concentrations, NaCl <2.0%, Na_2SO_4 <3.4% increase the solubility of hemihydrate or supersaturation, decreasing the working and setting times. K_2SO_4 also forms **syngenite $K_2(CaSO_4)_2H_2O$**, which very rapidly crystallize, i.e. increases the rate of crystallization. Uncalcined gypsum or anhydrite, increase the number of nuclei of crystallization and decrease setting time.

2. **Retarders:** Borax in small quantities is a very effective retarder. Borates, citrates, acetates, sodium chloride more than 2.0% prevent the rate of crystal growth by their salts, **enveloping** the growing spherulites **poisoning of nucleation**. Similarly, sulphates of Al, Fe, Cr, etc. and tartrates, retard the crystal growth. **Hydrocolloids, saliva, coagulated blood, etc. retard,** specially the setting of the surface of the casts, producing a soft chalky surface.

Applications

- To get longer working time and shorter setting times as required by technicians, **accelerators and retarders are added together**. The effect is represented graphically (Fig. 4.6).
- **Balanced gypsum products:** Both accelerators and retarders decrease the setting expansions. Hence, to get a minimum setting expansion, without changing the working and setting times, K_2SO_4 and borax can be added in the ratio 10:1 (e.g. 4% K_2SO_4 + 0.4 borax). These are added to the powder or better to mixing water which then becomes the **anti-expansion solution**.
- Both accelerators and retarders interfere with the growth and intermeshing of spherulites and decrease the strength slightly. Hence, to get maximum strength and setting expansion, less impurities or chemicals are to be added, as in type V die stone.
- Set gypsum impurity particles are sticking to plaster bowl/spatula, decrease the setting times. Addition of powdered gypsum can decrease setting time.

NORMAL AND HYGROSCOPIC SETTING EXPANSIONS

Minimum dimensional changes during setting of gypsum products are required for impression, cast and die materials, whereas, large setting expansion is

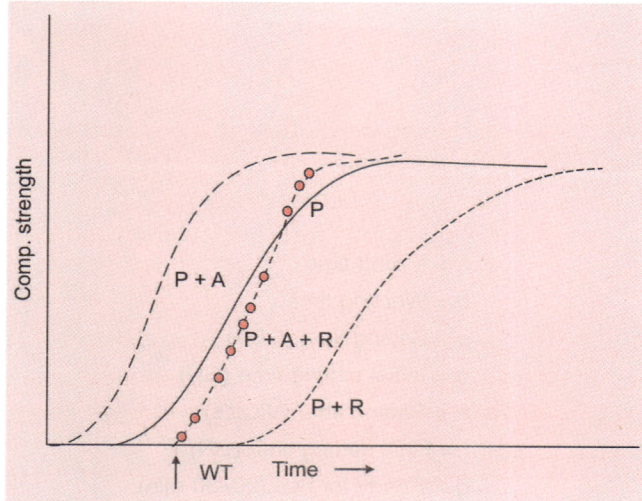

P = Supplied plaster or GP

P + A = Plus accelerator

P + R = Plus retarder

P + A + R = Plus accelerator + retarders (W.T.h , S.T. i)

Fig. 4.6: Variation of working and setting times with respect to accelerators and retarders

needed for investment and divestment materials for compensating casting shrinkages.

Calculation of initial volumes and final volumes during the setting reaction shows **volume shrinkage of about 7.11%**. Voids created by the escape of trapped excess water and the **pushing force** exerted by the outgrowing spherulites cause a **porous mass**. Hence, experimental measurements show a **resultant expansion**. However, the adhesion of setting gypsum products, to the supporting solid surface (like a glass slab/tile) prevents the actual expansion to a certain extent. The actual or unrestricted setting expansion can be measured by **floating** the mix on a large **pool of mercury** and measuring the distance between two marks on a line drawn on the surface of the mix, at various intervals.

As the powder is wetted, dissolved and set, first volume contraction takes place until the initial setting. But the technician can easily compensate by adding extra mix. Hence, this initial shrinkage has no much significance. The large expansion taking place after initial setting, and slight shrinkage taking place after a final set due to loss of excess water are of importance for the technician. These dimensional changes are represented in Fig. 4.7.

Normal Setting Expansion (NSE)

This is mainly due to the outgrowing spherulites pushing each other and hence should depend upon the spherulites concentrations.

Factors increasing normal setting expansion (NSE) are
- Lower W/P as the number of spherulites/unit volume is more.

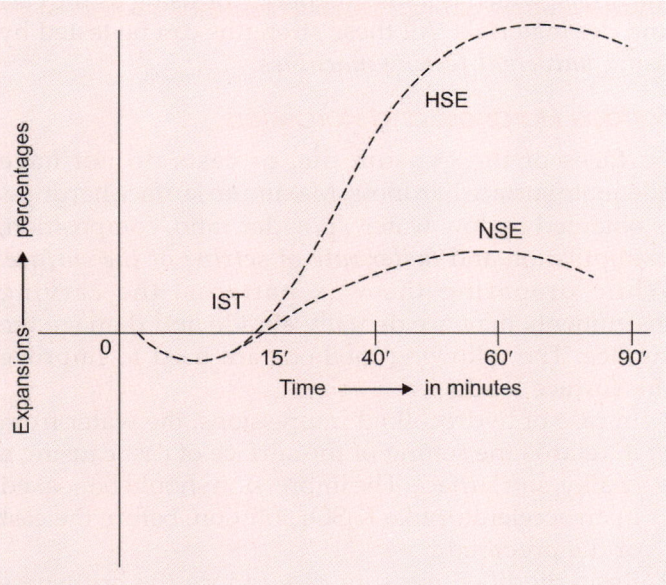

Fig. 4.7: NSE and HSE

- Longer time of mixing as more nuclei of crystallization are formed by fractured spherulites.

Factors decreasing normal setting expansion (NSE) are
- Higher W/P
- Shorter mixing time
- Chemical accelerators make the material to attain rigid structure more quickly so that spherulites cannot exert outward thrust. Hence, **accelerators decrease** the normal setting expansion.
- Chemical retarders envelope and prevent the outgrowing spherulites to expand and decrease NSE.

Hence, any chemical impurities, **accelerators or retarders decrease the normal setting expansion**.

Note: Balanced gypsum products

Accelerators decrease setting time and retarders increase setting time, but both **decrease setting expansion**. By adding $K_2SO_4 = 4\%$ and borax = 0.4% approximately in the ratio 10:1 it is possible to **minimise setting expansions without changing setting times**. Such gypsum products are said to be **balanced**. Type I, type III and type IV are balanced. If water containing these chemicals are used for mixing, it is called **anti-expansion solution**. As per ADA No. 25, the **maximum NSE for Types I, II, III, IV, and V are 0.15%, 0.3%, 0.2%, 0.1% and 0.1–0.3% respectively** (*refer* to Table 4.2).

Hygroscopic Setting Expansion (HSE)

After the initial setting, the actual setting expansion takes place due to the outward thrust. During setting, expansion is opposed by other crystals. If the cast or die, is immersed in water or added with more extra water, **after initial setting**, it sets with expansion more than double of NSE. This is because, more water enters into the voids of the setting mass by capillarity, i.e. into the growing spherulites which help the spherulites to exert more outward thrust. This is known as **hygroscopic setting expansion** (Fig. 4.8).

The HSE can be increased by
1. decreasing W/P ratio
2. mixing for a longer time
3. minimising chemical impurities
4. immersing in water **after initial set, for a longer time**
5. adding **more extra water** after the initial set.

In the **casting procedure, large setting expansion for gypsum or phosphate bonded investments is required to compensate large casting shrinkages**. The controlled water adding technique, immersing the invested casting ring in water for some time or supplying extra water by wetted ring-liners, etc. methods are used to get the desired setting expansions.

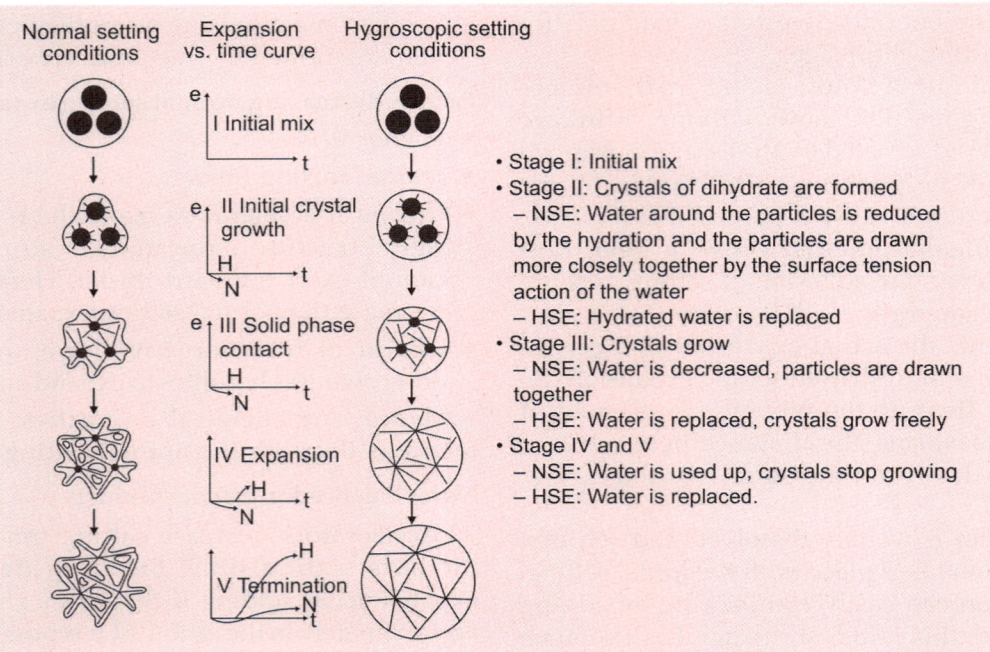

Fig. 4.8: Comparison of normal and hygroscopic setting mechanisms and expansions

Strength of Gypsum Products

The strength is the ability to resist fracture or the maximum stress, a material can withstand, before fracture. For brittle gypsum products, compressive strengths are usually considered. The strength is due to the **interlocking** of the growing spherulites, which increases with time as well as the number of spherulites per unit volume.

Wet (1 hour) strength: It is the compressive strength, at the end of one hour when the cast is in wet condition, i.e. all the mixing water is still present. Since the cast is used within this time, the gypsum products should have minimum one hour strength as per ADA specification No. 25 (*refer* to Table 4.2).

Dry strength corresponds to the compressive strength after drying completely in 24 or 48 hours. Strength increases later slightly more, **gradually as the reactions tend to complete**.

Factors increasing the strength are
- Lower W/P: Accordingly Types I to V, have W/P ratio is in the decreasing order and strength is in increasing order.
- Optimum mixing time: Prolonged mixing, interferes the interlocking effect and decreases strength.
- Smaller particles: Dissolve faster, form more nuclei and better interlocking.
- Minimum chemical impurities: The accelerators and retarders slightly decrease strength as they interfere the growth of spherulites
- Fresh stock has higher strength.

For the normal applications of gypsum products, the ADA No. 25 has prescribed the minimum compressive one-hour, wet strengths as, 4.0, 9.0, 27.5, 34.5 and 48.3 MPa for Types I, II, III, IV, and V respectively. Dry strengths are about 10–20, 20–30, 40–60, 60–80, 90–100 MPa for the above.

The **tensile strengths** are very low only **about $1/_{10}$th** of the compressive strengths and are slightly affected from the above factors. Similarly, they have very **low shear strengths and flexure strengths**. These show that the gypsum products are very **brittle** materials, which is a disadvantage for using as the cast and die materials. All these strengths can be tested by using *universal testing machines.*

Surface Hardness and Hardeners

Surfaces of the gypsum die, or casts do not have adequate surface hardness. Maximum surface hardness is obtained by low water /powder ratio, composition, manipulation and *faster rate of setting of the surface.* While preparing the wax patterns, the carving instruments may accidentally abrade and damage the surface. The following methods are used to **improve the surface** hardness:

1. In case of hydrocolloid impressions, the water from it, retards the setting of the surface of cast causing a chalky, soft surface. The impression should be soaked in an accelerator like K_2SO_4 solution, before the cast or die prepared.
2. Resin-modified gypsum dies reduce the brittleness of the surface.

3. Surface coatings can seal the surface porosities, improving the surface integrity and resistance to damage. For example, immersing in **certain acrylic solutions,** this can be done.

These surface hardener solutions may contain acrylics with acetates, citrates, polyesters, nitrocellulose, alcohol, etc. Sometimes oxides of metals, like bismuth, titanium, iron, barium, or silica may be present, in small quantities.

These surface coatings make the carving instruments easily glide over the surface and prevent damage while carving.

Care of Gypsum and Gypsum Products, Models and Dies

As all these are hygroscopic, they absorb moisture forming an envelope of calcium sulphate dihydrate on the hemihydrate particles. Due to the lower solubility of this dihydrate envelope, the dissolution and hence setting time becomes longer for old-stock. The strength also decreases.

Hence, the following precautions are to be used

1. Gypsum products are stored in a dry condition, in sealed closed plastic lined bags or containers.
2. Only required amount should be taken out at a time.
3. Large stock should not be purchased at a time.

Care of dies and models

1. During the laboratory procedure, sometimes the cast is to be wetted by immersing in water. The water quickly gets absorbed. Dihydrate gets dissolved from the surface causing inaccuracy. In such case, the cast can be immersed in water, saturated with gypsum (by adding a small amount of gypsum to water earlier). This is slurry water.
2. The cast should not be stored, at high temperatures above 70°C, (to prevent the calcinations), and also in moisture contact.
3. Suitable precautions are followed for infection controls (by treating the impressions with suitable sterilizers).

Short notes: 1–5 Model answers for 4–5 marks, to be answered in 8–10 min

Short Note 1

Impression plaster

Type I: β-CaSO$_4$ hemihydrate (classified as non-elastic, irreversible, mucostatic impression material, powder–water system).

This is calcium sulphate: β-hemihydrate obtained by modifying the model plaster, or POP (Type II), by adding small amounts of:

- Uncalcined gypsum and calcium sulphate anhydrite to decrease the setting time to 4 ± 1 min (ADA 25).

- Accelerators and retarders: To control working and setting times.
- Balancing chemicals (4% K$_2$SO$_4$ + 0.4% borax): To reduce the setting expansion to a minimum, i.e. 0–0.15% (ADA 25).
- Potato starch or sugar to form **soluble plaster** for dissolving and separation of the cast from an impression.
- Colouring pigments (alizarin S) to identify margins.

Properties

- Setting action: When mixed with water (W/P = 55–75%) it forms the calcium sulphate dihydrate, a rigid mass.
- Setting time is made short, 4 ± 1 minutes to minimise distortion of an impression.
- Setting expansion is minimized (<0.15%) to get good dimensional accuracy.
- Fine particles help to get an exact reproduction of finer details.
- Low strength: 4–5 MPa helps to separate impression from the cast by fracturing.

Impression techniques

- For edentulous cases without severe undercuts: Similar to other non-elastic impression materials, but apply **separating medium** before pouring cast.
- For partially dentulous cases with one or few teeth, or edentulous case with severe undercuts: After the impression sets, carefully **fracture** it by **hammering**, (to remove the impression), join the broken pieces, apply separating medium, pour the stone cast. After setting, immerse in boiling water to **dissolve** the impression.
- Also used as a **wash** or **secondary impression**.

Advantages

- Mucostatic impression
- Accurate reproduction of finer details
- Negligible dimensional changes.

Disadvantages

- Non-elastic—cannot be used for dentulous cases
- Bad taste—disliked by patients
- Messy work

Due to the availability of elastomeric and hydrocolloid impression materials, which can be used more **conveniently,** this impression plaster has become almost outdated.

Short Note 2

Model–dental plaster

Type II: β-CaSO$_4$ hemihydrate
(Briefly describe manufacturing method, composition, and setting actions to enrich the answer).

Properties

- Large W/P = 40%–55%,
- Setting time is adjusted to about, 12+ 4 min ADA 25.
- Large setting expansion <0.3% but has no much significance.
- Low compressive strengths >9 MPa (in 1 hour) and 20–30 MPa on drying is adequate for use.
- Low surface hardness and abrasive resistance.

Uses

Due to the low cost and adequate mechanical properties, it is used in dental laboratories for

- Large sized models and casts of edentulous cases
- Mounting plaster in articulations
- Edentulous cast bases
- Sometimes orthodontic study models (special white varieties)
- Flasking of wax patterns in complete denture fabrication with the stone cast.

Advantages: Adequate strength for large, models, flasking materials, etc. Easy to recover denture after curing.

Disadvantages: Cannot be used for dentulous casts, hard models.

Short Note 3

Dental stone, autoclaved—α-CaSO$_4$ hemihydrate, hydrocal
Type III: Class I
(Briefly describe manufacturing method, composition and setting action, to enrich the answer).

Properties

- Low W/P = 28%–35%
- Setting time: 12 $\pm$ 4 min (ADA)
- Setting expansion is reduced to <0.2%
- Compressive wet strength >20.7 MPa
- Dry strength: 40–60 MPa.
- Tensile, shear and flexure strengths are low and hence it is a brittle material
- Surface hardness is 60 RHN.

Uses

Due to larger strength and better dimensional stability it is used for:

- Hard casts or models of dentulous cases required for preparation of wax patterns for complete and removable acrylic partial dentures.
- Flasking materials for the wax patterns, specially for partial dentures.
- Binder for gypsum-bonded investment used for casting and soldering procedures.

- Bases for stone dies
- Orthodontic study models.

Short Note 4

Type IV: Die stone—densite improved class II stone (α-CaSo$_4$.½ H$_2$O)
Briefly describe the manufacturing method, composition and setting action.

Advantages

Simple technique of die preparation, adequate strength, less expensive and very suitable for laboratory procedures.

Disadvantages

Low surface hardness, brittle inadequate strength for die preparation, hygroscopic material.

Properties

- Low W/P = 22–28%
- Lowest setting expansion <0.1%
- Higher compressive strength, wet strength >34.5 MPa, and dry strength 60–80 MPa
- Surface hardness is about 80 RHN. To resist the abrasion by sharp carving instruments used to carve wax patterns, it requires higher surface hardness. This surface hardness increases faster than the increase of compressive strength due to the earlier drying of the surface, which is an advantage. Surface hardness can be improved further by immersing the die in surface hardener solutions (containing K$_2$SO$_4$, borax or cellulose-resins).
- Can be electroformed by copper or silver to resist surface abrasions.
- Die—dimensions can be increased by special paints, resin-nail paints, or resin coatings. This is required for availing **cement space** or to compensate larger casting shrinkages in base metal casting procedures.

Uses

Dimensionally stable, hard, common die material, compatible with all impression materials.

Short Note 5

Type V: High strength–high expansion die stones (α-CaSo$_4$·½ H$_2$O)
Briefly describe the manufacturing method: Composition and setting action.

Properties

- To obtain high strength, W/P is to be reduced to very low value = 19–20%.
  This is done by using surfactants or wetting agents like **lignin sulphonate**. Wet strength >48 MPa, and

dry compressive strength is about 80–100 MPa. Surface hardness is about 90 RHN.

- Large setting expansion: Chemical accelerators and retarders are minimized, and W/P ratio is also reduced.

Setting expansion is about 0.1% to 0.3%.

This can contribute for large compensation of casting shrinkages taking place in the casting of base-metal alloys.

Uses

- Enlarged hard dies
- Gypsum-bonded investment and divestments
- Dies for divestment casting techniques

Special Gypsum Products

- **Synthetic gypsum products**—α or β varieties can be obtained as by-products in **phosphoric acid manufacturing process**. These are more expensive but have slightly better properties. Properties do not depend on the nature of the ore (*see* colour plate 7, Fig. 4.2).
- **Extra white**, smooth dental stones: These are used for special orthodontic study models. Treating the models with soap solutions, a glossy smooth surface can be obtained.
- **Articulating-mounting plaster requires fast setting properties**. In addition, these plaster and stone have low setting expansions, low strength for easier trimming and separating the cast.
- **Resin-modified plaster or die stones** are prepared for reducing the brittleness and improving surface abrasion resistance.
- **Silicone–stone** combinations can reproduce the surface details more accurately.
- **Many varieties** with controlled amounts of consistencies, working times, setting times and short ready for use times, etc. are available to suit the different applications.

Manipulation of Gypsum Products

1. **Selection of suitable material and instruments.**
2. **Proportioning:** As far as possible minimum amounts of W/P ratios are to be used, by weighing the powder and measuring the volumes of water to get the best results. Plaster and stone dispensers are used by experienced technicians. The properties such as setting time, strength, setting expansion are technique-sensitive. Hence, difficult to get a reproducible mix.
3. **Mixing**
- **Hand mixing:** Clean parabolic flexible rubber bowl and stiff steel spatula are used. **Powder is sifted** (to minimize air trapping) into the water in the bowl. The spatula is moved around at constant speed for a definite time, 40–60 sec., until a **creamy mix** of **homogeneous consistency** is obtained. It is **vibrated** on an electrical-vibrator for few seconds (*see* Colour Plate 8, Fig. 4.5).
- **Mechanical-hand mixing:** A rotatable mixing pad (spatula) fitted to the plastic lid of the bowl, is used for mixing. The mixing time can be slightly less (*see* Colour Plate 8, Figs 4.3a and b).
- **Mechanical-Electrical mixing:** This method is specially useful for mixing investment materials. The mixing bowl is a cylindrical vessel. The mixing pad is rotated by connecting the shaft, to an **electric motor**. The vessel also can be **evacuated** through a side-tube to reduce the air bubbles accumulated on the wax pattern. The speed and the time of rotation can be adjusted by a rheostat and the **timers** to get a **reproducible mix** (Fig. 4.9) (*see* Colour Plate 8, Fig. 4.4 and Colour Plate 29, Fig. 15.4).

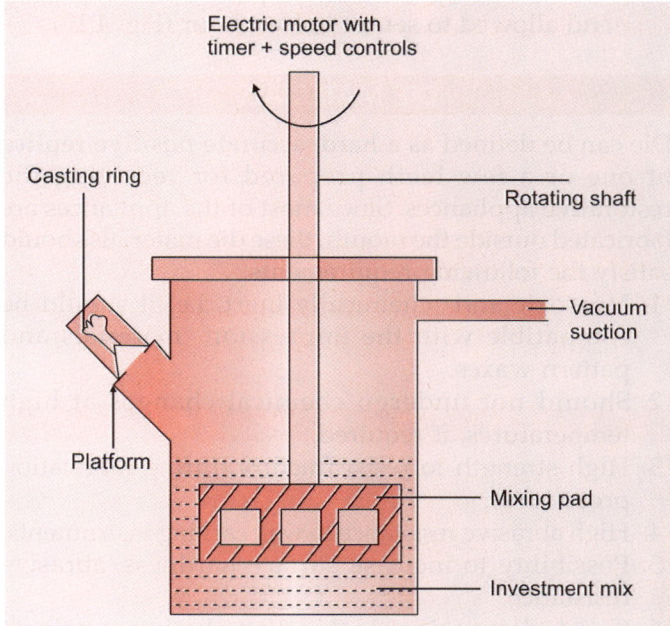

Fig. 4.9: Equipment for vacuum mixing and investing (*see* Colour Plate 8, Fig. 4.4)

4. **Preparing cast:** A small amount of mix is teased through the sides of the impression and vibrated to flow on the floor of the impression for wetting and to sweep all the trapped air bubbles. Remaining mix is then poured with vibration, and allowed to set.
5. **Preparing a base**
   - A plaster mix is then made and placed on a glazed tile. Over this, the initially set, cast is inverted, and excess is removed from the sides, shaped and allowed to harden.

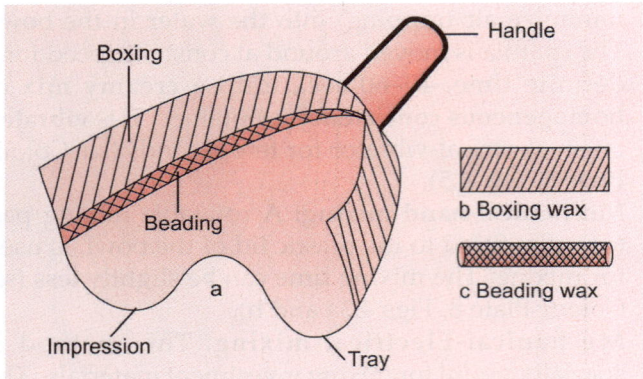

Fig. 4.10: a. Boxing of Impression, b. Boxing wax, c. Beading wax

- **Boxing method:** The impression can be contoured first by **beading wax rod** and then **boxing wax sheet** of about 3.0 cm width. The plaster or die stone mix is poured; first small quantity to cover the teeth portion of impression, vibrated, and then the remaining mix or fresh plaster mix is poured and allowed to set for half an hour (Fig. 4.10).

DIE MATERIALS

Die can be defined as a **hard, accurate positive replica** of one or a few teeth prepared for receiving the restorative appliances. Since most of the appliances are fabricated outside the mouth, these die materials should satisfy the following requirements:

1. Nontoxic and chemically inert, i.e. it should be compatible with the impression materials and pattern waxes.
2. Should not undergo chemical changes at high temperatures, if required.
3. High strength to resist fracture during fabrication procedures.
4. High abrasive resistance to wax carving instruments.
5. Possibility to increase surface hardness/abrasive resistance.
6. Good dimensional stability during setting/ hardening.
7. The possibility of **changing die dimensions** as required.
8. Accurate reproduction of the finer details of the impressions, without compressing or distorting the impression.
9. Good flow, and low viscosity, before setting.
10. The ability for electroforming with silver or copper.
11. Suitable working and setting times.
12. Ability to withstand high temperatures without changing dimensions, if required to be heated.
13. A suitable colour for contrast.
14. Simple techniques with minimum inexpensive equipment.
15. Inexpensive.
16. Long storage life.

Methods to change (increase) die dimensions

Small amounts of setting expansions of die materials may compensate the thermal and other shrinkages of impressions. The following methods are used to change the die dimensions:

- Manipulative variables for gypsum products.
- Coating the surface with certain paints (nail paints, resin paints dissolved in organic solvents, etc.).
- Coating with a thin layer of polymerizing resins. For example, die can first be wetted with self-cured monomer, then dipped in the polymer powder and repeated
- Electroforming with silver or copper
- Special resin paints of different colours (silver/gold) are used for coating alternately, to produce adequate space for cementation. Enlargement of dies are needed to compensate casting shrinkages and to provide **cementing spaces.**

Die Materials used

1. **Type IV stone, improved Class II stone, densite**
   The powder is mixed with water and poured into impression. The $CaSO_4.\frac{1}{2} H_2O$ is converted into hard $(CaSO_4.2H_2O)$ die.

Properties
- Low water/powder ratio
- Very small setting expansion <0.1%
- Adequate strength, wet strength >34.5 MPa and dry strength 60–80 MPa
- Surface hardness = 82 RHN

Advantages
- A very simple method for die fabrication
- Compatible with all impression materials
- Adequate mechanical properties
- Can be electroformed

Disadvantage
Brittle material can get abraded, by wax carving instruments accidentally.

2. **Type V: High strength–high expansion die stones**
Powder mixed with water and poured into the impression to get enlarged dies.

Properties
- High setting expansion 0.1–0.3%
- Large wet compressive strength >47 MPa, and dry strength 80–100 MPa and surface hardness 90 RHN
  This is more suitable for preparing hard enlarged dies in divestment technique and also for GBI investment

material as required to compensate for larger casting shrinkages in casting procedure of base metal alloys.

3. Epoxy resin dies

These are basically polyethers with **aziridine/oxirane** terminal groups

$$-\overset{|}{C}-\overset{|}{C}-$$
$$\underset{O}{\diagdown\diagup}$$

Epoxy polymers are prepared by reacting epichlorohydrin with Bisphenol-A or hydroxyl groups (glycols, glycerols, resorcinols), glycidyl methacrylates.

$$2\ Cl-CH_2-\overset{\overset{\displaystyle H}{|}}{C}-\overset{\overset{\displaystyle H}{|}}{\underset{\underset{\displaystyle O}{\diagdown\diagup}}{C}}-H + HO-\bigcirc-\overset{\overset{\displaystyle CH_3}{|}}{\underset{\underset{\displaystyle CH_3}{|}}{C}}-\bigcirc-OH \rightarrow$$

These are highly viscous liquids (sometimes solids). On further polymerizing with amines, polysulphides or polyamides, hard epoxy resin die can be obtained. Supplied as paste and liquid amine activator. Recently a fast setting material is supplied as paste and liquid in cartridges for use in automixer devices. This can be injected through a delivery tip into the impression or centrifuged.

Advantages

- High resistance to chemical attacks
- Very tough and hard
- Good structural adhesion.

Disadvantages

Toxic (carcinogenic) material and should not have skin contact. Mould-release material is to be used for polysilicone impressions.

This can be used to prepare dies from only rubber base impressions.

4. Self curing acrylic resins are dispensed as self cure-polymer powder + monomer liquid

Advantage

Less brittle, easy to prepare dies.

Disadvantage

Low compressive strength, abrasive resistance and large polymerization shrinkages.

5. Zinc-silicophosphate cement (synthetic porcelain): powder–liquid (phosphoric acid).

The large compressive strength of about 170 MPa and good surface hardness, but undergoes shrinkage during setting.

6. Ceramics

Have large hardness, high abrasion resistance, able to withstand high temperatures and are useful in fabricating porcelain articles. Difficult to get accurate dimensions, due to firing shrinkage.

7. Silver amalgam

Has high strength, and negligible dimensional change. Since large condensation force is required, it can be condensed only on nonelastic-rigid impressions, but cannot be used for hydrocolloid or elastomeric impressions.

8. Metal-sprayed dies:
Low fusing—bismuth-tin alloy, of a melting point around 140ºC, can be melted and injected on certain impressions to form a metal layer which is then poured with die stone. This method cannot be used for thermoplastic impressions.

ELECTROFORMED DIES

To improve the abrasive resistance of the die surface, one method is to form a thin film of a metal, like copper or silver. This is done by electroplating the **impression** with copper or silver, then pouring die stone.

Tube impression is quite suitable for a single tooth. **Metalizing agents like graphite, copper powder or silver dust**—suspension is coated over the impression for electrical conduction. This is made cathode and anode is a copper plate, for copper plating (Fig. 4.11).

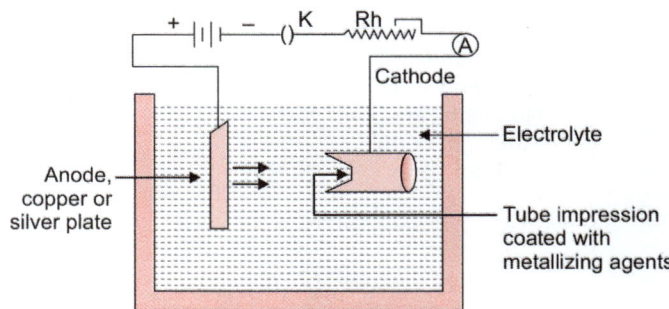

Fig. 4.11: Electrolytic bath for electroforming dies

The electrolyte is a solution of copper sulphate, sulphuric acid and phenol sulfonic acid (to improve the throwing power) in water. A small direct current of **15–50 mA** is passed for **8–10 hours**, to get fairly thick electroplating. It is washed, poured with die stone. The small setting expansion of die stone, cause firm mechanical bond with the copper film. Copper plating can be done for impression compound, but not on hydrocolloids and polysulphides.

For silver forming, the metalizing agent, such as silver dust suspension is first applied. The anode is silver plate, and the electrolyte is a solution of silver cyanide, potassium cyanide and potassium carbonate, i.e. **AgCN, KCN, K₂CO₃** in water. A small direct current of **5–10 mA** is passed for 12–15 hours and the die is poured.

As KCN and its vapours are **dangerously toxic,** the instruments are placed in a closed chamber and operated by **remote control**. Silver forming is prescribed to elastomers. Impression compound (as alkaline electrolyte softens it), and hydrocolloids cannot be electroplated.

These electroformed dies have not become popular and not commonly used.

Gypsum Products: Practical Exercises

Aim: To study the effects of variations of water/powder ratios, mixing times, chemical accelerators and retarders on the gloss disappearance and setting times of gypsum products by indentation method using Gilmore needles. **Procedure:** Weigh 50 gm of any gypsum products, types 2, 3, 4, and find their gloss disappearance and setting times for different variables, tabulate the observations and give inferences.

Table 4.1a Variation of setting times with respect to W/P ratio (mixing time: 60 sec)

Volume of water used W ml	$\frac{Water}{Powder}$ = (W/P) 100	At the instant of addition powder a	Gloss disappe-arance b	Small Gilmore needle c	Big Gilmore needle d	GD time e	Initial ST f	Final ST g	Inference
20	40%								
25	50%								Setting
30	60%	9–10'	9–16'	9–18'	9–24'	6'	8'	14'	times
35	70%								increase
40	80%								

Table 4.1b Variation of setting times with respect to accelerators (NaCl) and retarder (borax), W/P ratio: 30/50, i.e. 60% and mixing time = 60 seconds

Chemical (W/P = 60%)	%	a	b	c	d	e	f	g	Inference
+0.25 gm NaCl	0.5%								Setting time
+0.5 gm NaCl	1.0%								decreases
No chemical	0%								with more acc.
+0.25 gm borax	0.5%								Setting time increases
+0.5 gm borax	1.0%								with more retarders

Table 4.1c Variation of setting times with respect to mixing time, W/P ratio constant (60%) and mixing times: 40, 60, 80, 100 seconds

	Spatulation	a	b	c	d	e	f	g	
W/P = 30/50	40 sec.								Setting time decreases for longer spatulation time
	60 sec.								
	80 sec.								
	100 sec.								

Table 4.2　Resume of gypsum products

Properties	Types				
	I	II	III	IV	V
Common names	Impn. plaster, non-elastic, mucostatic	Dental plaster, POP	Dental stone–plaster, hydrocal, class I, autoclaved hemihydrate	Die stone, improved class II stone, densite	High strength, high expn. die stone
Manufacturing method	Dry calcination of gypsum $CaSO_4 . 2H_2O$	Dry calcination of gypsum $CaSO_4 . 2H_2O$	Wet calcination in steam press, closed vessel/autoclave	Boiling gypsum in 30% $CaCl_2$, 0.5% Na.Succ.soln. Wash at (100°C), dry	Boiling gypsum in 30% $CaCl_2$, 0.5% Na.Succ. Wash at (100°C) dry, powder
Composition	β-$CaSO_4 . \frac{1}{2} H_2O$ + uncalcined gypsum, Acc (K_2SO_4) retard-borax-balancing sugar/starch, colour	β-HH + uncalcined gypsum, K_2SO_4, ... borax, ...	α-HH + uncalcined gypsum, K_2SO_4..... borax..... balancing (4% K_2SO_4 + 0.4% borax), colour	α-HH + uncalcined gypsum, K_2SO_4...., borax, ..., balancing (4% K_2SO_4 + 0.4% borax), colour	α-HH + uncalcined gypsum and its anhydrite, α-HH unclaimed in purities. surfactant (lignin sulphonate) Min. K_2SO_4 + borax, colour
Setting reaction	$(CaSO_4)_2 . H_2O + 3H_2O \longrightarrow 2CaSO_4 . 2H_2O$ + Heat 3900 Cals/gm mol				
(Vicat-ST/min) ADA 25	4 ± 1	12 ± 4	12 ± 4	12 ± 4	12 ± 4
MAX. N.S.E. EXPN	0.15%	0.3%	0.2%	0.1%	0.1–0.3%
Water/Powder %	50–75	45–50	28–35	22–28	19–20, (Min. 18.6%)
Wet-strength, MPa	2–6	>8.5	>27.5	>34.5	>48
Approx. dry, CS MPa	10–20	30–50	60–80	70–90	70–100
Crystals, monoclinic	Spongy irreg.	Spongy irreg.	Prismatic reg. crystal	Fine prismatic reg. crystal	Fine prism. reg. crystal
Applications	Impression—edentulous arches (nonelastic mucostatic)	Edentulous casts, models, flasking, articulation	Hard edentulous casts flasking—wax denture binders for investments	Hard dies of tooth/teeth (wax pattern in casting procedures)	Enlarged dies, divestment

MODEL QUESTIONS

I. Long Essays   (20 minutes each)

1. What is gypsum? Describe the methods of manufacturing and uses of various gypsum products used in dentistry.
2. Define the term "water/powder" ratio and explain the setting action, methods of determining the setting times and factors affecting setting times of gypsum products.
3. Describe the method of measuring the setting expansion of gypsum products. Explain the terms normal and hygroscopic setting expansions and the methods of controlling them.
4. Define the terms cast and die. Give the ideal requirements of die materials. Describe the various die materials available for dentistry, their advantages and disadvantages.

II. Short Essays   (10 minutes each)

1. Strength of gypsum products
2. Impression plaster
3. Dental stone
4. Die stones
5. Electroformed dies
6. Manipulation methods of gypsum products
7. Accelerators and retarders
8. Normal and hygroscopic setting expansions
9. Compare dental stone and dental plaster or die stones

III. Brief Answers   (5 minutes each)

1. Balanced gypsum products
2. Type V die stone
3. Metalizing agents
4. Gilmore needles or Vicat penetrometer
5. Epoxy resin dies
6. Surface hardeners
7. Die enlargement
8. Spherulites

MCQs

1. Chemical formula for GP
   a) $CaSO_4$
   b) $CaSO_4 . \frac{1}{2} H_2O$
   c) $CaSO_4 . H_2O$
   d) $CaSO_4 . 2H_2O$
2. Dental stone is manufactured by
   a) Fritting
   b) Sintering
   c) Dry calcination
   d) Autoclaving
3. Lattice structure of calcium sulphate hemihydrate is
   a) Simple cubic
   b) Hexagonal
   c) Orthorhombic
   d) Monoclinic
4. Approximate W/P for dental stone is
   a) 18.6%   b) 27%   c) 35%   d) 60%
5. Gilmore needles are used to measure
   a) Setting times
   b) Setting expansion
   c) Strength
   d) Surface hardness
6. Vicat needle measures setting time by
   a) Indentation
   b) Penetration
   c) Gloss-disappearance
   d) Compression
7. Setting time of dental stone (ADA 25) in minutes
   a) 4 ± 1 b) 8 ± 2 c) 12 ± 4 d) 16 ± 6
8. The suitable best accelerator for GP is
   a) K_2SO_4 b) NaCl >6% c) Borax d) Hydrocolloids
9. Setting time of GP decreased is by
   a) Hot water
   b) Cold water
   c) More water
   d) Mixing for longer time
10. To increase working time and decrease setting time of GP, add
    a) Accelerator
    b) Retarders
    c) Accelerator + retarder
    d) More water
11. Maximum setting expansion of die stone is
    a) 0.1%   b) 0.15%   c) 0.2%   d) 0.3%
12. Normal setting expansion is decreased by
    a) Accelerator
    b) Retarder
    c) More water
    d) All of the above
13. Minimum wet strength of dental stone in MPa is
    a) 9   b) 20.7   c) 34.5   d) 48.3
14. Main consideration for selection of die material is
    a) Biocompatibility
    b) Cost
    c) Thermal expansion
    d) Strength and hardness

Answers

1-b, 2-d, 3-d, 4-c, 5-a, 6-b, 7-c, 8-a, 9-d, 10-c, 11-a, 12-d, 13-b, 14-d.

Dental Polymer—Resins

POLYMERIZATION: STRUCTURE, PROPERTIES

In this plastic age, synthetic resins having varied properties have become part and parcel of our life and dentistry is not an exception. Except for few resins of natural origin like rubbers, silk, cotton, etc. most of the others are synthetic. These polymers with large molecular size, is built up from many (poly) small parts (mers) or chemical repeating units. Most of these polymers are named, according to these polymers, e.g. polyethylene, polyvinyl chloride, polystyrene, polyacrylates, etc.

MONOMERS

These are simple chemical compounds or repeating units—reacting to form a polymer, e.g. ethylene, acrylic acid, itaconic acid, methyl methacrylates, etc.

OLIGOMERS

These are chemical compounds having two reactive groups or combinations of two units, e.g. ethylene glycol dimethacrylate, bisphenol glycidyl methacrylate, unsaturated low molecular weight polymers, etc. which usually act as cross-linking agents.

POLYMERS

Chemical compounds of huge organic or inorganic molecules formed by a large number of repeating smaller chemical structural units (mers), e.g. polyethylene, polyvinylchloride, polymethyl methacrylates, etc.

POLYMERIZATION

It is the repetitive process of chemical reactions between the small chemical structural units (mers), growing into giant molecules with long chained structures, having thousands and millions of mers.

CLASSIFICATION OF POLYMERS USED IN DENTISTRY

A large number of these polymer resins, used in dentistry can be broadly classified according to:

1. **Chemical repeating units (mers)** (Fig. 5.1)
   Polyvinylchloride, polyacrylic acids, polyacrylates, polyurethanes, polysulphides, polysilicones, polyethers, etc.

2. **Types of polymerizations**
   - Step-growth (or condensation) polymerization: Polysulphides, condensation polysilicones, etc.
   - Addition (or free radical) polymerization: Addition polysilicones, polymethyl methacrylates.

3. **Activating energies (or curing methods)**
   - Thermal (heat)
   - Chemical
   - Ultraviolet rays
   - Visible light

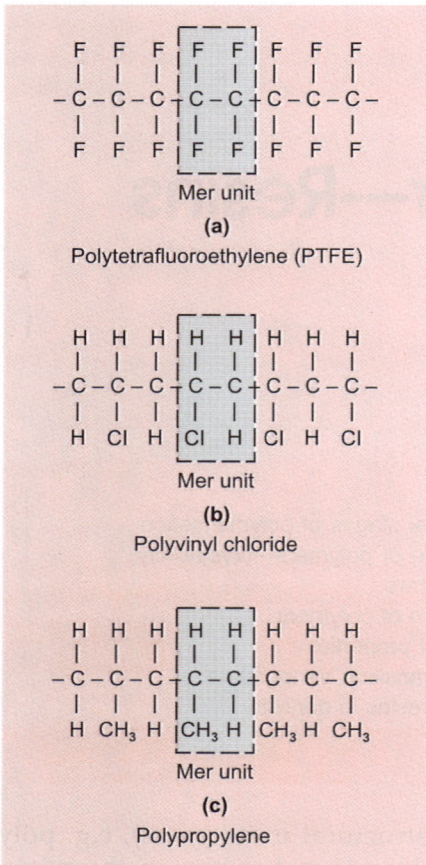

Fig. 5.1: Chemical repeating units (mers)

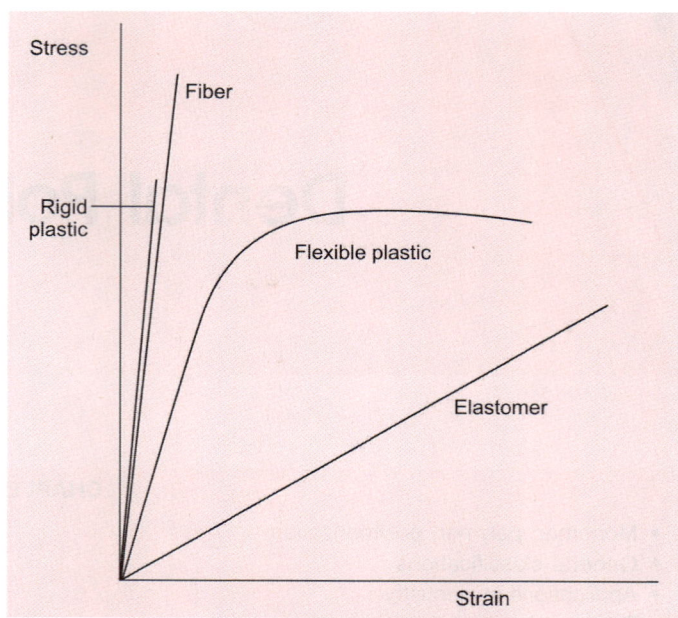

Fig. 5.2: Elastic behaviours of polymers

4. **Physical states**
   - Liquids
   - Gels
   - Elastomers
   - Flexible—fibrous
   - Rigid solids—plastics

5. **Compositions and spatial organizations**
   - Homopolymers—linear, branched
   - Copolymers: Random linear, branched, block, graft, cross-linked.

6. **According to the mechanical properties**
   - High strength, low elasticity
   - Low strength, high elasticity
   - High crystallinity, high cross-linking, high Tg
   - Low crytallinity, low cross-linking, low Tg

7. **Thermal behaviours**
   - *Thermoplastic:* Reversible, soft and mouldable at high temperatures (above Tg), soluble in organic solvents.
   - *Thermoset:* Irreversible, hard set by chemical changes, on heating do not soften but decompose, insoluble in organic solvents.

8. **Internal structure:** Crystalline, noncrystalline, semicrystalline.

9. **Dental applications**
   - Impression materials (elastomers, hydrocolloids)
   - Denture base, relining, repair materials (PMMA, PVC, polycarbonates), record base (cold cure PMMA)
   - Artificial teeth (cross-linked PMMA)
   - Temporary crowns, veneers, crowns, and bridges
   - Die materials: (PMMA, epoxy resins)
   - Maxillofacial reconstructions: Polysilicones, PMMA, PVC
   - Restorative composite resins: Anterior, posterior, pit and fissure sealants, bis GMA.
   - Restorative cements—resin cements, zinc polyacrylates, glass ionomers
   - Adhesives, bonding agents
   - Orthodontic functional appliances, space maintainers, elastics.
   - Instruments, laboratory facilities, clinical facilities (hand gloves, rubber dams, spatulas, etc.).

FACTORS AFFECTING THE PROPERTIES OF POLYMERS

- Molecular weight and chemical structural units of monomers
- Degree of polymerization or conversion factor and molecular weight distributions
- Copolymerization and spatial organizations
- Crystallinity
- Temperatures
- Compositions: Plasticisers, fillers, cross-linking agents, etc.

Degree of Polymerization

During polymerization, the chains grow until they are terminated by collisions with free radicals. This produces polymers of different numbers of repeating units and of different molecular weights. The mechanical properties depend on this extent of polymerization. Different polymer chains have different numbers of repeating units or molecular weights.

Degree of polymerization can be defined as average number of mers in the polymer chain, and also as average molecular weight of polymer chains, i.e. Mw. The degree of polymerization, Mn of denture base resins may vary from 8,000 to 40,000 units. However, the average mol.wt. represents, more predominantly, the polymers of higher mol. wt., i.e. $Mw > Mn$. When all the polymers have an equal number of mers, $Mw = Mn$. The ratio, Mw/Mn represents **polydispersity.**

Higher polydispersity indicates the presence of more polymers of higher molecular weights, which also increases the mechanical properties, softening or melting temperatures and lowers solubility.

Degree of polymerization or chain length becomes greater, with less free radicals created, and higher kinetic energy or temperature. For examples, the degree of polymerization is higher for heat cure acrylics, than cold cure acrylics, as the mobility of monomer (kinetic energy), is more at higher temperatures. Hence, the mechanical properties, etc. are about 10% higher for heat cure acrylics.

TYPES OF POLYMERS

Homopolymers have the same type of mers (M) joining and forming long, linear, or branched chains. The properties mainly depend on the monomer structure and degree of polymerization. The branched ones, may have slightly lower mechanical properties due to the separating effect of the backbone structures by the long branched structure in between. These can be represented as below, with M as a mer. For example, M is $CH_2 = CH_2$, or methyl methacrylates.

1. Linear polymer: MMMMMMMMMMMMMMMMM etc.

2. Branched polymer: MMMMMMMMMMMMMMMMMM........
$$
\begin{matrix} M & & M & & M \\ M & & M & & M \\ M & & M & & M \\ M & & M & & M \end{matrix}
$$

Copolymers

It is possible to **change the inherent properties** of the homopolymers, by suitably copolymerizing with mers of other chemical species and obtaining different spatial organizations. These comonomers (e.g. ethyl methacrylate, butyl methacrylate, etc.) can replace some of the methyl methacrylates, while monomers polymerise. Due to the comonomer structures, their concentrations and spatial organizations, the properties like Tg, strength, flexibility, solubility, etc. of the copolymers change. Copolymerization can also act as **internal plasticizers** by reducing the secondary bonding between the polymer chains.

The polymers of methyl, ethyl, butyl, and propyl methacrylates have their Tgs ≈ 120°C, 65°C, 38°C and 33°C respectively. By copolymerizing, materials of different Tgs, copolymers of different mechanical properties can be obtained. For example, a copolymer of PMMA containing 18% to 33% vinyl acetate, is available as thermoplastic sheet form. This can be softened by heating, to about 90°C and can be formed over a stone cast to produce athletic mouth protectors. Many oral appliances are made by copolymerized resins.

Spatial Organizations of Copolymers

Different spatial organizations of the comonomers, change many properties of the polymer resins like strengths, glass transition temperatures, solubilities, etc.

Consider a monomer M (say methyl methacrylate and a comonomer, E (say ethyl methacrylate).

These can copolymerize in different spatial organizations (Fig. 5.3).

Cross-linked polymer

When a cross-linking agent C, a dimethacrylate with two vinyl groups is added, the backbone chains are cross-linked by covalent bonding.

Also, *refer* to Figs 3.11d and 3.12

Ethylene glycol dimethacrylate is a common cross-linking agent, as two methyl methacrylate groups combined as M-R-M.

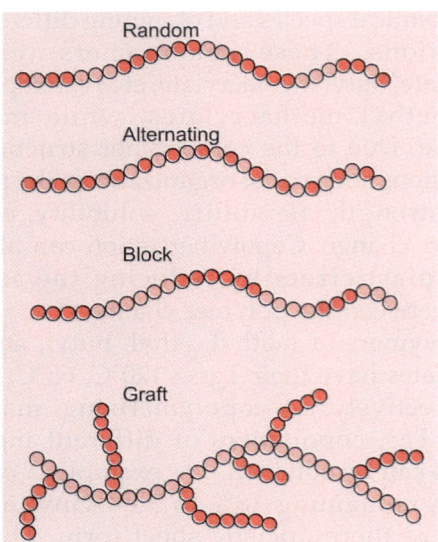

Fig. 5.3: Copolymers in spatial organizations

Such cross-linked network structures by strong covalent bonding, **resist separation** of polymer chains by thermal energies, solvents or mechanical deforming forces, so that they have higher strength, Tg, resistance to dissolution, etc.

Applications of Cross-linked Polymerizations

1. To improve the poor, inadequate physical properties of the acrylic denture base, and teeth, veneer, temporary crowns and bridges, etc., materials, they are suitably cross-linked usually by ethylene glycol dimethacrylate, or such other chemicals having two or more reactive groups.
2. **Composite** restorative resins are obtained by polymerizing an oligomer **BisGMA**, by chemical or light activations. This has two methyl methacrylate groups producing extensively cross-linked three-dimensional network, creating superior properties.
3. **Elastomeric** rubber base materials, polysulphides, polysilicones and polyethers are **cross-linked in a controlled manner**, to obtain adequate elastic recovery, tear strength, flexibility, etc. retaining Tg much below room temperature.
4. **Alginate** hydrocolloid impression material sol is converted into the gel by cross-linking with calcium ions.

Types of Polymerizations

1. **Step-growth (condensation) polymerization**
   The chemical reactions between bifunctional or trifunctional molecules, which become reactive,

simultaneously, and combine step by step forming dimers, trimers, ...polymers. In this step-growth polymerization, small molecules are repeatedly eliminated. Often there are some byproducts of small molecules like ammonia, water, alcohol, halogen acids, etc. The polymerization is not very fast due to the decrease in mobility as the polymerization proceeds. The degree of polymerization is also not very high, and low molecular weight only (10,000–20,000 only). For example:

$$n(H\text{-}A\text{-}H) + n(HO\text{-}B\text{-}OH) \rightarrow H\text{-}A\text{-}B\text{-}A\text{-}B\text{-}A\text{-}B..... BOH + nH_2O$$

Some **biological polymers** like collagen, proteins, carbohydrates, RNA, DNA, etc. belong to this category. Due to the production of byproducts, this type was named as condensation polymerization.

- **Polysulphide impression materials:** Step-growth of **bifunctional** mercaptan (SH) polysulphide increases viscosity. Cross-linking through **trifunctional** mercaptan results in the formation of rubber. The byproducts (water molecules) evaporate causing internal porosity, surface pits, and large polymerization shrinkages. (For reactions refer polysulphides, condensation polysilicones.)

- **Step-growth polymerization without by-products:** The reaction between diols and diisocyanates, forming polyurethanes.

$$HO - R_1 - OH + O = C = N - R_2 - N = C = O \rightarrow$$
$$HO - R_1 - O - C - N - R_2 - N = C = O, \text{ etc.}$$

As the structural changes take place, the polymer has **different chemical properties**, and the **molecular weight is less** than the total number of molecules involved if there are byproducts. At present in dentistry as well as in industries, addition polymerizations are mostly made use.

2. **Addition (ionic, ring opening and free radical) polymerizations**

- **Ionic addition polymerization:** Addition of molecules take place by hydrogen ion transfer from one to other. The polysilicone–rubber is formed by transfer of 'H' ion from hydrogen terminated polydimethyl siloxane to $-CH = CH_2$, i.e. vinyl terminated polydimethyl silane.

$$H - R - H + CH_2 = CH - R - CH = CH_2 \rightarrow H - R - CH_2 - CH_2 - R - CH = CH_2, \text{ etc.}$$

Where R is
$$\begin{bmatrix} & CH_3 \\ & | \\ - & Si - O - \\ & | \\ & CH_3 \end{bmatrix}_n$$

Key Box 5.1 Polymerization of expoxy resin die materials

- **Ring opening addition polymerization:** The monomer has two oxirane terminal rings, which are opened by amines or alkyl benzene sulphonates.

  For example, epoxy monomer reacts with difunctional amines, polymerizing to **epoxy resin die material** (Key Box 5.1).

  For example, polyether impression material. Polyether and alkyl benzene sulfonate react and form polyether rubber (refer elastomers), by opening the amine ring terminal groups by Key Box 5.1.

- **Free radical addition polymerization**

  Addition polymerization begins from an **active centre, like a free radical**, R$^{\bullet}$, adding monomers rapidly one after the other, forming a long chained giant molecule. **Free radical is an atom or group of atoms, having one unpaired electron.** The monomer-repeating unit, should have unsaturated group, a double bond, vinyl group, C = C, like ethylene, vinyl chloride, acrylics, acrylates, etc. When the free radical collides such as monomer,

it attracts one electron from one end leaving the other electron unpaired at the other end. After this initiation, it goes on combining and adding other mers by successive activation (Key Box 5.2).

- When, R$_1$ is H, monomer is ethylene, which polymerises to polyethylene or **polythene**
- R$_1$ is Cl, monomer is vinylchloride, which polymerises to polyvinylchloride or **PVC**
- R$_1$ is styrene, it polymerises to polystyrene or **polyster**
- R$_1$ is COOH, monomer is acrylic acid, which polymerises to **polyacrylic acid,** etc. (Key Box 5.3).

  The methyl (CH$_3$) group of methyl methacrylate can be replaced by ethyl, butyl, propyl, etc. to obtain the respective copolymers. A mixture of these monomers can form copolymerization.

  This activation and polymerization takes place **very rapidly** building into huge giant molecules with several thousands or millions of mers. The propagation of polymerization or growth of chains take place **indefinitely until terminated by**

- Exhaustion of all monomers
- Collision with another free radical or with another growing chain.
- Transfer of (hydrogen ion) energy to another molecule, making it to grow further.

Main features of addition polymerization are

- Very rapid almost instantaneous process
- High degree of polymerization
- Molecular weight of polymer equals the molecular weights of all monomers in it.
- Same chemical properties of monomers, but different physical properties.

Key Box 5.2 Successive activation

Key Box 5.3 Polymerization of PMMA

Key Box 5.3 Polymerization of PMMA

Similarly methyl methacrylate monomer

$$
\begin{array}{cc}
H & CH_3 \\
| & | \\
C & = C \quad \text{polymerizes, being initiated by } R^{\bullet} \text{ to} \\
| & | \\
H & C = O \\
& | \\
& OCH_3
\end{array}
$$

polymethyl methacrylate—the common denture base resin, i.e.

Chemical Stages of Addition Polymerization

The four stages of addition polymerization are induction (initiation), propagation, chain-transfer and terminations.

1. **Induction and initiation**

   Free radicals are produced by dissociation of certain chemicals, like benzoyl peroxide, using different activating energy systems like heat, chemicals, ultraviolet or visible light of particular wavelengths. The free radical produced ($R^{\bullet}$), then combines with a monomer M and initiates (starts) polymerization. **This interval is known as induction period.**

Key Box 5.4 Thermal activation of benzoyl peroxide (BPO)

Systems of activations

- **Heat activation:** The common initiator, **benzoyl peroxide,** when heated above 50°C or 60°C, dissociates forming free radicals (e.g. heat cure acrylic denture base material) (Key Box 5.4).
- **Chemical activation:** When certain chemicals like tertiary amines (N-N-dimethyl-*p*-toluidine) are added, the **dissociation temperature of benzoyl peroxide, depress below the room temperature** and liberate the free radicals as above. This refers to cold, self, chemically curing or autopolymerising resins.

- **Ultraviolet light activation:** The initiator **benzoin–methyl ether** is irradiated with ultraviolet rays of wavelength, $\lambda = 375$ nm, to liberate free radicals. Such system is not used now a days, due to health hazards of UV light.
- **Visible light activation:** Initiator is a **diketone like, camphoroquinone, with an accelerator N-N-dimethyl-p-toluidine** (or dimethyl aminoethyl methacrylate, DMAEMA), liberates free radicals when visible light of **wavelength, $\lambda = 468$ nm** is used, at ordinary temperatures. This system has become **very common and popular** for composite resins (and compomer restorative materials) as it gives easy control over setting).

The initiation of polymerization, takes place when this free radical attracts one unpaired electron of monomer and combines with it (Key Box 5.5).

Key Box 5.5 Initiation of polymerization

2. **Propagation:** The radical monomer complex, $RM^{\bullet}$ acts as a free radical and combines with another monomer by activation and forms a dimer $RM^{\bullet} + M \rightarrow RMM^{\bullet}$

   The process repeats one after the other, **continuously and rapidly** building up a long polymer chain,

   $RMM^{\bullet} + M \rightarrow RM_2M^{\bullet}$, etc. $\rightarrow RM_nM^{\bullet}$ (Key Box 5.3)

   This takes place almost **instantaneously,** until all the monomers are exhausted theoretically or terminated.

   For methyl methacrylate resins the reaction is exothermic and liberates **heat = 12,500 cal/gm mol.**

3. **Termination**

   a. The growing polymer chains terminate by collision with another free radical or with another growing polymer

   $$RM_nM^{\bullet} + R_1^{\bullet} \rightarrow RM_n\,MR_1, \text{ or}$$
   $$RM_nM^{\bullet} + R_1M_kM^{\bullet} \rightarrow R\,M_{n+k+2}\,R_1$$

   If these free radicals are not produced in adequate numbers or neutralised **(inhibited)** by impurities, the polymerization process is **retarded.**

Key Box 5.6 Termination by chain transfer

b. **Chain transfer:** The active-free radical energy of the growing chain can get transferred to another monomer or another already terminated polymer. The first polymer chain gets terminated and the next one starts growing, by this **hydrogen ion** transfer $RM_nM^{\bullet} + M \rightarrow RM_n = M + HM^{\bullet}$ (Key Box 5.6).

Inhibition of Polymerization

Certain impurity atoms can react with the free radicals or neutralize the growing chains. These inhibit or retard the polymerization process. The termination of polymerization may take place before acquiring large molecular weight or exhaustion of all the available monomers.

Small amounts of **hydroquinone** (or methyl ether of hydroquinone), about **0.006%**, added to denture base acrylic monomer liquid, prevents the spontaneous polymerization of the liquid, due to some stray radicals produced by some ionizing agents and improves its shelf-life. It also **retards** the polymerization process and gives **adequate working time** for mixing and packing. **Eugenol**, atmospheric oxygen, etc., can easily react with the free radicals. That is why **eugenol** cement base and certain cavity varnishes are contraindicated for composite resin restorations and certain bonding agents. As inhibitors interfere with the process of polymerization, the composite resin restoration is covered with cellulose matrix bands and glass ionomers are **coated with cocoa butter or varnishes** immediately after restoration. Otherwise, the atmospheric oxygen will inhibit the polymerization. The monomer liquids also are preserved in air tight **amber-coloured** dark bottles or containers.

Structure of Polymers

The short-range van der Waals attractive forces, form secondary bonding between the homopolymer long chains and align them causing certain **crystallinity**. This increases hardness, tensile strength and glass transition temperatures.

The long range—primary bonding between the monomers, comonomers, etc. cause cross-linked structures, co-polymerization, branched and long side chains. These, cause highly **disordered, coiled structure** **of tangled mass** (i.e. like cooked spaghetti or noodles). The polymerized material has amorphous structure with certain localised crystallinity. The properties of a polymer depend also on the **degree of crystallinity.**

The degree of crystallinity decreases by
- Copolymerization
- Long branched or side chains
- Plasticisers

General Properties of Polymers

1. **Mechanical properties**—resistance to deformations are more for higher
   - Degree of polymerization
   - Molecular weight and structure of the monomer
   - Cross-linking and spatial organizations.

2. **Rheological properties:** When a deforming force is applied, the long-linear chains slip one over the other causing **irreversible strain or plastic flow**, as they occupy the new positions in crystalline parts. The linear polymers have higher plastic (viscous) flow.

   The amorphous nature with coiled structures, very easily undergo elastic deformation (un-coiling like a spring), which is a reversible strain.

   As the actual polymer structure has certain crystallinity, the deformation produced is a combination of elastic and non-elastic strains. This **viscoelastic property** causes time-dependant deformations and elastic recoveries. That is why elastomeric impression materials have time-dependent incomplete elastic recoveries. Greater amount of **cross-linking** decreases the crystallinity and makes the material **more rigid or less flexible or of lower creep.**

3. **Solvation (dissolution) of polymers:** The polar bonding between polymer chains, causes adsorption of water or solvents, which later diffuse or get absorbed. This is known as **sorption.** The sorption causes **separation of the polymer chains,** due to which it **swells and softens**. This causes dimensional changes (expansion) in acrylic denture. This is measured by using a disc of standard dimensions, by first drying completely and weighing, W_1 gm, then immersing in water for 7 days and finding the

increase in weight (W_2-W_1) gm. As per ADA specification, it should be less than 0.8 mg/cm². If the same disc is again dried and weighed W_3 gm, the decrease from the initial weight W_1-W_3 gives the solubility, which should be <0.04 mg/cm².

The dimensional changes due to solvation are less for polymers having less sorption, that is for:

1. Long-linear chains and of a higher degree of polymerization
2. Greater cross-linking (as highly cross-linked polymers, show less/solvation or softening effect)
3. Greater crystallinity (as the crystalline structure has **physical cross-linking effect**)
4. Greater polydispersity (i.e. higher molecular weight or degree of polymerization).

Elastomers have lower **Tg** and hence **higher softening effect** than rigid plastics. Similarly, polymers with longer **side chains** and **copolymers** with large pendant groups have a higher tendency for separation of chains. Hence these have higher solvation effect and greater dimensional changes.

In the case of acrylic dentures, repeated drying and wetting cause dimensional changes, internal stress-relaxation and crazing of dentures. To minimize these, the denture is kept **either in the mouth or immersed in water** (when not in use, specially at night).

4. **Plasticizers**
These are substances of small molecular sizes incorporated into polymers to:

1. Increase the flexibility, softness, and flow
2. Decrease the softening (glass transition) and melting temperatures.

Plasticizers incorporated, function as external and internal plasticizers.

External plasticizers
These act sometimes, like solvents which enter into the substance and help slipping of the atoms. These neutralize the secondary bonding between the polymer chains or intermolecular forces. This decreases the resistance for deformation between the polymer chains, or it acts like **lubricants**. Ideally, these should have very **large chemical attraction, high boiling point, and insolubility**. As it is very rarely found, the plasticizer **leaches** out of the structure gradually, but at a faster rate at higher temperatures and decrease the flexibility. That is why plastic household articles kept in hot sunlight soon become brittle. **Dibutyl phthalate** is the common such plasticizer used with acrylic resins and elastomers.

Internal plasticizers
These are **comonomers,** entering the system during co-polymerisation by covalent bonds forming long side chains or large pendant molecules, separating the long polymer chains. **These do not leach out.** For example, some higher esters like butyl or octyl methacrylates added to methyl methacrylates, copolymerize and increase the flexibility.

5. **Thermal properties**
Physical properties of polymers are greatly affected by temperature changes due to their internal energies (inter-molecular and inter-chain forces) and structures.

Thermosetting resins
Polymerization by chemical changes takes place by the irreversible reaction. These are usually cross-linked hard set materials. They do not soften or melt but **decompose** (infusible) when heated further. **They are insoluble and have high impact strength, rigidity, abrasion resistance, and good dimensional stability.**

Thermoplastic resins (Note on Tg)
These begin to soften above their glass transition temperatures, Tg, at which the polymer chains, get debonded from each other and easily slip one over the other. These are then mouldable and retain the shapes, on cooling below Tg. Thermoplastic resins soften and melt on heating and can dissolve in organic solvents, (e.g. acrylic resins).

Theory: There is a strong intermolecular covalent–primary bonding between the monomers of a polymer chain. The **valency electrons** continuously **move back and forth along these chains forming** different electron charge densities. This induces corresponding opposite charge densities in the adjacent chains for balancing. This causes the hydrogen-polar bonding, by van der Waals and London forces forming weaker secondary bonding between the adjacent chains.

When the polymer is heated above a certain temperature, Tg, the weaker secondary bonds between the chains are broken, and they *begin to slip* one over the other, exhibiting the thermoplastic properties.

The Tg is lower when the polymer has
1. Shorter chains (DP), e.g. cold cure acrylics
2. Lower polydispersity
3. Impurities and copolymerization with large pendant groups, separating the chains more
4. Copolymers with long side chains, which rotate and separate chains
5. Less crystallinity
6. Plasticizers
7. Highly cross-linked and ordered (block, graft) and crystalline polymers have **higher Tg.**

Elastomers have controlled an amount of cross-linking and have **Tg, below the room temperature**. That is why, they behave as viscoelastic rubber-like materials.

Thermal conduction

Polymer resins are good insulators (K = 0.0003 to 0.0005 cgs units) of heat and electricity, due to a lack of conducting free electrons. This property is quite suitable for restorative composite resins (not for acrylic dentures) and is widely made use in industries specially in electrical gadgets, and insulations.

Thermal expansion

Long-chained polymer structures produce large thermal expansion. Linear polymers like acrylic denture base resins have α= 80–120 ppm/°C. Highly cross-linked rigid composite resins have lower values, 25–60 ppm/°C. Slightly cross-linked rubber-base elastomers having Tg < room temperatures, have an morphous structure and high α = 150–225 ppm/°C. Amorphous waxes have still higher values for α = 300–700 ppm/°C, varying with temperatures. **High thermal expansion is due to vibrations of mers along the direction of chains.**

Acrylic Resins in Dentistry

There are mainly two types of acrylic resins, which are derivatives of ethylene, having vinyl (C=C) groups. These undergo addition polymerization forming **transparent organic glasses.**

One series, derived from the **acrylic acid** unit, are **alkenoic** acids. These are used in glass ionomer and zinc polycarboxylate adhesive cements (Key Box 5.7).

The –COOH group can form chemical bonding with calcium of tooth materials, i.e. $COO^- Ca^-$ of enamel and dentin. Bonding by cross-linking is greater with acrylic acid units having more COOH groups.

The polarities of the carboxylic groups of these polyacids cause water sorption which tends to separate the polymer chains, decreasing the strength and rigidity.

The second series is the derivatives of methacrylic acids, $CH_2 = C (CH_3) COOR$. There are many esters of this group which are used in dentistry and industries. For example the ester radical R in the methacrylic acid $CH_2 = C (CH_3) COOR$ can be methyl, ethyl, propyl, butyl, etc.

These polymers are **thermoplastic** materials having different Tgs depending on the structural units and chain lengths. These are copolymerized and frequently used in various fields (Key Box 5.8).

Polymethyl methacrylate is the most common resin used in denture fabrications. The monomer **(mol. wt. = 100) is a volatile clear liquid, with MP = –48°C, BP = 100.8°C** at one-atmosphere "bar" pressure. Addition polymerization is done by using thermal, chemical or light energy activation. Suitable colours, can be added, and mechanical properties-like flexibility can be adjusted with plasticizers. The polymer is an organic glass and is a very common material in dentistry used for complete and partial dentures, artificial teeth, denture repairs, lining, etc. In industries and in everyday life, the plastic articles are obtained by slightly modifying this (for properties: *Refer* to denture base resins).

Multifunctional Acrylic Resins

Several multifunctional methacrylate resins like dimethacrylates, trimethacrylates, etc. are used to obtain polymers of superior mechanical properties. These cross-links the methacrylate polymer chains, by

Key Box 5.7	Structures of alkenoic acid mers
Acrylic acid unit	H – C – H | H – C – COOH
Maleic acid unit	H – C – COOH | H – C – COOH
Itaconic acid unit	H – C – H HOOC – C – COOH
Tricarboxylic acid unit	H – C – COOH | HOOC – C – CH$_2$ – COOH

Key Box 5.8	Tgs of different poly 'R' methacrylates

Poly 'R' (methacrylates):	Tg°C
Methyl	125
Ethyl	65
N-propyl	38
Isopropyl	95
N-butyl	33
Isobutyl	70
Phenyl	120

direct combination of two methyl methacrylate monomers. Ethylene glycol dimethacrylate is a common cross-linking acrylic oligomer.

Bisphenol glycidyl dimethacrylate (BisGMA), triethylene glycol dimethacrylate TEGDMA, urethane-dimethylacrylate (UDMA), etc. have two terminal double bond vinyl C = C groups, which cross-link the other monomers, to form a more rigid three-dimensional matrix.

Penta-P is a phosphate-containing monomer with five methacrylate groups. This acts as acid etching, as well as a bonding agent.

MODEL QUESTIONS

I. Short Essays   (10 minutes each)

1. Define the terms monomer, polymer and polymerization and classify the polymers. Give few applications of polymers in dentistry.

2. Define the degree of polymerization and polydispersity. Give the spatial organization of copolymers.

3. Write a note on cross-linked polymers and give two examples.

4. Explain step-growth and addition polymerization with one example to each.

5. Write a note on stages of polymerization.

6. Thermal properties of polymer resins.

II. Brief Answers   (5 minutes each)

1. Degree of polymerization
2. Inhibition of polymerization
3. Plasticizers
4. Glass transition temperature
5. Structure of polymers
6. Solvation of polymers
7. Acrylic resins in dentistry

Prosthetic Applications of Polymer Resins

DENTURE-BASE RESINS

A complete denture is a removable dental prosthesis (oral appliance) that replaces the entire dentition and associated structures of the maxilla or the mandible. This contains artificial teeth attached to the denture base, which is supported through the contact with the underlying oral tissues, teeth or implants.

A partial denture can be defined as a removable dental prosthesis, that replaces missing teeth and associated tissues.

Prior to 1937, the denture-base materials used were vulcanite, vinyl plastics, nitrocellulose, phenol formaldehyde, etc. Acrylic denture bases became very popular, within a decade with almost 98% use, due to its biocompatibility, aesthetics and simple fabrication techniques. Due to its inadequate mechanical properties, other polymers like polystyrene, epoxy resins, polycarbonates, nylon, polyurethanes were tried. Recently **butadiene rubber and fibre reinforced** acrylic resins are experimented to achieve higher impact strength and fracture resistances. Highly plasticized acrylic resins, polysilicones, polyurethanes have experimented for soft denture reliners, maxillofacial reconstructions, etc.

Dentures have to serve the primary functions of **mastication** and enhancing the **aesthetics**. It should be able to endure the following **hostile oral environments.**

1. Chemical attacks from slightly acidic or alkaline foods and beverages.
2. Large dynamic masticating forces (0–100 kg)
3. Attrition due to abrasions from opposing teeth or hard food.
4. Temperature fluctuations (0–60°C) of beverages.

Ideal Requirements of Denture-base Materials

1. **Biological–chemical** compatibility
   - Nonpoisonous, nontoxic, nonirritant, nonallergic
   - Noncarcinogenic
   - Chemically inert, but resistant to chemical attacks
   - Hygienic (should not be a seat for the growth of microorganisms like *Candida albicans*)
   - No bad taste or foul smelling.

2. **Physical–mechanical** requirements
   - Low density and low weight for better retention
   - Low creep for resisting time-dependent deformations
   - High proportional limit, elastic limit and yield strengths to resist permanent deformations.

- High modulus of elasticity to resist deformation
- High modulus of resilience to absorb dynamic masticating energies.
- High compressive, tensile, shear and flexure strengths and toughness to resist fracture.
- High impact strength to resist fracture from dynamic forces.
- High polishability as well as abrasive resistance
- High fatigue strength for long-life.
- High craze—resistance for higher strength, and resist fracture.

3. **Thermal compatibilities**
   - High distortion and softening glass transition (Tg) temperatures for resins.
   - High thermal conductivity for the patients to feel the hotness and coldness, and the real taste of food.
   - Low coefficient of thermal expansion for dimensional stability
   - Able to withstand frequent changes of oral temperatures (0–60°C).

4. **Aesthetic requirements**
   - Transparent and colourless
   - Able to incorporate desired colour pigments and shades
   - Colour stability—colour parameters should not change in long time service
   - Colour parameters should be the same for all wavelengths of incident light.

5. **Other requirements**
   - Simple fabrication techniques with inexpensive laboratory equipments and auxiliary materials
   - Long storage life
   - Easily available

Properties of Polymethyl Methacrylate Denture-base Resins

1. **Biocompatibility**
   - Nontoxic, nonirritant, noncarcinogenic
   - Chemically inert, and stable in oral conditions
   - Hygienic in well-polished conditions
   - No taste or foul smell
   - Very few patients may be allergic to residual monomers present, more, in cold-cure acrylics.

2. **Physical and mechanical properties of (heat cure acrylics)**
   - Density............................. 1.19 gm/cc
   - Proportional limit .... 27–45 MPa
   - Compressive strength............. 75 MPa
   - Tensile strength.................. 65 MPa
   - Shear strength....................122 MPa
   - Transverse strength..............85 MPa

- Modulus of elasticity............ 2500 MPa
- Fracture toughness............0.7–1.6 MPa $\sqrt{m}$
- Impact strength (Charpy)........0.98–1.27 J/m^3
- Fatigue strength (endurance limit).... 17 MPa (1.5 million cycles)
- Surface hardness..................18–20 KHN
- Water sorption.........0.6 (<0.8, ADA 12) mg.cm^{-2}
- Solubility in distilled water...........0.02 (<0.04, ADA 12) mg·cm^{-2}

3. **Thermal properties**
   - Thermal conductivity = K = 0.0006 cal/sec/cm^2/unit temperature gradient
   - Coefficient of thermal expansion = α = 80–120 ppm/°C
   - Heat distortion temperature = 80°C
   - Softening, glass transition temperature = Tg = 120°C
   - Moldable temperature = 120–200°C
   - Melting (depolymerization) temperature = 450°C

4. **Optical properties**
   - Transparent organic glass
   - Opaque for UV light
   - Suitable colour pigments (shades) can be added
   - Good colour stability (slightly poor for cold-cure acrylic).

Suitability of Polymethyl Methacrylate Material for Denture-base Fabrication

1. *Biocompatibility is very satisfactory,* and it is hygienic, not foul smelling, no taste. But slightly allergic to few patients, due to more residual monomer (5%) only in cold-cure acrylics.

2. *All mechanical properties are inadequate.* This cannot withstand large masticating dynamic forces. Fractures easily by careless handling or accidental falls. Poor abrasion resistance, i.e. acrylic teeth undergoes abrasion (attrition) by opposing natural or ceramic teeth. To compensate this *poor mechanical properties,* dentures should have about *2–3 mm thickness,* but it becomes *heavy* and retention of mandibular denture decrease.

3. *Low thermal conductivity and high coefficients of thermal expansion* causing dimensional changes and distortions are *disadvantages.*

4. *Aesthetic qualities are quite satisfactory.* Suitable colour pigments and **nylon fibres,** can be added to **imitate blood veins.** Due to oxidation of amine activators, cold-cure acrylics do not have good colour stability, and **gradual yellowing** takes place.

5. *Fabrication techniques, are not very much complicated.* Simple, inexpensive pieces of equipment and laboratories, only are required. Suitable precautions are to be followed in every stage of fabrication.

Materials and auxiliary materials are not very expensive compared to casting procedures.

6. *Adequate service time about six years and good shelf life for the materials*

Even though the mechanical, and thermal properties are not very suitable, biocompatibility, aesthetic considerations and fabrication simplicity, have made this material popular and acceptable.

Classification of Denture-base Materials

A denture can be defined as a dental prosthesis replacing the dentition and associated structures of maxilla and mandible. Complete and partial resin dentures, cast fixed and removable partial metallic dentures are fabricated as per the clinical requirements. Classification can be done according to:

1. **Materials**
   - Metallic alloys: Gold alloys, chromium-nickel alloys, titanium alloys, and 18-8 stainless steel
   - Nonmetallic resins:
     Earlier: Vulcanite, bakelite, polycarbonates, nylon, etc.
     Present: Polymethyl methacrylate—unmodified, or modified with carbon, nylon, fibers and butadiene–styrene rubbers, etc.

2. **Fabrication techniques**
   - Wax elimination casting (noble and base metal alloys)
   - Forging (stainless steel)
   - Polymerizing (resins)

3. **Clinical use**
   - Alloys: Fixed and removable cast partial dentures, metal-ceramic bridges
   - Resins: Complete and removable partial dentures, temporary crowns and bridges, denture liners, maxillofacial reconstructions, etc.

Classification of the Resins for Prosthetic Applications

1. **Materials**
   - Earlier: Vulcanite, bakelite, polycarbonates, nylon, etc.
   - Present: PMMA—unmodified, PMMA—modified with carbon, fibres, nylon, butadiene-styrene rubbers, etc.

2. **Fabrication techniques**
   - Compression moulding
   - Injection moulding
   - Fluid—pour and cure technique

3. **Methods of polymerization (curing)**
   - Thermal energy by heating
   - Chemical—autopolymerization

- Microwave energy
- Light energy

4. **Applications**
   - Complete denture: Heat or cold-cure unmodified or modified acrylics
   - Removable partial denture: Heat or cold-cure or flexible soft acrylics
   - Temporary crown and bridges, veneers: Cross-linked acrylics (shaded)
   - Repairing and rebasing: Cold-cure or heat cure acrylics
   - Relining: Cold-cure acrylics, polysilicones, plasticized resins
   - Maxillofacial reconstructions: Plasticized acrylics, PVC rubber polysilicones
   - Athletic mouth protectors: Acrylics, polycarbonates.

Classification of Denture Liners

1. **Materials**
   - Polymethylmethacrylate
   - Highly plasticized PMMA
   - Polysilicones

2. **Processing techniques**
   - Heat curing
   - Chemical curing
   - Light curing

3. **Applications**
   - Hard liners: PMMA—for better fit
   - Long term soft-resilient liners: Heat or cold-cure polysilicones, highly plasticized PMMA—for relieving pain
   - Short-term soft-tissue conditioners: Highly plasticized PMMA, polysilicones—for fast healing
   - Chairside: Liners for patients use for the better fit.

COMPLETE DENTURE FABRICATION PROCEDURES

Fabrication of acrylic complete dentures involves series of clinical steps followed by laboratory procedures to obtain well-fitting dentures with optimum mechanical, etc. properties.

PRELIMINARY STEPS

1. **Clinical step:** After the teeth extraction, and bone contouring, the patient is advised to wait for about three months for complete healing and resorption of the soft tissues. Obtain the primary impression of oral structure with impression compound (*see* Colour Plate 9, Fig. 6.1).
   Laboratory procedure: Pour the dental stone cast, in the impression, to get a **primary** cast. Adapt modeling-wax sheet spacer and prepare cold-cure

acrylic special tray (wait for 24 hours for better dimensional stability of the tray). **Trim** the **special tray** about **2 mm** short of sulcus (*see* Colour Plate 9, Fig. 6.2).

2. Perform border—moulding (tracing) with a green stick compound. Then, the spacer is removed. Zinc oxide eugenol impression paste is used to obtain the final wash or secondary impression, This gives mucostatic impression with accurate reproduction of finer details of oral structure (Figs 6.3 and 6.4).

   Laboratory procedure: The **master cast** is obtained by pouring dental stone. Prepare the base plate (i.e. recording base) with shellac base plate or cold-cure acrylics. Construct occlusal rims on the recording base (Figs 6.6 and 6.7).

3. Conduct **jaw relationship, vertical** and **horizontal orientations**, as well as **centric relations.**

   Laboratory procedure: Mount the cast in the recorded relationship, in the articulator. Assemble the artificial teeth in this wax denture-base (Figs 6.8 and 6.9; *see* Colour Plate 14, Fig. 6.21).

4. The unprocessed wax denture is **tried in** the mouth and conduct bite registration using bite registration materials (polysilicones, bite registration waxes, ZnOE pastes, etc.).

LABORATORY PROCEDURE OF DENTURE FABRICATION

Compression moulding technique

1. FLASKING: MULTIPLE MIX METHOD

The casts with the wax dentures are removed from the articulator and cleaned. Prepare dental stone (or plaster) mix, fill the lower half of the flask, place the cast and wax denture, in the mix and remove the excess mix, without creating undercuts in the land area of the stone mount.

Allow the stone plaster to set for 30 minutes. Apply a thin coating of alginate separating medium solution or vaseline. Place the upper half of the flask (without lid). Prepare the second stone/plaster mix, fill, until the **tips** of the teeth are **just visible**, and wait until it sets (again vaseline may be applied). Prepare a third stone (or plaster) mix, fill the flask completely, close **the lid,** clamp the flask and press until the lid is properly seated. Allow it to set for 30 min. **This three-mix flasking technique helps deflasking without causing damage to the denture and teeth** (Fig. 6.7, page 129).

2. DEWAXING

The clamp is slightly loosened (to allow wax expansion) and placed in boiling water for about 5 minutes. Two halves are separated, the baseplate is removed, wax is completely eliminated by flushing with boiling water and allowed to dry for about 20 minutes (*see* Colour Plate 10, Figs 6.6 to 6.10).

3. SEPARATING MEDIUM (TIN-FOIL SUBSTITUTE/COLD-MOULD SEAL)

To separate the plaster surface from the acrylic dough, an impervious separating medium (thin film) is formed in between them. Thin tin-foil was adapted earlier, which was found to be time consuming and inconvenient. Certain paints, cellulose lacquers, soap or starch solutions, were tried. At present, **alginate sol** is found to be the most convenient and effective, separating medium (Table 6.1).

The stone surfaces in the flask **except the exposed teeth surfaces** are applied with one or two layers of thin coatings of separating medium with a painting camel hair brush. It reacts and forms a thin transparent gel-film of calcium alginate. This gel-film is **impervious to MMA monomer, as well as water and prevents their diffusion across.**

Table 6.1	Composition of Stellon-cold-mould seal
1. Soluble salt of Na/K/NH$_4$ alginate	= 2–3%
2. Alcohol (for evaporating and drying)	= 3%
3. Glycerine for suitable viscosity	= 7%
4. Preservatives, colour	= small amounts
5. Water (balance 85–88%)	= 85–88%

Setting reaction

$$Na_n \, Alg + \frac{n}{2} CaSO_4 \rightarrow Ca_{\frac{n}{2}} Alg \, (gel\text{-}film) + \frac{n}{2} + Na_2SO_4$$

Purpose of application is to prevent

- Diffusion of water from wet plaster into the unpolymerised dough which later causes **voids,** resulting in **crazing.**
- Diffusion of monomer from the dough into plaster which polymerize and cause, **rough** surface and **adhesion** of plaster to acrylic, and to get plaster-free denture.

Precautions

- Perform complete dewaxing
- Apply, carefully two or three thin coatings without trapping air
- **Do not apply to the exposed teeth surface**, as thin film prevents the **chemical bonding** of teeth with denture
- Apply, when the plaster mould is still hot for quick setting.

Table 6.2	Composition and functions of polymer powder and monomer liquid

Polymer powder

1. Transparent prepolymerized fine powder or beads of polymethyl methacrylate	To dissolve in the monomer to form a dough which reduces polymerization shrinkage
2. Copolymers (PMEA, PEMA)	To increase the solubility of powder, reduce dough time and brittleness
3. Benzoyl peroxide	0.5 to 1.5% acts as initiator, and provide free radicals
4. Dibutyl phthalate	To act as a plasticizer
5. Barium or bismuth salts	To act as radio-opacifiers
6. Colour pigments (HgS, Fe_2O_3, CdSe)	These are locked to polymer beads for aesthetics
7. Died organic nylon or acrylic fibres	For the natural appearance of tissues (light veined)/surfaces

Monomer liquid

- Methyl methacrylate monomer
- Comonomers like ethacrylates, butacrylates, etc. : To improve mechanical properties
- Ethylene glycol dimethacrylate: 1–2% cross-linking agent to increase strength
- Hydroquinone ………….. 0.006% acts as an inhibitor—to increase shelf-life

4. HEAT-CURE ACRYLIC DENTURE-BASE RESIN

This is supplied as a fine powder or transparent beads of pre-polymerized PMMA resin. The liquid is mainly, methyl methacrylate monomer which is protected in an amber coloured bottle.

Manufacturing of these spherical beads is done by suspension and bead polymerization technique. Methyl methacrylate monomer and its co-monomer with a benzoyl peroxide initiator, and an emulsifier (or a colloid) is dispersed in water. This is carefully heated in a flask to about 60–70°C, which causes polymerization. Due to the surface tension of water these form spherical beads dispersed in water. This is separated dried and used as denture base powder, which has in addition, the following components (Table 6.2).

To prevent evaporation and polymerization by some stray ionizing agents, the liquid is stored in *air tight amber-coloured bottles.*

- **Note 1:** In case of cold-cure acrylic resins, the monomer contains, in addition, *tertiary amines like N-N-dimethyl paratoluidine as the chemical activator.*
- **Note 2:** To improve the **impact strength,** the powder may be added by inorganic fibres like $ZrSiO_2$, or glass particles, or fibres coated with vinyl silane—coupling agents, or whiskers of SiC, BN, Al_2O_3, etc.

Properties of methyl methacrylate monomer liquid
- Highly volatile, a transparent liquid of molecular structure
- Molecular weight = 100
- Melting temperature = –48°C at one atm pressure

- Boiling temperature = 100.8°C at one atm pressure
- Density at 20°C = 0.945 gm/ml
- Heat of polymerization = 12,500 cal/mole
- Polymerization volume shrinkage = 21%

5. MANIPULATION OF DENTURE-BASE RESINS

During polymerization of the monomer, large volume shrinkage of about 21% takes place. The linear dimensional change of about 7%, causes misfit of the denture. When prepolymerized polymer powder, is mixed with monomer liquid in the **ratio 3:1, by weight, and then polymerized, the volume** shrinkage is reduced to one-third, i.e. about 7% or linear shrinkage to about 2%. The powder dissolves in liquid and forms a "dough" which is **convenient** for packing the mould, under compression.

Physical stages (changes) of mixing: Polymer–monomer interactions

Monomer liquid, as much as required, is taken in a non-conducting thick porcelain mixing jar with a lid and the powder is added **in the ratio 3:1 by weight, or 2.5:1 by volume** (or until all the powder added gets wetted completely). It is quickly mixed, and the lid is closed, to prevent evaporation of monomers.

Five physically distinct stages of mixing observed are:

1. **Wet sandy stage:** The liquid first wets the powder particles. Interaction is at the molecular level. The mix appears grainy, or non-cohesive, like wet sand.

2. **Stringy or sticky–tacky stage:** Surface particles of powder dissolves in liquid. The polymer chains begin to uncoil and disperse in liquid. Mix become sticky or stringy (producing **cobweb**-like fine threads), when held between fingers.

3. **Dough stage:** The powder further dissolves forming a homogeneous, soft, 'dough' like mass. This is a nonsticky mouldable mass. **Packing is conducted at this dough-stage.**

4. **Rubbery or elastic stage:** The dispersion of polymer chains and evaporation of monomer, takes place resulting in a rubbery or elastic stage. Packing should be accomplished before this stage begins.

5. **Stiff stage:** The mass becomes stiff on further standing. Monomer evaporation causes **dry surface** which appears as if it has polymerized **(pseudo-polymerization).**

Dough forming time or dough time can be defined as the time interval from the beginning of mixing until the dough stage is just reached. This dough time is about **5 to 10 min.** According to ADA specification No. 12, it should be **less than 40 min.**

The dough time is shorter if
- Molecular weight of the polymer (degree of polymerization) is smaller
- Copolymers (which increase solubility) are present
- Plasticizers are present
- Temperature is higher
- Powder/liquid ratio is lower

Hence, to prolong the dough time or to delay packing, the mix can be stored in a refrigerator. To shorten dough time, the mix can be placed in warm water bath **(at <40°C).**

Working time is the time interval, in which dough stage is retained, i.e. from the end of sticky stage to the beginning of the rubbery stage. The trial closures and final closures are to be completed during this period. As per ADA specification No.12, working time should be **more than 5 minutes.**

6. PACKING

It is the careful, **complete filling** of the mould space without air trapping. Under-packing, with less dough, causes a lack of pressure and air trapping porosities. Over-packing (with excess dough) increases the denture thickness, and may cause displacement of teeth.

Method of Packing

As soon as the dough-stage is reached, it is kneaded, rolled and bent into U shape, which is carefully placed on the tooth surface in the upper half of flask and is **slightly overfilled.** Thin polythene sheet is covered and the two-halves are assembled.

Trial Closures

The assembly is pressed using a mechanical press, slowly in increments, to allow the excess dough to come out, as much as possible. Then, the halves are separated and the polythene sheet is carefully removed. Using a blunt instrument, the excess dough on the **land surface,** i.e. **flash,** is carefully removed without pulling from the denture position. This is the first trial closure which can be repeated, again and again, using fresh polythene papers 3–4 times until the **flash no longer comes out.**

Final Closure

The polythene sheet is removed, any broken investment pieces found, are removed and finally assembled. Large pressure is applied to get **metal-to-metal contact.** It is then transferred to a **carrier clamp** and kept under pressure on the table for **bench curing for about 30 min.**

Bench Curing

After packing, the flask under pressure is allowed to remain on a bench for **about** 30 minutes. During this time, *the dough becomes more homogeneous,* by diffusion of all monomers. *Otherwise small irregular (microporosity)* voids are formed throughout, due to volume shrinkages of unmixed monomer present, during polymerization.

Packing of chemically curing acrylic denture base
The polymerization begins as soon as the powder (containing initiator—benzoyl peroxide) and monomer liquid (containing the activator—amine) are mixed together. This causes **a decrease of dough time as well as working time.**

Hence, the number of **trial closures are reduced,** most to two, that is packing is to be done faster (*see* curing method).

7. POLYMERIZATION (CURING)

This takes place in four stages, **initiation (induction), propagation, chain transfer, and termination** (*refer* to stages of polymerization, **polymers**). The initiator, benzoyl peroxide decomposes into free radicals when the temperature of the packed flask is raised in a water bath, above 55°C or 60°C.

Free radicals combine with monomers, **initiating** polymerization (R°+M → RM°). The process continues or **propagates** rapidly until terminated by chain transfer, or coupling with other growing chains or free radicals. This exothermic reaction liberates large amount of heat, **12,500 cal/mole.** As the dough is surrounded by nonconducting thick stone-plaster investment, this heat produced cannot be conducted quickly back to the water bath. Hence, the temperature of the polymerizing dough, **shoots up** (rises more, at thicker portions), **much above the outside water** bath temperature. If this packed flask is kept in the water bath, which is heated to boil the water (100°C) the temperature of acrylic can very quickly rise above the boiling point of monomer **(100.8°C)**, and rise even to 150°C or more, at thicker sections in the middle of the mould (Fig. 6.1).

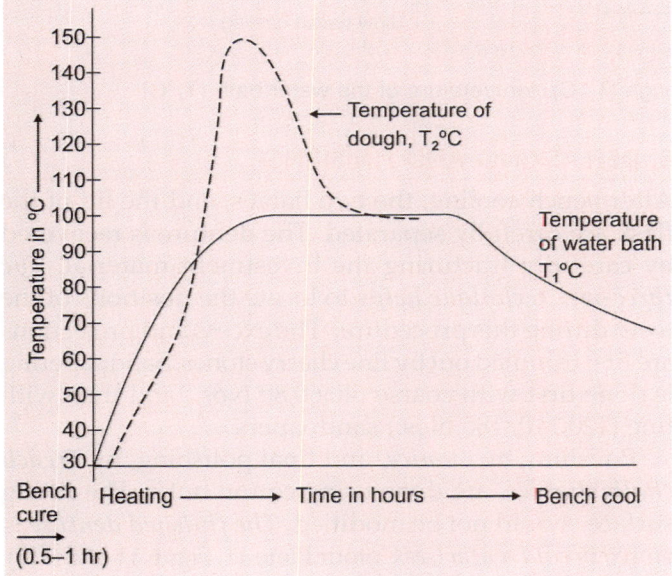

Fig. 6.1: Wrong curing cycle: The temperature of acrylic dough is (---- T_2°C) temperature of the water bath (— T_1°C). When water is heated and boiled (at 100°C)—cause boiling monomer porosity

The remaining monomer boils and converted into its vapour, forming **regular voids** known as **boiling monomer porosities.** The porosities are more at the bulkiest portions, away from the flask walls. In the case of dentures the porosities are formed at the **lingual side of bulkiest-posterior teeth setting portion.**

Hence for polymerization, a suitable curing cycle is to be adopted to **limit the rise of temperature** of the **dough well under 100°C.**

Curing Cycles

These are the methods for **complete polymerization** of heat cure acrylics, by raising the temperature of the packed flask and cooling down to room temperature. To eliminate boiling monomer porosity due to

exothermic polymerization, the temperature of the heating system (water bath) is to be kept much below the boiling point of monomer **(100.8°C)** and retained for a long time for maximum polymerization **(slow curing)**, and then cooled.

- **Slow curing:** After bench curing for about 30–60 minutes, the flask assembly is placed in a water bath and the temperature is slowly raised to **about 70°C and kept constant for about 8 hours, using a thermostat devise.** The temperature of the water bath and temperature of acrylic dough of a sample (placed in the middle) are represented by the continuous and dotted lines respectively (Fig. 6.2).

  The acrylic monomers begin to polymerize, releasing a large quantity of heat at about 60°C and temperatures rise as shown. But it cannot go beyond say 90–95°C, as that of the water bath is at a lower temperature and **excess heat generated is conducted from acrylic, back to water bath.** Thus boiling of the monomer is avoided (*see* colour plate 14, Fig. 6.22).

- **Bench cooling:** After keeping it at 70°C for about 8 hours, the heating source is switched off, and it is allowed to cool by itself in the water bath or left on the bench overnight. **Sudden cooling** of the flask, say, under running cold water tap, causes the outer investment first to contract, **producing the internal stresses** in the soft polymerized denture. **The relaxation** of this internal stresses in service, cause **crazing** resulting in the early fracture.

- **Fast curing method:** This is commonly adopted to save the curing time. The temperature of the water bath is raised to about 70°C and kept **constant for about 1 hour.** During this time about 90% of the monomer polymerizes and corresponding **heat produced is conducted back** to the water bath itself. It is heated further to boil the water for about 30 min or 60 min, when the remaining monomer polymerize with negligible heat or temperature rise as shown by the dotted line in the diagram. Afterward bench cooling is done overnight (Fig. 6.3).

  Improper temperature control causes internal and subsurface porosities in the denture, specially at the **bulkiest** (molar teeth) **portion at the lingual side due to lack of conduction of heat.**

  If **cooling also is to be done fast,** the flask assembly after curing is kept outside water bath on the bench for about 30 min. and then cooled under running cold water tap for 15 min. before deflasking. During this 30 min. cooling, the temperature inside, may decrease **below the distortion** temperature (80°C), the material becomes hard and reduces the chance of creating internal stresses (or crazing).

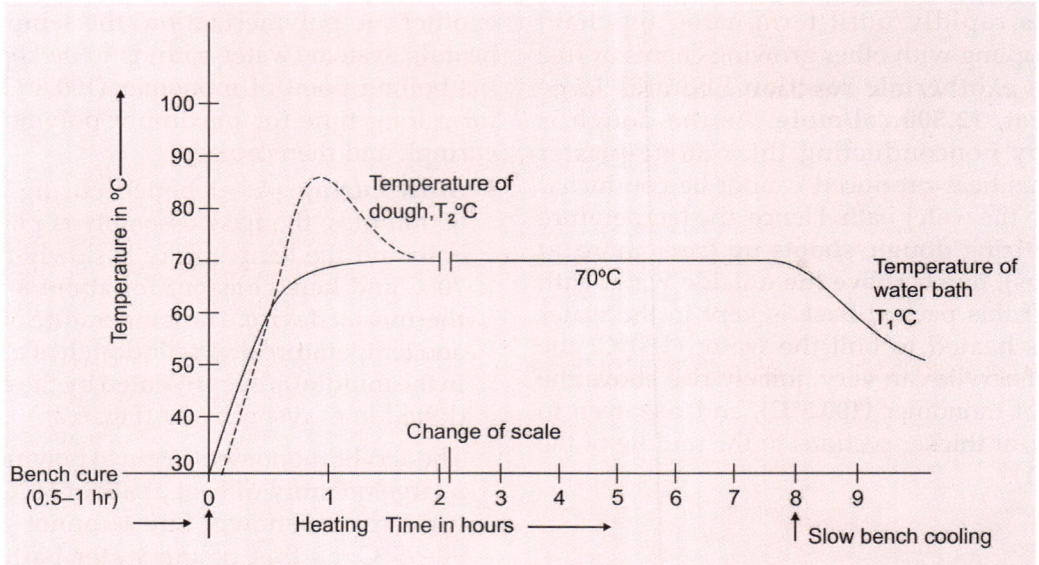

Fig. 6.2: Slow curing cycle: Temperature of acrylic dough (T_2°C), temperature of the water bath (T_1°C)

Programmed, temperature controlled curing units are used nowadays (see Colour Plate 14, Fig. 6.22).

Note 2: Microwave curing

Slightly modified resin and a nonmetallic flask are used. After packing and bench curing, the flask assembly is placed in *a microwave oven kept at low temperature (70°C–80°C) for about 1–2 hours.* Due to *greater penetration of microwaves,* the curing is done *homogeneously and at a faster rate, without causing internal boiling monomer porosities.* The mechanical, etc. properties do not improve, and the fitting is not very good.

8. DEFLASKING AND FINISHING

After bench cooling, the two halves, and the lid of the flask are carefully separated. The denture is recovered by carefully fracturing the investment material. *The three-mix technique helps* to locate the positions of the teeth during this procedure. The excess and projections are first trimmed out by fine cherry stones. Sandpapering is done first with coarse (40,60,80 Nos.) and then with fine (120,140, 180 Nos.) sandpapers.

Polishing by *pumice*, and final polishing, by *French chalk slurries,* are done using cotton buffs. The fitting surface should not be modified. *The finished denture is stored in cold water (see* Colour Plate 11, Figs 6.11 and 6.12).

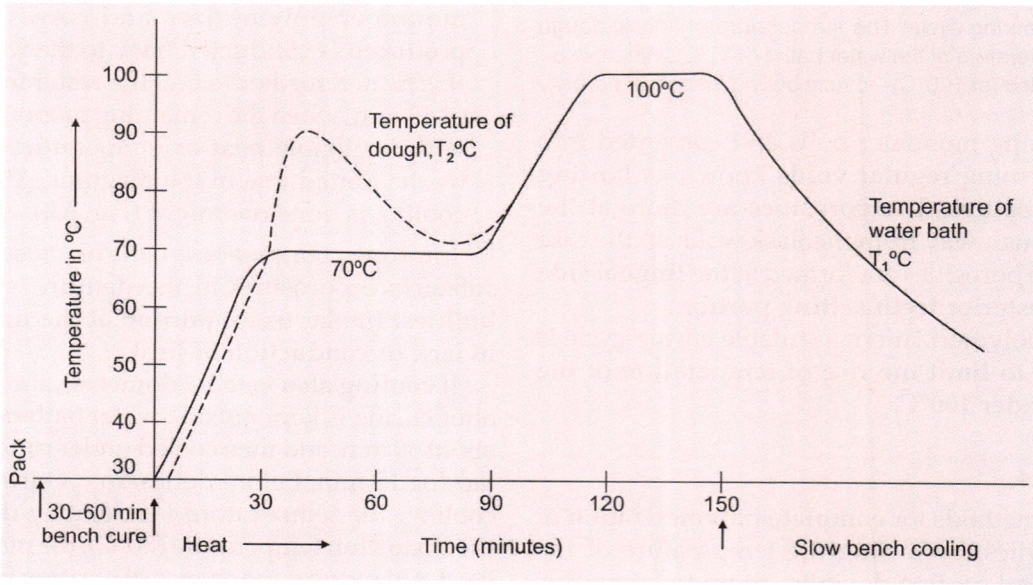

Fig. 6.3: Fast curing cycle: Temperature of acrylic dough (T_2°C) temperature of water bath (T_1°C).

Clinical Step

The dentist has to check the final fitting of the denture before delivering and ask the patient to visit after 2 or 3 days in case of small ill-fitting. The *patient is to be advised*, to keep the denture always *immersed in cold water,* when it is outside the mouth (specially while sleeping at night) and also *not to drop* on the wash basin or floor during cleaning, to avoid fracture.

SELF, COLD–CURED (CHEMICALLY ACTIVATED) ACRYLIC RESINS

These are usually supplied as powder–liquid systems having almost similar compositions, as heat cured acrylics with chemical activator *dimethyl-p-toluidine in the liquid.*

Composition for cold-cure denture-base resins (Table 6.3)

Table 6.3 Composition of cold-cure denture-base resins	
Powder	**Liquid** (in the amber-coloured bottle)
PMMA: Fine powder or beads	Methyl methacrylate— monomer
Copolymers	Comonomer
Benzoyl peroxide—initiator	N-N-dimethyl paratoluidine as activator
Dibutyl phthalate—plasticizer	Ethylene glycol for dimetha- crylate cross-linking
Colour pigments	Dibutyl phthalate—plasticizer Hydroquinone as inhibitor

Manipulation procedure

The initial clinical and laboratory procedures are the same, until packing. The powder and liquids are similarly mixed (with 3:1 ratio by weight).

As soon as these are mixed in the mixing jar, the benzoyl peroxide in presence of an amine is activated and begins to release free radicals. *Polymerization is initiated and gets propagated.* Due to this, the *dough time becomes shorter*. Also, the *working time* is reduced such that only *one or two trial closures* are possible.

Immediately after final closure, enough pressure is applied, and the flask assembly is kept in a *pressure chamber for curing.* The exothermic polymerization increases the temperature only up to about 50° to 70°C (Fig. 6.4). The polymerization requires about *1 or 2 hours* and then it cools down. There is no chance for the occurrence of boiling monomer—internal porosities unless the *article prepared is too thick*. The article is recovered and finished, by the same method.

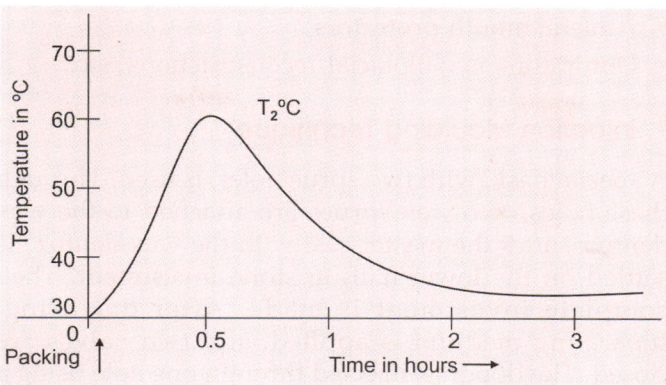

Fig. 6.4: Cold curing cycle: Temperature of acrylic dough ($T_2°C$)

Properties

Due to lower curing temperature the kinetic energy of mers is lower, the diffusion becomes less. This causes *a lower degree of polymerization* and molecular weight or chain length becomes shorter. *All the properties become inferior.*

Disadvantages of self-cure over, heat-cure acrylic

- The residual monomer is more, i.e. 5% which may cause greater allergic reactions
- All mechanical properties, compressive, tensile, flexure, impact, fatigue strengths, modulus of elasticity and resilience, surface hardness, etc. are *reduced by about 10%*. Sorption and solubilities are also slightly higher.
- The softening **glass transition temperature is slightly lower.**
- **The colour stability is also poor.** This is due to oxidation of amines, causing **yellowing** of colour gradually.

However, the main **advantages** of this chemically cured acrylics are:
- The **simpler** laboratory-curing procedure, which even does not require any heating equipment
- **Less**—internal boiling monomer **porosities**
- Less dimensional change and **better fit,** due to lower thermal shrinkage.

Note: To **overcome** the above many drawbacks, the denture containing flask, after cold-curing is sometimes kept in **a boiling water bath for 30 min. and then cooled.** This reduces residual monomer and slightly improves mechanical properties.

Applications of cold-cure acrylics

- Denture repairs
- Special trays
- Soft and hard denture relining
- Orthodontic appliances, functional removable, etc.

- Athletic mouth protectors
- Obturators, maxillofacial reconstructions, etc.

1. Injection Moulding Technique

A special flask, with two sprue holes, is used. Through these holes, two wax sprues are attached to the wax denture, after the master cast with the wax denture is settled on the lower-half, in stone investment. Then complete investment is made. After dewaxing, separating medium is applied, and two halves are closed. The dough is injected through one hole using **a high pressure-injecting device** until the excess dough begins to come out, from the other hole. After bench curing (for 30 min) it is placed in a water bath and polymerized. Extra dough may have to be injected to compensate the volume shrinkage during polymerisation. Except for slightly improved clinical accuracy, no other advantages have been noticed (*see* Colour Plate 11, Figs 6.13 to 6.17).

2. Pour and Cure—Fluid Resin Technique

This is a chemically activated resin supplied as a powder and liquids having similar compositions as the cold-cure denture-base resin. But, on mixing, it forms a **thin dough** which can be poured into the mould space prepared in a special flask.

Technique

The completed wax denture is attached with two wax rod-sprues. With the cast, it is placed on the lower half of the special flask, with holes, and closed. **Agar-agar investment** is melted and poured into it and allowed to set or gelate. The two halves are separated. The wax denture and sprue rods are pulled out. The teeth are separated, cleaned and fitted in agar in their positions.

The thin dough is prepared, and poured through one sprue, until, all trapped air is vented out and excess comes out through the other hole (**similar to injection moulding technique**). It is kept in a **pressure chamber** for 30–60 minutes for polymerization. The smooth denture **is recovered,** and the sprue excess is removed. Very **minimum polishing** is needed and can be delivered to the patient in a **short time**.

Advantages

- The simpler and quicker technique with lower cost
- Finishing and polishing a minimum procedure
- Less thermal change—cause better fit
- Less damage to artificial teeth while deflasking.

Table 6.4	Comparison of heat-cure and cold-cure acrylic denture resins	
Considerations	*Heat-cure*	*Cold-cure*
1. Composition	Powder–liquid system	In addition, liquid contains chemical activator—dimethyl paratoluidine
2. Activator	Heat (above 60°C)	Chemical activator
3. Initiator	Benzoyl peroxide	Same for chemically cure [*Note*: benzoin methyl ether for UVC, camphoroquinone for VLC (in liquid)]
4. Residual monomer	Less—better biocompatible	Higher—may cause some allergic reactions
5. Mechanical properties	Superior due to higher degree of polymerization (or mol. wt) stronger, higher impact strength, lower creep	Lower by about 10% / Fractures more easily abraded more easily
6. Porosity	More, due to boiling monomer	Less
7. Distortion and dimensional change	More	Less, better fit for chemical cure but more for pour and cure
8. Curing temperature	More than about 60°C	Room temperature
9. Processing time	Longer	Shorter
10. Processing procedure	Complicated	Simpler—no flasking is required in many cases
11. Equipment	More expensive thermostat controlled water bath	No heating equipment
12. Aesthetic	Better	Colour may slowly change due to oxidation of amines

Disadvantages
- Poor bonding of acrylic teeth to denture
- Shifting of teeth due to soft investment
- Larger polymerization shrinkage
- Air trapping
- Decrease in vertical dimensions
- Same disadvantages as the cold-cure acrylic dentures—higher residual monomer, lower mechanical properties, higher solubility, etc.

3. Light Cure Denture-base Technique

This is a single component system supplied as a **sheet and rope forms in light proof pouches**.

This has composite resin-like compositions
- High molecular weight acrylic resin monomer
- Urethane dimethacrylate—cross-linking agent-matrix
- Microfine silica inorganic fillers
- Acrylic resin particles—organic filler
- Camphoroquinone—initiator
- N-N-dimethyl paratoluidine—accelerator
  As visible light of wavelength $\lambda = 468$ nm is used as activator, **opaque investment-flasking technique cannot be used.**

Outline of technique
- The finished waxed-up trial denture is kept ready and visible light curable resin sheet is adapted on the denture over the occlusal surface of teeth to form a template. This template is exposed to visible light and cured for 10 minutes in a light chamber. The heat, during this curing time, softens the wax. With the teeth in the template, the wax denture and cast are placed in boiling water, and complete dewaxing is done.
- Separating medium or **releasing agent** is applied on the cast. Light-activated denture base sheet (and ropes) are adapted on the cast and cured (like a base plate).
- Another strip or sheet is placed under the teeth, which are repositioned, and kept in contact with the previous base, and anatomical form is carved to develop final shape and cured in a light chamber. Finally, denture is removed from the cast and finished. The method is more complicated, expensive, and no improvement of properties.

Modified denture-base materials
- **High impact strength** rubber modified acrylics: **Butadiene–styrene** rubber is included, to obtain higher resilience, abrasive resistance, impact strength, toughness, etc.
- **Rapid processing heat cure acrylics:** This can be cured by placing the packed flask, directly immersing in boiling water, immediately after packing for short time, without producing porosities.
- **Fibre reinforced** acrylics have higher impact strength.
- **Soft foldable/flexible dentures—for partial dentures (VALPLAST):** It is a type of nylon and thermoplastic, which is injection molded above 300°C. The retention of acrylic teeth with Valplast is by mechanical means by drilling holes in acrylic teeth.
- **Biocide-releasing polymers:** Silver nanoparticles were added to PMMA at different quantities but less effective for a longer time.
- **Antimicrobial polymers in acrylic denture base resins (polymeric biocides):**
  The absence of ionic charge, *hydrophobic interaction* and mechanical attachment favors biofilm formation and growth of the microorganism (*Candida albicans*) lead to tissue irritation and denture stomatitis. Antimicrobial polymers (e.g. MDPB 12-methacryloyloxy-dodecylpyridium bromide) *incorporated to PMMA by copolymerization*.

Critique of Heat-cured Acrylics and its Suitability for Denture-base Material

Only the aesthetics, biocompatibility and simpler fabrication techniques are the plus points, whereas, the mechanical and thermal properties are not very satisfactory.

1. **Biocompatibility**
   Completely polymerized acrylic resin is chemically inert, and non-toxic. Very rarely patients have allergic reactions. Toxicity is more in cold cure acrylics as the residual the monomer present is more (about 5%) than that in heat-cured acrylics (0.5%). Technicians come into contact with the monomer (MMA), benzoyl peroxide, hydroquinones, etc. while manipulating the dough (packing) and sensitization of the fingers causing dermatitis, is more frequently observed. It is tasteless, hygienic and not foul smelling.

2. **Physical and mechanical**
   - Even though density is low (1.19 gm/cc), due to poor mechanical properties, thick (2 mm–3 mm) dentures are to be prepared, which have greater weight and less retention. (Stainless steel denture base is lighter.)
   - Proportional limit (27 MPa), compressive strength (75 MPa), tensile strength (65 MPa), flexure strength (85 MPa) impact strength (0.98 to 1.27 J/m^3), modulus of elasticity (2,500 MPa) are not satisfactory. Careless handling, large dynamic masticating forces, and accidental falls cause a fracture.
   - Low surface hardness (18–20 KHN) and poor abrasive resistance, cause abrasion of denture and attrition of acrylic teeth by opposing natural or porcelain teeth.
   - Large polymerization shrinkage as well as thermal shrinkage during fabrication, cause dimensional inaccuracy and misfit.

- Viscoelastic nature may cause dimensional changes creep in long time service.
- Low fatigue strength and endurance limit (1.5 million cycles at 17 MPa) show a limited service-time or life, around 5 to 6 years.
  Note: Chemically, i.e. self-cure acrylics, have mechanical properties, about 10% lower than those for heat-cured acrylics due to the lower degree of polymerization.

3. **Thermal**
   - Low thermal conductivity causes the patient inability to feel the real taste (hotness or coldness) of food.
   - A higher coefficient of thermal contraction (80–120 ppm/°C) results in large shrinkage while cooling polymerized denture from about 85°C down to oral temperature (37°C) and adds up to total dimensional inaccuracy. (As this thermal shrinkage is smaller in cold-cured and light-cured dentures, have slightly better fit).

4. **Aesthetics**
   - Colourless and transparent **organic glass**
   - Any colour pigments, **vein-like coloured nylon fibres** can be added to get a natural appearance.
   - Good colour stability for heat-cure acrylics. But chemically cured acrylics gradually become more **yellowish** due to oxidation of residual amines.

5. **Other considerations**
   - Fabrication technique is time-consuming but not complicated-like alloy casting techniques
   - Simple equipment and cheap auxiliary materials
   - Shelf life of monomer liquid is limited
   - Not very expensive.

DEFECTS OF DENTURES

Fabrication of denture involves **a series of steps** and unless suitable precautions are followed, several defects may occur (all remedies are suggestive).

1. **Dimensional changes due to inherent properties** of the materials during fabrication, by water sorption, solubility, creep, etc. which cause misfit or poor retention.
2. **Fabrication defects** such as surface roughness and irregularities, internal porosities, and crazing. These cause poor aesthetics, unhygienic, and week dentures, etc.
3. **Processing stresses:** Crazing

1. Dimensional Changes

These are caused by polymerization shrinkage, thermal shrinkage, expansion by water sorption and creep due to viscoelastic properties.

- **Polymerization shrinkage:** Theoretical calculation from the densities of monomer (0.945 gm/ml) and polymer (1.19 gm/cc) shows a polymerization—**volume shrinkage of 21%** or linear shrinkage 7%. To reduce this large shrinkage prepolymerized powder is added to monomer at about 3:1 ratio by weight such that the shrinkage becomes about 7% by volume or 2% by linear. However, this is further reduced because:
  - There is a chance for the inclusion of slight excess dough material, due to high pressure, while packing.
  - The temperature during polymerization is around 85–90°C which is slightly above Tg, and hence initially the polymerized material is in soft condition. While cooling, the investment cools earlier, due to which this soft resin is not allowed to undergo shrinkage, or the shrinkage is inhibited by adhesion to mould walls. These two factors slightly compensate the polymerization shrinkage, down to around 0.4%.

- **Thermal shrinkage** is again effective below Tg only. The large coefficient of thermal shrinkage, nearly 80–120 ppm/°C may produce about 0.7% linear contractions when cooled from Tg to 37°C. This shrinkage also adds up to the polymerization shrinkage, causing dimensional inaccuracy and misfit (nearly 0.9–1.0%). In the case of cold-cure or light-cure acrylic dentures, as the range of temperatures of cooling (after curing) is smaller, this inaccuracy or misfit is slightly lower.

- **Water sorption:** When the acrylic denture is kept in water or mouth, the polarity of polymethyl-methacrylate causes adsorption of water molecules by van der Waals force. These water molecules enter into the polymer system by diffusion. **This sorption of water**, causes slight separation of polymer chains and increase the dimension in about a week or even up to about 17 days. **To measure this sorption**, an acrylic disc of standard dimensions is prepared and completely dried to reach a minimum weight (W_1 gm). It is then kept immersed in water (at 37°C) for 7 days and again weighed (W_2 gm). The increase in weight ($W_2–W_1$) mgm. per unit area of the surface, measures the **sorption.** It is about **0.6 to 0.7** mg/cm^2 (ADA specification No. 12 is <0.8 mg/cm^2). The water thus absorbed, enters into the space in between the polymer chains and forces them apart, so that it.
  - Acts as a *plasticiser and reduces the strength.*
  - Causes an expansion of about **0.2%** linear, which slightly compensates the thermal and polymerization shrinkages.

– On drying later, it causes relaxation of the internal stresses. Repeated drying and wetting of acrylic denture, causes crazing (microcracks). The total dimensional changes, appear large about 0.2 to 0.9%. However, this has *no much clinical significance regarding the fit, as the soft oral tissues can accommodate these changes*.

- **Solubility:** The solubility of acrylics in water or saliva is very negligible, *<0.04 mg/cm² as per ADA specification No. 12.* The disc weighed (W_2 gm) after keeping in water for 7 days, is again completely dried and weighed (W_3 gm) (refer: water sorption). The loss in weight ($W_1–W_3$) mgm, per unit area of the surface of the disc in 7 days duration is considered as the solubility. The cold-cure acrylic has slightly greater solubility than the solubility of heat-cure acrylics. As both of these are very low values these have **no clinical significance.**

- **Creep:** *It is the time-dependent deformations (flow) of viscoelastic materials under constant static or dynamic* loads. Many materials exhibit this property when they are near to their fusion temperatures. Acrylic polymer resins have Tg about 85°C which is not very high, and hence they behave-like viscoelastic materials.

The creep rate is more when the

- Temperature is higher
- Dynamic masticating forces are higher
- Residual monomer is more
- Plasticizers are more
- Degree of polymerization is less
- Cross-linking is less

Due to the above factors, the cold-cure acrylics have higher creep value. This creep rate has significance in long service, due to dimensional changes.

2. Denture Fabrication Defects and Remedies

Some of the properties of acrylic resins specially the mechanical ones are not entirely satisfactory. Hence, several possible defects should be remedied to get better fit, strength, aesthetics, etc.

a. **Rough surface** causes unhygienic condition by collection of food debris, poor aesthetics by scattering of light and irritation or abrasion of the soft tissues coming into contact. If the tissue side of denture is polished, it may not fit well. The **causes** which can be remedied are the following: (remedies are suggestive)

- Rough wax pattern
- Coarse powder particles of the cast and investment flasking materials
- High water/powder ratio and inadequate mixing of plaster stone

– Air trapping due to inadequate vibration of plaster mix
– Inadequate wetting of hydrophobic wax denture surface. (It can be washed or coated with a detergent, a surfactant or debubblizer solutions for better wetting)
– Incomplete and rapid dewaxing
– Improper application of separating medium
– Late or too early packing—before dough stage is reached or after
– Lack of pressure during packing or curing.

b. **Internal porosities:** Porous dentures lack strength and aesthetic qualities. Various types of porosities are to be considered. Their causes and remedies are the following:

- **Irregular voids:** If the monomer liquid and polymer powders are *not mixed properly,* or the liquid has not diffused properly to make the dough homogeneous, larger polymerization shrinkage takes place, at the sites of higher monomer concentrations. This causes irregular voids. *Bench curing* for about 30 min. allows the monomer to diffuse, homogeneously.

- **Opacity (micro-irregular voids):** This is caused due to *inadequate pressure* during the polymerization period. If the pressure is not applied, fine *micro-irregular voids*—porosities are created due to polymerization shrinkage, throughout the entire volume. This scatters and prevents the refraction (passage) of light resulting in opacity and poor aesthetics.

- **Regular voids: Boiling monomer porosity:** A large amount of heat *(12,500 cal/gm mol.)* is liberated during polymerization. As soon as polymerization begins to propagate, this heat generated adds up to the heat supplied and increases the temperature, of the polymerizing resin, **much above the outside temperature,** i.e. that of the water bath (or atmosphere in cold-cure system). Hence, if the temperature of the surrounding water bath is raised to high value, say 90°C or 100°C, i.e. the boiling point of water, the temperature of the acrylic dough can shoot up, even to 140°C or 160°C at thicker regions. This makes remaining monomer liquid to boil (BP = 100.8°C) and the vapour produced later cause **regular voids,** known as boiling monomer porosity. In the case of dentures, such porosities occur more at **thicker posterior–lingual side regions,** where the temperatures are higher.

The remedy is, not to allow the temperature of acrylic dough inside the flask to rise beyond say 90°C or 95°C. For this, proper curing cycle, i.e. slow curing at about 70°C for 8 or 10 hours, or careful fast curing methods are chosen (*refer* to curing cycles).

- **Regular voids: Sub-surface porosity:** These are regular boiling monomer porosities, forming **well below the surfaces.** The exothermic polymerization heat raises the temperature more at bulkier parts. **This heat produced cannot get conducted immediately to outside cooler surrounding water bath, as both resins and the plaster investments are poor conductors** of heat. That is why, the temperature of the resin rises more at the bulkier part as well as in the **far away middle portion** of the flask, and makes the remaining monomer boil at these regions. This sub-surface porosity is formed at the lingual side of the bulkiest—posterior parts of the denture, and sometimes in the thicker palatal portion of the mandibular denture. **The remedy is also slow curing at lower temperatures.**

- **Regular large voids air inclusion porosity:** This occurs due to trapping of air while packing the resin dough. Proper kneading of the resin dough before packing and application of high pressure are the remedies (Fig. 6.5).

3. Processing Stresses (Crazing)

Internal stresses of various types, are induced during the fabrication as well as in service, in different parts of denture. This is due to the *inhibition of dimensional changes,* which otherwise might have taken place. These internal stresses, cause *separation of polymer chains* and produce, many *microcracks. During relaxation, in service, these microcracks slowly increase in length, breadth, and depth.* This is known as crazing and the affected region appears *chalky or hazy,* loses strength and aesthetics and *finally, fracture takes place.* Main reasons for the internal stresses and crazing (all remedies are suggestive) are:

- **Rapid cooling after curing:** The outer portion of investment cools earlier and contracts initially. The soft denture (which is slightly, above its Tg), is adhering to the mould walls. This frictional adhesion of two materials of different coefficients of thermal contractions, and both being nonconductors, inhibit the contraction of acrylics. The internal stresses cause separation of polymer chains, and microcracks (remedy: Cool the flask by itself, i.e. **bench cooling overnight).**

- **Porcelain teeth in acrylic dentures:** Porcelain teeth and acrylic dentures have a vast difference in their coefficients of thermal expansions of about 7 to 8 ppm/°C and 80–120 ppm/°C respectively. When the oral temperatures fluctuate by hot or cold food, the teeth and denture expand and contract differently creating **internal stresses at their interface.** The microcracks/crazing is formed in the weaker denture around the porcelain teeth (*remedy:* **Select acrylic teeth for acrylic dentures).**

- **Separating medium:** If not applied correctly, water from plaster enters into resin dough. This goes out later creating voids, which become centers of stress concentrations and relaxations (remedy).

- **Internal porosities** (Fig. 6.5) also act as stress-concentration regions (remedy: Minimise internal porosities).

- **A chemical attack** by eugenol, alcohols, etc. (remedy: Minimise their contacts).

- **Solvent actions:** Increase the size of microcracks rapidly due to their tendency to push apart the polymer chains.

- **Repeated drying and wetting** of denture in service accelerates the internal stress relaxation, and cause crazing. (The patients are advised to keep their dentures in water when not used, i.e. at night.)

- **Cross-linked acrylic resins** have higher resistance to the separation of polymer chains and hence **decrease crazing as well as a creep.**

- Dimethacrylate system resins (like BisGMA) have a highly **cross-linked** three-dimensional structure and resist crazing.

- **Silicate cements,** which can absorb water into its gel structure, and relax on repeated wetting and drying also undergo crazing and hence was contraindicated to mouth breathers.

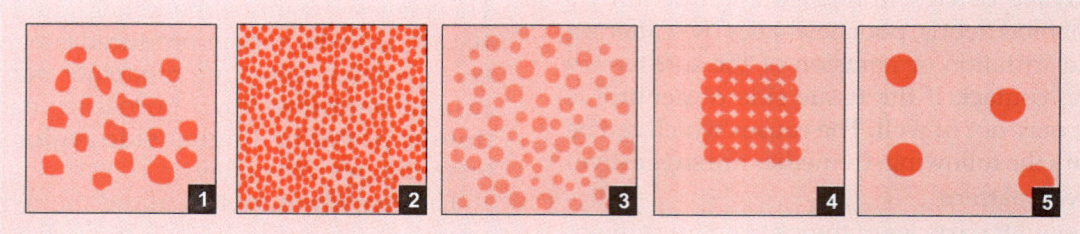

Fig. 6.5: Internal porosities. 1. Large irregular voids (inhomogeneous mixing of dough), 2. Small irregular voids (lack of pressure—opacity), 3. Regular voids (boiling monomer), 4. Regular voids (subsurface porosity—lack of heat conduction), 5. Large regular voids (air inclusion in dough)

Miscellaneous Resins and Techniques

1. Denture Reliners

Mainly three varieties of relining materials are used for different clinical situations. In all, extra materials are lined on the tissue surface of the dentures as required.

A. Hard liners

Due to the resorption and shrinkage of the tissues, after the teeth extraction, the denture prepared gradually becomes lose or misfitting. This requires an additional layer on the tissue side of the denture for a better fit.

- **Requirements** (ADA specification No. 17): These are same as those for a denture base materials. Also, it should **chemically bond** with the old denture base, and retain dimensional stability.
- **Materials used:** Usually cold-cure acrylics and sometimes heat cure acrylics with compositions similar to denture base resins, are used.
- **Techniques of fabrications:** Using the old misfitting denture as a **special tray, alginate impression** of the modified oral structure is obtained, and a dental stone cast is prepared. The stone cast and the old denture with the alginate impression are invested in the flask. After setting, the two halves are separated, and the **alginate impression material is completely removed**. Separating medium is applied. The polymer powder and monomer liquids are mixed. The resin dough is packed in the space between the stone cast and denture (i.e. in the space earlier occupied by the alginate impression). After curing, the denture is recovered, and slight finishing is done (colour plates 12 and 13, Figs 6.18a to j).

Cold-cure acrylic is preferred due to

- Simpler technical (curing) procedure
- Less distortion or warpage of denture. In heat cured denture relining procedures the polymerization shrinkage of the liner, causes **warpage** of the old denture when reheated to temperatures > Tg.
- Repeated heating of old denture causes distortion if heat-cured material and procedure is used.
- The strength of cold-cure acrylic is adequate, for the liner.

Modifications

- Some special relining fixtures (or mounting assembly) can be used. The method does not require elaborate flasking procedures.
- Some manufacturers supply cold-cure acrylics or polysilicone liners—chairside materials which the patients with adequate knowledge, can use himself.
- Visible light cured materials are also supplied.

B. Long-term soft resilient liners/soft resilient liners:

Long-term permanent soft liners and short-term tissue conditioners (Part C, page 128) are very soft cushion-like materials, lined on tissue side of dentures. These absorb the large dynamic, *masticating energies* and distribute, as required by the clinical situations. For obtaining these resilient properties, highly plasticized resins or elastomeric materials are used by addition of *plasticizers* like *dibutyl or dioctyl phthalate*. The polymer chains are reduced in length and are also separated more. They can slip easily one over the other (i.e. flexible) and also can recover from the large elastic deformations (i.e. resilient).

Requirements of soft liners: *In addition to* those for denture bases and those for hard liners, the following properties are required:

- Hygienic, i.e. they should not collect food debris and become foul smelling or seat for the growth of microorganisms like *Candida albicans* (e.g. as polysilicones)
- Large modulus of resilience (cushion-like property)
- Permanently resilient (i.e. plasticizers should not leach out)
- Chemically bond with acrylic denture bases
- Dimensionally stable, i.e. should not absorb oral fluids and swell
- Easy to trim and polish, to form a clean surface.

Materials used for long-term permanent soft liners

a. Polysilicones

- Chemically activated material is similar to condensation impression materials, supplied as a two-paste system.
- Heat-cured system is supplied as a single paste or gel.

The techniques are similar to denture relining. *The old denture* is provided with a *relief space*, by removing the material of some thickness from the tissue surface of denture. Alginate impression is obtained. Flasking, removal of alginate material, packing of the soft resilient liner in the space by a compression moulding technique, and then curing is done in pressure-chamber or heated water bath.

Advantage

Have permanent high resilience. Sometimes, **rubber—polymethyl methacrylate—cements** are used for **bonding** with a denture.

Disadvantages

- Poor bonding to acrylic denture
- Difficult to trim or polish
- The pores of the material can collect fluid or food debris which can be a *seat for the microorganisms*

or promote the growth of fungus (Candida albicans). To overcome this some antimycotic or antifungal agents can be used.

- Poor dimensional stability due to absorption of fluids
- Strength of denture decreases by reducing the denture thickness for providing relief space.

b. **Polymer resins:** These are highly plasticized polymethyl methacrylates and both chemically, and heat-cured resins are available. *The external plasticizers like dibutyl or octyl phthalates* are added in large quantities. These may leach out in service due to temperature fluctuations in the mouth, and gradually turn *brittle.* Higher methacrylates like polyethyl or butyl methacrylates have lower Tg and require less plasticizers. Copolymerization (internal plasticizer) can be done to decrease Tg.

These plasticizer molecules are quite large, that they push the polymer chains apart, reduce the entanglement of chains; so that the chains slip one over the other easily. That is, it becomes soft, flexible, elastically recoverable and very resilient. These polymer resins can **bond** with the acrylic denture, but gradually lose resilience and **become stiffer.**

c. **Highly plasticized** polyvinyl chlorides and acetates have been tried. These also become stiffer.

d. **Plasticized polyurethanes,** polyphosphazenes were also tried but, without much success.

None of the above materials satisfy all the requisites and it is quite difficult to choose suitable material.

C. **Short-term resilient liners—tissue conditioners**
In certain clinical situations, the denture may obstruct easy blood circulation, in some inflamed, irritated mucosa or distorted parts of the soft tissues. To enhance the healing of the affected part some "massaging" effect is required for a few days, by a soft, resilient liner until the tissues become **normal**. These short-term soft liners are sometimes called **tissue conditioners.** Materials used are chemically cured, polymethyl methacrylate or higher methacrylates with large amounts of plasticizers. These are supplied as a powder of polymethyl methacrylates or its higher copolymers. *The liquid is not methyl methacrylate monomer.* **The liquid has large molecular sized plasticizer, some aromatic esters like butyl phthalate, butyl glycolate or dibutyl phthalates of about 50 to 80% in alcohol or ethanol.** When these are mixed, the plasticizers decrease the entanglement of the polymer chain thereby increasing the softness, and decrease Tg.

Tissue conditioners can be formed directly in the patient's mouth. Suitable relief space is prepared in the denture. The powder and liquid are mixed and packed *directly on the denture,* which is held firmly in the patient's mouth in position for self-curing. After a few minutes, the excess is removed.

Since this is only a temporary lining, good *bonding* to the tissue side of denture *is not required.*

Recently a new technique for soft liners is studied. A viscous silicone liquid is filled in an envelope of thin polyethylene film. This liner has an advantage of continuous adaptation to the denture base.

Problems faced in fabrication and use of soft liners
- Poor mechanical bonding–debonding from dentures
- No permanent resilience: Due to leaching of plasticizers and stiffening in service
- Dimensional instability: Due to the absorption of oral fluids
- Poor hygiene: Collect food debris, become foul smelling, and promote the *growth of microorganisms like* Candida albicans.
- Difficulty in polishing, and maintain cleanliness
- The decrease of strength of the denture due to forming of *relief space.*

2. Denture Rebasing Technique

In certain clinical situations, the denture base gets abraded and damaged, whereas, the denture teeth remain without any damage. In such cases, new denture base can be done by rebasing technique.

The material used is the same as **heat cure** acrylic resins.

Method
Using the old denture as tray obtain the alginate impression of the oral structure and prepare the stone-cast. Mount these in a device known as **reline jig.** The positions of teeth are carefully indexed with respect to their occlusal surface. The teeth are removed and positioned in the jig. On the cast, the denture base-plate and occlusal rims are adapted. The teeth are then fixed according to their indices. The finished wax denture is then processed and acrylised in the conventional method.

The rebasing technique is not used frequently as the procedure is similar and time consuming like the fabrication of new denture. However, if the patient **cannot attend the clinical procedures,** this can be adopted.

3. Denture Repair Resins (ADA No.13)

Due to poor mechanical properties and low impact strength ($0.98 J/m^3$-$1.25 J/m^3$) the denture may fracture easily by mishandling or accidental drops. Instead of repeating the whole, time-consuming procedure, the broken denture can be repaired (Fig. 6.6).

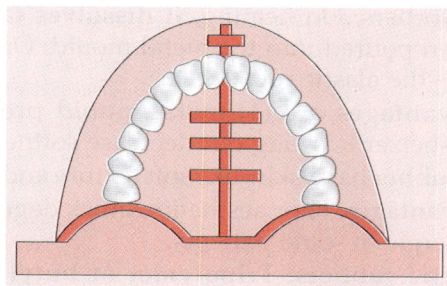

Fig. 6.6: Denture repair (color plate 13, Fig. 6.19)

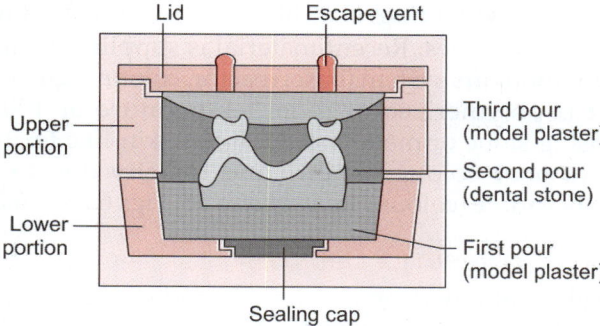

Fig. 6.7: Flasking the wax by multiple mix method

Selection of materials

Even though heat-cure acrylic resin has better mechanical properties; cold-cure acrylic resin is preferred due to the following reasons:

- The repairing procedure is simpler and less time-consuming.
- Thermal shrinkage of the repair cold-cure acrylic is smaller.
- Repeated heating and cooling may cause warpage of the denture if heat cure acrylic is used.

Method

Fractured pieces are joined together using **sticky wax,** and a stone-cast is prepared. Sticky wax is eliminated by flushing with hot water. Sharp corners at the fractured sites are trimmed and few cross-link lines of 2 or 3 mm length are cut, to provide enough space and bonding for the repair resin. The cast is coated with a separating medium (*see* Colour Plate 13, Fig. 6.19).

The repair sites are wetted with few drops of monomer and the polymer powder is sprinkled on it. This dissolves and forms a dough. Repeat this until a little excess dough is formed (to compensate polymerization shrinkage). It is then allowed to cure in a pressure chamber. The excess is trimmed, polishing is done, and the repaired denture is kept immersed in water until delivery.

4. Resin Special Trays and Baseplate Materials

The rigid metallic stock trays of particular standard sizes are not very suitable for individual patients. Hence, custom-made special trays are prepared.

The **material** used is cold-cure acrylic resins, supplied as monomer liquid and fine polymer powder or beads. The powder, also contains some inorganic fillers like **French-chalk or zinc oxide** powder to improve the workability.

Method

A preliminary impression is taken, and a stone-cast is prepared. A spacer like a wax sheet of a thickness of about 2–3 mm is adapted on the cast.

The acrylic dough is rolled into a thin sheet of a uniform thickness of about 2–3 mm, using a **template** and then closely adapted over the spacer on the cast and allowed to self-cure. It is better to wait for 24 hours to attain better dimensional stability. Then the spacer is removed, and the special tray is used. Sometimes suitable tray-adhesive is applied to bond with rubber base impression. **Urethane dimethacrylate trays** also can be prepared similarly.

Advantages

- The distortions of the impression due to relaxation of internal stresses induced by setting shrinkage and thermal shrinkages are minimized, as the **impression has a uniform thickness.**
- **Less wastage** of expensive impression materials.

Disadvantage

Cannot be reused for any other patient.

Note: **Earlier, shellac base plates** of uniform thickness were used by warming over a flame and adapting over the spacer on the cast. But acrylics have better dimensional accuracy.

5. Maxillofacial Reconstruction Materials

These are used for **correction or replacements** of the defects of the **craniofacial complex,** such as *ear, nose, eye orbits,* etc. resulting from cancer surgeries, accidents or congenital deformities. These are fabricated mainly for aesthetics and sometimes for functions. Many materials have been tried for fabrications, but none satisfies all the stringent requirements.

Requirements

- **Biocompatible** with the skin nontoxic, chemically stable and hygienic
- **Skin-like soft, flexible texture,** with high tear strength, resistance to abrasion, elastic movements under stresses.
- **Elastic** properties should be permanent, i.e. plasticizers should not leach out.
- Able to withstand **thermal fluctuations**, ultraviolet and infrared radiations.
- **Aesthetically** most suitable, and stable. Should be able to incorporate suitable matching colour shades like oil paints, earth pigments, etc.

- The above properties should **not degrade in service necessitating frequent replacements**.
- **Fabrication technique** should be simple using simple inexpensive equipment.

The fabrication methods involved are quite complicated, technique sensitive (like colouring) and require highly expensive equipment in many cases. An ordinary patient may find it difficult to afford the prosthesis and its frequent replacements due to **degradations.**

Outline of fabrication

Many steps of fabrication are common to most materials and sometimes are modified. An **alginate impression is taken, a stone master cast** is prepared, the suitable wax pattern is carved on the **master cast,** invested, dewaxed, packed with the materials—**dough, putty or paste consistencies** and polymerized. Suitable colour pigments are added to the dough **(internal colouring)** before packing. Sometimes, the inner part of the semitransparent prosthesis is painted with oil paints **(external colouring)**, which method is not good due to poor colour stability.

Materials used

a. **Polysilicones:** Both **heat curing** and room temperature vulcanizing **(RTV)** types are used. The **RTV** type is a single paste system, of similar compositions as addition polysilicone impression materials. Suitable (intrinsic) colour pigments like **dry earth, rayon fibres, oil paints,** etc. are added to the pastes. Fabrication is done using a stone or metal moulds, at room temperature. This has **good flexibility, skin-like texture, tear strength, etc.** However, the properties gradually **change** in service.

Heat curing variety has still better mechanical properties. This is supplied as **high viscosity putty consistency,** containing moderately low molecular weight poly dimethyl vinyl siloxane, 2–4 dichlorobenzoyl peroxide (initiator) and silica fillers. Colour pigments are to be intrinsically added by using an **expensive rolling milling machine**. It has properties better than RTV type.

The disadvantages are (1) expensive milling machine (2) metal mould (3) higher curing temperature (180–220°C) (4) sometimes unhygienic (5) difficult to polish and trim.

b. **Plasticized polymethyl methacrylate** or higher methacrylates. The fabrication method is simpler, curing is done at room temperature, using a stone mould.

Disadvantages are (1) prosthesis is heavy (2) low flexibility (3) gradual hardening due to leaching of plasticizer. Hence, it is not suitable.

c. **Plasticized PVC:** Supplied as finely divided **PVC particles suspended in a solvent**. This also contains small amounts of cross-linking agents and ultraviolet ray absorbers. On heating, **it dissolves (at 150°C)**, and then poured into the metal mould. On cooling, it forms the elastic prosthesis.

Disadvantages are (1) metal mould preparation (2) plasticizer leaching out decrease softness.

d. **Latex rubber** has a skin-like soft texture and low cost. **Disadvantages:** Poor aesthetics, quick degeneration, and allergic to some patients.

e. **Synthetic rubbers: Tripolymer of butyl acrylate, methyl methacrylate, and methyl methacrylamide.** This has good aesthetics (temporary), obtained by extrinsic colouring, skin-like softness, **but short life.**

f. **Polyurethanes:** Recent material is supplied as **three components** system (base, reactor, colour pigments). It is polymerized at room temperature or 100°C, using stone or metal mould. It has skin-like texture, but poor colour stability and **toxicity due to di-isocyanate** (colour plates 14 and 15, Figs 6.23 to 6.26).

6. Artificial Teeth for Dentures

Acrylic teeth: Both anatomical 33° and non-anatomical zero degree acrylic resin teeth—sets are available in **various colour shades and sizes for selection**. These are commonly selected due to the chemical bonding and **higher fracture resistance** compared to porcelain teeth.

These are prepared from heat cure acrylic, supplied as a powder and liquid forms. Larger amounts of **cross-linking agents, glycol or other dimethacrylates** are included to improve mechanical properties and decrease crazing. Suitable colour shades are also added. **Split brass-moulds** (similar to those used to prepare porcelain teeth) are used for packing the dough of suitable shades. It is possible to make the labial side and incisal portions more transparent, by packing this dough of more transparent material in the labial half of mould, and more opaque dough in the lingual half of mould. After, heat curing, polishing and finishing are done.

CAD-CAM and 3D printing techniques are also used for the fabrications of artificial teeth.

Mechanical bonding of teeth with acrylic denture is improved by

1. Removing the glossy ridge-lap surface of teeth
2. Roughening the bonding surface
3. Cutting small grooves or holes in the bonding surface.

Chemical bonding of teeth is improved by

1. Wetting the ridge-lap surface with methyl methacrylate monomer liquid.
2. Coating with a mixture of methylene chloride and MMA liquid to the necks or ridge-lap area, five minutes before use.
3. Complete dewaxing by flushing with hot water or using a detergent.
4. Avoiding coating of separating medium on the bonding surface of teeth.

The bonding of acrylic teeth to acrylic denture is **predominantly chemical** and hence bond—strength is better than the porcelain teeth (Table 6.5).

7. Porcelain Teeth (Colour Plate 14, Fig. 6.21)

The superior permanent **aesthetic** quality, higher resistance to abrasion and biocompatibility are the main criteria for fabrication and selection.

The manufacturing method of teeth is more complicated. **Split brass moulds of two or three sections are used**. Two halves have the semi-mould spaces corresponding to the labial and lingual sides of the teeth of different sizes. Porcelain powders of suitable shades corresponding to more opaque dentin, more transparent enamel (labial side) and incisal (transparent) porcelain powders are chosen, and mixed with special liquids to form slurries. Enamel porcelain is packed (1 or 2 mm thick) on the labial half, dentin porcelain on the lingual side half and transparent slurry are packed at the incisal tip of the moulds. Small **base metal rings** are inserted in the anterior teeth as provisions for fixing the gold plated retention pins and also some **wax provisions for diatoric or rhetoric holes,** in posterior teeth. **Two parts are pressed together and fired up to the low bisque stage.** The teeth are removed, placed in quartz trays and **fired under vacuum or in diffusible gases,** in an electric furnace, cooled under pressure, finished and glazed. To overcome the large shrinkages, the mould spaces should be larger.

Porcelain teeth also are supplied in various shades and sizes. Mechanical retention is achieved by rhetoric or diatoric holes, in the posterior and rarely in the anterior teeth. Gold plated base metal alloy pins are fitted to the small alloy rings inside anterior teeth (Figs 13.9a to c).

Main disadvantages are

1. Brittleness—low fracture resistance to impact forces
2. High cost
3. Clicking sound when opposite teeth contact
4. Abrasion of opposing natural teeth.

8. Composite Resins Artificial Teeth

The recent advances in artificial teeth are the development of **composite teeth** to overcome the drawbacks of acrylic and porcelain teeth with better mechanical and aesthetic properties (*refer* to page 190).

9. Temporary Crown and Bridge Resin—Restorations

The procedure for preparing permanent metallic crown and bridges involves several steps and requires a few weeks after the teeth preparations. During this interval, the **teeth may decay further or drift**, which will cause misfit of the appliance. Temporary acrylic crown and bridges are provided to avoid these.

The most common material used is chemically cured acrylic resin, of similar composition as resin teeth. This is supplied as monomer liquid and polymer powder in various shades (A, B, C, D, E, F, G, etc.) for selection to match the tooth colour.

Before preparation of the teeth, a stone cast is obtained and an acrylic tooth is waxed in the gap. A thin polystyrene sheet is softened by heat and closely adapted on this to form a **template**. After the preparation of teeth, the cold-cure acrylic dough is prepared; the template is packed and placed in position. Patient

Table 6.5	Comparison of acrylic and porcelain teeth	
Properties	*Acrylic teeth*	*Porcelain teeth*
1. Biocompatibility	Adequate	Excellent, chemically inert
2. Aesthetic	Adequate	Excellent
3. Colour stability	Adequate	Permanent
4. Crazing	If not cross-linked	Very rare
5. Surface hardness	Low (20 KHN)	High (460 KHN)
6. Abrasive resistance	Low, wears out by opposing teeth	High, abrades opposing natural teeth
7. Toughness	Higher, resilient, flexible (greater fracture resistance)	Brittle, fractures easily by impact and shearing forces or trauma
8. Natural feel	Silent	Clicking sound
9. Bonding to acrylic denture	Chemical	Mechanical pins, rhetoric or diatoric holes
10. Thermal expansion	High—same as acrylic denture (80–120 ppm/°C)	Low (7–8 ppm/°C), cause crazing of denture
11. Finishing	Easy to grind and polish	Difficult to fit in small inter-arch spaces
12. Water sorption	Cause dimensional change	Dimensional stability is more
13. Fabrication	Simple method	Complicated (expensive)

has to apply the pressure, with the opposing teeth. During polymerization, cooling with water spray is done many times. After curing it is taken out, the excess is trimmed, polished and cemented temporarily.

If heat-cure acrylic is used, after the teeth preparation, the suitable wax pattern of crown and the bridge is carved, flasked, dewaxed, and acrylised. In case of light curing resins, curing is done in a light chamber.

Chemically or light-cured (BisGMA) composite resins are used nowadays.

Note 1: Acrylic Veneers

Acrylic veneers can be prepared by methods similar to that of the heat-cured acrylic crown. For acrylic veneering of metallic crowns and bridges, wax patterns are formed on the roughened labial surface, invested, dewaxed completely, the suitable bonding agent is applied, the acrylic-dough is packed and cured.

Note 2: Acrylic Occlusal Splints

Heat or chemically cured acrylic resin (similar to denture base) material is used with a similar procedure for the preparation of splints in the treatment of patients having TMJ syndrome.

Note 3: Acrylic Inlay Patterns

Chemical-cure acrylic resin is sometimes used to prepare inlay or crown patterns for the casting procedure. Powder and liquid are applied alternately on the prepared teeth-die, allowed to cure and trimmed for the required shape. Sprue can be fitted, before investment. This requires **long burn-out time**. This method has the advantage of overcoming the distortion of the wax patterns.

Note 4: Denture Cleansers

For long service and good hygiene, the dentures are to be frequently cleaned and always kept immersed in water when not kept in the mouth.

Several types of denture cleaning materials can be used. These are **household cleansers, bleaches, vinegar, dentifrices (paste or gel forms), mild detergents, etc.** Cleaning with toothbrushes using dentifrices may damage the surface texture in the long-time. Hard abrasives should not be tried.

Immersion type denture cleansers

Special denture cleansers marketed are in the form of powder or tablets. These contain detergents, sodium perborate, and flavors. When dissolved in water it forms alkaline peroxide and gives out oxygen, which dislodges the debris. Hypochlorite and such chemically reacting solutions are contraindicated to base metal alloy removable cast partial dentures.

MODEL QUESTIONS

I. Long Essays (20 minutes each)

1. Explain the term complete denture and classify the denture base materials. Briefly outline the compression moulding technique of denture fabrication.
2. Describe the ideal requirements of denture base materials. Give the properties of heat cure PMMA denture-base resin and explain how far these, satisfy the requirements.
3. Explain the chemical stages of polymerization and the curing procedure required to obtain non-porous, non-crazing denture.
4. Give the compositions of cold-cure acrylic denture materials and explain the compression moulding technique of fabrication. Give the advantages and disadvantages of cold-cure over, heat-cure resins.
5. Describe the ideal requirements of denture reliners. Outline the relining procedure. Describe any two permanent, resilient relining materials, their advantages and disadvantages.

II. Short Essays (10 minutes each)

1. Multiple mix flasking
2. Separating media
3. Curing cycle
4. Injection moulding technique
5. Fluid resin technique
6. Dimensional changes in dentures
7. Internal porosities in acrylic denture
8. Crazing of dentures
9. Denture repair
10. Denture relining
11. Long-term resilient liners
12. Short-term soft liners—tissue conditioners
13. Maxillofacial reconstruction materials
14. Crown and bridge resins
15. Special tray acrylic resins
16. Acrylic and porcelain artificial teeth

III. Brief Answers (5 minutes each)

1. Flasking
2. Physical stages of mixing of acrylic powder and liquid
3. Dough time
4. Trial closures
5. Bench curing
6. Bench cooling
7. Surface roughness of dentures
8. Sub-surface porosity in dentures
9. Denture finishing
10. Cold-cure acrylic denture curing
11. Acrylic veneers
12. Denture rebasing
13. Denture cleansers

Biocompatible Aspects of Dental Materials

Biocompatibility is the property of the materials which remain harmoniously with the living tissues. These should not react and produce any toxic or injurious effects on the biological functions. This property is measured on the basis of localized cytotoxicity such as pulp, mucosal and systemic responses, allergenicity, hypersensitivity, estrogenecity, etc. The dental materials also may undergo biological degradations, like loss of mechanical properties, corrosion, discolourations, etc. in oral environments.

Earlier the main criteria for selection of restorative materials were the mechanical properties, thermal and chemical stabilities, and aesthetic qualities. But the recent trend of selection is mainly based on their biocompatibilities. Several *in vivo* and *in vitro* tests are to be conducted to estimate the biohazardous properties of the materials used for placing in the oral cavities, as well as auxiliary materials used by technicians. These tests are required to take suitable precautions, and to avoid such materials. Many such materials, like silver amalgam, beryllium, and nickel in base metal alloys, asbestos, silica—abrasive dust, monomers and polymer resins, etc. have been identified.

Dynamic Interactions between the Body and the Foreign Materials Introduced

Biocompatibility can also be defined as the interaction between the body tissues and the foreign materials placed in the oral cavity. Whenever, a restoration is placed in contact with the body tissues, a tenacious interface is formed between the material and the tooth pulp, through the dentin, periodontium, periapical areas of the oral cavity in general.

The dynamics of the interactions through this interface determines the biological responses of the materials and the tissues. The materials can cause localized and systemic responses depending on the duration and concentration of the exposure, the excretion rate of the substances and the site of exposures.

Adverse Effects from Dental Materials

The biological reactions of some materials are toxicity, hypersensitivity (allergic), inflammatory, mutagenic, estrogenic, etc.

Toxicity

This is a dose-related potential of a material resulting in cell or tissue deaths. Certain materials may continuously release or leach, some substances (like mercury, nickel, beryllium, etc.) into the body which can cause over toxicity above a certain amount.

Hypersensitivity and Allergy

Hypersensitivity is the abnormal reaction that occurs when the body is exposed to foreign materials. These

133

materials sensitize the immune system, so that when the person is repeatedly exposed to the same material, the body responds with a hypersensitivity reaction which is not dose-dependent.

The allergic or hypersensitive reaction develops only in persons whose immune system recognize the material as foreign. The allergic reactions can manifest as a localized reaction in the tissue which is directly in contact with the material. Allergy can be a systemic manifestation in the form of itching, skin eruptions, sneezing, erythema, breathing difficulties, etc.

According to Gell and Coombs' classifications, the allergic reactions or immune responses can be:

Type I   : Immediate
Type II : Cytotoxic hypersensitivity
Type III : Immune complex hypersensitivity
Type IV : Delayed, cell-mediated hypersensitivity, etc.

The allergic reactions are due to the individual's immune systems, recognizing a substance as foreign materials and are initially dose-independent.

Inflammation

This is a complex phenomena, involving the *host's immune system to overcome the external invasions.* The inflammation may be caused by toxic or allergic materials and sometimes may preceed toxicity. The pulpal and periodontal diseases are mainly due to long-term infections.

Mutagenic Reactions

These are caused by the materials or its components *altering the base-pair sequence of DNA in cells (i.e. mutation).* Some resin-based restoratives, sealants, ions of metals (Ni, Be, Cu, etc.) are found to be mutagens. Fortunately, these *may not be carcinogenic,* as the immune system supplies a lot of cellular energies and mechanics to repair the mutated DNA, etc.

Estrogenicity

It is the ability to produce materials like *xeno-estrogens,* to act in the body as *estrogens (i.e. female sex hormones).* The resin, *Bisphenol-A,* the starting substance of BisGMA, composite restorative materials and few other resins are found to be estrogenic.

In most cases, the surface characteristics, such as compositions, roughness, etc. and the corrosion degradation products, mainly affect the biocompatibilities.

Osseointegration and Biointegration

Both of these take place due to the dynamic interactions between the body and the materials. These are the key phenomena in the implantology, for stabilizations. **Osseointegration is the formation of a living body tissues within 10 mm space from the implant material surface, without any fibrous-connective tissues.** Materials which allow osseointegrations are, CpTi, Ti-6Al-4V alloy, tantalum, and few ceramics. These do not easily undergo biodegradation. The oxide layer may promote adsorption, adhesion and deposition of materials in the extracellular matrix, for the bone formation and maturation.

Biointegration refers to certain materials-like bioglasses which undergo biointegration with the bone directly without any intervening space. For this, the surface of the material should undergo some modifications (plasma coating) or *degradations.*

Immunotoxicity

The oral immune system is slightly different than those in other locations. Certain allergenic materials like nickel or chromium may induce immunological tolerance. Immunotoxicity is due to the *alterations in the cells of immune systems,* by the materials. This will cause either an increase or decrease of cellular functions. For example, mercury, palladium, the dentin bonding agent—*HEMA, etc. may indirectly cause changes in the cellular functions.*

The biocompatibility aspects (responses) depend upon the following factors

- **Chemical and physical nature** of substances (i.e. acidity, solubility, disintegration, leaching of ions, etc.).
- **Compositions**, which may include biohazardous materials (like mercury, nickel, beryllium, etc.).
- **Oral health conditions**, chronic medical problems, requiring long-term treatments like radiation, chemotherapies, etc.
- **Age** of the person
- **Products of corrosion** of alloys or degradation of materials
- **The context of placement** of restorations, e.g. a crown and bridge alloy shows different biological responses when used as an implant.
- **Surface characteristics:** Rough surface, may accumulate food debris which acts as a seat for the microorganisms to grow and produce certain biohazardous materials causing inflammations, etc.

Biocompatibility Requirements

Certain substances released from some dental restorative materials may produce biological responses at the localized sites like the pulp of the tooth, periodontium, root apex, or nearby soft tissues such as buccal mucosa, tongue, etc.

These can enter into the body system by several routes. Hence, biocompatibility requirements are: They should not:

- Sensitize and produce allergic reactions
- Be harmful to the tooth pulp or soft tissues
- Contain toxic diffusible substances which get released and enter into the circulatory systems
- Be carcinogenic
- Undergo biodegradations
- Show estrogenicity; and contain xenoestrogens
- Create immunotoxicity, i.e. they should not alter the cell structures of the immune systems, by changing the cellular functions.

However, implant materials should be bioactive and cause osseointegration or biointegration.

Evaluation of Biocompatibilities

Before adopting any methods for biocompatibility tests, the following aspects must be carefully considered:

- Location of the material.
- Nature of the tissues, i.e. soft or mineralized hard tissues, surrounding the foreign material.
- Exposure of the material to the oral situations, blood, saliva, tissue fluids, etc.
- Types of contacts, direct or indirect, through a barrier-like epithelium.
- Duration of contact, i.e. from few minutes in case of impression materials, to several years, in case of permanent alloy or resin restorations.
- Chemical nature—compositions, degradations, and corrosion products of restoratives.
- Physical conditions, like stress, fatigue resistance, wearing, abrasion.
- Surface modifications, coated, electroplated and surface characteristics.

Methods of Evaluation of Biocompatibilities

Biocompatibility tests are conducted, mainly in three stages for screening and eliminating the biohazardous materials, which may damage the oral tissues, if used.

- Group I : Primary screening tests
- Group II: Secondary—animal tests
- Group III: Preclinical—usage tests

For final acceptance for use, the materials should pass through all these tests successfully.

Group I: Primary—in vitro Screening Tests

a. **Cytotoxicity tests:** The dental materials, fresh or in a cured state, are placed directly in contact with tissue culture cells or on the membrane overlying the tissue culture cells. If the initial products are cytotoxic, the manufacturer can modify them.

b. **Genotoxicity tests:** Mammalian or nonmammalian cells, bacteria, yeasts or fungi are used to investigate the changes in gene mutation, chromosomal structures, DNA or genetic changes, with the dental materials, or their extracts or devices.

Advantages

- Can be conducted in controlled experimental conditions
- Large scale screening can be done
- Methods are relatively fast, inexpensive and can be standardized.

Disadvantages

- Lack of relevance *in vivo* usage conditions as the cytotoxicity measured in osteoblast cell culture is nonrelevant, as the materials are not in contact with osteoblast *in vivo*.
- The lack of immune, inflammatory and circulatory systems *in vitro* test.

Group II: Secondary—Animal in vivo Screening Tests

These tests are done by using dental materials in contact with the tissues of healthy laboratory animals, like mice, guinea pigs, hamsters, monkeys, sheep, etc. Several tests to mucous membrane—immune sensitization, bone responses, mutagenicity, carcinogenicity, etc. are done for checking allergy, inflammations, and other sublethal chronic biological responses.

- **Systemic toxicity tests** are done by administering the materials to rats directly or intravenously.
- **Skin irritation tests** are done by placing the materials in contact with the shaved skin of the animals to check erythema and edema.
- **Skin sensitization tests** are done similarly to check allergic responses.
- **Inhalation tests** are done by spraying the aerosol preparations around the head of the animals in a chamber periodically. If an animal dies in a few minutes or hours, the materials are considered as very toxic.
- **Implantation tests:** Materials are implanted in subcutaneous tissues or muscles of animals of suitable sizes. Inflammations, etc. are checked in 2 to 3 month periods.

Advantage

In vivo tests are quite reliable as the biological responses are investigated directly.

Disadvantages

- Expensive and difficult to control the experiment in long duration.
- Reliability of the fact whether the animal represents the human species fully.
- Ethical concern of animal sacrifice.

Group III: Preclinical Usage Screening Tests

Only when the material passes through the group I and group II tests, these preclinical usage tests can be conducted on *sub-human primate—dogs, pigs, etc.* for clinical trials. Materials are placed in the relevant locations for studies.

- **Pulp and dentin usage tests:** These are sometimes, initially conducted on subhuman primates—dogs, ferrets, pigs, etc. as clinical trials. Materials are placed in class V cavity preparations, using ZnOE as controls. After sacrificing the animals, specimen is checked in 7 days or 28 + 3 days or 70 + 5 days intervals, making thorough investigations for various responses, like, *microleakage, inflammations, secondary dentin formations, etc.*
- **Pulp-capping and pulpotomy usage tests:** The material is placed in contact with the exposed pulp and calcium hydroxide is used as a control. Testing is done, in 7 days or 70 + 5 days. Formation of secondary dentin and pulp responses are studied
- **Endodontic usage tests:** Materials are placed by replacing the pulp chamber and root canal materials. ZnOE is used as a sealer control. Testing is done for 1 or 3 months. *The degree of inflammations in periapical tissues is studied.*

Clinical Usage

The dentist should not be carried away by the marketing literature regarding the materials, supplied by the manufactures. Before using any new materials introduced, he should make a thorough study of the details of the biocompatibility tests conducted by the manufacturer. The advantages and risks of these new materials should be communicated to the patients.

BIOCOMPATIBILITY OF VARIOUS DENTAL MATERIALS

1. *Reactions of restorative materials on the pulp*

Restorative materials may directly affect pulpal tissues or cause sublethal changes in pulpal cells which make them more susceptible to bacterial or neutrophilic damages.

- **Microleakage**
  Many restoratives do not chemically bond perfectly with the tooth structure. Debonding occurs during thermal fluctuations and the marginal gap created, collect food debris or saliva. The bacteria and bacterial products such as liposaccharides can cause pulpal irritations. Also, the restorative materials can cause pulpal irritation through microleakages.

- **Dentin bonding**
  Bonding of restoratives to the dentin involves the biocompatibility issues more seriously. The dentinal tubules and the odontoblasts are the extensions of the pulp. During the cavity preparation, the smear layer is formed enveloping the exposed dentin, which may act as a protective layer. If this smear layer is removed, greater pulpal irritation will be caused due to:
  - Diffusion of material through the dentinal tubules
  - Diffusion of bacteria and bacterial products in the microleakages, through the dentinal tubules.
  - Diffusion of acids (etchants) used to remove smear layers.

  It has been proved that dentin is a very efficient buffer of proteins due to which most acid ions cannot pass through if the dentin layer remaining has at least about 0.5 mm thickness. Recent studies have shown that the acid ions cannot penetrate more than 100 μm (microns) thick dentin layer. But still, the odontoblast process in the dentin tubules get affected.

  Most of the dentin bonding agents have shown cyto-toxicity. The resin based restorative materials require protective liners or bonding agents which show least cytotoxicity (like HEMA).

- **Glass-ionomer cements**
  The pulpal reactions is found to be very mild and the usage tests have shown that the inflammatory cell infiltrate is minimum or absent after one month. This is because
  - Polyacrylic acid is a very weak acid
  - Large sized acid molecules (ions) cannot pass through the dentin tubules.
  - It forms certain complexes and seals dentin tubules (*refer* to biological properties of GIC).

- **Liners, varnishes and nonresin cements**
  Calcium hydroxide is marketed in many forms from saline suspensions to modifications with zirconium oxide, titanium oxide, resins, etc. *Calcium hydroxide in suspension is extremely cytotoxic.* Initial exposure of dentin causes necrosis to a depth of 1 mm or more. The alkaline pH helps to coagulate any hemorrhagic exudates of superficial pulp. Then the necrotic inflammatory cells infiltrate into a subnecrotic zone. The inflammatory reaction remains for few weeks. Necrotic zone undergoes dystrophic calcification which stimulates dentin bridge formations. *If the resin is incorporated, it becomes less irritating. Reparative dentin bridge is formed more quickly without pulp necrosis.*

- **Polycarboxylate cements**
  Polyacrylic acids, above 1% concentrations, appear to be cytotoxic. Zinc and fluoride ions leaching can also cause cytotoxicity. However, the buffering and protein binding can neutralize this. Polycarboxylate cements induce mild to moderate inflammatory responses in pulpal tissues in few days and only mild chronic inflammations later. Reparative dentin formation is minimal. Hence, it can be used in cavities with dentin layer on the floor.

- **Zinc oxide cements**
  Show slightly to moderate inflammatory responses in the first week, and reduced mild chronic reaction, with some reparative dentin formation in deep cavities in 5–8 days.

- **Bleaching agents**
  These are used on non-vital and vital teeth. These contain some peroxides, which are capable of passing through the exposed dentin and cause cytotoxicity. This response is more at higher concentrations.

2. *Responses of few metals*

- **Nickel**
  Nickel is an important component of most of the base metal alloys, like, Ni-Cr, Ni-Ti, stainless steel, etc. The Nickel ions (Ni^{2+}) can leach out from these metal appliances like crowns, fixed and removable partial dentures, orthodontic appliances, etc. This leaching out is more in the acidic environments and is also more for Ni-Cr alloys. These cause hypersensitivity and sometimes, non-specific inflammatory reactions. Nickel is one of the most allergic toxic metals. It is also found to be mutagenic. Nickel sulphide, in industries, is found to be a respiratory carcinogen. Similarly nickel carboxyl [$Ni(CO)_4$] used in industries is extremely toxic.

- **Beryllium**
  This is used in small amounts (1%–2%) in the base metal alloys, Cr-Co, Cr-Ni, etc. to reduce the melting point and brittleness. Metallic beryllium (BeO) and ionic beryllium (Be^{++}) are found to be carcinogenic. Acidic environments enhance release of Be^{++} ions from base metal alloys. Beryllium dust inhaled (during grinding of base metal alloy appliances or in factories) reach the alveoli of lungs, causing chronic inflammatory conditions, known as berylliosis. This occurs only for patients who are allergic to Beryllium.

- **Chromium**
  There is no documentary evidence of toxicity. However, technician or clinician must take precautions during grinding of base metal appliances.

- **Cobalt**
  Cobalt has not yet been proved as allergic until now. Co-Cr alloy (without Ni) are considered as biocompatible.

- **Platinum**
  The documented evidence of toxicity is quite rare.

- **Gold**
  Generally considered as an inert and noblest biomaterial. However, certain allergic reactions, dermatitis has been reported at the area of contacts with jewelry in few cases.

- **Mercury and silver amalgam**
  Refer to Chapter 12: Mercury health hazards.

3. *Orthodontic materials*

  In orthodontia, different materials are used such as nickel-based alloys, latex based elastic bands, and acrylic resins. These are considered as allergic materials. *In vitro* experiments showed non-cyto-toxicity of orthodontic wires. The bands were found to be cytotoxic because of the silver and copper based brazing alloys used to prepare the bands. The materials used in fixed orthodontic appliances are metallic alloys and nonmetalli ceramics, composites and polycarbonates. Many alloys used in orthodontics, like stainless steel, nickel titanium, titanium molybdenum alloys, etc. are placed in patients mouth for 1–2 years and undergo several corrosion phenomenon. These corrosion products of zinc are known to cause acute toxicity or subacute effects such as glossitis, metallic tastes, bleeding and inflamed or hypertrophied gingiva, which cannot be chemically distinguished from gingivitis of bacterial etiology.

4. *Responses of other materials*

- **Latex**
  In dentistry, the latex has been used in gloves, rubber dams, orthodontic elastics, etc. The latex hyper-sensitivity is a problem for both dental personnel and patients. The concern for this problem is increasing in recent days. Hypersensitivity to latex-containing products may occur as a true latex allergy or reactions to accelerators and antioxidants used in latex processing. The reactions vary from *localized rashes, swelling to more serious wheezing and anaphylaxis. Dermatitis of hands* is the most common adverse reaction. Severe reactions can occur when latex products come into contact with mucous membranes. Allergenicity of latex depends on how the latex was collected, preserved and processed.

Both natural and synthetic latex are known to cause allergic reactions.

• **Acrylic resins**

Acrylic resins are reported to cause allergic reactions when used as denture base restorative material or provisional fixed partial denture resins. The primary risk of this material is an allergy in the form of contact dermatitis, or even anaphylactic reactions and their risk are highest for dental professionals because of the frequent exposure to unpolymerised monomers. There is ample evidence that resins release unpolymerized component into the biological environment, although the release involved is not well-documented. The reaction may start shortly after insertion or manifested after a period of time.

• **Composite resins**

The pathologic mechanism may be related to contact allergy to formaldehyde formed in resin composite restorations. This formaldehyde found in (visible light, UV light and chemically cured) composite resins mainly produce *lichenoid lesions on oral mucosa.*

• **Eugenol**

Eugenol containing products—oil of cloves or eugenol with zinc oxide to form zinc oxide eugenol which are used as a temporary restorative material, base material, impression material (paste) or periodontal pack. Eugenol is highly soluble and is continuously released from zinc oxide eugenol which can lead to short-term saturation of oral environment with eugenol concentration, sufficient to cause cytotoxicity. ZnOE is considered as the least damaging restorative material and possesses sedative effect. Despite advantageous properties of eugenol, sensitivity is manifested as a positive inflammatory response to eugenol in some patients.

• **Impression materials**

Polyether impression materials have been known to cause allergic problems. Allergic reactions can be decreased if adequate care is taken by thoroughly mixing the material to avoid the contact of aromatic sulphonic ester catalyst with mucous membranes.

MODEL QUESTIONS

I. Long Essays (20 minutes each)

1. Explain the term 'biocompatibility' of dental materials and describe briefly adverse effects from dental materials.
2. What are the factors, which affect the biocompatibility aspects? Give the requirements of biocompatible materials.
3. Briefly outline the evaluation of biocompatibility of dental materials for acceptance to clinical uses.

II. Short Essays (10 minutes each)

1. Adverse effects of dental materials
2. Microleakage
3. Mercury toxicity
4. Preclinical usage tests for dental materials
5. Osseointegration and biointegration
6. Biomaterials
7. Biocompatibilities of base metal dental alloys.

III. Brief Answers (5 minutes each)

1. Latex hypersensitivity
2. Beryllium toxicity
3. Primary tests for biocompatibilities
4. Hypersensitivity and allergy
5. Nickel toxicity
6. Biocompatibilities of alloys used in orthodontia.

Restorative Materials: Dental Cements

Dental restorative materials are used to replace the missing parts of the tooth or teeth. The loss of the tooth materials can be due to:

- Decay or caries
- Attrition, abrasion, or erosions
- Trauma of accidents
- Developmental defects

Large varieties of materials used for this purpose may be metals, alloys, inorganic and organic substances. These are selected according to clinical situations.

Dental cement is a general term for the materials, which harden on placing in the teeth cavities. These are filling materials, adhesive materials, for binding the prosthesis to teeth, bases, liners, sealants, etc.

Conservative methods are applied in dentistry by selecting suitable materials and manipulating properly, to replace these missing parts. However, there are no **all-purpose single restorative materials**, which satisfy all the requirements for the different clinical situations. Hence, two or more materials of different properties are selected and ingeniously manipulated to avail most of the requirements. Materials can be selected according to their applications in the various treatment procedures such as:

- Temporary restoratives—lasting for few days to weeks

- Intermediate restoratives—lasting for few weeks to months
- Permanent restoratives—lasting for more than five years
- Cementing—luting, temporary and permanent materials
- Pulp protecting agents
- Insulating bases
- Cavity liners and varnishes
- Root canal treatment materials
- Pit and fissure sealants, etc.

Brief Explanations

1. **Temporary restorative materials**

   These are used to protect the teeth from further decay, during the treatment period of few days or weeks, in cases of RCT. These are also used for reducing the **postoperative sensitivity** before a permanent restoration is placed. The general ideal requirements for restorative materials have to be slightly modified as follows: These should have:

   - Ability to promote the healing process
   - Obtundent property to reduce postoperative sensitivity
   - Low compressive strength **less than 35 MPa** to facilitate removal.

- Good marginal sealing property
- Antibacterial and cariostatic properties, etc. Materials used are **calcium hydroxide, zinc oxide eugenol (type III).**

2. **Intermediate restorative materials**

These are required if the fabrication procedure requires a longer time (few months) in case of complicated procedures, for patients with rampant caries. These materials have higher strength than temporary restoratives.

Materials used are improved zinc oxide eugenol cements with a polymer resin, or alumina and EBA modifications. Sometimes zinc phosphate cements, zinc polycarboxylates, glass ionomer cements, zinc silico-phosphate cements, etc. are also used.

3. **Permanent restorative materials**

These should last **life-time theoretically.** Materials and methods are selected according to clinical situations, such as anterior, posterior, metallic, non-metallic, etc. These require very strong, bonding to tooth structures, high strength, etc. properties. Hybrid composites, GIC for non-stress bearing areas are used as nonmetallic restorations. Direct filling gold, silver amalgam, HN, N, PBM alloy castings, CAD-CAM techniques have been also tried successfully.

4. **Cementing or luting materials**
   - **Temporary:** These are **interface** materials between the tooth structure and permanent alloy casting fabrications. **The temporary cementing agents** are used for the trial of the appliances for few days for approval by the patients. These should have **lower strength <75 MPa** for easy dislodging during permanent cementation. Materials used are **ZnOE (type I)** or sometimes **calcium hydroxide.**
   - **Permanent cementing materials** should have higher strength (>75 MPa), a thin film thickness (<25 microns), suitable consistency, ability to chemically bond with tooth and metal appliances, etc.

     Materials used are modified ZnOE, $ZnPO_4$, zinc polycarboxylate cement, GIC (type I), zinc silicophosphate, resin cements, etc.

5. **Pulp protecting (capping) agents—low strength bases: Delicate pulp** well-protected by tough dentin and enamel. It is very sensitive to various external insults like chemical, thermal, electrical, mechanical trauma, etc. Due to severe tooth decay, excavations, traumatic fractures, etc. pulp may, just about to get exposed. In such cases the pulp protecting agents, having obtundent, and ability to form reparative dentin, properties are used. These are ZnOE (type I),

or $Ca(OH)_2$ cements, which are sometimes known as **low strength** bases.

6. **Insulating cement bases of high strength**

These are placed directly on the cavity floor to protect the pulp when a dentin layer more than 0.75 mm thickness is present over the pulp, these are known as **high strength bases.** Materials used are ZnOE (type III), $ZnPO_4$, zinc polycarboxy-late cement, GIC (type II), etc.

7. **Cavity liners**

These are thin suspensions of $Ca(OH)_2$, ZnOE or GIC III applied as a coating on the exposed dentin to neutralize the penetrating acid ions from the acidic restoratives.

Cavity varnishes: These are natural or synthetic gums dissolved in organic solvents like acetone, ethanol, chloroform, etc. used to protect the cavity walls from microleakages.

8. **Root canal treatment—endodontic materials**

These are permanent restoratives intended to obturate the pulp space of the tooth. This treatment is required to provide a long-term retention of permanent restorations and to give a sound **dentin support** for the functional crown. The treatment involves removal of the pulp, sterilization of root canal, cleaning (preparing) root canal and filling with **gutta-percha or silver points.** Zinc oxide eugenol is then used as root canal sealant.

9. **Pit and fissure sealants**

Small pits, fissures or some cracks on the occlusal surface of deciduous and permanent teeth collect food debris which initiates the decay. As a protective measure these are sealed by materials which have good flow, adequate strength, aesthetic, thermal insulating, properties. Microfilled, visible light-cured—thin composite resins, GIC type III are commonly used.

IDEAL REQUIREMENTS OF RESTORATIVE MATERIALS

Since these materials are used for functional and aesthetic restorations in the oral cavity, they should have the following general requirements.

1. **Biological properties**
   - Biocompatible with the pulp and other tissues.
   - Bacteriostatic—resist the growth of bacteria or micro-organisms
   - Cariostatic and anticariogenic
   - Obtundent and promote healing effect.

Chemical properties
   - Chemically inert, should not be acidic or alkaline.
   - Resistant to tarnish and corrosion in case of metallic appliances.

- Resist dissolution and disintegrations in oral fluids.
- Should not absorb saliva, or any oral fluids which may decrease the properties.
- **Chemically bond with tooth structure and metallic restorations** when used as interface-cementing material.

2. **Rheological properties**
   - Good flow properties, constant low viscosity during manipulation.
   - Adequate adjustable working times and short setting times for the conveniences of dentists and patients respectively, i.e. **dentists' command set properties.**
   - Shear thinning or pseudoplastic property to assist proper cementation.
   - Suitable film thickness, **<25 μm** for luting and about **25–40 μm** for bases.
   - Dentist should be able to adjust the consistencies, working and setting times.

3. **Mechanical properties:** These requirements depend upon the types and positions of restorations like class I, II, III, IV, V cavities, anterior and posterior restorations, etc. But generally they should have:
   - High proportional or elastic limit or yield strengths to **resist permanent deformations.**
   - High stiffness or modulus of elasticity to resist any dimensional changes. However, ideally, the modulus of elasticity should be similar to that of dentin (14,000–18,000 MPa).
   - Large adequate compressive strength to resist fracture from large dynamic masticating forces. For the temporary cement <35 MPa to assist removal, intermediate restoratives 35–100 MPa and for permanent restoratives >300 MPa those of enamel or dentin.
   - Good resilience and not brittleness to avoid fractures.
   - Good abrasive resistance and surface hardness nearly same as tooth enamel **~340 KHN**. Otherwise either the softer restoratives get abraded or the harder restoratives (like ceramics) abrade the opposing tooth.
   - **High fatigue strength** and endurance limits for long service.
   - Good bond strength rather chemically bonding to teeth to prevent marginal leakage and **minimize the removal of tooth material during cavity preparations.**

   The chemically adhesive cements like GIC satisfy the requirements of **minimum cavity preparations.**

4. **Thermal properties**
   - Should have the **same** COTE of enamel (and dentin) nearly **11.4 ppm/°C** to minimize micro-

leakage during thermal changes or cycling in the oral cavity.
   - **Very good insulators** to protect the pulp from thermal insults. However, most permanent metallic restorations, DFG, silver amalgam, HN, N, PBM alloy castings are good conductors of heat and electric ions and **require thermal insulating bases**.
   - **Low thermal diffusivities**
   - Should not soften or show viscoelastic properties at the oral temperatures.

5. **Aesthetic requirements**

   These are of **prime importance for anterior restoratives.**
   - Transparent or translucent and ability to incorporate any desired shades or opacifiers.
   - Same refractive index as tooth material.
   - Have same colour parameters, i.e. **hue, chroma and value** as a tooth for correct colour matching.
   - The colour parameters should not change or undergo **discolouration**.

   Note: Perfect colour matching of any optically isotropic restorative material is impossible due to highly optically anisotropic (due to inhomogeneous distributions of dentinal tubules and enamel rods) nature of the tooth structure (*refer* to "problems of colour matching" page 46).

6. **Other requirements**
   - Should be radio-opaque for detection of secondary caries, overhanging restorations, and imperfect filling, i.e. air trappings.
   - Simple manipulation techniques without sophisticated equipment.
   - Properties should not have technique sensitivity.
   - Long storage life, readily available and less expensive.

   As all these requirements are not satisfied by any material, complicated restorative procedures and fabricating techniques, with many (direct and also sometimes auxiliary) materials of different properties are used ingeniously to avail maximum required properties.

CLASSIFICATION OF RESTORATIVE MATERIALS

Classification is required for quick decision for the selection of materials and procedures according to the required clinical situations.

1. **According to the nature of materials**
   - *Metallic restoratives*
     - Indirect castings of HN, N, PBM alloys.
     - Direct filling materials—direct filling gold, silver amalgam.

- *Non-metallic restoratives*
  - Ceramics (PJC, veneers, inlays, etc.)
  - Composite resins
  - Dental cements
  - Metal-ceramics

2. **According to lifespan**
   - Temporary restoratives lasting for a few days to a week: ZnOE, acrylic crowns.
   - Intermediate restoratives: Lasting for few weeks to months, modified ZnOE, ZnPO$_4$, zinc polycarboxylate cement, acrylic crowns, and bridges.
   - Permanent restoratives: Alloy castings, DFG, dental amalgam, posterior composite resins, modified GIC, ceramics.

3. **According to the placements**
   - Anterior restoratives—tooth coloured, aesthetics is the main criteria: Ceramics, GIC, composite resins, metal ceramics, compomers, etc.
   - Posterior restoratives—large strength is the main criteria: HN, N, PBM alloy castings, silver amalgam, hybrid composites, modified GIC, metal ceramics.

4. **According to the methods of hardening**
   - Solidification (of molten alloys)—castings of HN, N, PBM alloys, ceramics, gutta-percha.
   - Chemical acid–base reactions: ZnOE, ZnPO$_4$, zinc polycarboxylate cement, GIC.
   - Polymerizing reactions: Composite resins, acrylics (chemical, VLC system), compomers.

5. **According to the applications**
   - *Metallic restorations* obtained by casting methods. Inlays, crowns, fixed partial dentures (crowns and bridges), removable partial dentures, pontics, abutments, etc. Direct filling materials: Pure gold foils and silver amalgams.
   - *Nonmetallic restorations*
     - Pulp protecting agents
     - Cement bases
     - Cavity primers, liners, varnishes
     - Cementing or luting materials
     - Tooth filling materials
     - Root canal sealants
     - Pit and fissure sealants.

CLASSIFICATION OF DENTAL CEMENTS—NON-METALLIC RESTORATIVES

These harden in the prepared tooth cavities by acid–base or polymerizing reactions. These are frequently used in conservative dentistry for selective applications, even though, they have many following drawbacks.
- Acidic or alkaline nature, causing pulp irritation.

- Low strength and mechanical properties—causing fractures.
- Poor abrasive resistance—causing wearing
- High solubility and disintegration—causing short life
- Poor chemical adhesion (except polycarboxylates)—causing debonding.

Hence, most of these (except composite resins) cannot be used for permanent restorations.
1. Classification of dental cements according to their functions (Table 8.1).
2. Classifications can be done according to composition and applications/Skinner's classification (Table 8.2).
3. Classification of dental cements according to their setting actions and reaction ingredients.

- **Zinc oxide cements**
  - ZnO + HE $\rightarrow$ ZnOE cement
  - ZnO + EBA $\rightarrow$ EBA cement
  - ZnO + H$_3$PO$_4$ $\rightarrow$ ZnPO$_4$ cement
  - ZnO + polycarboxylic acid $\rightarrow$ zinc polycarboxylate cement
- **Aluminosilicate glass cements**
  - (SiO$_2$+Al$_2$O$_3$) + H$_3$PO$_4$ $\rightarrow$ silicate cement
  - (SiO$_2$+Al$_2$O$_3$) + polycarboxylic acid $\rightarrow$ glass ionomer
  - (SiO$_2$+Al$_2$O$_3$) + resin $\rightarrow$ compomer
  - (SiO$_2$+Al$_2$O$_3$) + metals $\rightarrow$ modified GIC
- **Combinations**
  - ZnO + (Al$_2$O$_3$ + SiO$_2$) + H$_3$PO$_4$ $\rightarrow$ Zinc silicophosphate cement
  - ZnO + resins + HE $\rightarrow$ resin bonded ZnOE
- **Calcium hydroxide cement**

4. **According to the pH values**
   - Acidic cements (pH <7) Silicate, zinc silicophosphate, zinc phosphate, zinc polycarboxylates, glass ionomers, compomers.
   - *Almost neutral cement:* Zinc oxide eugenol and its modifications.
   - *Alkaline cement:* Calcium hydroxide (dycal).

ZINC OXIDE EUGENOL CEMENTS

These are obtundent, chemically neutral, physically low strength, thermal insulating opaque restorative materials having a long history. These are used for pulp protection, cement base, temporary restoration, and cementations. Modified forms can be used for permanent cementations of inlays and crowns.

Table 8.1 Classification of dental cements according to their functions

	Functions	Materials used
1.	Pulp capping	Calcium hydroxide, ZnOE
2.	Low strength bases	Calcium hydroxide, ZnOE
3.	High strength bases	Modified ZnOE, $ZnPO_4$, zinc polycarboxylate cement, GIC (III)
4.	Temporary cementations	ZnOE, $Ca(OH)_2$
5.	Final permanent cementation (luting)	Modified ZnOE, $ZnPO_4$ zinc polycarboxylate cement, GIC (I), zinc silicophosphate
6.	Temporary filling	ZnOE, modified ZnOE, zinc polycarboxylate cement
7.	Intermediate restorations (IRM)	$ZnPO_4$, resin bonded alumina modified—ZnOE, zinc polycarboxylate cement, $ZnSiPO_4$ cements
8.	Cavity liners	Calcium hydroxide suspensions, zinc polycarboxylate cement, GIC III
9.	Cavity varnishes	Gum or resins in organic solvents
10.	Pit and fissure sealants	Microfilled composite resins, GIC IV
11.	Cementation of orthodontic bands	Zinc polycarboxylates, zinc phosphate, composite or acrylic resins (for direct bonding)
12.	Root canal sealers	ZnOE, gutta-percha, zinc polycarboxylates

Table 8.2 Skinner's classification according to chemical composition and applications

	Materials	Primary applications	Secondary applications
1.	ZnOE I	Temp. cementation	Root canal sealing, pulp capping
	ZnOE II	Permanent cementation	Periodontic bandage
	ZnOE III	Temp. filling, base	Pulp capping
	ZnOE IV	Lining	Surgical dressing
2.	$Ca(OH)_2$	Pulp capping	Weak cement base, cavity liner
3.	$ZnPO_4$	Luting metallic restoration and orthodontic bands	Thermal insulating base, intermediate restorations root canal treatment
4.	$ZnPO_4$ with Ag or Cu	Intermediate restorations	Temporary filling of deciduous teeth
5.	Zinc polycarboxylate cement	Luting, bases	Cementation of orthodontic bands, intermediate restorations, root canal, sealants, lining
6.	Silicate (not used now)	Anterior restorations	Rampant caries of deciduous teeth treatment
7.	Zn-Si-Phosphate	Luting of a porcelain crown or veneers	Intermediate restorations, luting of alloy fabrications, orthodontic bands
8.	Glass ionomers (I)	Luting	Restoration of cervical erosion cavities.
	Glass ionomers (II)	Restoration	Pit and fissure sealant, core build up
	Glass ionomers (III)	Liner, base	
		Restoration	
	GIC metal modified, compomers	Posterior restorations	Luting orthodontic bands
9.	Composite resins	Anterior, posterior restorations	Pit and fissure sealants, veneers

According to ADA specification No. 30, they are classified into 4 types according to their uses

- Type I: Temporary cementation ...... comp strength <35 MPa
- Type II: Permanent cementation ...... comp strength >35 MPa
- Type III: Temporary restoration ...... comp strength >25 MPa
- Type IV: Cavity lining .... comp strength >5 MPa

Zinc oxide cements are dispensed as powder liquid systems (*see* Colour Plate 15, Fig. 8.1)

Conventional zinc oxide eugenol cements have a very low strength (3–40 MPa). Hence, to increase the strength of the cement, a slight modification is done in the composition. These are resins bonded and EBA+ alumina modified.

1. **Conventional ZnOE cements** (Table 8.3)
2. **Resin-modified zinc oxide-eugenol cements:** Natural or synthetic resins (methyl methacrylate resin) are added into the powder to increase the strength of the cement (Table 8.4).

Table 8.3 The composition of conventional ZnOE cement

Ingredients	Weight%	Functions
Powder		
1. Zinc oxide	69%	Reactive ingredient
2. White rosin	29.3%	Reduces the brittleness
3. Zn stearate	1%	Plasticizer
4. Zn acetate, CaCl$_2$	0.7%	Accelerator
Liquid		
1. Eugenol	85%	Reactor
2. Olive oil	15%	Plasticizer

Table 8.4 The composition of resin-modified ZnOE cement

Ingredients	Weight%	Functions
Powder		
Zinc oxide	70%	Reactive ingredient
Natural or synthetic resin	30%	
(methyl methacrylate resin)		Increases strength
Liquid		
Eugenol	85%	Reactor
Acetic acid	15%	Accelerators
Thymol	Small amount	Antimicrobial agent

3. **Ethoxybenzoic acid (EBA) alumina cement**
Fused **alumina** is added to the powder and **orthoethoxy benzoic acid** into the liquid to enhance the strength of the cement (Table 8.5).

Table 8.5 The composition of EBA alumina cement

Ingredients	Weight%	Functions
Powder		
Zinc oxide	60–70%	Reactive ingredient
Fused alumina	25–30%	Increases the strength
Rosin	balance	Reduces the brittleness
Calcium chloride	1.2%	Accelerator
Liquid		
Eugenol	37.5%	Reactive ingredient
Orthoethoxy benzoic acid	62.5%	Increases the strength

Setting Action

When the powder is mixed with the eugenol liquid, following chemical reactions take place, in the presence of moisture (similar to ZnOE impression pastes) (Fig. 8.1a).

1. $ZnO + H_2O \rightarrow Zn(OH)_2$
2. $Zn(OH)_2 + 2HE \rightarrow Zn$ eugenolate $+ 2H_2O$

In the first step, hydrolysis of ZnO takes place. ZnO combines with H_2O to form $Zn(OH)_2$.

In the second step $Zn(OH)_2$ combines with eugenol to form zinc oxide eugenolate (chelate compound) and releases H_2O.

It is an **autocatalytic acid–base reaction** in which H_2O is a by-product. Without H_2O the reaction will not proceed or does not exist. The chelate forms an amorphous gel that tends to crystallize and **binding unreacted particles** imparting strength to the set mass.

Structure of the Set Cement

The set cement consists of particles of ZnO embedded in the matrix of zinc eugenolate (Fig. 8.1b).

Properties

1. **Biological property**
Eugenol has an **obtundent** effect on the pulp. The release of eugenol by hydrolysis of zinc eugenolate matrix relieves pain in the pulp in deep cavities. Hence, **these** materials are most widely used as **pulp capping materials**, and to **reduce postoperative sensitivity**.

There are however disadvantages of eugenol. Eugenol is **cytotoxic and causes toxic cell reactions**.

This reaction can be represented as:

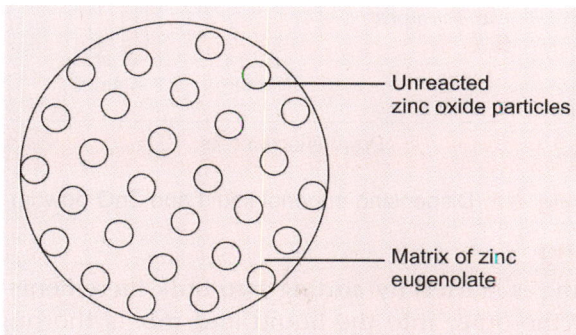

Acid + Base $\longrightarrow$ Zinc eugenolate (chelate compound) + $2H_2O$

Fig. 8.1a: Setting reaction of ZnO and eugenol

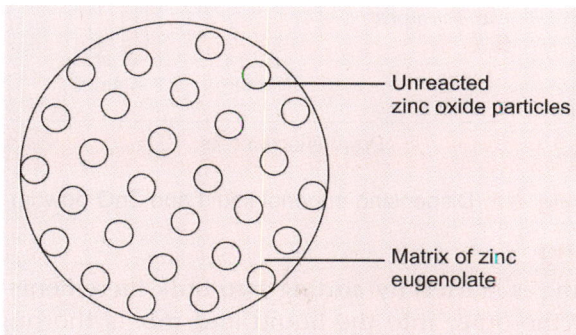

Fig. 8.1b: Structure of the set cement

Thus, direct contact of eugenol with soft tissues should be avoided since it is an **irritant**.

It has bacteriostatic property. These cements destroy the bacteria in or near the surface of the cavity and thus sterilizes the cavity to a limited extent.

These cements are non-acidic in nature pH 6.8–7.0 (neutral) and hence they can be easily placed at the base of the cavity very near to the pulp. It protects the pulp from the penetration of acid ions from restorative materials.

2. **Rheological property**

The cement material does not change its viscosity quickly during its placement into the prepared cavity. The dentist should get sufficient time to adapt and seal the margins. The material sets into a hard mass once it is completely placed inside the prepared cavity.

3. **Mixing and setting times**

Mixing time is about 1–1.5 minutes for all the three varieties

- *Setting times of*
  - Conventional ZnO eugenol cement: 4–10 minutes
  - Resin modified cement: 9 minutes
  - EBA alumina cement: 6–10 minutes

(Setting times can be determined by indentation methods).

Factors Affecting Setting Times

Setting time is decreased by

- Sintering of powder at 300°C for a longer time
- Smaller particle size
- Accelerators like calcium chloride, primary alcohols, glacial acetic acid
- Moisture
- Higher powder–liquid ratio
- Higher temperature, i.e. warm glass slab and spatula.

Setting time is increased by

- Larger particle size
- Retarders like glycol or glycerine
- Lower powder–liquid ratio
- Lower temperature without moisture contact, i.e. by **cooling the glass slab and spatula, but not below the dew point.** If cooled further, atmospheric-moisture condenses on the mix, which acts as accelerator.

4. **Consistency**

The consistency of the cements are measured by modified slump test (*refer* to zinc oxide eugenol impression paste and elastomers).

According to specification No. 30, the consistency should be minimum **of 30 mm** by standard testing method, for all the types ZnO eugenol cements.

5. **Film thickness**

For better retention of cemented appliances, cement thickness must be very low. Standard method measures this by applying a load of 2.5 kg on the standard mix placed in-between two glass plates. Film thickness should be **less than 25 μm** for types I and II.

6. **Solubility and disintegration**

This is measured from the percentage loss of weight of a standard disc, immersed in distilled water for 24 hours. The maximum allowable value is 2.5% for types I and II cements and 1.5% for types III and IV restoratives **(as per ADA specification number 30).** Actual values are less than these.

Approximate solubility values are
- Zinc-oxide eugenol cement   0.04%
- Resin modified cement   0.05%
- EBA alumina cement   0.03%

7. **Mechanical properties**
- Higher the strength of the cement greater is the retention of cemented restorations.
- Strength properties depend on mainly **composition and powder–liquid ratio** (Table 8.6).

8. **Thermal properties**

These materials have a **very low thermal conductivity, i.e. 0.0004** cal/sec/cm^2/°C/cm. These can act as thermal insulating or electrically insulating materials. (But these should be used in larger **thickness >2 mm.**)

The coefficient of thermal expansion value is **35 ppm/°C**, which is higher than tooth structure.

9. **Retention**

Zinc oxide eugenol cements do not adhere to the tooth structure chemically, and retention is by physical means. Retention depends on:
- The strength of the cement
- Stress imposed on restoration
- Consistency and film thickness
- Particle size

10. **Dimensional changes**

During setting it undergoes small, **negligible** volumetric shrinkage of about **2.5%.**

MANIPULATION OF ZINC OXIDE EUGENOL CEMENTS

Instruments required

Glass slab, narrow-bladed stainless steel spatula (or cement spatula).

Powder–liquid ratio (approximate) for
- Zinc oxide eugenol cement: 3 or 4:1
- Resin-modified cement: 6:1
- EBA-alumina cement: 7:1

The powder bottle should be **shaken well** for uniform distribution of powder particles and a suitable amount of powder is dispensed at one end of the glass slab using cement spatula. The powder is divided into two bulk increments, followed by smaller increments. (The reaction is not exothermic, and the pH is $\simeq$ 7.) Dispense required amount of liquid drops (2 to 3 drops) in the middle of the glass slab (Fig. 8.2).

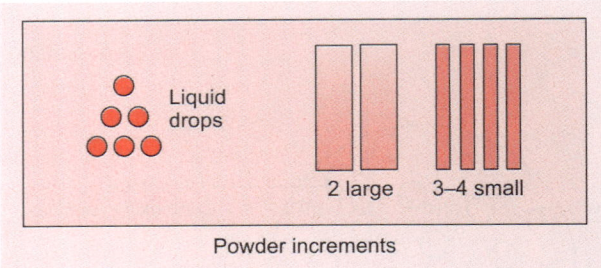

Fig. 8.2: Dispensing eugenol liquid and ZnO powder

Mixing

Mixing is started by adding two bulk increments one after the other into the liquid and mix is thoroughly spatulated. Then small increments are added one by one until required consistency is achieved. For luting consistency, the mix should be thinner and have a **creamy** appearance. For restorative consistency, the mix should be thicker, nonsticky, and should be able to roll it on the glass slab.

For EBA-alumina cement, the required P/L ratio is taken according to the manufacturer's instructions on a glass slab. The bulk increment is taken **and kneaded for 30 seconds**, followed by smaller increments and then stropped for 30 secs until a creamy consistency is developed.

Cementation technique

The mix is applied to the seating surface of the restoration and then placed on the prepared tooth. The

Table 8.6	Properties of ZnOE cements		
	Zinc oxide eugenol cement unmodified	Resin modified cement	EBA-alumina cement
Compressive strength	3–40 MPa	55 MPa	50 MPa
Tensile strength	0.3–6 MPa	4 MPa	4 MPa
Modulus of elasticity	220–5400 MPa	2500 MPa	5000 MPa
Powder–liquid ratio	3–4:1	5–6:1	7:1

restoration is held on the tooth under pressure until cement sets. The excess is carefully removed.

Contraindication

Zinc oxide eugenol cements are contraindicated for using in contact with:
- Composite resins (eugenol can dissolve the resin and make it soft)
- GIC restorations (leaching eugenol can diffuse and cause discolouration).

Uses

1. **Zinc oxide eugenol cements are used for**
   - Type I—temporary cementation
   - Type II—permanent cementation
   - Type III—temporary restorations
   - Type IV—cavity liners
     These cements can also be used as **pulp capping agents and root canal sealants.**
2. **Resin-modified ZnO eugenol cements**
   As these have higher strengths, they can be used for
   - Permanent cementations
   - Cavity lining agents
   - Temporary and intermediate restorations.
3. **EBA-alumina cement is used for**
   - Permanent cementation
   - Cavity liners and bases
   - Intermediate restorations.

Advantages

- **Obtundent**—suitable for use to relieve postoperative sensitivity, pulp protection from thermal, chemical and electrical insults.
- Good marginal sealing properties due to low dimensional changes during setting.
- Resist marginal leakage.
- Sufficient strength for cementation—only for modified ZnOE cement.

Disadvantages

- The low compressive strength of conventional cement is inadequate for permanent cementation (however, modified cements can be used for intermediate restorations, cement bases and permanent cementations).
- Eugenol is a solvent for resins. Hence, contraindicated to use as a base for composite resins.
- Eugenol leaches and may diffuse causing discolouration if used as a base for glass ionomer cements.
- Does not chemically bond with dentin, enamel or metallic restorations and not anticariogenic.

Recent Modifications

1. **Noneugenol cements**
   Since direct contact of eugenol can cause irritation to soft tissues, eugenol is completely replaced with material like **vanillate esters (hexyl vanillate)** and **orthoethoxybenzoic acid.**

Composition	
Powder	
ZnO	60–70%
Alumina	30%
Liquid	
Hexyl vanillate	12.5%
Rosin	6%
Ethoxybenzoic acid	81.5%

2. **Zinc oxide eugenol endodontic sealer**
   Good sealing capacity of ZnOE cement has been utilized in endodontic treatment, to seal the root canal and protect from marginal leakage. This is sometimes used alone (type II) or with gutta-percha or silver points or cores—type I.

   There are mainly three formulations

   Ricker's, Grossman's and therapeutic formulae, with zinc oxide and eugenol as main ingredients. Several ingredients, medicaments, etc. are added to
   - Increase the flow (or decrease viscosity) for proper penetration into the root canal
   - Adjust the setting time suitably, 15 min to few hours
   - Adjust the film thickness to proper values 80–500 mm
   - Increase the compressive strength 8 to 50 MPa to support the root which has been weakened during root canal preparation
   - Decrease solubility inside
   - Obtain radio-opacity (barium, bismuth salts)
   - Decrease dimensional changes.

ZINC PHOSPHATE CEMENT

These cements are mainly used as luting cements (type I) as well as thermal insulating base and intermediate restorative material (type II).

This is the oldest luting cement available, having a long track record which can be used as **a standard** for comparing new cementation materials.

Alternative names

- Zinc cement
- Zinc improved cement
- Zinc oxyphosphate cement
- Crown and bridge cement.

Table 8.7 The composition of zinc phosphate cement

Ingredients	Weight%	Functions
Powder		
Zinc oxide	90.2%	Reactive ingredient
Magnesium oxide	8.2%	Aids in sintering (reduces fusion temperature)
Bismuth trioxide, calcium oxide	0.2%	Imparts smoothness to the freshly mixed cement
Barium oxide	Trace	Radio-opacifier
Silicon dioxide (silica)	1.4%	Inert fillers, gives strength and also aids in sintering
Liquid		
Phosphoric acid	38.2%	Reactive ingredient
Water	33±5%	Controls the rate of the reaction
Aluminum phosphate or zinc phosphate	16.2 %	Buffers—stabilizes the pH of acids and they reduce the rate of reaction (retarders)
Aluminum	2.5%	Essential for cement formation and assist in the formation of an amorphous product, zinc aluminum phosphate for cohesion and strength
Zinc for cohesion	7.1%	Acts as moderator of the reaction, aids

Composition (*refer* to Table 8.7)

Dispensing

Dispensed in the form of powder and liquid in separate bottles. It can also be supplied in the form of **capsule** with pre-proportioned powder and liquid.

According to ADA specification, adapted in 1935, zinc phosphate cements can be classified into two types

- **Type I:** Fine grain, used as luting cement (film thickness is <25 mm)
- **Type II:** Medium grain, used as a thermal insulting base and intermediate restorative material (film thickness is <40 mm).

Manufacturing of powder

Sintering

The ingredients of the powder are mixed and heated at a temperature **of 1000–1400°C for 4–8 hours.** The cake formed is then powdered/ground into fine particles. The sintering helps to change the reactivity suitably.

Chemistry of Setting Action

When the powder is mixed with the liquid, the following reaction takes place.

$$3ZnO + 2H_3PO_4 + H_2O \rightarrow Zn_3(PO_4)_2 \cdot 4H_2O + \textbf{heat}$$

Zinc oxide + phosphoric acid → Tertiary zinc phosphate

(non-cohesive **Hopeite** crystals)

Recent studies confirmed the following reaction

ZnO + phosphoric acid ⟶ Zinc alumino-
(in the presence of Al and zinc phosphate buffers) phosphate gel + H_2O + heat

When the excess of zinc phosphate cement powder is mixed with liquid, wetting occurs and chemical reaction is initiated. The reaction is rapid and **exothermic** and pH increases gradually. The reaction is slowed down by the buffers present.

The exact nature of the final product of this reaction is uncertain. In the past, it has been thought that the tertiary zinc phosphate ($Zn_3(PO_4)_2 4H_2O$—Hopeite) as the final product. But recent studies explain the reaction in a simple way, i.e. when the powder and liquid are mixed, phosphoric acid attacks zinc oxide powder and releases zinc ions. The aluminum already present in the liquid, forms complex with phosphoric acid and this complex combines with Zn ions to form an **amorphous gel matrix** known as **zinc aluminophosphate gel**. The set cement consists of a matrix of amorphous zinc aluminophosphate that **surrounds unreacted zinc oxide particles**. The final structure is a cored structure (Fig. 8.3).

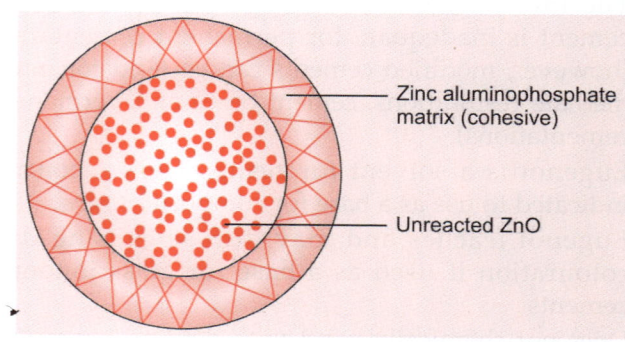

Fig. 8.3: Structure of set ZnPO₄ cement

Properties

1. **Biological property**

   Zinc phosphate cement is quite irritant to the pulp, particularly when used as cement base material. The freshly mixed cement is highly acidic with pH as low as 1.6–3.0. Even after 1 hr, the pH may be less than 4. This can give rise to **pulpal irritation and pain. The degree of irritation depends on the depth of the cavity or the thickness of dentin left**. To protect the pulp from irritation (or the dentin surface), **it should be covered with pulp capping agents such** as zinc oxide-eugenol cements or calcium hydroxide cements (or a varnish). These materials may neutralize the acidic effect. The pH of cement changes with respect time as:

pH at the end of 3 minutes	1.6–3.5
pH at the end of 1 hour	4.0
pH at the end of 24 hours	5.6
pH at the end of 7 days	6.8

2. **Rheological properties**

   - **Mixing time:** 1–1.25 min

   - **Setting time:** According to ADA specification No. 8, **it is 5–9 minutes**
     Type I—zinc phosphate cement: 5.5 minutes
     Type II—zinc phosphate cement base: 3.5 minutes
     Setting time can be defined as the time elapsed from the start of the mix until the **modified Gilmore needle** no longer indents into the mix.

Factors affecting setting time
Controlled by the manufacturer

- **Sintering temperature:** Higher the sintering temperature, the more slow the cement sets.

- **Particle size:** Finer the particle size, faster the setting.
- **Accelerators:** Small amount of water accelerates the setting.
- **Buffering agents:** Retards the rate of the reaction.

Controlled by the operator

- **Temperature:** Higher temperature shorter is setting time.
- **P/L ratio:** Higher P/L ratio, faster is the setting.
- The reaction is slowed down if the powder is incorporated into the liquid slowly (longer setting time).
  Setting time is seriously affected if the liquid bottle is exposed to the dry or humid atmosphere. **Loss of water** by evaporation to dry atmosphere **decreases pH and increases setting time. Absorption** of water from humid atmosphere increases pH and decreases setting time. Hence, the bottle should always be kept closed to retain the water content which is critical (33 ± 5%).

- **Consistency** is measured by finding the disc diameter, d, formed when 0.5 ml of freshly mixed cement is slabs in-between 2 glass plates and a weight of 120 gm in placed for 10 minutes (Fig. 8.4c).

  It depends upon the particular use of the material
  Type I: Luting cement **30–35 mm** (thin strand-like consistency, Fig. 8.4a).
  Type II: Base or intermediate restorative material hook-like consistency, Fig. 8.4b—disc diameters, d, 25–30 mm.
  Band or standard seating consistency = 30 mm.

- **The film thickness** is measured according to ADA specifications by loading 2.5 kg on the mix placed in between two glass plates (Table 8.8).

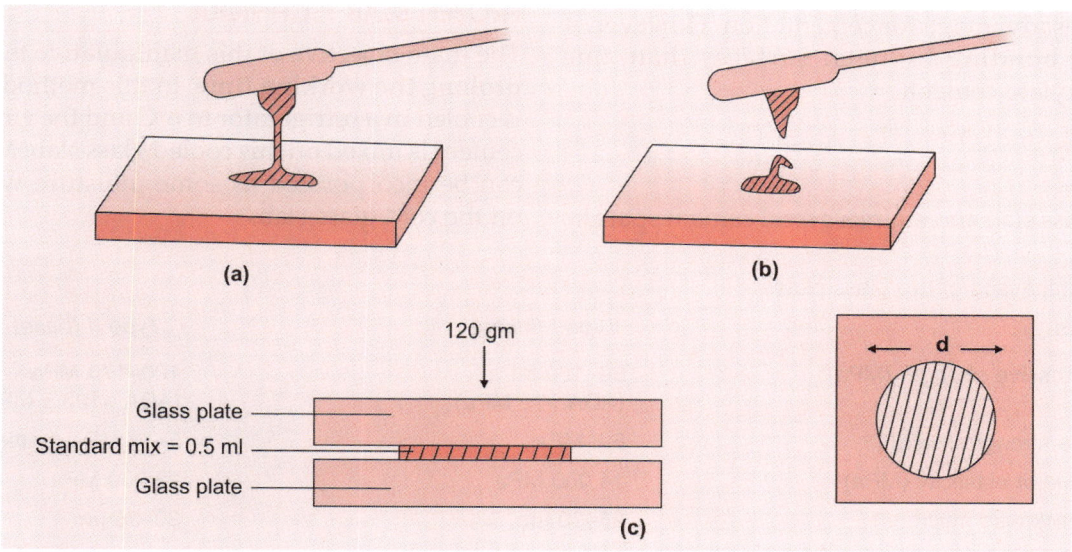

Figs 8.4a to c: (a) Cementation threading, (b) hook-like base consistency, (c) consistency measurement

Type 1:   20–25 µm (luting)
Type 11: 25–40 µm (base)

Thinner film is more advantageous specially for luting cements because

- It has better cementing-action or strength.
- It helps in complete seating of the restoration due to higher flow.

3. **Solubility and disintegration**
   According to ADA specification, it should be <0.2%. For the available zinc phosphate cements, the values are only ≈ 0.06% by weight in distilled water measured in 24 hours.
   Solubility is minimum for optimum powder/liquid ratio. Solubility also depends on the pH values of various media like citric acid, tartaric acid, etc.
   Longer time of initial wetting, greater is the solubility. To decrease the initial larger solubility, the cement can be **coated with a varnish**.

4. **Mechanical properties**
   Factors affecting strength
   P/L ratio: Higher P/L, greater the strength, up to an optimum value 4.8 gm/ml, above this strength decreases.
   Water content: Change in the water content of the liquid either loss or gain will reduce the strength.

5. **Thermal properties**
   It is a good thermal insulator and is suitable to be used as a thermal insulating base.

6. **Adhesion property**
   This does not form chemical bonding with enamel or dentin. The retention of cemented restoration depends on the mechanical interlocking of the set cement with the roughness of the surface of the cavity and the inner part of the alloy restorations. This is the main disadvantage for cementation. However, it has better bonding to metal surfaces than zinc polycarboxylate cement.

Manipulation

Instruments
Clean, dry glass slab and stainless steel cement spatula.

P/L ratio
   Type I: 2.8 gm/ml for luting consistency
   Type 2: 4.8 gm/ml for base consistency

Proportioning
A suitable amount of powder is taken on a glass slab with the help of cement spatula. It is divided into two small increments, two bulk increments, followed by smaller increments. Then two to three drops of liquid are taken in front of the small increments and **close the bottle immediately, to retain the water content or pH.**

Mixing (Fig. 8.5)
It is initiated by the addition of a small increment of powder to the liquid. This slow addition of powder to the liquid has the effect of delaying the setting slightly, creating **more working time and reduces initial acidity**. Spatulation is done by rotary motion over a large area of the slab, to **dissipate the heat of the chemical reaction** and slows down the setting action to a certain extent. A large amount of powder (bulk increment) is then added during the middle of the mixing to further **saturate the liquid quickly** with the newly forming complex, i.e. $ZnPO_4$. Finally, small increments of the powder are incorporated one by one until the desired ultimate consistency is reached. Mixing time is about 60–75 sec.

Cementation procedure
The mix is first applied to the **inner surface of pre-formed restoration** say a crown and then it is seated on the prepared tooth. The restoration is then kept **under pressure** and maintained until the cement sets, when excess flows out through a vent hole, sometimes drilled in the crown, which also prevents air trapping.

FROZEN SLAB TECHNIQUE

The main objective of this manipulative technique is to **prolong the working time**. In this method, a glass slab is cooled in a refrigerator to 6°C and the zinc phosphate cement is mixed on this cooled glass slab. **More powder** can be incorporated as some moisture will condense on the cold glass slab.

Table 8.8	Comparison of two glass plates		
	Properties	Type I (luting)	Type II (base)
1.	Compressive strength (MPa)	80–100 MPa (ADA >75 MPa)	100–170 MPa (ADA >103.5 MPa)
2.	Tensile strength (MPa)	5.5 MPa	5–14 MPa (brittle)
3.	Modulus of elasticity (MPa)	14,000 MPa	22,000 MPa
4.	Film thickness (microns)	25–30 µm	30–35 µm
5.	Consistency (mm)	30–35 mm	25–30 mm

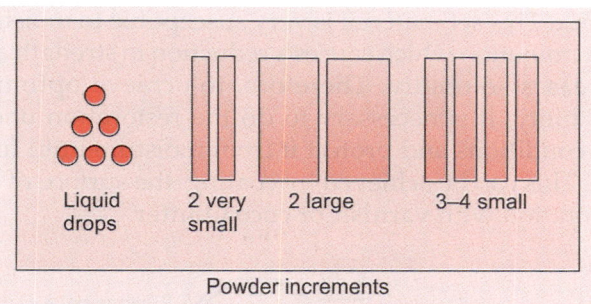

Fig. 8.5: Division of powder before mixing of $ZnPO_4$ cement

Advantages
- Increases working time
- Decreases setting time
- Greater P/L ratio can be achieved, but mechanical properties remain almost the same.

Uses
This technique is most widely used in orthodontia where a series of **orthodontic** bands have to be cemented, one after the other, with one mix, which should have longer working time.

Precautions required during mixing zinc phosphate cement
- The liquid bottle should be kept closed when not in use to prevent water loss, as the loss of water will lower pH and slows down the reaction, increases setting time.
- The liquid bottle which appears cloudy should be discarded.
- Liquid and powder should not be interchanged with those of different batches.
- Last 1/5th portion of the liquid should be discarded (as pH might have changed)
- Liquid should be dispensed on the slab just before mixing.
- The consistency of the mix should be checked after adding each increment of powder.
- Cement mix should be applied to the inner surface of the preformed restorations or casting before it is seated on the prepared tooth cavity (otherwise cement may set on the tooth before the restoration is seated).

Uses of zinc phosphate cements
- It is primarily used as permanent cementation material to fix preformed restorations or castings (inlays, crowns, bridges, etc.).
- Used to fix orthodontic bands.
- Used as a thermal insulating high strength base.
- It is also used as a temporary or intermediate restorative material.

Advantages
- It has adequate compressive strength and same modulus of elasticity of dentin to resist fracture and deformation/under stress.
- Easy manipulation procedure, and less critical technique.
- Sets sharply to relatively hard mass from a fluid consistency.
- Lower solubility than silicate cement.

Disadvantages
- Pulpal irritation due to its high initial acidity. Hence should not be placed directly on exposed dentin.
- Lack of anticariogenic property.
- It is a brittle cement, poor tensile strength.
- **Lack of chemical adhesion** to the tooth.
- Soluble in oral fluids.
- Not aesthetic.

MODIFICATIONS OF ZINC PHOSPHATE CEMENT

1. **Hydrophosphate water settable zinc phosphate cement**

   This cement is supplied as single component powder system. The liquid used is distilled water. The phosphoric acid liquid is freeze-dried and converted to solid form (powder). These solid acid phosphates are blended with conventional zinc phosphate powder.

   The acidity is the same as that of the conventional zinc phosphate cement. Compressive strength, film thickness, solubility, and disintegration are inferior to that of conventional zinc phosphate cement and is mainly used as luting cement and thermal insulting bases. It is not popular.

2. **Fluoride cements:** Fluoride containing $ZnPO_4$ cements are obtained by adding a small percentage of **stannous fluoride** and made antibacterial or anticariogenic. Such cements are known as fluoride cements. These cements have high solubility but the anticariogenic property is not so good **as leaching of fluoride ions decrease in one or two days**.

3. **Germicidal cements (silver or copper cements)**

   Silver salts or copper oxides are sometimes added to the powders of zinc phosphate cement to impart antibacterial/antiseptic properties to the cement. The cement is black in colour when cupric oxide (CuO) is added, red when cuprous oxide (Cu_2O) is added, white when cuprous iodide (Cu_2I_2) is added and green when cupric silicate ($CuSiO_3$) is added. Due to its higher initial acidity, the cement is used only in rare cases, such as in rampant caries of deciduous teeth.

4. **Zinc silicophosphate cements (*refer* to silicate cements).**

SILICATE CEMENTS

Silicate cement is the **earliest of direct tooth coloured** restorative material available since the beginning of 20th century. This cement disappeared as soon as the composite restorative resins were introduced into the dentistry. Silicate cement is **highly acidic** even after months and has a higher degree of solubility and hence this cement cause severe damage to the pulp or exposed dentin and therefore, not used now and replaced by multipurpose glass ionomer cements. But this cement should be studied because it was the first cement which had **fluorides in it and had anticariogenic** property, which opened the doors for other fluoride-containing cements.

The silicate cement is dispensed as powder liquid system and also in pre-proportional capsules (like silver amalgam).

Compositions of silicate cement powder and liquids (Table 8.9).

Manufacturing of Powder

The ingredients are **fused and solidified by quenching**. This **fritting** causes many microcraks and makes easy to powder into fine particles. The liquid is protected in air-tight closed bottles.

Setting action

When the powder and liquids are mixed, the H⁺ ions attack the glass powder displacing Al, Ca, F, and Na⁺ ions. As a result of this attack, there is a **degradation of the glass network to form a hydrated silicious gel** around the powder particles. The ions liberated from the surface of the glass particles combine with H_2PO_3 ions and subsequently precipitate as phosphates and fluorides. As the pH rises, this reaction causes the cement to set and the resulting matrix is an amorphous solid, i.e. **hydrated aluminum phosphate and fluoride**

matrix. This set material is very susceptible to moisture contamination which causes a reduction in strength and increases solubility. Therefore, to achieve optimum durability, it is necessary to do the restoration under dry conditions and protect it from moisture until fully sets. This can be achieved by coating the surface of the restoration with **varnish or cocoa butter.**

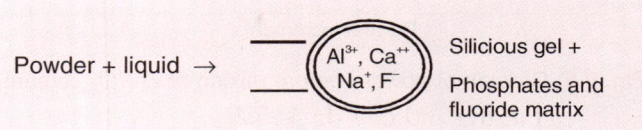

Structure of set cement (Fig. 8.6)

The set cement consist of unreacted glass particles covered with a layer of hydrated **alumina-silica gel** and they are embedded in the matrix of insoluble fluorides and phosphates.

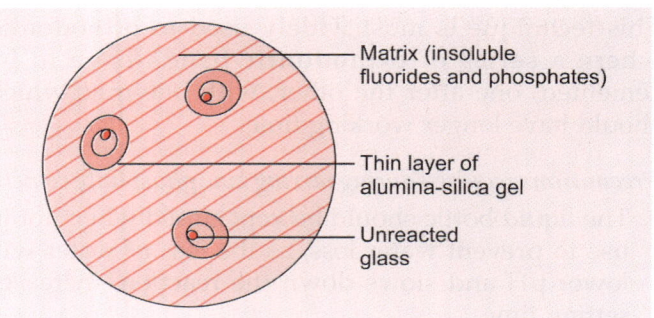

Fig. 8.6: Structure of set silicate cement

Properties

1. **Biological property**
   - *Effect of silicate cement on pulp*
     Highly irritant to the pulp. Silicate cements irritate pulp when placed in freshly cut dentin unless a base protects it. In terms of **pulp response,** it is

Table 8.9	The compositions of silicate cement powder and liquids		
	Ingredients	Approximate weight%	Functions
	Powder		
	• Silica SiO_2	40%	Gives strength translucency
	• Alumina Al_2O_3	30%	Reacts with phosphoric acid
	• Na_3PO_4, K_3PO_4, CaO	5–7%	Provide Al, Ca, K ions to form a matrix
	• Fluorides (CaF, NaF, KF, lite)	23%	Flux, decreases melting and fritting temperatures, contributes anticariogenic property
	Liquid		
	• Phosphoric acid	45%	Reactor
	• Buffers—$AlPO_4$, $ZnPO_4$	15%	Control setting time
	• Water	40%	Controls pH and setting times

classified as a **severely irritant**. The irritating properties are due to phosphoric acid which can penetrate through a thickness of dentin as great as 1 mm to 1.5 mm. Sometimes the irritation of pulp is sufficiently severe to cause **pulp death.**

Also, the pH has significant value even after a month
- pH at the end of 3 minutes: **2.8**
- pH at the end of 1 hour: 3.7
- pH at the end of 24 hrs: 5
- pH at the end of 48 hrs: 5.2
- pH at the end of 7 days: 5.2
- pH at the end of 28 days: **5.8**

The pulp must be protected by using a $Ca(OH)_2$ cement base. Cavity varnish should be applied **only to dentin and not to enamel** because of the penetration of fluoride into enamel is prevented and thus there is no effect of anticariogenic property.

- *Anticariogenic property*
  This is due to the presence and release of fluoride ions from the restorative materials. The silicate cement restoration is quite **soluble** in the oral fluid releasing fluoride ions from the restoration. These fluoride ions are responsible for decreasing the chances of decay of an adjacent tooth, i.e. fluoride uptake by the enamel adjacent to the restoration can occur, and **this reduces enamel solubility.** The anticariogenic properties may be due to two important reasons.
- *Physiochemical mechanism:* Fluoride ions released during the setting and subsequent dissolution from the silicate cements react with the adjacent tooth to form a very strong structure that is more **resistant to acid decalcification.** The fluoride is able to replace the hydroxyl group of the hydroxyapatite present in enamel to form an acid-resistant structure called **fluorapatite**, which cannot be quickly dissolved and thus **caries (demineralization)** is prevented.

  Hydroxyapatite + F $\longrightarrow$ Fluorapatite

  $Ca_{10}(PO_4)_6(OH)_2 + F \longrightarrow Ca_{10}(PO_4)_6F_2$

- *Biological mechanism:* The available fluoride at the surface of the restoration and the cement-tooth interface serves as an **enzyme inhibitor.** The fluoride which is coming out of silicate restoration can enter the bacterial cell present in the plaque and **inhibit the carbohydrate metabolism, thus preventing the production of acids.** Hence, the caries formation is prevented.

2. **Rheological properties**
   - Mixing time: 1 minute
   - Setting time: 3 to 8 minutes
3. **Mechanical properties (approximate)**
   - High compressive strength = 200 MPa (hardest of inorganic cements)
   - Low tensile strength (brittle) = 15 MPa
   - Large abrasive resistance surface, hardness = 80 KHN
4. **Solubility and disintegration**
   Solubility = 0.7% in distilled water. Solubility is much higher in citric, tartaric, acetic acids and **is highest in citric acid of pH = 4.**
5. **Aesthetic property**
   Initially good, but disintegration and solubility takes place faster at the boundaries of restoration which collects food debris and form **a dark cement line.**

Manipulation

Instruments required

Clean glass slab and a non-abradable, i.e. stellite (Cr-Co-Ni alloys), agate spatula or plastic spatula.

Reason to use a plastic spatula instead of stainless steel spatula

Since the silicate powder (glass) is a hard abrasive material, this can abrade the stainless steel spatula and release carbon, iron and other impurities from steel which can contaminate and discolour the mix and restoration.

Manipulation

Use a clean glass slab and **agate or stellite spatula.** Take a suitable amount of powder and divide into **two parts.** Later part is again divided into 3 or 4 smaller parts for adjusting the putty consistency. Take two drops of liquid **(powder/liquid ratio = 4:1)**. Add the large bulk of powder and mix by **overlapping, folding or tapping** method **in a minimum area to retain gel structure.** Add increments one after the other, and get putty, glossy consistency (0.5 ml mix placed in between two glass plates, and pressed by 2.5 kg, should form a disc of 2.5 cm diameter). The plastic spatula can be used on folding technique does not get abrade.

Place it in the tooth cavity **isolated** from the moist mouth, **using a rubber dam.** Smoothen by covering with a **cellulose matrix** band, allow to set, and apply a coating of **cocoa-butter or varnish.** All these procedures are to be followed as the cement has **gel structure**, which may get disturbed by **moisture contamination** causing syneresis inhibition and a decrease in strength. This is avoided for the first two days by the coating and thereafter it should not get dried—to minimize crazing.

Silicate cement restoration should not be given to **mouth breathers**.

Precautions

Precautions to be observed are similar to zinc phosphate cement manipulation procedures.

If dentine is exposed, $Ca(OH)_2$ base is to be applied to **protect the pulp**, as the acid ions can pass through dentinal tubules are **causing pulp death**.

Contraindications

1. Posterior restorations and stress-bearing areas like class I, class II cavities
2. Zinc oxide eugenol base should not be used (as diffusing eugenol **cause discolouration**).
3. Cavity varnishes should **not be applied on enamel** surface where silicate cement is applied to retain anticariogenic property.
4. **Mouth breathers** should not be given silicate cement restorations.
5. Stainless steel spatula should not be used.

Applications

Now it is not used due to its severe irritant properties. Formerly used for
- Anterior restorations class III, V
- Patients with high caries index
- Intermediate restorations

Merits
- Anticariogenic property
- Good initial aesthetics
- High compressive strength (200 MPa).

Demerits
- High acidity for a long time and severe irritant causing pulp death
- Colour changes due to syneresis, imbibition and solubility (dark margins—cement lines are formed)
- Lack of chemical bonding with the tooth.

ZINC SILICOPHOSPHATE CEMENT, ADA 21

This cement is the combination of $ZnPO_4$ cement and silicate cement (hybrid variety). **The main objective** of combining both these cements, **is to obtain** the good aesthetics and anticariogenic properties of silicate cements, lower initial solubility and acidity of $ZnPO_4$ cement.

Alternative names
- Synthetic porcelain
- Silicate zinc cement
- Zinc silicate cement
- Filling synthetic porcelain.

Special properties
- **Anticariogenic property**
- Translucency similar to that of porcelain and hence used as **luting cements** to fix preformed **porcelain restorations** (porcelain jacket crown—PJC).

Dispensing

Dispensed as powder and liquid in the air-tight bottle with a nozzle.

According to ADA specification No. 21, these are classified into 3 types
Type I: Luting or cementation material
Type II: Temporary posterior filling material and IRM

Table 8.10	The composition of zinc silicophosphate cement	
Ingredients	Weight%	Functions
Silica	25%	Provides translucency, strength, and hardness
Alumina	25%	Reactive ingredient
ZnO	15%	Reactive ingredient
MgO	10%	Increases strength
CaO	10%	Imparts smoothness to the mix
Calcium fluoride and sodium fluoride	15%	Anticariogenic property, decreases fusion temperature (flux)
Liquid		
Phosphoric acid	50%	Reactive ingredient
Zinc phosphate and aluminum phosphate	3–5%	Buffers (stabilize the pH of acids)
Water	45%	Controls the rate of the reaction

Table 8.11 Properties of zinc silicophosphate cements

Properties	Type I (luting)	Type II IRM, temp. posterior restoration
1. Consistency (mm)	25 ± 1	25 ± 1
2. Film thickness (μm)	25	25–40
3. Setting time (min)	5-9	3–8
4. Compressive strength (MPa)	140	170
5. Tensile strength (MPa)	6	7
6. Surface hardness (KHN)	70	70
7. Thermal conduction	Insulator	Insulator
8. COTE (ppm/°C)	9–10	9–10
9. Solubility (% in 24 hrs)	0.1–0.3%	0.1–0.3%

Type III: Luting and restorative cement (dual purpose cement). The composition of zinc silicophosphate cement (Table 8.10.)

Manufacturing of Powder

The ingredients of the powder are heated at 1400°C and fused to form an acid-soluble glass. The fluoride salts melt at a lower temperature and dissolve the other ingredients. These **fluorides** are known as **ceramic fluxes.** Aluminum phosphate can also be used as a flux. It also furnishes additional aluminum to the glass. After thorough melting at fusion temperature, the fused mass is cooled quickly by quenching. This causes the glass to crack which helps in grinding the material to a fine powder. This process is known as **fritting.**

Setting reaction

Zinc aluminosilicate glass + H_3PO_4 → zinc aluminophosphate silicate gel.

Properties

The properties of zinc silicophosphate cements are **intermediate** between those of silicate and zinc phosphate cements.

Biological property

It is more closely approximated to that of zinc phosphate than that of silicate cement.

It is irritating to the pulp because of the acidity and prolonged low pH after setting. Therefore, pulpal protection is necessary for all vital teeth. **It is anticariogenic:**

- pH at the end of 3 min: **3.2**
- pH at the end of 1 hr: 5.4
- pH at the end of 24 hrs: 6.1
- pH at the end of 48 hrs: 6.3
- pH at the end of 7 days: **6.5**

Mechanical and thermal properties are described in Table 8.11.

Manipulation

The method is very **similar** to that of **silicate cement.** Powder/liquid ratios are 2–2.5 gm/ml and 3.5–4.0 gm/ml for type I and type II cements, respectively. Similar precautions are to be observed.

Merits of zinc silicophosphate cements

Compared to zinc phosphate cement. This has:

- Higher strength and abrasive resistance
- Anticariogenic due to fluoride leaching
- Better mechanical bonding, specially with ceramics
- Higher translucency is similar to ceramics.

Demerits

- Higher initial acidity
- Prolonged acidity causing more pulp sensitivity
- More brittleness
- Higher film thickness.

Uses

It was used for cementation of aesthetic restoratives like ceramic (PJC) crowns. However, at present, it is not used much due to the availability of better resin and GIC materials.

ZINC POLYCARBOXYLATE CEMENT, ADA 61

It was the first dental cement which had chemical bonding with tooth structure (adhesive dental cement) formulated by **Dr. Smith in 1968,** while trying to find out a cement which had the strength of zinc phosphate and biological acceptability of zinc oxide eugenol cements (*see* Colour Plate 15, Fig. 8.1).

It is now most widely used as a thermal insulating base and also as luting cement to fix metallic crowns, bridges and orthodontic bands.

Alternative names
- Zinc polyacrylate cement
- Zinc poly C
- Zinc poly F
- Hy bond, Polycarb

Special properties
1. Direct chemical bonding with tooth structure. **It is a real cement**.
2. Excellent biocompatibility and kind to the pulp.

Dispensing
1. Dispensed as powder and liquid system with a measuring scoop and paper pad for mixing.
2. It is also be supplied as a single component system, i.e. powder which can be mixed with distilled water.

Composition of powder
Zinc polycarboxylate cement powder is shown in Table 8.12.

Composition of liquid
This is an **aqueous solution** of polyacrylic acid of moderate molecular weights 25,000–50,000, with about **32–45% in water**. This reacts with ZnO and sets, also forms chemical bonding with tooth enamel and dentin, through Ca^{2+} and collagen, respectively.

This also may contain some of its **copolymers, itaconic acid** and **tartaric acids** to reduce the high viscosities.

Water settable—anhydrous polycarboxylate cements
This is a single component system. The **polyacrylic acid is freeze-dried** and incorporated in the same powder. When the powder is mixed with distilled water, the polyacrylic acid dissolves in water and then reacts in the same manner. There is no much difference or improvements in the properties, and hence it has not become popular.

Setting and Bonding Reactions to Tooth Enamel and Dentin
1. **Setting reaction:** When the powder is mixed with polyacrylic acid, the Zn^{++} cations cross-link the polymer chains through COO^- groups forming zinc polyacrylate matrix, as represented in **a** (page 157).
2. **Bonding to tooth enamel:** When the mix is placed on the tooth enamel, **which is rich in Ca^{++} ions,** chemical bonding (adhesion) takes place forming calcium polyacrylates, through the COO^- groups not involved in the setting reaction. These undergo a complex reaction with the Ca^{++}, by ionic bonding with the Ca^{++} ions acting as bridges. This is represented in **b**.
3. **Bonding to dentin:** Dentin is a composite material containing almost equal volumes of calcium hydroxyapatite and organic material. The organic material has mainly collagen, with carboxylic and NH_2 groups available for reaction and bonding.

This bonding to dentin takes place by two methods
1. **Hydrogen bonds** are formed between COO^- groups of polyacrylic acid and NH_2 groups of dentin collagen.
2. Ions diffusing from the cement allow cations bridges to be formed between the COO^- groups of polyacrylic acid and collagen. This is represented in **c**.

The inorganic component calcium and homogeneity of enamel is higher than that of dentin. Hence, the bond strength to enamel is greater. To improve the bonding strength to dentin, several methods have been used (*refer* to bonding agents).

All the above three reactions **a, b, c** can be represented, in a simple manner.

Properties
1. **Biological property:** It has good biocompatibility with pulp. The effect of polycarboxylate cement on

Table 8.12	The composition of zinc polycarboxylate cement powder		
Ingredients	Weight%		Functions
Powder			
• ZnO	80%		Principle reactor
• MgO	10%		Decreases calcination temperature
• $SiO_2 + Al_2O_3$	2–8%		Increases strength
• Stannous fluoride	4–5%		Improves mixing and physical properties, modifies setting time, may impart anti-cariogenic property, initially only

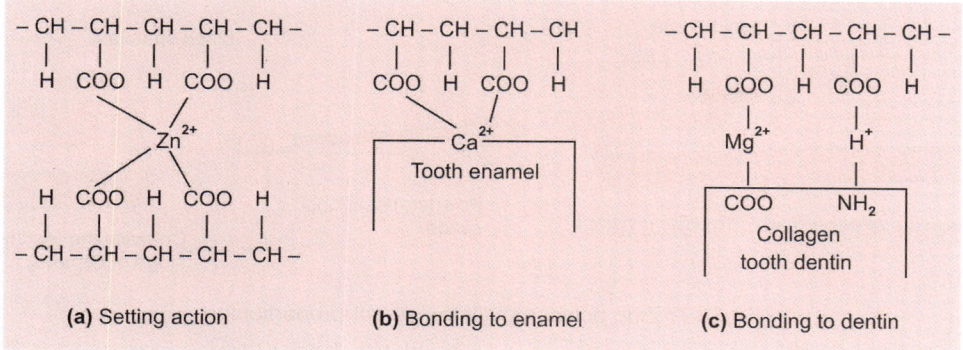

Setting and bonding reactions of zinc polycarboxylate cement to tooth structure

soft and calcified tissues is found to be **mild**. The effect on the pulp is similar or less than that of zinc oxide eugenol cement.

Causes for the mildness of zinc polycarboxylate cements towards pulp
- Polyacrylic acid is a **weak acid** compared with phosphoric acid
- **The rapid rise** of pH towards neutrality. Polyacrylic pH of the cement liquid is approximately **1.7**. However, the liquid is rapidly neutralized by the powder, thus the pH of the mix rapidly rises as the reaction proceeds. The approximate values, at the ends of:

2 minutes pH	3.42
5 minutes pH	3.99
30 minutes	5.03
1 hr	5.08
1 day	5.94–6.5

- **The larger size** of polyacrylic acid molecules as compared to phosphoric acid molecules may **limit its diffusion** through the dentinal tubules.
- The attraction towards proteins (enamelin, amelogenin) may also limit its diffusion through the dentinal tubules or **complexes formed may block exposed dentinal tubules. Excellent biocompatibility** to the pulp is the major factor to the popularity of the cement.
- Fluoride-containing materials release fluoride ions which is taken up by the neighboring enamel and cause anticariogenic effect. But the effect in this cement is not so good as silicate cements as the fluoride ions cannot leach out for a long time.

2. **Rheological properties**
- Mixing time is only 30–45 seconds
- According to ADA specification **No. 61,** this should have setting time <9 minutes.
- Setting time for the commercial products, for luting purpose = 6–9 min
- Setting time for the commercial products for base cement = 3–5 min

The rate of setting is faster (setting time is shorter) if
- The P/L ratio is more
- The temperature of mixing spatula and slab is higher
- The particle size is smaller
- The reactivity of zinc oxide is more.

The best method of prolonging the setting time is by **cooling the glass slab** and spatula but not below the dew point.

Film thickness
According to ADA specification No. 61, it should have film thickness less than 25 μm. But the commercial products have a film thickness between 21 and 35 μm.

The mix appears to be more viscous but flows under pressure to film thickness of approximately 25 μm. This can be classified as **pseudoplastic** materials, i.e. it undergoes thinning with increased shear rate during seating of restoration.

3. **Mechanical properties**
- The compressive strength of luting = 55–85 MPa and of base cement = 70–95 MPa
- The tensile strength of luting cement = 8–12 MPa and of base cement = 9–14 MPa
- Modulus of elasticity of luting = 5–6 GPa and of base cement = 4–5 GPa

4. **Adhesion/bond strength and bonding**
Polycarboxylate cement displays good adhesion to enamel and dentin through **calcium chelation (chemical bonding)**. The cement also binds to stainless steel, amalgam, chromium-cobalt alloys, etc. The bond strength to enamel is about **3.45 to 13.1 MPa.** The bond strength to **dentin is only 2.07 MPa.** Zinc polycarboxylate cement is not superior to zinc phosphate cement with respect to retention of cast gold restorations, but retention can be enhanced by **electroplating the inner surface of restoration with tin.**

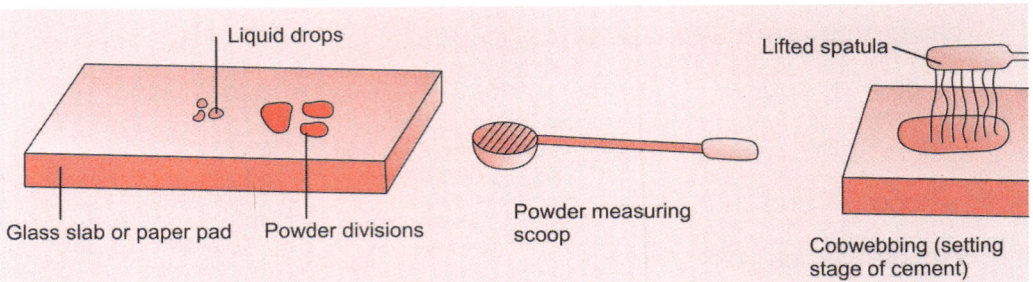

Fig. 8.7: Zinc polycarboxylate cement proportioning

5. **Solubility and disintegration**
   According to ADA specification No. 61, solubility and disintegration in distilled water at the end of 24 hrs should be **<0.2%** by weight. Solubilities for commercial products for luting cements is only 0.06% by weight and for the base cements is 0.2% by weight, and not high.
6. **Thermal properties**
   These are good thermal insulating materials and can be used as thermal insulating bases.
7. **Aesthetics**
   These cements cannot be used as anterior restorative material as the set cement is **opaque** due to concentration of unreacted zinc oxide.

Manipulation

Instruments required are glass slab or paper pad, stainless steel or plastic spatula.
Powder-liquid ratio for luting cement = **1.5 gm/ml**
Powder-liquid ratio for base cement = **2.3 gm/ml**

Proportioning

The required amount of powder is dispensed on the glass slab by using the measuring scoop provided by the manufacturer and the powder is divided into **1 bulk and 2 small increments.** Take 2 or 3 drops of liquid as suggested.

Mixing

Mixing is initiated by the addition of bulk increment and followed by smaller increments as the mixing proceeds. The mixing is continued until a homogeneous mass is formed. The mixing is done by **folding, overlapping and tapping techniques to protect the gel structure formed**. It should be completed within 30 seconds to provide sufficient working time to carry out cementation or base operation. Proper mix of polycarboxylate cement is somewhat thicker in appearance but has a **shiny, glossy appearance, which indicates that polyacrylic acid is still available to bond to the tooth structure,** otherwise, no retention will occur. A proper mix of polycarboxylate cement forms a thin strand when pulled up with a spatula in case of luting consistency or hook-like in case of base consistency (Fig. 8.7).

Cementation

The mix is applied to the seating surfaces of casting as well as on the prepared surfaces of the tooth, and the cast restoration is **firmly held under pressure** until the cement sets. Cementation should be done before the cement loses its **glossy appearance.**

If the cement mix shows **tackiness or cobwebbing** it has already started setting and should be discarded.

Precautions taken during manipulation

- Polyacrylic acid liquid should not be stored in refrigeration because the low temperature causes the liquid to **gel or thicken.**
- The liquid should be dispensed only just before the commencement of mixing. Exposure of the liquid to the atmosphere even for short periods, results in evaporation of water causing significant increase in viscosity.
- Cementation should be done before cement loses its glossy appearance **or before** starting of **cobwebbing**.
- Instruments should be cleaned before cement loses its glossy appearance using alcohol or boiling in NaOH solution.
- **The tooth surface and casting surface should be clean and dry** to achieve a good bond with the tooth surface. Tooth surface can be cleaned by pumice slurry followed by thorough rinsing and drying. The casting surface must be made rough for better retention by sandblasting or it should be electroplated with tin.

Uses

- For cementation of cast-alloy restoration like metallic crowns and bridges.
- For cementation of porcelain restorations and orthodontic bands.
- For thermal insulating bases
- For temporary filling materials.

Merits

- Excellent biocompatibility when the pulp is not exposed
- Chemical bonding to the tooth (enamel and dentin)
- Freshly mixed cement exhibits shear thinning or pseudoplastic properly
- Good thermal insulating materials
- Easy manipulation methods.

Demerits

- Accurate proportioning is required for optimum properties
- Need for a clean surface to utilize adhesion potential
- Short mixing and working times
- Lower compressive strength than zinc phosphate cement
- Soluble in oral fluids
- Anticariogenic properties, is not good when compared with silicate or glass ionomer cements
- **Does not bond** chemically with porcelain or noble metal or base metal castings.

Zinc phosphate cement has better mechanical bonding property, with metal restoration and no chemical bonding with tooth enamel, whereas the chemical bonding of zinc polycarboxylate cement is much stronger with enamel. Hence, bond failures takes place for $ZnPO_4$ cement at enamel interface and for zinc polycarboxylate cement at metal restorations interface (Figs 8.8a and b).

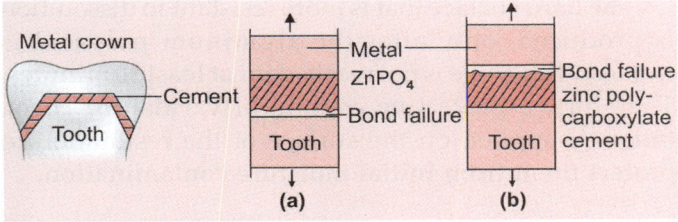

Figs 8.8a and b: Bond failures. (a) $ZnPO_4$; (b) zinc polycarboxylate cement at enamel and metal surfaces respectively

GLASS IONOMER CEMENTS (GICs)

This cement is termed as **glass ionomer cement** since the powder is **glass,** and the setting and bonding reaction to the tooth involves **ionic bonding.**

Glass ionomer cement consists of basic glass and an acid polymer which sets by **an acid–base reaction** between the components.

GIC is a product formed when **ion-leachable glass** combines with an aqueous solution of polyacrylic acid. GIC is **adhesive, tooth coloured, restorative materials** which was originally used for restoration of **eroded areas.** But in the recent days, the cement has been developed by many folds and has become **multi-purpose cement**. This cement has combined properties of silicate cement and polycarboxylate cements.

GIC was prepared by Dr. Wilson, Dr. Kent in 1972 and their first clinical use was reported by Dr. McLean and Dr. Wilson in 1975 and released for use as ASPA cement (Fuji) with polyacrylic acid, citric acid conditioner, powders of three shades, and two colour pigments.

Alternative names

- ASPA cement (aluminosilicate polyacrylate cement)
- Glass polyalkeonates
- Glass ionomer cement
- Ionofill
- Chemfill

Special properties

GIC has desirable characteristics of both silicate and zinc polyacrylic cement

- Excellent biocompatibility with the pulp
- Direct chemical bonding to the tooth structure
- Anticariogenic properties due to release of fluorides
- Porcelain-like translucency which is derived from the glass
- Favourable bioactive properties
- Can also be used as a **bone substitute** for maxillo-facial surgery and **as a cement for hip joint replacement**

TYPES OF GLASS IONOMER CEMENTS
(*see* Colour Plate 16, Fig. 8.3)

- **Type I:** Luting cements
- **Type II:** Restorative cements
- **Type III:** Cavity liners, cement bases
- **Type IV:** Fissure sealants
- **Type V:** Orthodontic cements
- **Type VI:** Core build-up material
- **Metal modified GIC**
  - Silver alloy admix or miracle mix cement
  - Glass cermet cement (Ketac silver)
- **Resin-modified GIC compomer, dicure, tricure systems.**
- **Fuji VII:** Excellent material for prevention of caries, the world's first **high fluoride non-resin containing autocure GIC.**
- **Fuji VIII and Fuji IX:** These materials are new, high viscosity GICs launched in the 1990s—**atraumatic restorative materials** (ART) (also referred to as **gaediatric or paediatric materials**).
- **Pit and fissure sealants**

Dispensing

- Powder–liquid system
- Single component powder (distilled water)
- Preproportioned capsules.

Table 8.13 Composition of GIC powder

Ingredients	%	Functions
Silica	29%	Does not take part in the reaction but increases hardness and translucency
Alumina (Al_2O_3)	16.5%	Reacts with polyacrylic acid to form aluminum polyacrylate matrix
Aluminum fluoride	7.3%	a. These act as a flux and reduce fusion temperature
Calcium fluoride	34.3%	b. Improves the working characteristics
Sodium fluoride	3%	c. Provide anticariogenic property
Aluminum phosphate	9.9%	Controls the setting time

Manufacturing of powder is done (by fritting)

The ingredients of the powder are fused at 1000°C to 1500°C and then fused mass is immersed into the water. The sudden cooling produces cracks which facilitate later grinding of the powder (Table 8.13).

The composition of liquid (polyalkenoic acid)

- This contains **45–50% aqueous solution of polyacids** containing polyacrylic acids, and its copolymers like **itaconic acid, maleic acid, and tricarboxylic acids,** with a small amount of tartaric acid. These poly-alkenoic acids have many reactive COOH groups (page 111, Key Box 5.7) to chemically bond with tooth enamel Ca^{++} and dentin collagen, and form stronger bonding and harder materials. These decrease the viscosity of the liquid, and tendency to undergo thickening by gelation due to intermolecular hydrogen bonding.
- Tartaric acid increases working time, decreases setting time and prevents thickening of the liquid, during storage.

Water settable GICs

Polyacrylic acid with copolymers is **freeze-dried and** mixed with glass ionomer powder. The liquid for cement formation is either distilled water or an **aqueous solution of tartaric acid.** When the above-blended powder is mixed with water, it goes into the solution to reconstitute and the setting reaction then proceeds in the same manner as for conventional powder–liquid system.

The advantages of these types of cements are very low viscosity in early stages of mixing and rapid set at mouth temperature. These cements are stronger and have longer shelf-life.

Setting reaction

When the acid is mixed with powder, a paste is formed, that rapidly hardens into a solid mass bound by polysalt gel. Polysalt binds unreacted glass particles in a cement matrix. During the early stages of mixing Ca^{++} ions are released more rapidly and are primarily responsible for reacting with polyacids to form calcium polysalt gel (initial set). This calcium polyacrylate has the properties of being carvable like amalgam. At this stage, the ionomer system is highly susceptible to moisture contamination or water sorption.

If water comes into contact with this surface before hardening the calcium and aluminum cements forming ions will be washed out and lost for the cement formation. The damage is permanent and water will be absorbed, the cement will lose its translucency and the weakened surface is formed (low strength) which can get eroded easily.

The hard surface that is more resistant to dissolution is produced, only after the **aluminum polyacid** is formed. This stage is not reached for **at least 30 minutes**. Therefore, a protective coating of **varnish or cocoa butter** is applied on the surface of the restoration to **protect them from initial moisture contamination.**

Role of Water in GIC

Water is the most important constituent of cement liquid. It serves as reaction medium initially, then slowly hydrates the cross-linked matrix and thereby increases the material strength.

Water present in GIC can be termed

- Loosely bound water
- Tightly bound water

During the **initial reaction period**, the water present in the cement can be easily removed by desiccation and this is termed loosely bound water.

If freshly mixed cement is isolated from the ambient air the loosely bound water will slowly become **tightly bound water** over a while. This phenomenon results in a cement which is **stronger** and less susceptible to moisture.

Bonding Reactions to Tooth Enamel and Dentin
(Refer to Zinc Polycarboxylate Cement)

1. Bonding to enamel: Same as that for zinc polycarboxylate cement.
2. Bonding to dentin: Similar to that for zinc polycarboxylate cement (*see* page 16, reactions B and C).

Properties of GIC

1. **Biological properties**
   - Biocompatibility when the pulp is not exposed
   - Anticariogenic
   - Bioactivity (osseointegration)
   - Direct bonding with tooth

   - *Biocompatibility*
     The effect of GIC on soft and calcified tissues is found to be mild

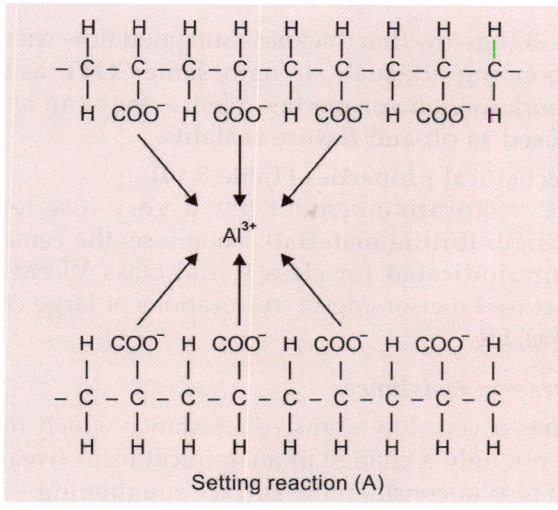

Setting reaction (A)

Causes for mildness (similar to zinc polycarboxylate, cement)

- Polyacrylic acid is a **weak acid** initially, and it becomes even weaker with time.
- **The rapid rise** of pH towards neutrality. pH of the liquid is approximately 1.7 at the time of initial mixing but the powder rapidly neutralizes it and thus the pH of the mix rises quickly as the setting reaction proceeds.

At the end of 2 minutes	**2.33 pH**
At the end of the 20 minutes	4.18 pH
At the end of 1 hr	4.55 pH
At the end of the 1 day	**5.67–6.0 pH**

- The **larger size** of polyacrylic acid molecules may limit its diffusion through dentinal tubules to the delicate pulp.
- Dentin is an excellent buffer to all acids which can neutralize the effects of polyacrylic acid
- *The attraction for proteins:* Polyacrylic acid forms **complexes with proteins** present in enamel **(enamelin and amelogenin)** which may limit its diffusion through dentinal tubules.
  However, if the thickness of dentin is less than 0.5 mm it is important to protect dentin from direct contact with the unset materials by placing Dycal, $Ca(OH)_2$—cement base.
- *Anticariogenic property* (also *refer* to silicate cements). Fluorides contribute to the caries inhibition in the oral environment by two mechanisms.
- *Physiochemical mechanism*
  GIC releases fluoride ions. These ions react with the hydroxyapatite crystals of the adjacent tooth structure to form **fluorapatite which is more resistant** to acid-mediated **decalcification**.

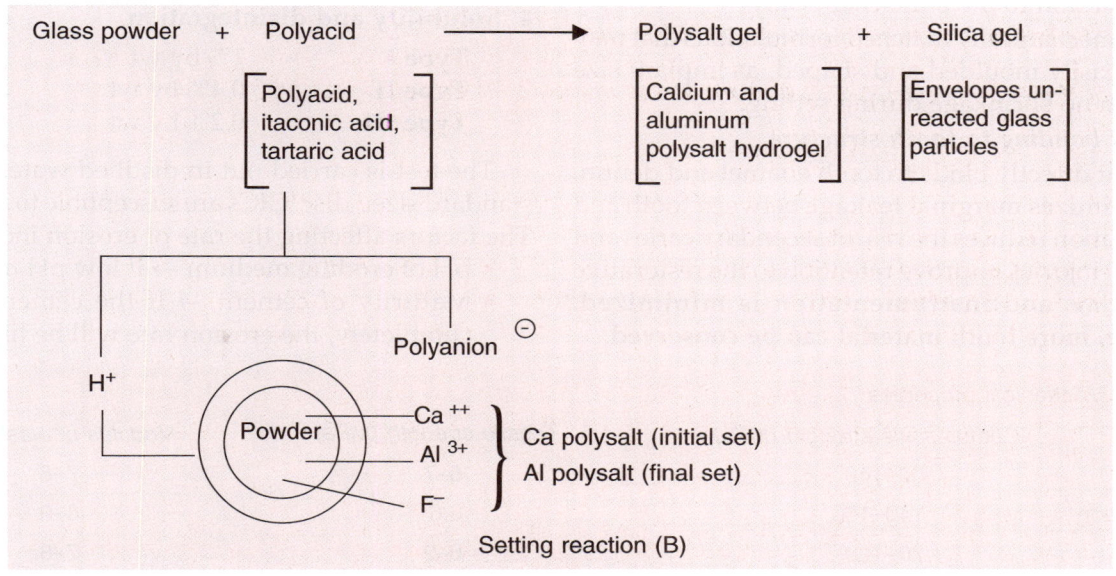

Setting reaction (B)

Hydroxyapatite + Fluoride → Fluorapatite, $Ca_{10}(PO_4)_6F_2$

Fluorides also enhance **remineralization of** carious and noncarious enamel. Fluorides act as a catalyst for uptake of calcium and phosphate ions.

Carious enamel is more porous and allows greater penetration of fluoride ions in higher concentration which contributes to the formation of acid resistant crystals and reduces the risk of caries development.

- *Biological mechanism*

  Fluoride ions **inhibit or alter the carbohydrate metabolism of acidogenic bacteria** which are responsible for caries formation. Fluorides released from restorations, diet, topically applied gels, gingival fluids, toothpastes, fluoride gels, etc. enter as hydrogens fluoride (HF) into acid producing microorganisms, **plaque, microflora and accumulate intracellularly.** The extracellular pH decreases and hydrogen fluoride gets dissociated into H^+ and F^- ions in the intracellular fluid. The ionic fluoride then induces **enzyme inhibition** leading to a slower rate of acid production, and thus carbohydrate metabolism is altered in such a way to reduce acidogenicity. Hence, **acid production by microorganisms is reduced, and** caries formation is prevented.

- *Bioactive property (osseointegration)*

  GIC can be used as bone-substitute in **maxillofacial** surgeries or in hip joint **replacements (orthopaedics)**. The additional properties which make GIC more attractive as a bone substitute are:
  - Nonexothermic setting reaction
  - Bioactivity due to the release of **osteoconductive ions**
  - Adhesion to the bone chemically
  - Biomechanically matched formulations that may be easily moulded and shaped, as implant size with no shrinkage during setting.

- *Direct bonding to tooth structure*

  Since it directly binds to tooth enamel and dentin, it **minimizes marginal leakage** between tooth and restoration reduces the risk of secondary caries and pulpal injuries improve retention to the restorative materials and **instrumentation is minimized. Hence, more tooth material can be conserved**.

2. **Rheological properties**
   - Mixing time = 30 seconds (follow manufacturer's instructions)
   - Working time = 1½ minutes

   - Setting times

Type I	6–9 minutes	
Type II	3–5 minutes	
Type III	4–5 minutes	

   Working and setting times can be modified by
   - Cooling the glass slab and spatula increases the setting time.
   - Higher P/L ratio decreases setting time and vice versa
   - The smaller particle size of powder decreases setting time and vice versa

   - *Film thickness*

Type I	25–30 μm
Type II	30–40 μm

   GIC has low film thickness and good flow chemical bonding, adequate strength, **same COTE as tooth** and aesthetic properties. Hence, they can also be **used as pit and fissure sealants.**

3. **Mechanical properties** (Table 8.14)

   GIC restorative cement has a very low tensile strength **(brittle material)**. Therefore, the cement is **contraindicated** for class II and class VI cavities, fractured incisor edges, restorations of large cuspal areas, etc.

   Abrasive resistance

   It has a very low abrasive resistance which results in, not only a change in anatomical form **(wearing)** but also in considerable **surface roughening**. Surface hardness Type II is 48 **KHN.**

4. **Solubility and disintegration**

Type I	1% by wt
Type II	0.4% by wt
Type III	0.2% by wt

   The test is carried out in distilled water by using a standard sized disc. GICs are susceptible to acid erosion. The factors affecting the rate of erosion include:
   - pH of eroding medium → If low pH more erosion
   - Maturity of cement → If the cement is not set completely, the erosion rate will be higher.

Table 8.14	Mechanical properties		
Types	**Compressive strength (MPa)**	**Tensile strength (MPa)**	**Modulus of elasticity (GPa)**
I: Luting	90–140	6–7	7–8
II: Restoration	140–150	6.6	8–9
III: Liner	70–100	6–9	7–8

- Time of contact with acid → if acids come into contact with the cement before it is completely set, the erosion rate is higher.

  Resistance to dissolution and disintegration is improved by **initial varnish protection**.

Adhesion

GIC bonds well to enamel, dentin, stainless steel, tin oxide plated platinum and gold alloys. Clean and smooth surface is required for optimum bonding. The bond strength to enamel is **~ 12 MPa**, the bond strength to dentin is only **~1.23 MPa**. The bonding to dentin requires the **removal of smear layer,** which is the debris generated by cutting the tooth surface specially dentin covering cavity surface. Bond strength can be improved by pretreatment of the dentin with conditioning liquid or surface active agents, to remove the smear layer.

Conditioning liquid

Previously **50% citric acid** was used but was found to be pulpal irritant. The most popular conditioner used clinically is **10% polyacrylic acid** applied to the tooth surface for **10 seconds** followed by **washing** and gently drying without dehydration. This treatment increases the surface energy of the tooth and allows the cement to come into more intimate contact with it.

6. **Thermal property**

   The thermal properties are almost similar to dentin. They have adequate thermal insulation properties and help to protect from thermal hot or cold sensations, COTE of GIC is about 13–16 ppm/°C, quite close to the values of the tooth (8–11 ppm/°C), which reduces marginal leakage.

7. **Aesthetics (appearance)**

   It is highly translucent with the considerable amounts of unreacted glass core. So, it has good aesthetics and can be used as anterior restorative material.

Manipulation

Instruments required: Glass slab or paper pad and plastic or agate spatula.

Powder/liquid ratios: P/L

Type I: 1.25–1.5 gm/ml

Type II: 3 gm/ml

Type III: 1.5 gm/ml (for cavity lining and 3 gm/ml for base).

Higher the P/L ratio, lower is the solubility, shorter is setting time, and higher is the strength.

Proportioning

Take the required amount of powder (1 scoop) (follow manufacturer's instructions) on one side of the glass slab, and divide the powder into one bulk and two small increments (Fig. 8.7, refer to zinc polycarboxylate cement). Place 2 drops of liquid for luting, or one drop for restoration, on the same side, near the bulk.

Mixing

The larger portion of the powder (bulk increment) is mixed into the liquid with a **plastic spatula** followed by smaller increments. Mixing is done by **tapping, folding or overlapping methods**. The total mixing time is 30–45 seconds. The luting cement is a fluid similar to $ZnPO_4$ cement mix. The restorative mix should have a putty-like consistency and a glossy surface. **The glossy surface indicates the presence of unreacted polyacrylic acid which can bond with the tooth surface.**

Cementation

Type I—luting: The seating surface of casting is coated with the mix, and the rest is applied on the prepared tooth surface. The casting is placed on the tooth and kept under pressure until the cement sets. When the cement sets, the flash is removed by breaking the cement away at the margin. The **coating of varnish** is immediately applied to the exposed cement margin. Cementation should be done before the cement loses its glossy, shiny appearance (*see* Colour Plate 17, Figs 8.4a to g).

Restoration

Type II—restorative cement: Conditioning the cavity prior to placement of cement is done by applying 10% polyacrylic acid on the surface of the tooth for 10–15 seconds and then washing and drying without desiccation (dehydration). Upon completion of mixing the cement is immediately packed into the prepared cavity by using a plastic carrier and contoured with cellulose matrix band. Sometimes preshaped matrix packed with the mix is sometimes applied, and it is left in that place for approximately 5 minutes.

Functions of matrix bands are

1. To ensure adequate adaptation to the tooth structure.
2. Smooth surface on set cement.
3. To protect the cement from the moist environment during the initial set, and prevent evaporation of liquid.
4. To get the correct shape.

   After the removal of the matrix, the surface is covered with a water-insoluble varnish. This is necessary to protect the cement from water sorption. During the finishing procedure, only the gross excess is removed and the final finishing and polishing are done after 24 hours. After removal of the excess cement, once again coat with varnish to provide initial protection to marginal areas.

Precautions

1. Polyacrylic acid should not be stored in the refrigerator, (causes gelling)
2. Stainless-steel spatula should not be used (*refer* to silicate cement)
3. Adequate care should be taken during proportioning for optimum properties and liquid should not be dispensed until proportioning is complete.
4. Clean surface must be obtained to make the best use of the adhesion properties.
5. Cementation must be done before cement loses its glossy appearance.
6. After completion of the restoration, a varnish coating must be applied.

Advantages

- Chemical adhesion to tooth structure, minimizes marginal leakage
- Anticariogenic property due to the release of fluoride ions from restoration
- Excellent biocompatibility with pulp
- Porcelain-like translucency
- Favourable bioactive properties
- COTE almost similar to tooth structure
- Good thermal insulator
- Freshly mixed cement has pseudoplastic property
- The manipulative procedure is simple.

Disadvantages

- Low wear resistance
- Low fracture resistance and low tensile strength
- Moisture sensitivity, susceptibility to moisture uptake
- Initial slow setting

Uses

Type I—luting cement: For cementation of metallic crowns, bridges, porcelain restorations, orthodontic bands (*see* Colour Plate 19, Figs 8.7a to f).

Type II—restorative cement

- Restoration of class V and III cavities
- Restoration of abraded and cervical eroded areas **without any cavity preparation** (*see* Colour Plate 18, Fig. 8.5).
- Restoration of deciduous teeth
- Repairing defective margins in restorations

Type III—GIC: Designed for **lining** the cavities, also used as cement **bases** and **pit and fissure sealants.**

Modified GIC

- The miracle mix and glass cermet cement which are metal modified GICs can be ideally used for **core build up** where there is residual dentin support. These materials can also be used in restoring the deciduous tooth.
- Resin-modified GIC can be used as a **liner** under composite resin restoration.

Note: Core build up (*see* Colour Plate 18, Fig. 8.6)
The fabrication of core is an important step which is often necessary prior to crown preparation to achieve a satisfactory form for resistance and retentions.

Special uses

GIC can also be used as **bone cement or bone substitute** for maxillofacial surgery and **hip joint replacements.**

Contraindications

- GIC is brittle and hence contraindicated for class II and class VI cavities for replacement of **lost cusp-areas**.
- Cannot be used as the amalgam replacement material
- Should not be used in contact with the zinc oxide eugenol cements.

MODIFICATIONS OF GIC

GIC has been modified by the addition of metal powder or resin fibers in an attempt **to improve strength, fracture resistance, and abrasion resistance.** Two methods of modifications have been tried. They are: 1. Metal modified, 2. resin modified, varieties.

1. **Metal modified GIC: There are two types of metal modified cements**

1A. Miracle Mix GIC (Silver–Alloy Admix)

This was the first approach where GIC powder was modified by incorporating additional powder particles for reinforcements. In this cement, **spherical amalgam alloy** powder is mixed with type II—GIC powder and the liquid an aqueous solution of polyacrylic acid. This cement was developed by **Dr. Siemens,** clinically under the name **miracle mix** and introduced as an amalgam substitute for safety against mercury. The properties of miracle mix **were far inferior** to those of dental amalgam. The problem with the miracle mix was that the **silver–tin alloy particles did not adhere strongly** into the cement matrix but acted as a filler to **improve the mechanical properties of GIC slightly.**

Properties
- Compressive strength 150–180 MPa
- Tensile strength 10 MPa
- Chemical adhesion to tooth structure takes place
- Anticariogenic property—present
- Finishing of the restoration can be done after 15–20 minutes.

Uses
- **Core build-up** material (*see* Colour Plate 18, Fig. 8.6)
- Treatment of **high caries incidences.**

Drawbacks
- **Poor aesthetics**, due to silver-tin amalgam alloys
- Inferior mechanical properties, when compared to amalgam
- Low abrasion resistance.

  (Note: Amalgam alternatives, posterior composites, miracle mix GIC, glass cermet cement were tried as amalgam alternatives).

1B. Glass Cermet Cement

The solution to the problem of improving resistance to abrasion and strength was the development of cermet ionomer system by **Dr. McLean in 1985.**

  Cermet cement contains glass + metal powder sintered to high density that can be made to react with an active solution of polyacrylic acid to form a cement.

  Ceramic powder + metal modifiers → **cermet cement** (ceramic) + (Au or Ag) metal → **(ceramic-metal)**

Powder manufacturing process
Manufactured by intimate mixing of the glass and the metal powder (Au or Ag) which are then compressed in a hydraulic press **(pelletizing)** at high pressure. The compressed pellets are **fused at about 800°C** and then ground into fine powder. Commercially, available cements contain fine **Ag powder particles of less than 3.5 nm** and colour has been improved by the addition of **5% titanium dioxide.**

Advantages (similar to GIC)
- Excellent biocompatibility
- Anticariogenic property
- Higher compressive strength = 180–200 MPa
- Tensile strength = 6–7 MPa
- Improved abrasive resistance
- Chemical adhesion to tooth structure
- Shorter setting time than the conventional GIC cement
- Low thermal conductivity (higher than GIC)
- COTE similar to tooth structure.

Disadvantages
- Low fracture resistance due to brittleness
- More opacity, poor aesthetics.

Manipulation method
Supplied in **disposable capsules** that contain glass metal powder and **dry polyacrylic acid.** A foil envelope within the capsule contains distilled water. The mixing is done in a high-speed vibrator, the distilled water comes in contact with powder and polyacrylic acid, goes into solution form, and conventional acid–base reaction takes place. The mixed cement is used according to the operators requirement. The structure of cement consists of **unreacted glass particles to which silver is fused** and held together by a metal salt matrix.

Uses
- **Ideal material for core build up** (*see* colour plate 18, Fig. 8.6)
- Restoration of deciduous teeth
- Can be used as a lining under composite resins for chemical bonding.

2A. Resin Modified Glass Ionomer Cement (RMGIC)/Hybrid Ionomer
(*see* Colour Plate 20, Fig. 8.8; Colour Plate 21, Fig. 8.9 and Colour Plate 22, Fig. 9.3)

Conventional and metal modified GIC is **moisture sensitive and have low early strengths.** These drawbacks are due to **slow acid–base** setting reaction. To overcome these drawbacks, some polymerizable functional groups (resins) have been added to impart additional curing process and allow the bulk of matrix to set through acid base reaction in the **dual cure system.**

Alternative names
- **Resin ionomers (resinomer)**
- **Compomers** (combination of composite resins and glass ionomers)
- **Hybrid ionomers**
- **Dual cure** glass ionomers (material set by acid–base reaction and light activated polymerization reaction).

Tricure glass ionomers
- **Acid–base** reaction has advantages: Fluoride release, chemical adhesion, and biocompatibility.
- **Light curing** polymerization reaction has advantages of improved physical properties, **command setting properties**, immediate finishing, and extended working time.
- **Chemically curing** polymerization reaction has advantages of **bulk placement** and controlled working and setting times.

Conventional light curing glass ionomer offers improved characteristics. However, to ensure whether light penetrates throughout the entire material, the material has to be **placed in increments and cured.** But in **tricure system** the additional chemical cure polymerization makes **bulk placement** possible, assuring optimum cure, even when the light does not reach the entire bulk. Hence, **no incremental procedure** is required, which also saves time.

Commercial names

Dyract—light curing compomer restorative material—Vitremer-Tricure system.

Composition of powder

Contains ion-leachable glass with fluorides + resin matrix (BisGMA) + coupling agents (organosilanes) + initiators (light initiators and chemical initiators or both).

The initiator for chemical curing is benzoyl peroxide. Initiators for light curing is camphoroquinone with dimethyl para-toluidine as an accelerator.

Liquid

An aqueous solution of polyacrylic acid 30–50% with some carboxyl groups, modified with methyl methacrylate and HEMA (hydroxyethyl methacrylate) chemical activator (N-N-dimethyl *para*-toluidine), light accelerator dimethyl aminoethyl methacrylate or camphoroquinone.

It is also dispensed in disposable capsules and paste (syringe) forms.

Properties of Tricure Resin Modified Glass Ionomer Cement (RMGIC)

- Releases fluorides   Anticariogenic
- Pulpal response   Mild (biocompatible with pulp)
- Compressive strength   105 MPa
- Tensile strength   20 MPa
- Surface hardness   40 KHN
- Chemical adhesion to tooth structure
- Exhibits greater degree of shrinkage on setting as a result of polymerization
- This material is susceptible to dehydration and also absorbs water which produces significant dimensional changes, **reduction in translucency** because of significant difference in the refractive indices between powder and resin matrix.

Uses

- Liner under composite resins
- Core build-up material
- Fissure sealants
- Cement base materials
- Cementation materials for orthodontic bands.

GIC—Cavity Liner

Mainly used for pulpal protection under composite resins. Supplied as conventional powder–liquid system, similar to Type II—GIC.

Light cure glass ionomer system—powder–liquid and also a single paste component in disposable syringes.

The Composition of Light-cured System

Powder

Acid soluble glass + resin matrix + photoinitiators + accelerators.

Liquid

The aqueous solution of polyacrylic acid or copolymers which have pendant methacrylate groups + HEMA monomers.

The powder and liquids are mixed according to the manufacturers' instructions, coated on the cavity walls, and exposed to resin curing lights. It undergoes addition polymerization reaction, chemically bonds with tooth structure and seals the exposed dentin surface.

2B. Polyacids Modified Resin Composite (Compomer)

Shortly after the introduction of RMGICs, "compomers" were introduced to the market. These materials are said to provide the combined benefits of composites (the "comp" in their name) and glass ionomers ("omer"). These material designed to combine the aesthetics of resin composites and fluoride release and adhesion of GIC Examples: Dyract and Compoglass.

These materials have two main constituents: dimethacrylate monomer(s) (bisglycidyl ether dimethacrylate (bisGMA), urethane dimethacrylate (UDMA), triethylene glycol dimethacrylate (TEGDMA) with two carboxylic groups (*water-free polyacid liquid monomer* with initiator-camphoroquinone) present in their structure, and filler that is similar to the ion-leachable glass present in GICs. The ratio of carboxylic groups to backbone carbon atoms is approximately 1:8. There is no water in the composition of these materials, and the ion-leachable glass is partially silanized to ensure some bonding with the matrix. These materials set via a free radical polymerization reaction, *cannot bond to hard tooth tissues (do not contain water), and have significantly lower levels of fluoride release than conventional GICs.*

Based on their structure and properties, these materials belong to the class of dental composites. Often, they have been erroneously referred to as "hybrid glass ionomers" or "light-cured GICs" or "resin-modified glass ionomers" along with the "genuine" resin-modified GICs. The proposed nomenclature for these materials as polyacid-modified composite resins, a nomenclature that is widely used in the literature may over-emphasize a structural characteristic of no or a little consequence.

2C. Giomers

Giomer = Glass ionomer + composite

Giomers are a relatively new type of restorative material. The name "giomer" is a hybrid of the words "glass ionomer" and "composite", which pretty well describes what a giomer is claimed to be. Although glass-ionomer restorative materials such as Ketac-Fil (3M ESPE) and Fuji Type II (GC America) have some very significant properties, such as fluoride release, fluoride rechargeability, and chemical bonding to tooth structure, they also have well-known shortcomings. Their esthetic property is less than ideal and make them a poor second choice to resin composites for restoring aesthetically demanding areas. Also, they are sensitive to moisture contamination and desiccation, which can present the clinician with challenges during their placement.

In the continuing quest for improved glass ionomer-like restoratives, manufacturers have developed and introduced a new class of materials called "giomers." As noted earlier, the term implies they are combinations of glass ionomers and composites. Their manufacturers claim they have properties of both glass ionomers (fluoride release, fluoride recharge) and resin composites (excellent esthetics, easy polishability, biocompatibility). Giomers are distinguished by the fact that, while they are resin-based, they contain *pre-reacted glass-ionomer (PRG) particles*. The particles are made of fluorosilicate glass that has been reacted with polyacrylic acid prior to being incorporated into the resin. The pre-reaction can involve only the surface of the glass particles (called surface pre-reacted glass ionomer or S-PRG) or almost the entire particle (termed fully pre-reacted glass ionomer or F-PRG). Giomers are similar to compomers and resin composites in being light activated and requiring the use of a bonding agent to adhere to tooth structure (Brand name— Shofu's Beautiful, supplied in syringes.) This PRG technology was applied to the filler component of resin composite materials to provide a bioactive result that released and was recharged with fluoride-like a traditional glass ionomer cement—all the while maintaining the original physical properties of the resin composite system.

SANDWICH TECHNIQUE

GIC: Chemical bonding to tooth enamel or dentin, prevents marginal leakage, increases biocompatibility and acts as dentin bondings agent

+

Composite resins: Restorative material replacing enamel or dentin adheres to GIC as mechanically bonding by an acid etching technique, superior mechanical properties.

In this technique, GIC acts as enamel or dentin bonding agent and composite resin as a restorative material. Bonding between resin and GIC surface is due to penetration of resin into surface irregularities of etched enamel and cement surface. The setting of resin gives mechanical interlocking. This technique is particularly applicable to cervical and posterior composite restorations (Fig. 8.9).

Advantages of GIC Liners

- Minimizes marginal leakage
- Anticariogenic property present
- Direct bonding to tooth structure
- Combined setting
- Adequate strength for posterior cavities.

Recent Advances in GIC

1. **Fuji VII:** Excellent material for prevention of caries. **The worlds first high fluoride, non-resin auto-cure glass ionomer cement.**
2. **Fuji VIII and Fuji IX:** These materials are new high viscosity GICs introduced in the 1990s. These materials were mainly developed for use in **atraumatic restorative therapy (ART)** which refers to the restoration of the tooth with minimum cavity preparation or **minimum instrumentation.**

These materials are also called **paediatric or gaediatric restorative materials.**

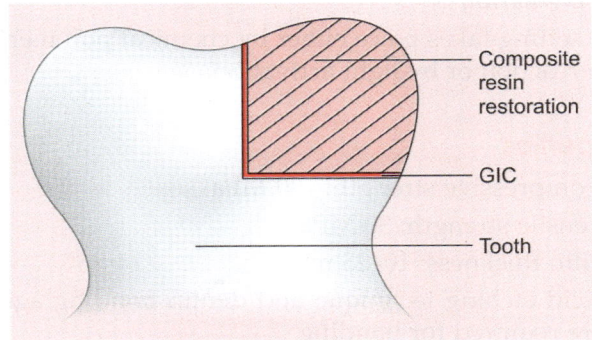

Fig. 8.9: Sandwich technique, GIC + composite resin

Advantages
- Easily packable and condensable
- Early moisture sensitivity is reduced
- Nonsticky
- Rapid finishing, can be done immediately
- Improved wear resistance
- Low solubility in oral fluids.

Indications
- **Fuji VII** is an ideal material for molar restorations in deciduous teeth and also used as **core build** up material.
- **Fuji VIII** has good aesthetics and can be used as an **anterior restorative** material.
- **Fuji IX** is mostly used as a **posterior restorative** material.

ACRYLIC RESIN CEMENTS

Synthetic resin cements based on methyl methacrylates have been available since 1952. These materials were widely used for the cementation of inlays, crowns and other appliances. Since 1986, these resin cements have retained popularity because of their use in the cementation of porcelain veneers, cast crowns and orthodontic bands.

Classification
- Type I: Unfilled resins
- Type II: Filled resins

Powder contains
Very fine beads or powder of methyl methacrylate polymer, inorganic fillers like $CaCO_3$, quartz, mica, coupling agent organosilanes and initiator benzoyl peroxide-like composite resins.

Liquid
The liquid is methyl methacrylate monomer and N-N-dimethyl *para*-toluidine, activator and cross-linking agents.

Setting action
The setting takes place either by chemical polymerization reaction or by light activation.

Properties
- Compressive strength: 180 MPa
- Tensile strength: 30 MPa
- Film thickness: 10–25 mm
- Acid etching technique and dentin bonding agents are required for bonding
- Bond strength to enamel: 7.4 MPa

- Biological properties—irritation to the pulp, therefore pulp protection via $Ca(OH)_2$ base is necessary
- Solubility—insoluble in oral fluids
- Polymerization shrinkage is high
- Adhesion properties: They do not adhere chemically to tooth structure and lead to **marginal** or microleakage, also due to large COTE.

Manipulation of Resin Cements
Chemically curing
Two components are mixed on paper pad (mixing time is $\sim$ 20–30 seconds), and then used as required for cementation. Removal of excess cement is difficult and is delayed until the cement has polymerized.

Enamel acid etching technique for retention of direct filing resin restoration has lead to the use of resins for bonding orthodontic bands and brackets directly to the tooth surface.

Light curing material supplied as single component system should have the time of exposure of light towards the resin more than 40 seconds.

Short Note on Luting Cements
These are materials supplied usually as powder–liquid system, and are used for temporary and permanent cementations (or fixing) of permanent metallic restorations like inlays, crowns, bridges, etc.

Requirements: These should have biocompatibility, anticariogenic property, low film thickness (<25 microns), suitable strength for temporary cementation <35 MPa, permanent cementation >75 MPa, chemically bonding to tooth and metallic crowns, bridges, etc.

Materials used for cementation
- Zinc oxide eugenol type I is used for temporary cementations due to its low strength.
- Zinc oxide eugenol modified with alumina and EBA (*ortho*-ethoxybenzoic acid) type IV has higher strength and is used for permanent cementation.
- Zinc phosphate cement is used for permanent cementation of *ortho*-bands, metal crowns, inlays, etc. as it has high strength and low film thickness. It adheres well to the metal surface but no chemical bonding with the tooth.
- Zinc silicophosphate cement is translucent. Hence, it is used for ceramic crowns.
- Zinc polycarboxylate cement has chemical bonding to the tooth but poor bonding to metal. It is used for cementation of metallic crowns, bridges, ceramic crowns, etc. as it can chemically combine with the tooth.
- GIC type I is suitable for cementation of ceramic crowns and veneers.

- Resin cements are used for cementation of *ortho*-resin bands.
  Methods of cementation (option)

CAVITY LINERS, VARNISHES, AND CEMENT BASES

PULP-PROTECTING MATERIALS

Pulpal irritations are caused by
1. Chemical irritation........ by the passage of chemicals from restorative materials to the pulp.
2. Marginal leakage.......... due to poor bonding of restorations—percolation.
3. Thermal sensitivity........ due to passage of heat, and thermal fluctuations.
4. Galvanic shock/pain..... due to the presence of two dissimilar metals coming into contact.
5. Trauma...................... accident, biting forces

  Therefore, pulpal protection requires consideration of chemical, thermal, electrical protections, mechanical support to overlying restorations and pulpal medications. Thus, the cavity **liners, varnishes and bases are designed** as materials to **protect** the **pulp against thermal, electrical, chemical and mechanical trauma insults** and must also give mechanical support to the above restoration.

Cavity Liners

These are the materials used to coat the walls and floors of the prepared cavity to protect the underlying dentin and pulp from the chemical and thermal insults. There are two types of cavity lining agents:
1. Cavity liners
2. Cavity varnishes.

Ideal requirements of cavity liners
- Bacteriostatic
- Low solubility, chemically neutral or slightly alkaline
- Provide electrical and thermal insulation
- Prevent discolouration of tooth structure
- Prevent penetration of chemical ions from the restorative materials to dentin and pulp, i.e. good insulators
- Prevent marginal leakage at the tooth restoration interface
- Anticariogenic property
- Chemical bonding to tooth structure.

  Cavity liners are used to provide a **barrier against the passage of irritants from cement** or other restorative materials and to reduce the penetration of oral fluids at the **restoration-tooth interface** into the underlying dentin and protect the dentin and pulp from the harmful effects of the above agents. They also provide some

therapeutic benefits to the pulp and **reduce the sensitivity** of freshly cut dentin.

Dispensing and composition
- **Suspension or liquid cavity liner:** Suspensions of $Ca(OH)_2$ or zinc oxide eugenol in organic solvents such as methyl ethyl ketone, ethyl alcohol or an aqueous solution of ethyl cellulose. Upon evaporation of volatile solvents, the liner forms a thin film on the surface of the prepared cavity.
- **Paste form cavity liners**
  - **Two-paste system** (base + reactor)
    For example, $Ca(OH)_2$ (Dycal), zinc oxide-eugenol liner (type IV)
  - **Single paste with solvent:** For example, $Ca(OH)_2$ paste and a solvent, methylcellulose.
  - **Single paste system:** Light-activated $Ca(OH)_2$, Dycal
  - **Powder and liquid system:** For example, glass ionomer liners (type III and zinc oxide-eugenol liners (type IV).

Properties of $Ca(OH)_2$ liners
- They are *alkaline*, pH ≃ 12
- Promote the growth of *secondary or repairative dentin*
- They are very effective neutralizers of phosphoric acid
- Material of choice for **pulp capping** in cases of microscopic pulp exposures
- The material of choice for liners in the deepest portions of the cavities
- They do not have sufficient, hardness and strength, so they cannot be used alone in deep cavities. They are overlaid with one of the high strength bases such as zinc phosphate cement base or zinc polycarboxylate cement, etc.

Zinc oxide-eugenol liners
- Noted for its **sedative or obtundent** effect on the pulp.
- Considered as least irritating to the pulp of all the materials used in cavity restorations.
- Contraindicated for use under composite resins, because eugenol interferes with polymerization and defective restoration results (dissolution of resins).
- Should not be used under GIC or silicate cements as diffusion of eugenol causes discolouration of the restoration.

GIC liners—properties
- They are primarily used for pulp protection under composite resins as dentin bonding agents (sandwich technique)
- Minimizes marginal leakage
- Chemically bond to the tooth structure

- Biocompatibility with pulp
- Anticariogenic property present
- **Command setting properties for the light cured type**
- **Should not be placed directly on the exposed pulp.**

Uses

- **Liquid cavity liners** or **suspension liners** can be used mainly as cavity liners which neutralize H_3PO_4 (phosphoric acid) containing cements and these liners are most effective in protecting the pulp from **chemical irritation** than the inert cavity varnishes.
- **Paste liners:** Used extensively in deep cavities where pulp exposure is likely to take place.

Manipulation of liners

As they are fluid, these liners can be **painted on the walls and floors of** the prepared cavity by using cotton pledgets. **The solvents evaporate quickly and leave a thin layer of residue that provides protection for the underlying pulp.**

Cavity Varnishes

These materials are used to provide a **barrier against the passage of irritants** from the restorative materials and to reduce the penetration of oral fluids at the restoration-tooth interface into the pulp.

Composition

Consists of natural gum such as **Copal resin or rosin or a synthetic resin (nitrated cellulose) dissolved in organic solvents such as acetone, chloroform or ether**. When applied to the walls of the prepared cavities, the solvent evaporates and leaves a thin resinous film on the surface that protects the underlying tooth structure.

Functions

- Reduces the marginal leakage around most restorative materials and specially for **silver amalgam.**
- Protect the pulp from irritation by chemicals in the restorative materials.
- **Blocks the penetration of metallic ions** from amalgam restoration to the adjoining dentin and enamel and reduces tooth discolouration.

Note: These materials cannot give protection against electrical or thermal insults, because of low thickness and strength.

Contraindications

1. **For GICs** and silicate cements: Because it prevents the chemical adhesion and also reduces anticariogenic effects. Solvent supplied can be added for thinning.
2. **For composite resins:** Because it inhibits the polymerization mechanism of the resin and produce softening of the resin.

Manipulation

The usual technique involved is dipping small cotton pledgets held with pliers, into the varnish and then thoroughly painting all the cavity walls. Two or three successive applications should be made to reduce the possibility of **voids and produce more continuous layer**.

Precautions

1. The repeated opening of the bottle evaporates the solvents, and the unused varnish gradually becomes thicker. Extra solvents supplied can be added.
2. If cement base is acidic, varnish must be applied to the dentin first to protect the pulp from the acid in the cement.
3. If a base provides a sedative effect such as zinc oxide eugenol cement, $Ca(OH)_2$ base should be applied to the dentin first and then varnish over it.

CEMENT BASES

These are materials applied on the exposed dentin, as a sufficiently thick layer (0.75 mm–2 mm), to protect the underlying pulp from external insults like chemical, thermal, electrical and mechanical (such as condensation of amalgam or biting forces).

Ideal requirements

- They should be bacteriostatic, obtundent, anticariogenic
- Promote the formation of **secondary or reparative dentin**
- Provide **electrical, thermal insulation under metallic restorations, i.e. they should be good insulators**
- Prevent the penetration of harmful chemical ions from the restoration
- Should have sufficient strength to withstand condensation forces of amalgam, or biting forces.
- Thickness of approximately **1.5 mm** is needed for effective insulation.

Classification of Cement Bases

1. *According to strength properties*

Low strength bases	High strength bases
Ca $(OH)_2$ cement, and zinc oxide eugenol cement used for pulp capping	Kalginol, zinc phosphate cement, zinc polycarboxylate cement, GIC, etc. are used for thermal, electrical, chemical insulations and provide mechanical support to restorations, i.e. they should be a good insulator.

2. *According to its chemical nature or pH*
   Acidic: GIC, $ZnPO_4$, zinc polycarboxylate cements
   Neutral: Zinc oxide eugenol cements
   Alkaline: $Ca(OH)_2$ cement
3. *According to method of dispensing*
   Two-paste systems: $Ca(OH)_2$ cement and zinc oxide eugenol cements
   Powder–liquid system: Zinc oxide eugenol cements, $ZnPO_4$ cements, zinc poly-carboxylate cement, $Ca(OH)_2$ cement
   Single paste system: Light-activated $Ca(OH)_2$ cement

CALCIUM HYDROXIDE CEMENT (DYCAL)

Speciality

Forms of **reparative or secondary dentin** and this action appear due to its higher alkaline pH and remineralization action.

Dispensing

Compositions of chemically activated two-paste systems (Table 8.15).

Setting Reaction

Glycol salicylate + $Ca(OH)_2$ → Calcium disalicylate (chelate product)
The reaction is greatly accelerated by **moisture**

Composition of light activated single paste system (Dycal)

$Ca(OH)_2$ + $BaSO_4$ (radio-opacifiers) + urethane dimethacrylate + photoinitiators + accelerators

All these ingredients are dispensed in **ethylene toluene sulfonamide = 39.5%**.

Properties

- Stimulates the formation of **reparative secondary dentin** at the site of placement.

- pH (alkaline) $\sim$ 12 (10–13)
- Setting time: 2.5–5.5 minutes
- **Low compressive strength: 10–27 MPa**
- Low tensile strength: <1.5 MPa, hence cannot be used as a high strength base
- Good thermal insulator: Provides **thermal insulation** to a pulp if used in sufficient thick layers, but practically thermal insulation is provided by high strength bases.

Manipulation

Equal lengths of two pastes are mixed to a uniform consistency (colour), and used as required.

Uses

- As pulp capping agent
- Can be used as a liner in deep cavity preparation.

Advantages

- Promotes the growth of secondary or reparative dentin
- Neutralize strong acids
- Seals the exposed dentin surface
- Easy manipulation method.

Disadvantages

- Cannot provide thermal insulation at low thickness
- It has very low strength when fully set
- Dissolves under acidic condition
- Weakened by exposure to moisture.

Note: Other cement bases: If required briefly explain the properties of ZnOE(II), $ZnPO_4$, zinc polycarboxylate, GIC(II).

The conclusion of cement bases

The choice thickness of cement base material and its placement should depend on the depth and design of the cavity as well as the permanent restorative material chosen.

Table 8.15 The composition of $Ca(OH)_2$ cement bases (chemically activated system)

Base paste ingredients	Percentage	Functions
1. Glycol salicylate	40%	Reactive ingredient
2. Calcium tungstate	16%	Radio-opacifiers
3. TiO_2	14%	Fillers
4. Calcium sulphate	30%	Gives strength and colour to the paste
Reactor paste ingredients	Percentage	Functions
1. $Ca(OH)_2$	50%	Reactive ingredient
2. ZnO	10%	Reactive ingredient
3. Zn stearate	0.5%	Strength

Pulp Capping (Fig. 8.10a)

a. Direct pulp capping (Fig. 8.10b)
b. Indirect pulp capping (Fig. 8.10c)

Pulp capping is a clinical procedure of placing specialized material in contact with (direct pulp capping) or close to the pulp (indirect pulp capping) with the intention of encouraging the formation of reparative dentin and promote the healing of the pulp and protect it from external insults.

As the tooth decay or caries continues, it can reach very **close to the pulp.** The pulp also may just get exposed during **cavity preparations, trauma, etc.** The pulp contains nerves, blood vessels, etc. It is very sensitive and severe pain is caused due to thermal, chemical, electrical insults or trauma. Since the permanent restorative materials are either acidic or conducting metals, pulp protecting agents should be applied.

These pulp capping materials should be neutral (or slightly alkaline to neutralize acid ions migrating from restorations), very good insulators, and have adequate strengths.

Materials used for pulp capping are Ca(OH)$_2$ (Dycal), MTA (mineral trioxide aggregate) or ZnOE cement. Ca(OH)$_2$ is slightly alkaline and can promote the formation of secondary or reparative dentin. Since it has low strength and high solubility, it should be reinforced with harder cement bases, like zinc phosphate, zinc polycarboxylate or GIC. **Zinc oxide eugenol is neutral, and good thermal insulators, but contraindicated to glass ionomer, zinc polycarboxylate, and composite resin as eugenol is a solvent for resins.**

Mineral Trioxide Aggregate (MTA)

The first hydraulic calcium silicate-based cement (HCSC); mineral trioxide aggregate (MTA) was developed for use as a dental root repair material commercially available as ProRoot MTA, Endoseal, etc. It is formulated from commercial Portland cement, combined with bismuth oxide powder for radiopacity. MTA is used for creating apical plugs during apexification, repairing root perforations during root canal therapy, and treating internal root resorption. This can be used for root-end filling material and as a pulp capping material. MTA is composed of tricalcium silicate, dicalcium silicate, tricalcium aluminate, tetracalcium aluminoferrite, calcium sulfate, and bismuth oxide.

Manipulation: Powder/water ratio for MTA should be 3:1 (P:W). Mixing can be done on a paper pad or on a glass slab using a plastic or metal spatula to achieve a putty-like paste consistency. This mix should be cover with moistened cotton pellet to prevent dehydration of mix.

Immediately after mixing MTA has a pH of 10.2. After 3 hours of setting the pH increased to 12.5.[8] The pH of set MTA is almost similar to calcium hydroxide.

Characteristics properties
- Biocompatible with periradicular tissues
- Non-cytotoxic, but antimicrobial to bacteria
- Non-resorbable
- Minimal leakage around the margins.
- Very basic AKA alkaline (high pH when mixed with water).
- As a root-end filling material, MTA shows less leakage than other root-end filling materials, which means bacterial migration to the apex is diminished.
- The treated area needs to be infection-free when applying MTA, because an acidic environment will prevent MTA from setting.
- Compressive strength develops throughout 28 days, similar to Portland cement. Strengths of more than 50 MPa is achieved when mixed in a powder-to-liquid ratio of more than 3 to 1.
- Recently fast setting MTA is developed by using polyacrylic acid as an accelerator.

Drawbacks: Long setting times, difficulty with manipulation, limited resistance to washout before setting, and the possibility of staining the tooth structure.

Modification: Hydraulic premixed bio-ceramic paste is an insoluble, radiopaque and aluminum-free material based on calcium silicate, with a composition calcium

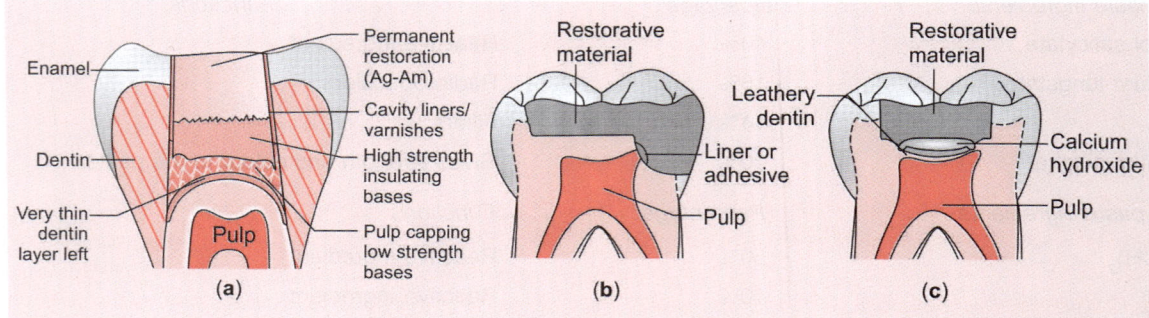

Fig. 8.10: a. Relative positions of liners (varnishes) bases and restorations, b. direct pulp capping, c. indirect pulp capping

silicates, calcium phosphate monobasic, calcium hydroxide, zirconium oxide, tantalum oxide, filler, and thickening agents. This material commercially available as Endosequence BC RRM and Endosequence BC RRM fast setting putty supplied in condensable putty or syringable paste which requires the presence of water to set and harden. Quickly setting cement could allow for a reduction in chair-side time and the number of visits needed per treatment. This cement is highly biocompatible and antibacterial (+12 pH) with improved physical and mechanical properties.

Applications: Root endo filling (retrograde fills), repair of root perforation, repair of root resorption, apexification, pulp capping, etc.

GUTTA-PERCHA (Table 8.16)

Gutta-percha is a naturally occurring polymeric material which is chemically known as *trans* isomer of **polyisoprene** (isoprene, $CH_2 = CH-C(CH)_3 = CH_2$) obtained from the **latex** of various tropical rubber trees similar to rubbers.

It is supplied in the form of small **narrow cones** of various sizes that is 15–80 numbers (15 means the tip

Table 8.16 Composition of gutta-percha

Ingredients	Weight%	Functions
• Gutta-percha	20%	Forms the matrix
• ZnO	60%	Fillers, improves the strength
• Waxes	5–10%	Plasticizers
• Barium sulphate	Trace	Radio-opacifiers

diameter of gutta-percha 15/100 = 0.15 mm and every one mm from the tip there is an increase of 0.02 mm in size) in various colours that indicates diameters. It is also supplied as rods of different colours of about 10 cm in length, 3 mm in diameter.

At room temperature, gutta-percha is in β form. When gutta-percha is heated to 50°C it gets converted to α form and when heated to 56–62°C it gets converted to γ form. During the conversion from β to α, there is an **expansion** and it contracts more during conversion from the α-β form. So, **thorough condensation** and good marginal adaption is necessary to avoid marginal leakage.

Gutta-percha is mainly used to **fill the pulp space of the root canal after** obturating the pulp.

Table 8.17 Properties of Fuji—GIC supplied by manufacturers, 2001

Properties		Fuji IX GP fast	Fuji IX GP regular set	Ketac-Molar quick	Ionofil Molar AC quick
Powder/liquid ratio (g/g)	0.36/0.1	0.35/0.1	0.26/0.09	0.46/0.125	
Extrusion volume (ml)		0.12	0.12	0.12	0.17
Working time at 23°C		1'15"	2'00"	1'00"	0'50"
Setting time at 23°C		3'00"	4'15"	4'30"	2'00"
Compressive strength (MPa)	After 2 hours	195 (8)	182 (8)	160 (13)	
	After 1 day	268 (10)	220 (9)	221 (25)	171 (20)
	After 1 week	274 (11)	230 (14)	188 (29)	
Modulus of elasticity (GPa)	After 1 day	8.6 (0.3)	8.3 (0.5)	6.2 (0.2)	5.4 (0.3)
Adhesive strength (MPa,1day)	Enamel	6.9 (1.6)	5.9 (1.7)	4.4 (1.0)	3.2 (0.8)
	Dentin	5.8 (2.2)	4.4 (1.6)	3.6 (0.7)	2.7 (0.3)
Diametral tensile strength (MPa,1 day)		23 (2)	22 (2)	16 (3)	
Surface hardness (VHN)	After 10 mins	31	31	30	
	after 1 hour	51	45	49	
	After 1 day	74	74	62	56 (5)
Radiopacity (mm)		3.7 (0.3)	3.7 (0.3)	2.3 (0.3)	
Batch #		01043166	0106075	002/010	01465E7

Properties

- It is nontoxic to the pulpal tissues
- Chemically stable in the root canal
- It is a brittle material in the β state. More brittle when aged
- It is dimensionally stable in ordinary conditions after proper compaction/condensation. This helps preventing marginal leakage, when a root canal is sealed.

$$\beta \text{ Gutta-percha} \xrightarrow{50°C} \alpha \text{ Gutta-percha} \xrightarrow{50°C–62°C} \gamma \text{ Gutta-percha}$$

Manipulation Techniques

1. **Warm up technique**

   A suitable conical gutta-percha is taken, warmed either with alcohol flame (or electrical method) by careful rotation and inserted into the cavity with the help of pluggers, **sometimes plugger itself is warmed for better insertion.**

2. **Cold up technique**

   Gutta-percha is inserted at ordinary temperature and condensed with the help of **slow rotating bur.**

3. **Injection technique**

   Gutta-percha when heated to about 70°C, becomes a fluid, It is taken in a syringe and injected into the root canal at about 50°C. This method is most suitable **if the root canal is curved.**

4. **Semi dissolved method**

   The gutta-percha cone is kept in either **chloroform or eucalyptus oil** and stirred carefully when it partially dissolves and forms a soft layer. Then it is introduced and condensed. So, it is also called **chlorapercha or eucapercha** (Fig. 8.11).

Advantages of the gutta-percha

- Inert and nontoxic

- Dimensionally stable if condensed well
- Easy condensation method
- Suitable thermoplastic and mechanical properties for root canal filling.

   Note: Gutta-percha is sometimes used for taking **functional impression** in the case of **cleft palate patients** for fabrication of oral appliances.

I. Long Essays   **(20 minutes each)**

1. Classify restorative dental cements. Give the compositions, properties and uses of ZnOE cements.
2. Describe ideal requirements of restorative cements. Add a note on zinc silicophosphate cement.
3. Describe the composition, properties and manipulation of silicate cements. Explain why it is replaced by glass ionomer cements.
4. Describe the composition, setting action, properties and uses of zinc phosphate cements.
5. Describe the composition, setting and bonding actions to tooth, properties, and uses of zinc polycarboxylate cement.
6. Explain the term glass ionomer cement. Give the composition, the chemistry of bonding to tooth enamel and dentin. Describe the mechanical properties and uses.
7. Give the composition of glass ionomer cements. Describe its biological and chemical bonding properties. Add a note on its modifications.

II. Short Essays   **(10 minutes each)**

1. Classification of cements
2. Zinc oxide eugenol cements
3. Zinc phosphate cement
4. Zinc polycarboxylate cement

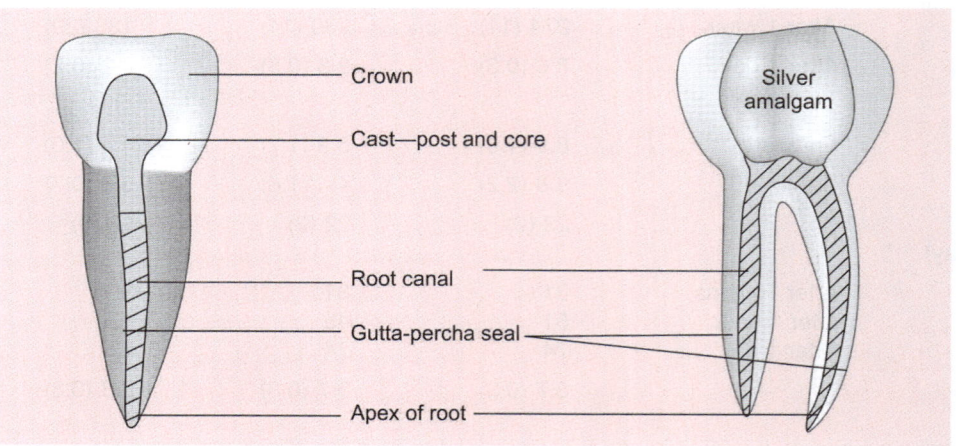

Fig. 8.11: Gutta-percha sealing in root canal treatment (RCT)

5. Cavity liners and varnishes
6. Modified glass ionomer cements
7. Pit and fissure sealants
8. Cement bases
9. Anticariogenic properties of cements
10. Zinc silicophosphate cements

III. Brief Answers (5 minutes each)

1. Temporary restorations
2. Intermediate restorations
3. Luting cements
4. Anticariogenic properties
5. Compomer
6. Cavity varnish
7. Dycal
8. Resin cements
9. Gutta-percha
10. Endodontic sealers
11. Film thickness of cements
12. Consistency of luting cements
13. Solubility and disintegration of cements
14. Manipulation of zinc phosphate cements
15. Frozen glass slab technique
16. Hydrophosphate cement
17. Germicidal cements
18. Mildness of polycarboxylate or GIC cements
19. Bond failures of cements
20. Miracle mix
21. Ketac silver or cermet cement
22. "Sandwich technique"
23. Water settable GIC
24. Loosely and tightly bound water

Composite Restorative Resins

Many varieties of resins have been developed as anterior restorative materials, mainly because of their aesthetic qualities. There are two types of direct filling resins.

Type I: Unfilled acrylic resins

Type II: Filled/composite resins

UNFILLED ACRYLIC RESINS

These resins were developed mainly because of two reasons

1. To overcome the drawbacks of silicate cements, such as high acidity (pulpal irritation), brittleness, moisture contamination degradations, high solubility, etc.
2. To formulate synthetic polymers which could be readily cured at mouth temperature by adding colour pigments and fillers, to resemble natural tooth in appearance.

Dispensing

These are supplied as a powder and liquid system.

Composition of powder

- Polymethyl methacrylate—fine particles of size more than 50 μm

- Benzoyl peroxide (initiator)
- Colour pigments to match the colour of natural tooth shades.
- Radio-opacifiers, heavy metals dust.

Composition of liquid

- Methyl methacrylate monomer
- Ethylene glycol dimethacrylate cross-linking agent.
- Dimethyl *para*-toluidine, activator.
- Hydroquinone, inhibitor of pre-polymerization.

Setting Reaction

When the powder and liquids are mixed, the polymethyl methacrylate powder dissolves in methyl methacrylate monomer, and polymerizes in the presence of benzoyl peroxide initiator which is activated by dimethyl *para*-toluidine to give **cross-linked** polymethyl methacrylate matrix and heat is liberated.

This is an exothermic addition polymerization reaction which results in **polymerization shrinkage**.

Cavity Primers/Conditioners

Cavity primers are the materials which can be used to coat the walls of the cavity when acrylic resins are used as restorative materials. The function of cavity primers is to **minimize the marginal leakage** and also act as etching agents to fix the restorative resin to the tooth structure.

For example, a solution of **itaconic acid or phosphoric acid ester of glycerine, dissolved in methyl methacrylate monomers.** This cavity primer is applied to the surface of the prepared cavity prior to the insertion of the resin. The intended purpose is to wet the hydrophilic surface of dentin and enamel to make it more attractive towards hydrophobic resins.

Manipulation of Resin Restoratives

Bulk pack or pressure technique

Sufficient quantity of liquid monomer is dispensed in a **dappen dish** and powder of appropriate shade is added uniformly to the liquid until an excess of dry powder remains on the surface. The mix is stirred/spatulated gently to minimize entrapment of air in the chemically activated material, which can introduce voids in the restoration and inhibit polymerization. When the material reaches a full dough stage; **the bulk is quickly inserted into the cavity and held under pressure by** means of matrix band and pressure is applied by matrix strip to prevent the resin from **pulling away from the cavity margins,** while it contracts due to polymerization shrinkage, causing detachment from cavity walls.

Brush technique/incremental technique/bead technique

It is done by applying the polymer-monomer mixture incrementally rather than by filling the cavity with bulk mass. A few drops of monomer are placed in a dappen dish, and a small amount of powder is placed in another dappen dish. The prepared cavity is first coated with a monomer liquid by using a brush. The tip of the pointed brush is then dipped into the monomer and lightly placed on the powder so that few particles attach to it to form a small bead or agglomerate of the powder particles and monomer. The mix is then carried to the prepared cavity and placed on the floor of the cavity. The fluid mix flows readily over the cavity already wetted by the monomer and begins to polymerize. The procedure is repeated until the cavity is slightly overfilled and then a protective film is placed over the surface to prevent evaporation of monomer and moisture or air contamination. This method helps polymerization to occur in increments. **Polymerization shrinkage (contraction) occurs towards cavity walls** and restoration does not get detached.

Properties, advantages and disadvantages

Advantageous properties

- Simple direct filling method

- Good aesthetic properties (initially), but undergoes yellowing due to oxidation of the residual amine activator, i.e. poor colour stability.
- Not expensive material.
- Suitable working and polymerization times.

Disadvantageous properties

- Pulp irritant due to a residual monomer which requires $Ca(OH)_2$ liners to protect exposed dentin.
- Large polymerization shrinkage, leading to marginal gap (and microleakage) and debonding from tooth walls.

Poor mechanical properties

(Compressive strength 65 MPa, tensile strength = 50 MPa, shear strength = 45 MPa, modulus of elasticity = 2,500 MPa)

- Low surface hardness (14–16 KHN) and abrasive resistance
- High COTE (80–120 ppm/°C) cause microleakage, and cavity primers, are to be coated.

In the absence of other anterior restorative materials (like composite resins) this material was tried for restoration of class III and class V cavities.

COMPOSITE RESTORATIVE RESINS

These resins were developed to overcome the drawbacks of unfilled acrylic resins such as low mechanical properties, large polymerization shrinkage, thermal shrinkage due to high COTE, low wear resistance, etc.

Composite resins have the following advantages

- Improved mechanical properties
- Reduced polymerization shrinkage
- Reduction in thermal shrinkage (COTE)
- Superior aesthetics
- Easy to manipulate
- Ability to be moulded at room temperature
- Better wear resistance
- Greater range of applications
- Dentists command set property for VLC composites.

Definitions of composites

The term composite refers to a three-dimensional combination of at least two or more chemically different materials, insoluble in each other, with distinct interphase separating the components.

or

The term composite may be defined as the compound of two or more distinctly different materials with properties that are superior or intermediate to those of the individual components which are chemically bonded by another interface.

CLASSIFICATION OF DENTAL COMPOSITE RESTORATIVE RESINS

Classification is required for the quick selection of material most suitable for the clinical situation.

1. **Earlier classification according to the filler particle size** is given in Table 9.1.

Table 9.1	Earlier classification according to the filler particle size
Category	*Filler particle size*
• Macrofilled composite (conventional/traditional composite)	8–12 µm
• Small particle composite	1–5 µm
• Microfilled composite	0.04–0.4 µm
• Hybrid composite	0.6–1 µm

2. **According to the method of activation**
   Chemically activated composites
   • Initiator benzoyl peroxide
   • Activator—N-N-dimethyl *para*-toluidine

   Light-activated composites
   UV light-activated composite resin:
   • Initiator—benzoin methyl ether
   • Activator—UV light of wavelength, 360 nm
   Visible light cured composites (VLC):
   • Initiator—camphoroquinone, diketones
   • Activator—visible light of wavelength 460–480 nm
   • Accelerator—tertiary amines (dimethylamino-ethyl methacrylate, N-N-dimethyl *para*-toluidine).

3. **According to the method of dispensing**
   Two-paste system: As base and reactor pastes dispensed in separate jars or cylinders, e.g. chemically activated composites.
   Single paste and liquid, e.g. chemically cured composites.
   Single paste system: Supplied in syringes in different shades, e.g. visible light activated composites, and UV light-cured composites.
   Disposable capsules, e.g. compomers.

4. **According to their applications**
   • Anterior composites (for class III and class V cavities)
   • Posterior composites
   • Core build-up composites
   • Pit and fissure sealant composites
   • Prosthodontic composite resins (veneering of gold or base metal-alloy crowns)
   • Glaze resin composites
   • Bonding agents

5. **A recent classification of composites based on their filler particle size and application** (Table 9.2).

Alternatives for BisGMA resin matrix
• BisGMA without OH groups
• Urethane dimethacrylate
• Polyfluorinated polymethyl methacrylate.

COMPOSITION OF DENTAL COMPOSITE RESTORATIVE MATERIALS

Dental composites are made up of three structurally different phases:
A. Organic resin phase—matrix
B. Inorganic filler particles phase dispersed in resin matrix to increase strength, hardness, etc.
C. Interfacial phase (coupling or keying agent)—adhesive agent that promotes adhesion between filler and resin matrix by chemical bonding.

A. Organic Resin Phase Matrix

• High molecular weight monomer
  For example, bisphenol glycidyl methacrylate (BisGMA)

This is normally formed by reaction between ethylene glycol and Bisphenol-A glycidyl methacrylate. This resin was first developed by **Dr. Bowen** in 1960 and hence it is termed **Bowen's resin.**

BisGMA undergoes free radical addition polymerization reaction to form a **highly cross-linked rigid resin** after setting. It has a polymerization shrinkage of only about 5%.

Drawbacks of BisGMA
• **Highly viscous** due to two benzene rings and OH groups, difficult to manipulate, and therefore requires diluent monomers.
• High water sorption
• *Low molecular weight monomer*
  For example, triethylene glycol dimethacrylate (TEGDMA) is added to reduce the viscosity of BisGMA and to obtain a reasonable consistency for convenient use (Fig. 9.2).
• Usually mixtures of **3 parts of BisGMA and 1 part of TEGDMA** are used in dental composites.

B. Different Types of Filler Phases

Inorganic filler phase
Fillers are hard and fine particles in the form of powder, beads, cylinders, etc. having high strength and chemical inertness.

Table 9.2 Recent classification based on the filler particle size and applications

Type of composites	Particle size	Uses
1. Traditional (large particle)	1–50 μm (glass)	High stress areas
2. Hybrid (large particle)	1–20 μm glass+ 0.04 μm silica	High stress areas requiring strength and improved polishability (class I, II, III, IV)
3. Hybrid (midfiller)	0.1–10 μm glass+ 0.04 μm silica	High stress areas requiring improved polishability (class III, IV)
4. Hybrid (minifiller or small particle)	0.1–2 μm glass+ 0.04 μm silica	Moderate stress areas requiring optimal polishability (class III and IV)
5. Packable hybrid	Midfiller/mini-fillers	Situations in which improved condensability is needed (class I and II)
6. Flowable hybrid	Midfiller hybrid	Improved flow due to its finer particles and needed for the situation in which the access is difficult (class II)
7. Homogeneous microfiller	0.04 to 0.06 μm silica	Low stress and subgingival areas that require a high luster of polish
8. Heterogeneous microfiller	0.04 μm silica + prepolymerised resin particles containing 0.04 μm silica (organic fillers)	Low stress and subgingival areas where reduced shrinkage is essential
9. Nanocomposite	Nanomer (single particles)—5 to 75 nm Nanocluster (group of nano-particles)—2–20 nm	Low and high stress bearing areas

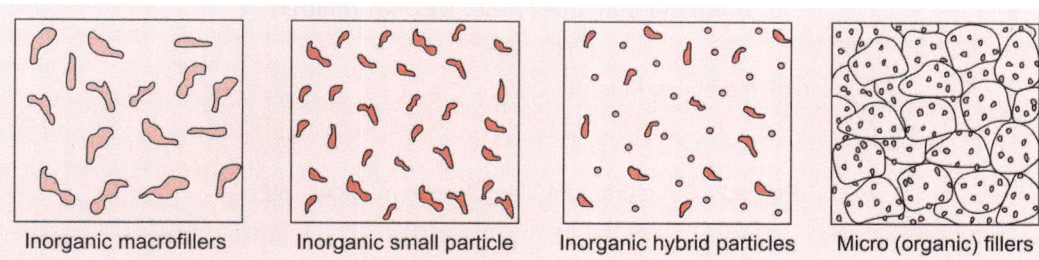

Inorganic macrofillers   Inorganic small particle   Inorganic hybrid particles   Micro (organic) fillers

Fig. 9.1: Different types of fillers

Inorganic filler materials

Ground quartz, precipitated or pyrolytic silica, aluminium silicate, lithium aluminum silicate, borosilicate glasses, barium glasses, etc.

By adding the filler particles to the resin matrix, the material strength and other properties improve **if the filler particles are well bonded to the matrix.** If the filler particles do not adhere well to resin matrix, it can weaken the material. Thus, an **effective coupling agent** is required to keep the resin matrix and filler particles **intact** for the success of composite resins.

The properties enhanced by the addition of fillers are

- **Improved mechanical** properties, i.e. compressive strength, tensile strength, modulus of elasticity, abrasive resistance, hardness, etc. if the filler is chemically bonded to the resin matrix.
- **Reduction in coefficient of thermal expansion** which reduces thermal shrinkage and hence marginal leakage.
- **Reduction in polymerization shrinkage** which also reduces marginal leakage.
- Less heat evolved during polymerization.
- Better aesthetic qualities.
- **For radio-opacity, barium or strontium glasses are used which facilitates the diagnosis of recurrent caries and postoperative sensitivities.**

Inorganic filler particles are present in **30–70 vol%** or **50–85 wt% of the composites.** Fillers used in composites may be produced by grinding, milling,

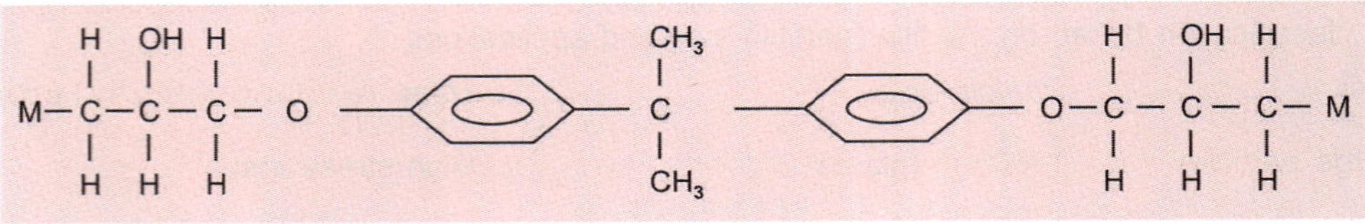

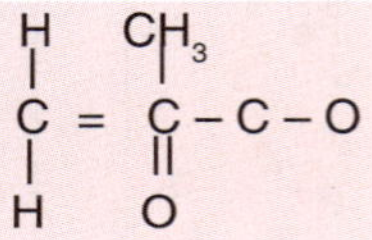

Fig. 9.2: Structural formulae of resin matrices, etc.

precipitation processes. The concentration, particle size and particle size distribution of the fillers used in a composite material, are the major factors controlling the properties.

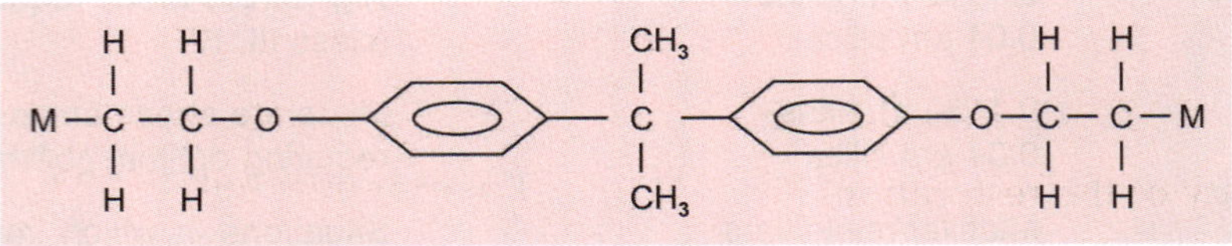

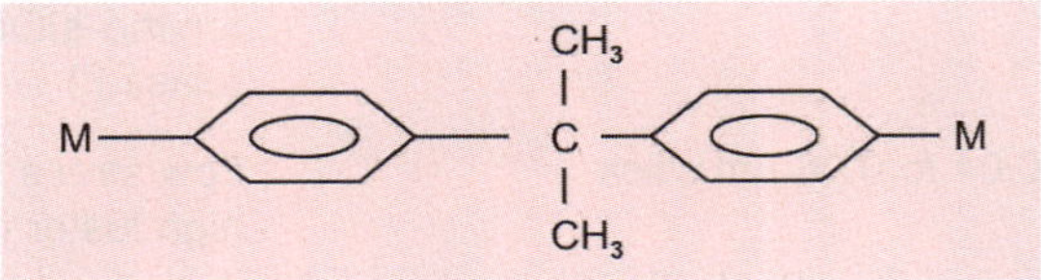

Pyrolytic/Precipitated/Colloidal Silica

These are obtained by precipitation or the pyrolytic processing of the silicon present as low molecular weight compounds such as $SiCl_4$. **The $SiCl_4$ is burned in O_2 and H_2** atmosphere to form macromolecule chains of SiO_2. These macromolecules are of colloidal size and constitute the inorganic filler particles. These are called **pyrogenic (born in a fire) silica particles.**

Organic filler phase

Silane coated colloidal silica is mixed with resin monomers and **chloroform** at a slightly elevated temperature. The filler is thoroughly mixed with the resin and the composite paste is heat cured using a conventional benzoyl peroxide initiator. The cured composite is then ground into powder. These pre-polymerised particles are often called **organic fillers,** which help polishing.

The composite resins are broadly classified into 4 groups based on the filler particle size.

1. **Macro/conventional/traditional composite** with ground glass fillers of particle sizes 8–12 μm.

   Drawbacks
   Difficult to polish due to plucking of hard fillers from soft resin matrix, which leads to rough surface and may cause surface staining.

   Advantage
   Has reasonably good mechanical properties.

2. **Small particle composites** containing ground quartz or barium glass of particle sizes (1–5 µm).

Advantage

Good mechanical properties with better finishing and polishing characteristics.

Disadvantage

The heavy metal glass fibres (barium glass) are softer and more prone to hydrolysis and leach in water. Then silica and quartz gradually soften and become more prone to wear and deterioration, which reduces the long-term durability of the restoration.

3. **Microfilled composites** are containing colloidal silica of particle size 0.04–0.6 µm.

Advantage

Easy to obtain **excellent polish** maintain smooth surface, and good aesthetics.

Disadvantage

Inferior mechanical properties due to small filler particles and less filler load, and higher COTE.

4. **Hybrid composite** (0.6–1 µm): Containing two different types of filler particles, e.g. colloidal silica + barium glasses, i.e. of different sizes (micro + small particles).

These materials were developed in an attempt to obtain the benefits of both types of fillers, i.e. **higher mechanical properties and polishability**.

C. Coupling Agent (Interfacial Phase)

Suitable adhesive bonding of the filler to the resin is essential for the strength and durability of the composite. Without coupling agent, composite resins have inferior mechanical properties. **The adhesive bonding between filler and resin matrix is produced by coupling agent**. Such agents may act as **stress absorbers** at the filler resin interface. This allows the more **flexible polymer** matrix to transfer stresses to stiffer filler with a suitable coupling agent.

A properly applied coupling agent can impart **improved physical and mechanical properties,** and provide **hydrolytic stability** by preventing water from penetrating along the filler resin interface.

The most common coupling agent used in the composite resin is **γ-methacryloxypropyltrimethoxysilane, titanates, zirconates, and vinyl silanes were earlier used.**

Coupling agent: γ-methacryloxypropyltrimethoxysilane

In the presence of water, the methoxy groups ($-OCH_3$) are hydrolyzed to silanol (Si-OH) groups that can bond with the resin when it is polymerized, thereby completing the coupling process.

D. Polymerization Inhibitors

Since dimethacrylate monomers get polymerized during storage by stray ionizing radiations, inhibitors are added to the resin systems to **minimize or prevent accidental polymerization of monomers**.

For example, **butylated hydroxytoluene (BHT**, 0.01 wt%) is a typical **inhibitor** used in dental composites.

This inhibitor extends the storage and stability of the resin, **delays polymerization thereby providing working time.**

E. Initiators and Activators

- **The chemically activated resins** are supplied as two pastes system, one of which contains the **benzoyl peroxide initiator** and the other **N-N-dimethyl-p-toluidine** (tertiary amino activator). When the two pastes are mixed, the amine reacts with the benzoyl peroxide to form free radicals, and addition polymerization occurs.

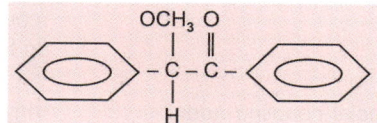

Benzoin methyl ether

- *UV light activated composites*

Initiators: Benzoin methyl ether

Activators: UV light of wavelength **360 nm**

The use of UV light-cured resins have declined because of, health hazards, slow decrease in intensity of UV light and low depth of cure.

- *Visible light activated composites.*

Initiators: Camphoroquinone (0.2 wt%) + tertiary amines (dimethyl aminoethyl methacrylate) (0.15 wt%). Tertiary amines act as an **accelerator**.

Activator: Visible light of wavelength **460–480 nm (or 468 nm).**

UV absorbers or stabilizers 2-hydroxy-4-methoxy benzoquinone

This material is added to improve colour stability by minimizing colour change in the material, when exposed to UV rays or sunlight.

Colour Pigments

To provide a natural appearance similar to patients teeth, dental composites must have visual shading and translucency. This can be achieved by adding various pigments. Metal oxides in minute quantities used are:

Barium oxide, titanium dioxide, aluminum oxide (0.001 to 0.007 wt%), etc.

General compositions of composite resins are given in Table 9.3.

Setting Mechanism

Composite resins set by additional polymerization reaction (for details; *refer* to polymerization). These can be chemically activated or light activated.

BisGMA + TEGDMA + initiators + activators + coupling agent coated inorganic fillers → cross-linked polymer matrix-composite resin chemically bonded to filter (Fig. 9.3)

Table 9.3	General compositions of composite resins		
	Components	**Materials**	**Functions**
A.	Organic phase resin matrix	BisGMA BisGMA without (OH) UEDMA PEPMMA TEGDMA	Highly viscous oligomers polymerize by cross-linking and bind fillers Diluent, to help manipulation
B.	Filler phases a. Inorganic	Quartz, pyrolytic silica, lithium aluminosilicate (β-eucryptite), Al-silicate, borosilicate, barium glasses	Increase strength, control opacity, decreases COTE and polymerization shrinkages
	b. Organic	Pyrolytic precipitated silica (0.04–0.06 microns), treated with coupling agent, and polymerized in BisGMA	Increase filler load in microfilled and hybrid composites. Increase polishability
C	Interfacial coupling agent	Vinyl silane or gamamethacryloxypropyltrimethoxysilane (titanates, zirconates also can be used)	Chemically binds filler particles and resin matrix Increases strength, resilience, decreases COTE and polymerization shrinkage
D.	Polymerization inhibitors	Butylated hydroxytoluene (BHT)	Increases shelf-life and working time of chemically cured resins
E.	Initiators and accelerators a. Chemical curing system	i. Initiator—benzoyl peroxide ii. Activator—N-N-dimethyl-p-toluidine	Produce free radicals by depressing the dissociation (ion forming) temperature, initiates polymerization
	b. Ultraviolet curing system	i. Initiator—benzoin methyl ether ii. Activator—UV of = 350 nm	UV rays activate initiator and release free radicals
	c. Visible light curing system	i. Initiator—diketone camphoroquinone ii. Accelerator—DEA-EMA iii. Activator—VL rays of λ = 468 nm	Visible light rays activate initiator and release free radicals
F.	Colour shade pigments	TiO_2, Al_2O_3, BaO	Control colour shades opacity and radio-opacities

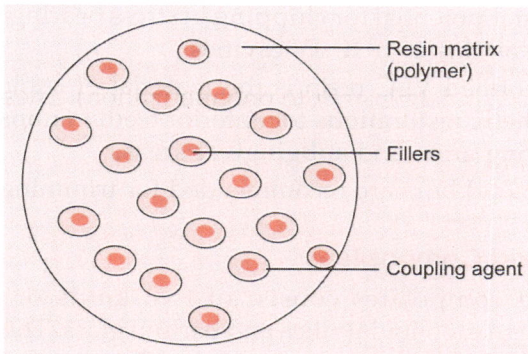

Fig. 9.3: Structure of composite resins

Reaction initiated by free radicals which may be produced by chemical or photochemical means, undergoes addition polymerization (without formation of by-products), with volumetric contraction of 2% (polymerization shrinkage), and is exothermic.

In the case of **chemically cured composite resins shrinkage is towards the centre** of the cavity, whereas in the case of visible light cured composite contraction is towards the external surface of restoration **closest to the light source,** i.e. away from cavity walls.

It is an exothermic reaction with a rise in temperature but the duration of the temperature rise is reasonably short.

The degree of polymerization (or degree of conversion) is uniform in the case of chemically cured composites but not uniform throughout the mass in case of light-cured composite resins. The concentration of unpolymerized groups is more at the base of the cavity, away from the light source as the depth of penetration is low.

The biological property of composite resins

The biocompatibility with pulp **is not satisfactory, and it requires pulp protection** with $Ca(OH)_2$ base. The other reasons for irritations are:

1. Polymerization shrinkage leading to marginal leakage
2. An acid-etching technique using with 37% H_3PO_4

3. The concentration of residual monomers at the floor of the cavity.

Properly polymerized composites are relatively biocompatible but the unpolymerized materials are potentially cytotoxic.

VARIETIES OF COMPOSITE RESINS

1. Conventional/Traditional Composites

These types of composites have comparatively large filler particles. These were developed in the 1970s. The most commonly used filler for these types is finely ground **amorphous silica or quartz filler.** The particle size of the filler averages from **8 to 12 µm,** but some particles of up to 50 µm may also be present. **Filler particle** load may vary from **70–80 wt%** (or 60–65 vol%.)

Clinical significance and considerations

- **Difficulty in finishing and polishing** is due to the presence of large sized filler particles which are harder than the matrix. During finishing and polishing attempts, softer matrix (surface hardness = 55 KHN) easily gets removed and the harder silica fillers (SH = 800 KHN) are **plucked out and lost.** Hence, the surface **becomes more rough.**
- The rough surface is also formed during finishing of the restoration or tooth brushing (Figs 9.4a and b).
- The tendency to discolour by the surface staining is due to the rough surface after finishing.
- A smooth surface can be obtained from a rough surface, by using a glazing agent (unfilled BisGMA). When applied to the surface of the finished restoration, it sets to form a smooth surface layer of about 100 µm thickness. However, this is a temporary measure since the resin coating is abraded away by tooth brushing. **Therefore, glaze must be reapplied regularly.**
- The strength properties are inferior to amalgam restoration and posterior composites.

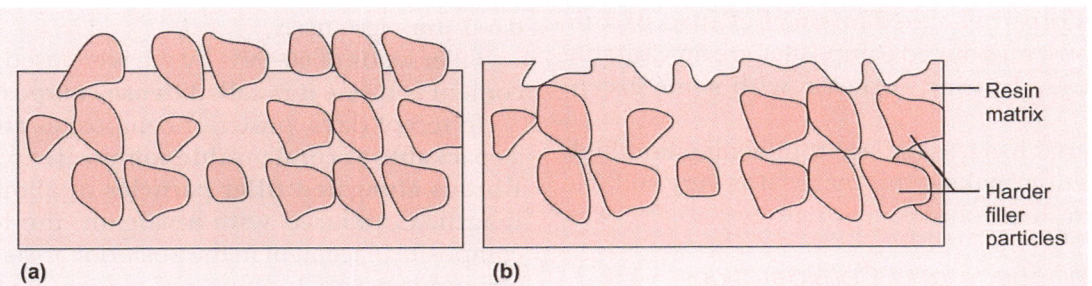

Figs 9.4a and b: Abrasive action on traditional composites. (a) Before polishing, (b) after polishing surface becomes more rough due to plucking of filler particles

2. Small Particle Filled (SPF) Composites

The filler particle size used in SPF composites is ranging from **1 to 5/μm (or microns)**. This broad particle size distribution facilitates a **high filler loading**. The SPF composites were mainly invented to improve the surface smoothness and retain or improve the physical and mechanical properties of traditional composites. The filler particle load is more and varies from **80 to 90 wt%** (or 65 to 77 vol%) when compared with traditional composites. The fillers usually used in SPF composites are **quartz** or **barium glass**.

Clinical Significance and Considerations

- Due to improved strength and higher filler loading, this is indicated for applications in the **large stress bearing areas such as class I and class II cavities.**
- **Reasonably smooth surfaces** can be achieved for anterior restorations (not as good as microfilled composites and hybrid composites).
- The **heavy metal** glass fillers used in SPF composites are softer and more prone to hydrolysis and leach in water than the amorphous silica and quartz. In long service they soften and become more prone to wear and destruction, which reduces the long-term durability of the restoration.

3. Microfilled Composites

The filler particle size used in these types of composites vary from **0.04 to 0.6 μm** and common fillers used are colloidal silica (pyrogenic/precipitated silica).

The filler load is **low 35–60 wt% or 20–55 vol%** because the colloidal silica particles form polymer like chains and increase the viscosity to produce undue thickening, even with very small addition of fillers. There are different techniques used to increase the filler loads. The most likely used technique is to **add organic fillers** (*refer* to fillers of the organic phase of dental composites).

By adding these **organic fillers** the total filler content can be boosted up to **80 wt% or 60 vol%**. These organic fillers **do not bond well** to the resin matrix, causing **wear by a chipping** mechanism. Because of this deficiency, most microfilled composites are **not suitable** for use in **stress bearing surfaces, with some exceptions.**

This material has less surface roughening and high translucency thus making this material as very suitable for anterior restorations.

Clinical Significance and Considerations

- These materials have **lower mechanical properties** because of smaller **filler particles and less filler load.**

- Greater potential for **chipping** in stress bearing areas such as classes I, II, IV cavities.
- Microfilled VLC resin is the material of choice for **aesthetic restorations** for anterior teeth in **nonstress bearing** areas and **subgingival areas.**
- Diamond burs are recommended for trimming.

4. Hybrid Composites

Hybrid composites consist of two kinds of filler particles, i.e. colloidal silica and barium glass. The filler particles size vary **from 0.6 to 1 μm**. These composites were mainly developed to obtain better surface smoothness and all the desirable properties provided by the two types of fillers. The filler load varies from **70 to 80% wt% (or 60–65% vol%)**. The microfillers (colloidal silica) contribute significantly to the properties and also provide increased surface area. The barium glasses (heavy metal) are sufficient for radiographic detection of secondary caries and various other diagnostic tasks.

Clinical Significance and Considerations

1. Widely used for anterior restorations including class IV cavities because of their surface smoothness and reasonably good strength.
2. The mechanical properties are slightly inferior to that of small particles filled composites yet widely used for stress-bearing areas (posterior restorations).

5. Direct Posterior Composites (Dense Composites)

Due to the increased demand in aesthetic dentistry and concern about the potential toxicity of mercury, there has been increased interest in the use of composites for class I and class II restorations. These are the resins developed with improved mechanical properties for restorations of posterior teeth, which could also give good aesthetics.

The fillers used were either **small particles fillers** or **hybrid variety** fillers, quartz or barium glass of particle **size 1–5 μm** were tried and also a **combination of colloidal silica and barium glasses of particle size 0.6–1 μm** were used.

Filler loads of **60–90%** by wt, were used. As the filler content is more, it is called **dense composites**.

In recent days, posterior composites are referred to as **packable or condensable composites** which contain **fibrous elongated filler particles of about 100 μm in length.** Compared with amalgam, the technique of composite placement in the posterior areas is more time consuming and tedious procedure, because of the highly plastic, paste-like consistency in the precured state. The **mechanical properties of posterior** composites are inferior to amalgam and cannot be fully compared with amalgam except for mercury toxicity which is a drawback for amalgam.

Properties

1. Fully polymerized material is biocompatible but the residual monomers left, can irritate the pulp. Pulpal protection should be given with **Ca(OH)$_2$ base**
2. • High compressive strength: 300–380 MPa
   • Tensile strength   : 45–70 MPa
   • Modulus of elasticity   : 5000–13000 MPa
3. Coefficient of thermal expansion : 25–35 ppm/°C
4. Water sorption: 0.1–0.85 mg/cm^2
5. **Radiopacity** due to the presence of heavy metal oxide glass fillers.

   These posterior composites are used in conjunction with a glass ionomer liner or a dentin-bonding agent to secure the best possible bond (and prevent marginal leakage).

Advantages

- Good aesthetics and has a natural appearance
- Adhesion to enamel, if acid etched
- **Light activated** materials have a **command set** properties
- Can be built incrementally which reduces polymerization shrinkage
- Compared with amalgam there are no health hazards.

Drawbacks

- **Poor wear resistance** which leads to occlusal wear.
- Difficult to finish and polish, because margins are not easily recognized.
- **It may irritate pulp by monomer left** due to incomplete polymerization.
- **More expensive** compared to silver amalgam.
- Polymerization shrinkage is large.
- Difficult to obtain predictable and reliable bonding to dentin.
- Marginal leakage is significant.

Uses

- Most widely used for **class I and class II** cavities.
- The material of choice when the patient has documented allergy to mercury.

6. Indirect Posterior Composite Resins

The main **drawbacks** of posterior composites are **polymerization shrinkage, technique sensitivity** and difficulty in obtaining a predictable, **reliable bond** to dentin or cementum margins. These problems lead to **marginal leakage** in class I and class II cavities.

In order to overcome these problems, indirect posterior composites in the form of **inlays and onlays** were tried.

The indirect composites for the fabrication of **inlays or onlays** are polymerized outside the oral environment and fixed to the tooth with resin cement. Indirect composite **inlays** and **onlays** reduce wear, and marginal leakage.

The composite resin systems can be used to prepare **direct composite inlays and indirect composite inlays.**

The direct composite resin inlay: Separating medium (glycerin) is applied to the prepared tooth cavity and resin inlay pattern is formed in it. It is light-cured for a short time and removed from the prepared tooth. This rough inlay is then exposed to additional light for approximately **4 to 6 minutes or heat-cured** at approximately **100°C for 7 minutes**. After this, the prepared tooth is etched, and the **inlay is cemented** on the prepared tooth with a **dual-cure** resin cement and polished.

The indirect composite inlay is prepared in the dental laboratory by technician. The first step is to record the **impression** of the prepared tooth which is taken by the dentist and sent to the laboratory. The inlay is prepared either by **heat curing or light curing** method. The laboratory method is keeping at **140°C temperature and 0.6 MPa pressure for 10 minutes**. High **degree of polymerization** obtained improves physical properties and resistance to wear. The polymerization shrinkage does not occur in the prepared teeth, which reduces marginal leakage and bond failures.

7. Flowable Composite Resins

The flowable composite resins are the **modified form of small particle filled and hybrid composites** which contain **less filler load** to provide a consistency that makes the material to flow readily, **spread uniformly and intimately adapt** to a cavity form to produce a desired contour of the tooth. The reduced filler content makes them highly **susceptible to wear**. But clinically they adapt well to the cavity. Because of their greater ease of adaptation and greater flexibility as a cured material, flowable composites are used for **class I and class II restorations where the access is difficult.** Flowable composites are also used as **pit and fissure sealants** mainly because of their high flowability.

The properties and clinical uses of flowable composite material match to those of **compomers.**

Manipulation of Chemically Curing Composites

These are dispensed in two separate jars or syringes or tubes as base and reactor pastes. An equal **volume** of two pastes are dispensed onto the mixing pad by using a disposable plastic spatula. In order to ensure proper polymerization, the components must be evenly dispersed throughout the mix. Mixing is done by spatulation with a plastic spatula until a homogeneous mix is obtained.

Mixing time is about 20–30 seconds.

Precautions

1. **Air should not** be incorporated during mixing.
2. **Stainless steel spatula should not be used** because fillers are sufficiently hard to abrade the metal spatula and can release some impurities which may discolour the restoration.
3. During dispensing care must be taken to avoid contamination of the paste of one jar with that of the other.

Insertion

A base of Ca(OH)$_2$ is required to protect exposed dentin from the possibility of irritation from the organic constituents of the resin and acid etchants.

Acid etching: To provide a bond with the composite resin and tooth structure the enamel portion of the cavity preparation is acid etched with etchant 37% H$_3$PO$_4$ for 15–20 sec. Acid is flushed away with water and surface is dried with a stream of air.

Apply a bonding agent to the etched enamel and dentin. It penetrates the irregularities to form **retentive mechanical tags of resins.** The mixed resin is inserted into the cavity by using the plastic instrument and the matrix should be placed immediately after insertion and held for 2 minutes under pressure, for proper marginal adaptation (Fig. 9.4).

Finishing: Gross reduction can be done with **diamond or carbide finishing** burs or **green stone** and final finishing is done with fine silica or alumina disc. The

final procedure can be usually started **5 minutes** after insertion. For conventional composite, a glazing agent should be applied to get a smooth surface.

Advantages

* The reaction takes place almost uniformly throughout the bulk of the material, curing is not generally dependent on the thickness of restoration.
* Easy manipulation with no elaborate procedures.

Disadvantages

* Short working time, since the reaction and increased viscosity occurs immediately when the two components come into contact.
* Air may be incorporated during mixing, which produces porosities or voids and inhibition of polymerization.
* The polymerization shrinkage is towards the center of the cavity leading to marginal leakage, due to detachment from cavity walls.

8. Light Activated Composite Resins

A. **UV light activated composite resins:** These are activated by external energy **UV** light of wavelength **360 nm.** A photoinitiator **benzoin methyl ether** undergoes photo-fragmentation producing free radicals which initiate reaction and the material sets by the addition polymerization reaction.

B. **Visible light-cured (VLC) composite resins:** These are the composite resins utilizing visible light for activation during polymerization. Here the diketone (camphoroquinone) absorbs radiation energy of wavelength 468 nm (or 460–475 nm, blue region of light) and is transferred to excited states. At this appropriate excited states, the diketone then combines with reducing agent **tertiary amine (dimethyl aminoethyl methacrylate)** to form an excited state complex, which breaks down to give reactive **free radicals** and reaction is initiated. Thus, it undergoes addition polymerization and material hardens.

Light sources used (curing lamps) (*see* Colour Plate 22, Fig. 9.5)

Hand-held light curing devices are usually used. These contain light sources which are equipped with a relatively short rigid light guides made up of optical fibers.

Remote controlled light sources are also available. Long flexible fibre optic chord is used to transmit light to the mouth.

There are 4 types of light sources which emit light radiations of **different intensities.**

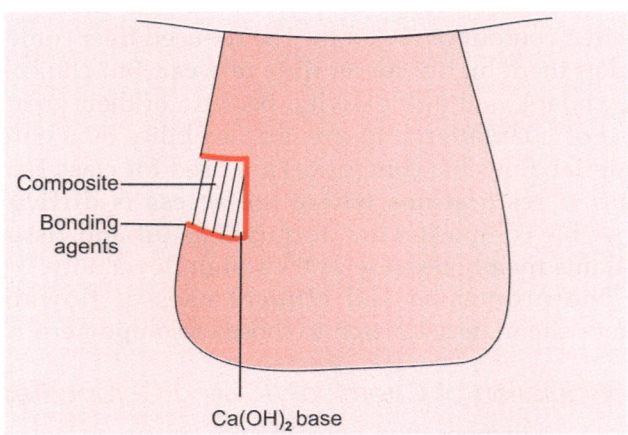

Fig. 9.4: Composite restoration

1. **Light emitting diodes (LED) lamps**
   These light sources emit radiation only in the blue part of the visible spectrum between 440 nm and 480 nm and they do not require any filters.
   This light source requires low voltage and can be **battery operated**. This does not produce any heat or sound.

   Drawback
   These produce lowest intensity radiations and require a **long time for curing**.

2. **Quartz-tungsten halogen (QTH) lamps**
   These light sources have quartz halogen bulbs with tungsten filament which radiates both UV light and visible light. So, **filters are required** to remove the unwanted UV wavelength and to emit only violet–blue range (~ 400–500 nm). The intensity of the bulb **decreases** with use. Hence, the light source has to be **calibrated often** to measure the output intensity.

3. **Plasma arc curing (PAC) lamps**
   These lamps use **xenon gas** that is ionized to produce a plasma, which is a **high-intensity white light.** It is to be **filtered** to remove heat and allow blue-light (~ 400–500 nm) to be emitted.

4. **Argon laser lamps**
   These lamps produce the **highest intensity** of light radiation of a **single wavelength.** Argon laser lamps produce a wavelength usually of ~ 490 nm.
   The widely used light source is **quartz tungsten halogen lamps** as it is cost-effective. Since it emits the lowest intensity of light and the efficiency of the bulb decreases with time, other light sources are **slowly replacing QTH lamps.**
   The curing lamps usually have an appropriate light filters, switches tuning devices and curing tips. (vary from 5 mm to 7 mm in diameter). The curing tip of the light source must be **held within 1 mm** of the surface to give **optimum penetration and short curing time.**

Depth and degree of curing

For the given radiation and material, polymerization requires a specific amount of light energy and it depends on:

- The characteristics of the light source (new bulb gives higher intensity).
- Distance between the light source and composite restoration.
- Exposure time (proper exposure time of minimum 40 seconds). The curing time is **inversely proportional to the intensity of light incident**, on the surface, i.e. the curing or exposure time should be **directly proportional to the square of the distance**. In other words if the distance of the tip of the light source is increased by 5 times, curing time increases by 25 times.

- *Composition:* Concentration of photoinitiators in the composite resins must be such that it will react at a proper wavelength and be present in sufficient concentrations.

Composite resins which undergo incomplete polymerization show

1. Inferior mechanical properties
2. Adverse bulk tissue reaction
3. Poor colour stability
4. Greater susceptibility to stains
5. Retention failures

Manipulation of UV or Visible Light Activated Resins

Bonding agent should be applied to the prepared tooth cavity. (The recent bonding agents contain etching agents in them, **etch and bond**.) In case of small cavities, the resin paste is packed into the cavity, moulded to proper contour and cured by passing light of proper wavelength. But in **case of deep cavities**, the restoration must be built up in **increments** since the depth of curing is limited. Each increment inserted is shaped to the desired form and then cured. Additional increments are then added, shaped and cured. The best method is to insert the material with a syringe. To ensure maximum polymerization and clinical success, a high intensity light unit should be used, and the light intensity should be evaluated periodically. Ideally, curing should be initiated at the tooth-resin interface so that the resin shrinks towards the cavity walls rather than away from these walls. The light tip should be **positioned as closely as possible** to the resin, the exposure time should not be less than 40 seconds and the thickness of the resin should not be more than 2.0 to 2.5 mm.

The light emitting from the curing units **can cause retinal damage** if focussed or seen directly for a long time. Direct focusing or seeing the light should be avoided and minimize observing the reflected lights for longer periods. Protective eye glasses can be used.

Finishing

The finishing procedure can be started, **5 minutes after curing.** The gross reduction can be made with **diamond or carbide finishing burs or green stones** and final finishing can be done with fine **silica or alumina** discs.

Advantages of (UV light and visible light cured) composites over chemically cured composites

1. **Command setting properties: Infinite working and short controlled setting time.**

Table 9.4 Properties of different varieties of composite resins versus tooth enamel and dentin

S.No.	Properties/ materials	Unfilled acrylics	Conventional traditional large particle macrofilled	Hybrid small particle	Hybrid all-purpose	Hybrid flowable	Hybrid posterior packable	Microfilled	Tooth enamel	Tooth dentin
1.	Particle size (microns)	—	8–12	0.5–3	0.4–1.0	0.6–1.0	Fibrous	.04–4	—	—
2.	Inorganic fillers (vol%)	0	60–70	65–77	60–65	30–55	48–67	20–59	—	—
3.	Inorganic fillers (wt%)	0	70–80	80–90	75–80	40–60	65–81	35–67	—	—
4.	Compressive strength (MPa)	75	250–300	350–400	300–350	105	300–380	250–350	380	300
5.	Tensile strength (MPa)	25–55	50–65	75–90	40–50	20	45–70	30–50	10	5
6.	Modulus of elasticity (MPa)	2500	8,000–15,000	15000–20,000	11,000–15,000	4000–8000	5000–13000	3000–6000	80000	18000
7.	COTE (ppm/°C)	95	25–35	19–26	30–40	—	25–30	50–60	11.4	8.6
8.	Water sorption (mg/mm^2)	1.7	0.5–0.7	0.5–0.6	0.5–0.7	—	0.1–0.85	1.4–1.7	—	—
9.	Surface hardness—KHN (kg/mm^2)	15–20	55	50–60	50–60	40	50–60	25–35	350–430	68
10.	Curing shrinkage (vol%)	8–10	2–3	2–3	2–3	3–5	2–3	2–3	—	—
11.	Radio-opacity (mm A1)	0.1	2–3	2–3	2–4	1–4	2–3	0.5–2	2	1

Viscosity does not increase until resin is exposed to light activation and then set in short time (ability to set rapidly after exposure to light source).

2. No mixing is needed
3. Less chance of incorporation of air into mix, i.e. porosity in the restoration is minimized
4. Less wastage of material
5. Amount of finishing required is less
6. Easy manipulation technique

Disadvantages of UV light activated composites

- Health hazard of UV rays **cause skin cancer or retinal damage.**
- **Limited depth** of cure as low as **1.5 mm** by exposure of UV light.
- Approximately 60 seconds is required to cure the composite resins to a depth of 1.5 mm.
- UV generators require several minutes for **warm up** before use.
- **Intensity** of the light source gradually **decreases with time** and hence **exposure (setting) time increases.**

Advantages of visible light cured (VLC) over UV light cured composites

- The VLC composite resin can be cured to a **greater depth of 2–2.5 mm** in a relatively short-time (20–40 seconds) but the thick mix and the dark shades of the material absorb more light. So, it requires longer curing time.
- **Health hazard is virtually eliminated.**
- **No warm up time** is needed for the proper operation of light source.
- **No decrease in the intensity** of light source because the output is constant.
- **Incremental technique** can be used to maintain adhesion to the cavity floor in deep cavities.

Drawbacks of light activated composites

- **The degree of polymerization is not uniform** throughout the mass of the material.
- **Polymerization shrinkage** is towards the external surface **closer to the light source**.

9. Prosthodontic Composite Resins

The composite resins like BisGMA or urethane dimethacrylate, either chemically, cured or light cured materials, are used for veneering (preparing the crown by giving a resin facing over a metallic casting). These composite resins have **superior mechanical** and aesthetic qualities compared to polymethyl methacrylate.

The bonding of composite resins to metal castings are done by micromechanical retention by using acid etching the base metal alloy and **using bonding agents such as 4 META, phosphorylated methacrylate, epoxy**

resins. Sometimes silica flame sprayed metal surfaces are also used for bonding purpose.

Advantages

- Easily repairable in early stage
- The opposite tooth wearing is minimum
- Fabrication technique is easier and simpler.

Disadvantages

- Poor mechanical properties are leading to distortion due to occlusal loading.
- Marginal leakage and staining.
- Poor abrasion resistance and wears out during tooth brushing.

Repairing of composite resins

The freshly prepared composite resin restoration, if gets fractured **can be easily repaired** by placing fresh composite resin mix which is cured over that. The fresh, composite resin combines with the old resin chemically as many unpolymerized monomer molecules in the old restoration still present, can combine with the freshly mixed material. However, **very old restorations cannot** be repaired by this method.

10. Preventive Resin Restorations (Pit and Fissure Sealants)

The decay of tooth usually begins from the occlusal surface by collection of food debris in the small pits and fissures especially in deciduous teeth. The preventive method adopted is to seal it with pit and fissure sealants like GIC or composite resins.

Composite resins either microfilled or with a low percentage of fillers are used along with bonding agents for this sealing. If the dentist feels that the chances of decaying is more due to unhygienic conditions, he can choose simple conservative methods with minimum cavity preparations. The above type of composite resins is applied using bonding agents to the carious lesions, continuing from pit and fissures, sometimes covering the entire occlusal surface. This is known as preventive resin restoration (PRR) technique.

11. Pit and Fissure Sealants (Fig. 9.5)

Pits are small pinpoint deep depressions in the enamel and sometimes extending to dentine of the tooth. Fissures are the micro crevices in the enamel and sometimes extending to dentin of the tooth, **usually located at the junction of development grooves**.

Small pits and fissures are found on the occlusal surface of the teeth of small children (deciduous dentition), where food debris gets collected which can lead to caries. To protect these teeth, the pits and fissures

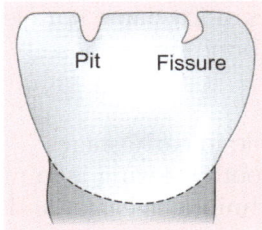

Fig. 9.5: Pit and fissure sealants

should be sealed with sealants, as conservative measures.

Requirements for pit and fissure sealants
- Should chemically bond with tooth structure.
- Chemically stable in the mouth, i.e. biocompatible.
- Sufficient mechanical properties to withstand masticatory forces.
- Should have high flow properties, i.e. low surface tension, low viscosity and low or zero angles of contact for bonding before setting.
- COTE should be similar to tooth structure (i.e. 11.4 ppm/°C)
- They should be good insulators of heat and electricity.
- Match with the tooth colour.

Materials used
- Glass ionomer cements—type III (which can bond chemically and has low COTE).
- Composite resins (flowable composites)—with less amount of fillers.

Pits and fissures are cleaned, applied with acid etchant, dried, washed, applied with bonding agents, and filled with restorative materials (i.e. composites). VLC composites are cured using visible light of wavelength 460–480 nm.

12. Composite Resins Artificial Teeth

These have been introduced recently to overcome the drawbacks of acrylic teeth. These are micro and hybrid filler varieties. These have higher mechanical properties and greater wear resistance. These do not have the disadvantages of ceramic teeth, namely clicking sound, brittleness, poor fracture resistance and bonding to the acrylic denture. Available in different shades and sizes. Comparison of properties of acrylic, ceramic, composite resin teeth (Table 6.5, page 131).

(Table 6.5, page 131).

MODEL QUESTIONS

I. Long Essays (20 minutes each)
1. Describe the compositions of various types of composite resins and give the functions of the ingredients and uses.
2. Describe the term composite resin and classify the dental composite resins. Add a note on small particle filler (SPF) composite resins.
3. Give the composition and properties of visible light-cured composite resins. What are its advantages and disadvantages?

II. Short Essays (10 minutes each)
1. Fillers and resin matrix of composite resins
2. Initiators and activators of composite resins
3. Microfilled VLC composite resins
4. Recent composite resins
5. Advantages of VLC over chemically and ultraviolet cured composite resins
6. Visible light sources for curing
7. Hybrid composite resins
8. Pit and fissure sealants
9. Sandwich technique
10. Manipulation methods of chemically cured/VLC composite resins

III. Brief Answers (5 minutes each)
1. Coupling agents
2. Fillers of composite resins
3. Organic fillers
4. Polishing of composite resins
5. Indirect composites
6. Prosthodontic composite resins
7. Flowable composite resins
8. Acid etching for composite resins
9. Repairing of composite resin restorations
10. Disadvantages of UV cure composite resins
11. Finishing of composite resins
12. Composite resin matrix
13. Dentists command set property
14. Preventive resin restorations
15. Composite resin artificial teeth

Bonding of Restorations

One of the main problems faced in the conservative dentistry is to achieve true adhesion of restorations to the tooth structure, e.g. enamel and dentin surfaces for longer retention and minimize microleakage and deterioration of cavity walls. Wetting of an adhesive to the adherend surface is the most important part of bonding.

Mechanisms of Bonding

1. Wetting of the enamel and dentin surfaces.
2. Micromechanical interlocking.
3. Chemical bonding.
4. Interpenetration is forming hybrid zones.

The Factors Improving Wetting

- **Clean surface** of adherend without any impurities or contaminations like oil of cutting instruments, moisture, debris, smear layer, etc.
- **The high surface energy** of adherend—acid etching increases surface area and energy.
- **The surface tension** of adhesive should be low. Many cements have higher surface energies than that of tooth enamel **(84 erg/cm^2).**
- **The angle of contact** should be low.

For successful true bonding of restorations

- **Microleakage** at the interface of restoration and tooth surface, should not take place.
- Maximum retention of the restoration

- The maximum healthy part of the tooth should be retained during cavity preparation, i.e. cavity cutting should be minimum.

BONDING TO ENAMEL

Enamel has a complex surface structure with enamel rods inside and more organic components on the surface. The surface energy of enamel, **84 erg/cm^2** is usually less than many restoratives, which do not help to wet. The surface has moisture and other contaminations which also decrease wetting and bonding. Mechanical bonding is achieved by forming microporous surface which increases area of contact and surface energies. This is done by **acid etching.** Chemical bonding is achieved by polycarboxylate cements and glass ionomers.

Acid etching

This technique was first used **in 1955 by Buonocore**, with the intention of reducing microleakage by improving marginal sealing of interfacial gap. This technique has become quite popular, and recently, mild acids are used to etch or remove the debris layer on the dentin surface also.

Mechanism

The common acid etchant, phosphoric acid aqueous solution or gel is placed on the tooth enamel. It reacts with the hydroxyapatite of enamel or the enamel rods and causes **selective dissolution.** Selective dissolution of **enamel rods is type I etching,** and dissolution of **peripheral areas is type II etching.** The microporosities formed on surface have about 6 μm width and 10–20 μm depth, depending on the dilution of acid and time of etching. When a restorative material with low viscosity is placed, it flows into the formed microtags, which mechanically bonds to it (Fig. 10.1).

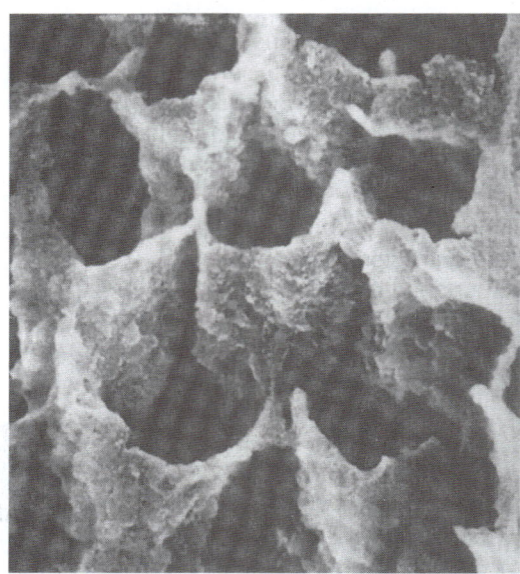

Fig. 10.1: Scanning electron microscope (SEM) image of the tags formed by penetration of resin into etched enamel (*see* Colour Plate 23, Figs 10.1a and b)

Etchants (*see* Colour Plate 23, Fig. 10.2)

The common etchant is phosphoric acid solution of **37%** concentration. **About 30 to 50%** aqueous solution, also can be used. Etchant with more than 50%, reacts with enamel, forms **monocalcium phosphate-monohydrate** which is insoluble and prevents further etching. The **recent trend** is to use H_3PO_4 of lower concentration, **15 to 30%** for forming deeper **tags.**

The etchants are used **as gels** or liquid in syringes. The gel is made by adding colloidal silica or polymer beads to the H_3PO_4 solution and applied with brushes. **Gel form is preferred as its flow is limited only to the etching area.** Sometimes other etchants and conditioner acids are also used for **cleaning** the surface debris or smear layer of the cavity preparations and **selective** dissolutions to form micropores.

Etching Technique Steps

1. **Cleaning** the enamel surface by pumice slurry and then washing with water.
2. **Etching** the surface by placing the etchant gel using brush or liquid by cotton pledget for 30–60 sec as per manufacturer's instructions.
3. **Washing** the etched surface by flushing with water carefully for 15 seconds.
4. **Drying** the surface with a mild stream of air.
5. **Bonding** agent is applied **immediately** before the etched surface gets contaminated with moisture, saliva, blood, etc.

Precautions

- Acid etchant should not come into contact with the exposed dentin surface as the acid ions penetrate through the dentin tubules. As a precautionary measure, $Ca(OH)_2$ cement can be applied over exposed dentin.
- **Delicate** etched surface has thin fragile sections. These should not be damaged by touching or contact with instruments.
- The etched surface should not get contaminated with blood, saliva, moisture or oils spray through instruments before the bonding resin is applied.

The etched surface has a **frosted whitish appearance,** if the acid etching is done properly. The etched surface has higher energy and increased wettability. Any contamination decreases the bond strength. Acid etching method has produced bond strength of about 15–25 MPa.

BONDING AGENTS

Bonding agent can be defined as a material of low viscosity, when applied, on the tooth surface, can form thin film after setting. This thin film is strongly bonded to tooth surface, on which the viscous composite restorative resin, is applied. This sets forming an integrated resin restoration.

Classification of Bonding Agents

1. *According to the bonding mechanism*
   - Mechanical bonding through acid etching (composite resins, BisGMA, TEGDMA, cyanoacrylates).
   - Chemical bonding by direct application (zinc polycarboxylate cements—GIC).

2. *According to the application*
   - Enamel bonding agents—thin composite resins, TEGDMA, cyanoacrylates, glass ionomers
   - Dentin bonding agents several dimethacrylate systems, NPG-GMA, cyanoacrylates, BisGMA, polyurethanes, 4-META, ferric oxalate systems, etc.

Enamel Bonding Mechanisms

These are mainly of two types. These are usually microfilled composites or BisGMA resins with small amount of (or without) fillers. After acid etching, the thin (low viscosity) composite is flown into the micropores, as a thin layer. This polymerizes by chemical or visible light actions. Over this the harder posterior, anterior or hybrid composites are applied and cured. The bonding agent and restorative resins have same chemical structure, and polymerise forming an integrated structure (Fig. 10.2).

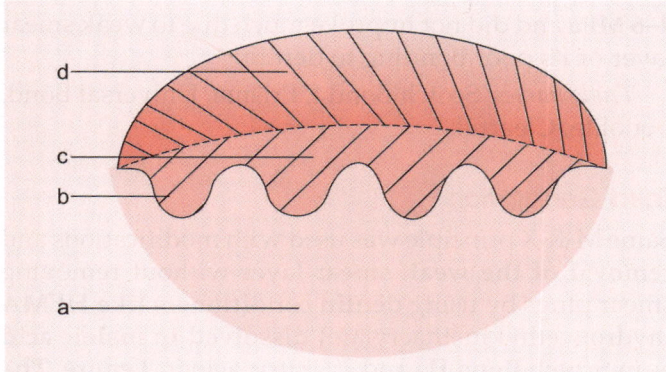

Fig. 10.2: Enamel resin restoration bonding. (a) Enamel surface, (b) acid etched tags, (c) bonding agent—resin or GIC 'sandwich', (d) restorative hard composite resin

Chemically bonding polyacrylate systems

The polyacrylic acid of zinc polycarboxylate cement or glass ionomer cements have their acrylic acid –COOH groups. These can react and bond with Ca⁺⁺ ions of enamel or collagen of dentin structures.

Sandwich technique

The chemically bonding material does not require cavity cutting but only removal of carious lesion completely. Initially glass ionomer cement is applied as chemical bonding agent and over that the stronger composite resin is applied.

Dentin Bonding

The enamel bonding techniques and agents did not yield good results for dentin. There are many more problems to be solved for bonding of resin restorations to dentin, such as:

1. Dentin surface has complex structure. Due to lower degree of calcification, **less calcium ions** are available for chemical bonding. Only 70 wt% inorganic hydroxyapatite and about 20 wt% of organic collagen can contribute to chemical bonding.
2. **Remaining water** about 10 wt% is a big obstacle. The **fluids** coming out of the exposed dentinal tubules, prevents the bonding of hydrophobic resin materials. Hence, bonding agents should contain hydrophilic –OH groups.

3. Presence of **smear layer** on the exposed dentin tubules.
4. Controversy regarding acid etching of dentin surface.
5. Dentin is biologically sensitive.
6. Surface energy of organic materials is quite low. This also discourage bonding.

Ideal requirements of bonding agents

- Biocompatibility, nontoxic, nonirritant, nonpoisonous
- Should not react with organic and inorganic constituents
- Suitable low viscosity to flow easily on the surface of adherend
- **Wet the tooth surface easily, i.e. low surface tension and angle of contact**
- Low film thickness
- Form strong permanent bond
- Good dimensional stability
- Should have both hydrophilic and hydrophobic reactive groups
- Similar COTE as tooth **(11.4 ppm/°C)**
- Low thermal conductivity
- Good shelf-life

The **intermediate linkage** between dentin and restorative resin, is known as dentinal or **dentin bonding agent.** Various types of chemical and bonding systems have been tried to have a proper solution to the problem. Development of bonding systems are spread out from generation first to generation seventh. Initial problems found in the generations 1st, 2nd, 3rd, 4th have been overcome in the modifications 5th, 6th and 7th generations (*see* Colour Plate 23, Fig. 10.3).

Acid Etching of Dentin

In 1979, Fusayama, used 37% phosphoric acid solution for etching enamel and dentin and showed that it did not damage the pulp and improved the bond strength. **In 1982, Nakabayashi** discovered formation of **a hybrid layer** of resin infiltrated dentin. Around 1990s the dentin etching procedure was almost accepted.

Principles of Dentin Bonding

Composite resins were developed by using a coupling agent which can bond chemically with the resin matrix at one side and the silica filler at the other side. This coupling agent contained at one end an unsaturated methyl methacrylate group (M, which is $H_2C = C(CH_3) – C(=O) –OCH_3$), to chemically combine with resin matrix and at the other end a silane group (X) to combine with silica fillers and a spacer structure R in between. This M-R-X bonding was very successful to get the composite resin of high strength, lower COTE and polymerization shrinkages. This principle was tried to bond the resin matrix of the restorative to the dentin. During the past years, this simple principle has undergone many modifications, aiming at obtaining a **permanent bonding.** According to the principles and techniques, many varieties or generations of bonding agents, have been invented.

First Generation

In this M is the same unsaturated methyl methacrylate group, X is an acidic phosphate group to react with Ca^{++} of dentin. The first product (1950s) contained glycerol phosphoric acid dimethacrylate (Fig. 10.3).

The composition was aimed only to bond with Ca^{++} ions and not with the organic matrix (collagen) of dentin.

This is not successful due to:
- Hydrolysis of bonding agent
- Large COTE
- Large polymerization shrinkages.

In addition, cyanoacrylates, N-phenyl glycine-glycidyl methacrylates (NPG-GMA) have also been tried without much success. (Bond strength was only about **2 MPa.**)

Trade name = Cosmic bond

Second Generation

It was proposed that smear layer (dentin debris of cavity preparation) may play certain role in bonding to dentin. The bonding agents were developed with the intention of using the resins for cervical, class V restorations with minimum cavity preparations.

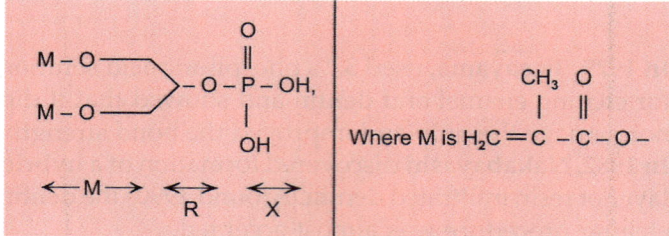

Fig. 10.3: Glycerol phosphoric acid dimethacrylate

The materials tried were
- Halogen (chloro) phosphoric acid esters of BisGMA, polyurethanes
- N phenyl glycine + glycidyl methacrylate (NPG-GMA)
- Phenyl-P (Fig. 10.4)
- 2 Methacryloxy phenyl phosphoric acid, etc.

Both the first and second generations were considered as **phosphate bonding system.** These also had same disadvantages. The bond strength was only

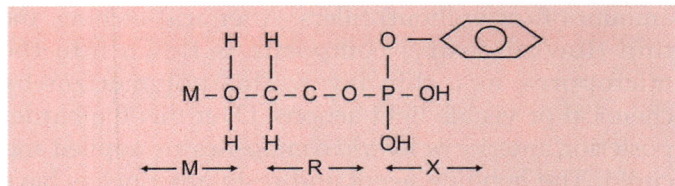

Fig. 10.4: Phenyl-P

4–6 MPa and did not improve much due to weak smear layer or its poor bonding to dentin.

Trade names: Scotch Bond I, Prisma, Universal Bond, Bonolite, Clearfill.

Third Generation

Same M-R-X principle was used with modifications and **removal of the weak smear layer** without removing smear plugs by using **dentin conditioners like HEMA** (hydroxyethyl methacrylate) **dissolved in maleic acid** as in **Scotch Bond II,** and 2% nitric acid in **Tenure. The Scotch Bond II** agent was chlorophosphoric acid ester of BisGMA.

These bonding agents were aimed at reacting with Ca^{++} of dentin. Attempts have been then made to bond the organic matrix, **collagen** which is about 20 wt% of dentin. For this **35% glutaraldehyde** in **HEMA and EDTA** as conditioner were tried. This was also not successful, as collagen, perhaps did not bond.

The procedure of bonding was followed by applying
- The dentin conditioner (to modify or remove smear layer)
- The primer bonding agent—a monomer dissolved in an organic solvent
- Unfilled resin adhesive
- Composite restoration on it.

Trade names
Scotch Bond II, Tenure, Mirage Bond, Prisma, Universal Bond, etc.

Fourth Generation

It was believed that opening of the dentin tubules by phosphoric acid etching, may cause pulp irritation and permanent damage. However, it was shown by scientists of Japan, that this belief was incorrect. Acid etching with dilute etchants can be done for removal of smear layers and smear plugs, and also **open the dentin tubules for mechanical bonding**. To minimise clinical procedures, the **total etching technique** (i.e. etching of enamel and dentin) could be conducted, and then the bonding and restorations are followed.

General steps for using the fourth generation bonding systems (3-step)

- **Total etching** of enamel and dentin surface with the conditioner (usually dil. phosphoric acid) for 15 sec. This removes the smear layer and exposes the collagen network.
- **Wash** it with water, carefully to remove debris and dry it. Desiccation should not be done as it collapses collagen network, and block dentin tubules. Moisten the surface and then.
- **Apply the primer coatings** (1 to 6 times) which infiltrates collagen and allow it to polymerise. Again dry thoroughly.
- **Apply the thin adhesive-bonding agent**, to enamel and dentin, to about **50 μm** thickness. The primers and bonding agents can be simultaneously cured by light.
- **Apply the composite resin** over this adhesive and cure it with light.

The total etching, drying, moistening, applying primers, etc. are quite critical. The demineralized collagen layers are very fragile and may collapse during this procedure (Fig. 10.4).

Trade names: All Bond II

Fifth Generation (Twp-Step)

The current bonding mechanisms have **micro-mechanical retention by:**
- **Penetration** into the partially opened dentin tubules
- Formation of **hybrid layer** by interpenetration into demineralized collagen fibril network.
- **Chemical bonding**

Perception of the complexity of clinical procedure lead the manufacturer to develop two steps, i.e. **etch and bond** systems. This is a two-component system. One component has etchant or conditioner and the other primer or adhesive. The etching is done for 20–30 sec, with phosphoric acid. Then primer and bonding (adhesive) agents are applied. Composite restoration is finally placed over it. This system contains hydrophobic and hydrophilic resins dissolved in volatile ethanol or acetone, which drives out water and brings the monomer into intimate contact with the exposed collagen fibres.

Trade names

Bond I
a. BisGMA + HEMA + acetone
b. 37% H_3PO_4 etchant + primers

3M Single Bond
a. BisGMA + HEMA + H_2O + ethanol + polyalkenoic acid-copolymer
b. 37% phosphoric acid etchant
   Prime and Bond, One Step Bisco.

Sixth Generation (Two-Step)

In this case acidic monomer is used to condition (not rinsed) and prime the tooth at the same time and supplied as mild and strong varieties. This bonds to dentin due to mineral content, but more prone to hydrolytic degradation.

Seventh Generation (One-Step)

These are single component system liquid, containing etchants for enamel and dentin, conditioners primer and bonding adhesives. This requires single application without washing. This generation attracted clinicians due to reduced clinical step.

Trade names: All Bond, ED-primer (both are VLC)

Examples of bonding agents
- Organic phosphates
- Polyurethanes

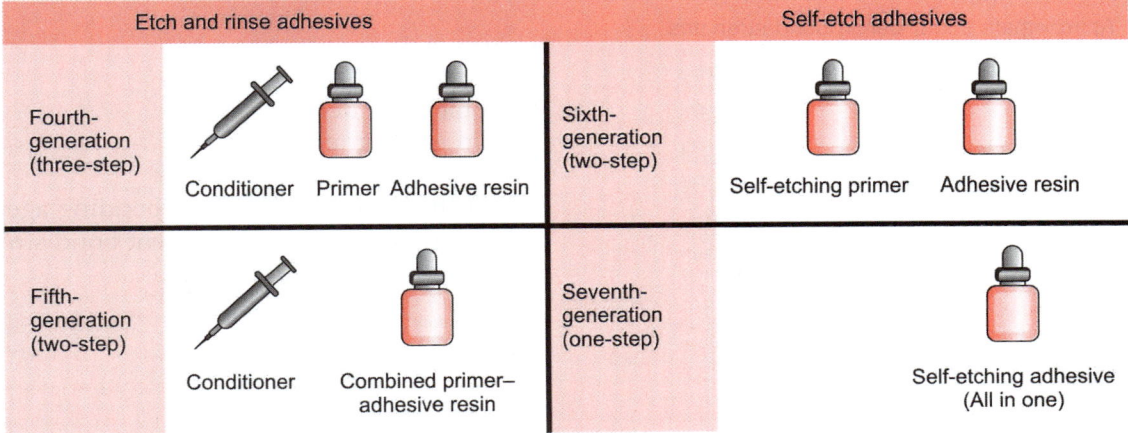

Fig. 10.4: Different generations of dentin bonding agents

- 4-Methacryloxyethyl trimallitate anhydride (4-META)
- HEMA + glutaraldehyde
- Ferric oxalate (NPG-GMA) + PMDM (pyromalletic dihydride, 2-hydroxymethyl methacrylate)
- HEMA + BisGMA + maleic acid
- Bisphenyl dimethacrylate
- Polyalkenoates.

Measurement of Bond Strengths

Bond strengths are measured by preparing standard specimens and applying shear or tensile forces until the debonding takes place. The bond strengths are expressed as force/area in MPa.

The values thus obtained (Tables 10.1 and 10.2), correspond to or indicative of the bond strengths *in vivo*. However, the values thus obtained for different specimens always have large deviations. This is because there are many variable parameters which cannot be controlled, in the experimental procedures (like cavity surface roughness, extent of acid etching, water present, drying, application of primers, adhesives, etc.). **Recently micro-tensile testing method** has been developed. This requires very small <1 mm^2 samples, and many samples can be prepared from the same tooth and the results are more reliable. The interfacial adhesive failure takes place and not failure within

Table 10.1	Approximate tensile dentin bond strength of bonding agents	
1.	Glass ionomer cement	1–3 MPa
2.	Polyalkenoic acids	2–4 MPa
3.	Polyurethanes	2–6 MPa
4.	4-META	4–8 MPa
5.	NPG-GMA	4–13 MPa
6.	HEMA + glutaraldehyde	11–17 MPa

Table 10.2	Approximate shear dentin bond strengths	
1.	Bisphenyl dimethacrylate (BPDM)	28 MPa
2.	HEMA + BisGMA	24 MPa
3.	HEMA + glutaraldehyde (5%)	17 MPa
4.	4-META	14 MPa
5.	Organic phosphonates	4 MPa
6.	Polyurethanes	3 MPa

dentin. Bond failures also have been studied after thermal cycling (from 0 to 65°C).

The interfacial marginal leakage between the tooth surface and the restorative also has been studied, by the extent of penetration of certain dies. This microleakage is due to polymerization shrinkage, dissimilarity in COTE and the ineffectiveness of bonding.

Amalgam Bonding

One of the main problems of silver amalgam restoration is its poor bonding and retention. Special cavity design with undercuts, pin-retention techniques, etc. have been tried.

As the resin bonding agents development progressed, new dentin bonding agents entered the field. The 4-META resin was found to have large bond strength with metal alloys and silver amalgam. Almost similar methods, like conditioning, acid etching, application of adhesive, etc. are followed, and **amalgam mix is immediately condensed by** usual procedure. However, the amalgam bonding with 4-META resin is found to be mostly **mechanical retention** and not chemical.

Glass Ionomer Cements

The polyacrylic or polyalkenoate system forms chemical bonding with Ca^{++} ions of enamel and also collagen of dentin. This is used to bond composite resins to the tooth structure by sandwich technique refer GIC or using its resin modified form—compomer.

MODEL QUESTIONS

I. Long Essay   (20 minutes)

1. Describe the problems of dentin-restoration bonding. Give an outline of the principles of bonding of the various generations of bonding agents.

II. Short Essays   (10 minutes each)

1. Enamel bonding
2. Problems of dentin bonding
3. Acid etching techniques
4. Total etch bonding technique
5. Fourth generation of dentin bonding agents
6. Measurement of dentin cement bond strengths
7. Dentin bonding principles

Direct Filling Gold

Gold, perhaps, has the longest history of more than 500 years, in the field of restorative dentistry as cavity filling materials. Even though in the modern dentistry, it is almost not used as such, **direct filling gold restoration is considered as a standard.**

Gold available in the purest form, four nines: 99.99% purity has the following **advantageous properties.**

- Excellent biocompatibility, corrosion resistance, and chemical inertness
- Highest ductility and malleability. It can be beaten into a very thin foil of submicron thickness
- Cold-welding (pressure welding)
- Undergoes high work hardening during compaction.

The disadvantageous properties are

- Inadequate mechanical properties for use in high-stress bearing areas
- Condensation perfection of attaining maximum density cannot be reached
- Requires very high clinical skill and a long time for filling
- High density (19.3 gm/cc) and high cost
- Poor bonding to the tooth and poor aesthetics
- High thermal and electrical conductivities

Varieties/types/classification of direct filling gold (Fig. 11.1)

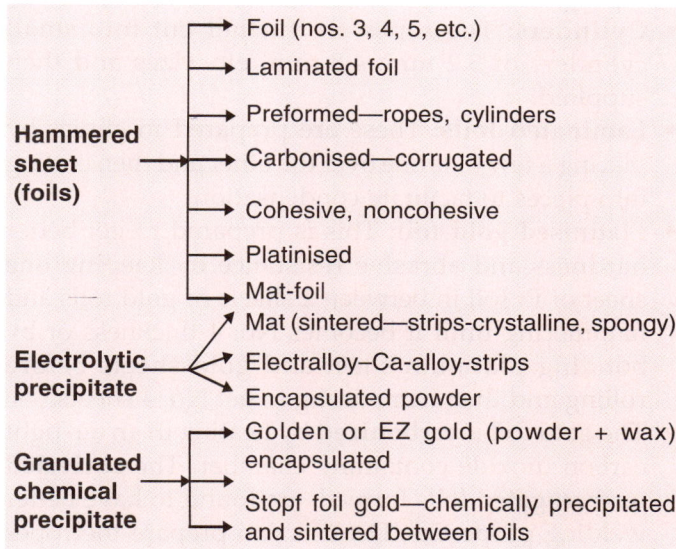

Fig. 11.1: Types and classification of direct filling gold (see Colour Plate 24, Fig. 11.1)

MANUFACTURING METHODS

1. Gold Foil (Fibrous Gold)

Very thin gold sheets are placed in-between some special papers or **chamois leather** as alternate layers, and subjected to continuous hammering (and sometimes intermittent annealing) until the extremely thin foil is obtained. It is then cut into small square pieces of 10 cm × 10 cm, treated in **ammonia gas** (noncohesive form), placed alternately in-between the sheets of a book and supplied to the dentist. The thickness of the gold foil is indirectly mentioned in certain numbers. For example, No. 3 gold foil weighs 3 grains (0.194 gm) and has a thickness = 0.38 microns, No. 4 gold foil weighs 4 grains (0.259 gm) and has thickness = 0.51 microns. Similarly, numbers 20, 40, 60, 90, etc. foils are also available.

Sub-types of gold foil
1. Sheet gold, cohesive and noncohesive
2. Ropes
3. Cylinders
4. Laminated foil
5. Platinised foil
6. Carbonized or corrugated foil
7. Mat-foil gold

- **Gold foil** is treated when with NH_3 gas to protect it from contaminations by other gases during storage. This is non-cohesive gold. NH_3 gas is driven out by heating, before use.
- **Ropes:** The 10 cm square pieces of No. 4 gold foil is cut into $^1/_4$, $^1/_8$, $^1/_{16}$, etc. small pieces and rolled into ropes mechanically.
- **Cylinders:** The ropes are further cut into small cylinders of 3.2 mm, 4.8 mm, etc. sizes and then supplied.
- **Laminated foils:** These are prepared in clinics by placing a few foils one over the other and then cutting into pieces to facilitate condensation.
- **Platinised gold foil:** This is prepared to get better hardness and abrasive resistance by keeping one sheet of Pt foil in between 2 sheets of gold foils and hammering until it becomes No. 4 thickness or by bonding platinum sheet and gold sheets before rolling and then hammering to get No. 4 sheets.
- The gold foil is **carbonized** by heating in an air-tight carbon dioxide containing chamber. The **shriveled or corrugated** foils formed, are found to have better welding properties. Dentists can prepare the ropes or cylinders from this.
- **Mat-foil gold** (refer electrolytic precipitate sub-types).

2. Electrolytic Precipitate: Subtypes (Fig. 11.2)
- Mat gold
- Mat-foil gold
- Electralloy
- **Mat gold (spongy, crystalline):** Microcrystalline gold powder is obtained from electrolytic precipitation on

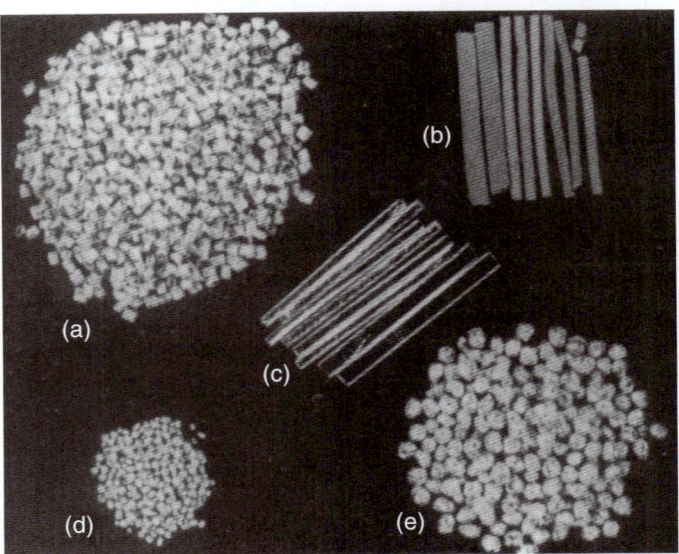

Fig. 11.2: Equal weights of (a) machine rolled cylinders, (b) mat gold, (c) electralloy RV, (d) EZ gold, (e) hand rolled pallets

the cathode gold plate surface. These dendritic structured crystal powder is heated to a temperature well below the melting temperature (1063°C) of pure gold for some time **(sintering)** and then formed into strips of about 3–6 mm width and 15 mm long. This sintering makes the crystals coalesce and grow together. This mat gold is sometimes called **spongy crystalline gold.**

- **Mat-foil gold:** The electrolytic precipitate powder is sandwiched, between No. 3 gold foils sintered and cut into strips. This variety is preferred by dentists for building up internal bulk, as compaction can be done more efficiently in a shorter time. But more voids are left out between the particles, after condensation.
- **Electralloy–calcium alloyed gold:** By using the anode plate of gold with 0.1% calcium, the calcium alloy electrolytic precipitate powder is obtained. This is sandwiched in-between the gold foils and sintered at high temperature (heating; maintaining at, well below the MP of gold when the crystals grow and coalesce). It is then formed into thin strips. This mat-foil electralloy has higher hardness.

3. Granulated Powdered Gold
- **EZ gold:** The chemically precipitated gold powder and atomized gold powder are first mixed with soft wax and made into small **pellets or cylinders** of different sizes (Fig. 11.3) **1–2 mm**, and then wrapped in No. 3, gold foil. The wax is removed by heating before using. The powder or atomized particles size should be less than 75 microns with an average 15 microns.

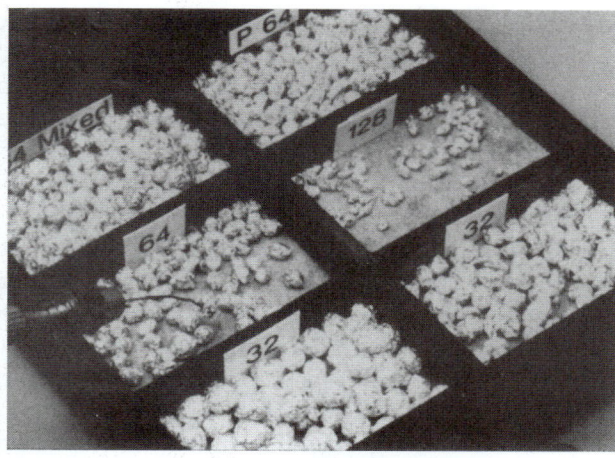

Fig. 11.3: Gold foil pellets of different sizes

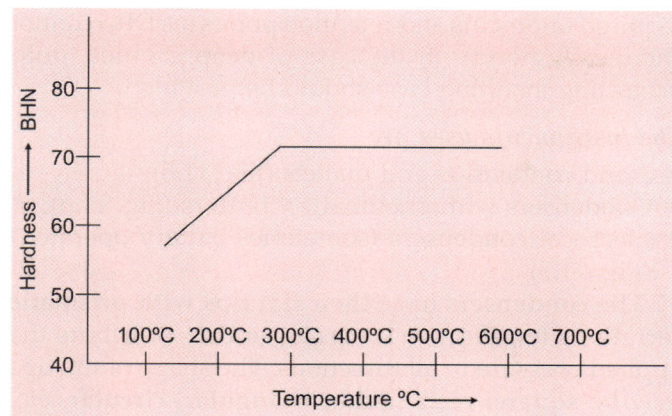

Fig. 11.4: BHN of condensed DFG foil, against desorption heat treatment temperatures

- **Stopf foil gold** is prepared by keeping chemically precipitated gold powder, in-between gold foils and then sintering into strips and pieces for use.

Manipulation of DFG: Clinical Procedures

Clinical indications for DFG restorations

To be used for small restorations at the **nonstress or small stress bearing areas** such as:

- Small occlusal grooves
- Buccal and lingual pits
- Small proximal lesions in the premolars
- Gingival erosions
- Small carious gingival lesions

Removal of Surface Impurities (Desorption Heat Treatment)

Cohesive and noncohesive gold

Cold welding takes place perfectly only if the surface of DFG-foil has a clean surface without any adsorbed gases impurities. Pure gold tends to adsorb moisture and gases like O_2, N_2, H_2, etc. These impurities cannot be easily removed unless heating to very high temperature near the melting point when DFG will get damaged. There is every chance, the stored DFG, foils, etc. can adsorb these impurities. Hence, the manufacturer treats the DFG with **ammonia** gas before supplying. This protects the gold surface from other contaminations. This noncohesive (**NH_3 gas treated**) DFG is supplied to the dentist.

Desorption heat treatment (formerly, wrongly, termed annealing and degassing)

If the DFG is heated NH_3 gas goes out, the welding becomes better and the hardness of compacted gold increases. The hardness becomes maximum when desorption is complete. For this, the temperature is to be raised **above 350°C** as shown in Fig. 11.4.

1. **Heating piece by piece:** It is one method of desorption heat treatments using well adjusted reducing blue flame of pure alcohol. The individual DFG pieces are carried by piercing through pointed instruments piece by piece and passed over the flame carefully and then compacting into the cavity immediately. The advantages are:
   - Selection of individual pieces
   - Control of time and temperature
   - Less contamination, during the interval of desorption and compaction.

2. **Heating bulk in a tray** by a gas flame or electric furnaces. The required type and amounts of DFG is taken in a ceramic tray and heated for a few seconds. This method appears to be more convenient to the clinician, but have many disadvantages:
   - The difficulty of selection of a particular type
   - Less control over the time and temperature
   - DFG pieces may join together if come into contact
   - As the compaction is to be slightly delayed for the bulk, further adsorption—surface contamination occurs in the interval which results in poor welding.

Precautions

- **Temperature** range should be between 350 and 700°C. It should become just red hot if directly heated.
- **Source:** Pure alcohol reducing pale blue region of the flame should be used.
- **Time** of heating should be properly controlled.
- **The only required amount** should be taken in the tray.

Compaction of DFG

This is the procedure of filling the prepared tooth cavity by cold-welding DFG. The cavity is first designed with required undercuts and retention points (as DFG cannot chemically bond). In the case of deep cavities, pulp protecting insulting base should be provided.

The instruments used are
- Hand condensers and mallets (Fig. 11.5).
- Condensers with pneumatic vibrators (Fig. 11.6).
- Electrical condensers (sometimes battery operated) (Fig. 11.7).

The condensers have their flat tips with prismatic serrations for effective swagging and to distribute the applied pressure in all directions. The shape of the tips may be **square, rectangular, triangular, circular**, etc. The instruments may be **straight, contra-angled or curved**. Size of the tips is about **1 to 3 mm** depending on the size of the cavity. Too thin tips can pierce and damage the restoration, whereas too large tips cannot be effective in producing sufficient pressure (i.e. force/area) (Fig. 11.8).

Brief procedure
- **Hand condensing**
  The gold foil is cut into small pieces of the required size, passed through the pure alcohol flame for degassing and then swagged by hand condenser on the cavity floor, without air trapping. Another piece is degassed similarly, placed on the previous swagged foil or stepped and hand condensed, by hammering, **point by point in a sweeping manner**. This is known as **'wedging'**. The entire portion is welded like this without **bridging to avoid air-trapping porosity** or voids. Similarly, the gold foils are **stepped** one over the other with the same precautions. The bulky portion filling is usually done using mat gold or powdered gold capsules pellets (after dewaxing). When the filling is almost complete, the top surface is again stepped, by condensing platinized or mat-foil golds to get better mechanical properties. Finishing is done by burnishing and using polishing agents like french chalk, pumice or rouge.

- **Mechanical/electrical condensers**
  To speed up the condensing procedure, pneumatic vibrators and battery operated condensers are used. The condensers are fitted to the vibrator—a hand piece-like instrument. As the condenser vibrates it hammers and welds. Studies have shown, there are no much improvements in the properties of mechanically compacted restorations (Colour Plate 24, Fig. 11.2).

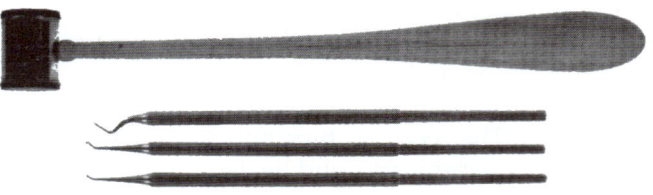

Fig. 11.5: Hand condensing mallet and condensers

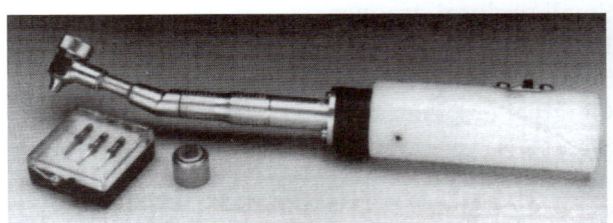

Fig. 11.6: Battery-operated condenser

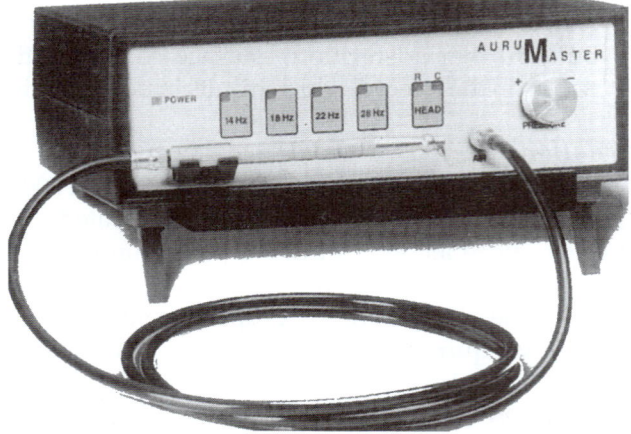

Fig. 11.7: Pneumatic condenser for gold foil condensation

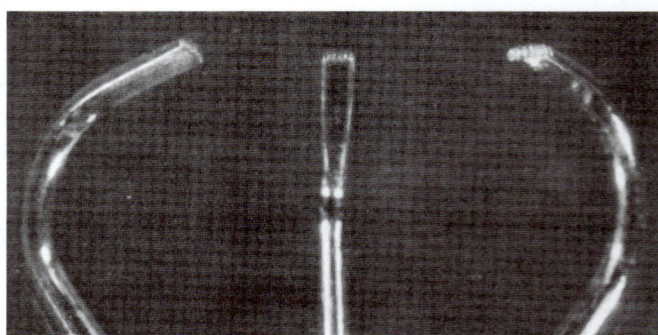

Fig. 11.8: Hand condensers with convex serrated faces

Table 11.1	Properties of direct filling gold			
Materials	Condensation techniques	Apparent density gm/cc	Surface hardness KHN (kg/mm^2)	Transverse strength, MPa
Gold foil	Hand	15.9	69	296
	Mechanical	15.8	69	265
	Combined	15.8	69	273
Mat-foil	Hand	15.0	70	96
	Mechanical	15.1	71	206
	Combined	15.1	75	227
Mat	Hand	14.3	52	161
	Mechanical	14.7	62	169
	Combined	14.5	53	169
Powdered	Hand	14.4	55	165
	Mechanical	14.5	64	155
	Combined	14.9	58	190

Properties of DFG Restoration (Table 11.1)

1. **Density:** Whatever, precautions and clinical skills are used during condensation, it is possible to achieve maximum density of only 14.00 to 16.00 gm/cc which is far below the real density of pure gold, 19.2 gm/cc. This shows still **large amounts air-voids** or porosities are left behind. These act as centers of stress concentrations, gradually distort and finally cause marginal leakage, caries and failure. The foil type DFG gives maximum density.

2. **Hardness mechanical properties:** As the compaction is continued, work hardening, causes an increase of hardness from about 24 KHN up to about 70 or 75 KHN which correspond to foil type and mat-foil or platinized DFG.

3. **Transverse strength:** Due to work hardening the transverse strength also increases to about **150–290 MPa**.

Approximate Properties of DFG

These mechanical properties are quite low and inadequate for the use of DFG in high stress-bearing areas. Hence, this is indicated only for low stress-bearing areas, of small sizes like class **I, III and V,** cavities, buccal and lingual pits, gingival erosions, etc.

It is said that DFG is a standard best material for restoration, if it is manipulated perfectly. Otherwise it becomes the worst restoration due to marginal seepage and failures. The expected skill is not possible to attain, **as the procedure is very technique-sensitive and time-consuming.** Since better stronger aesthetic materials like composite resins, GIC, metal ceramic, castable ceramics, etc. are nowadays available, the DFG restorations are very rarely used.

MODEL QUESTIONS

I. Long Essay   (20 minutes)

1. Classify the varieties of direct filling golds, Explain the compaction of direct filling gold. Give its merits and demerits.

II. Short Essays   (10 minutes each)

1. Types of direct filling gold
2. Gold foil
3. Desorption heat treatment
4. Direct filling gold compaction

III. Brief Answers   (5 minutes each)

1. Mat (spongy) gold
2. Mat-foil gold
3. Platinised gold foil
4. Powdered gold
5. Direct filling gold condensers
6. Properties of direct filling gold and its restorations.

Silver Amalgam

Amalgam is an alloy of any metal with **mercury.** Dental amalgam, as it is popularly known, is made by alloying pure mercury by mixing or triturating it with powder of an alloy of **silver-tin-copper.** On mixing, the metal components of the alloy powder dissolve in mercury and react to form a thick paste or plastic mass. This is **carried** into the prepared tooth cavities and **condensed** by applying pressure. The different metallographic phases produced, Ag_2-$Hg_3(\gamma_1)$, $Sn_{7-8}Hg$ (γ_2), $Cu_6Sn_5(\eta)$, gradually crystallize, binding the unreacted Ag_3Sn (γ), Cu_3Sn, or Ag_3Cu_2 (**ε**) phases to form a hard solid of composite structure.

GV Black had formulated this alloy, perhaps for the first time, in 1896. This, now known as, **low-copper** amalgam alloy, had, Ag = 65–68%, Sn = 27–29% and Cu = <6% by weight with a small amount of Zn. To overcome many drawbacks such as low one-hour strength, corrosion resistance, dimensional stabilities, etc. high copper amalgam alloys with copper 6–30% or 12–30% have been used since about 1970s. High strengths, adequate mechanical properties, and very simple direct filling methods have made this, a very popular permanent posterior restorative material in the last century. However, the considerations of toxicity and serious health hazards of mercury to the clinical personnel have made the researchers to try other metals like **gallium** instead of mercury. Modified visible light cure **Bowen's** hybrid composite resins have many desirable properties to replace the silver amalgam restorations.

SILVER–TIN SYSTEM (Fig. 12.1)

Silver and tin have densities 10.5 gm/cc and 7.3 gm/cc, and melting points 961°C and 232°C respectively. These can form substitutional solid solutions, Ag-Sn, beta (β) phase and intermetallic alloy Ag_3Sn, gamma (γ) phases, when the alloy contains 26–29% tin by weight. Alpha and delta phases (α, δ) also are formed at the extremities. During solidification, the β disordered solid solution formed in the liquid, when cooled below 724°C, begins to grow as dendritic crystals. For a critical composition of 26.8% tin, the tin atoms **go around** (peritectic) and form ordered intermetallic alloy known as gamma (γ) phase at 480°C. This **peritectic transformation** formula is represented as (*refer* to page 258, Chapter 17):

Liquid + disordered β phase $\xrightarrow{\text{Cooled below 480°C}}$ ordered γ phase

Depending on the rate of solidification, different proportions of γ phases are formed around β phase.

Figures 8.4a to g: Crown and bridge cementation steps

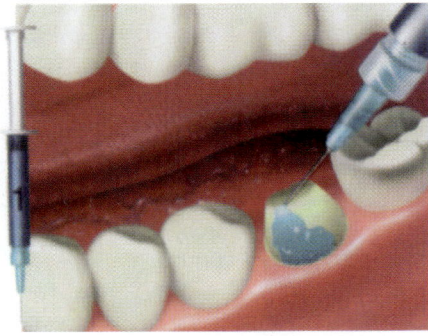

Fig. 8.4a: Application of etchant

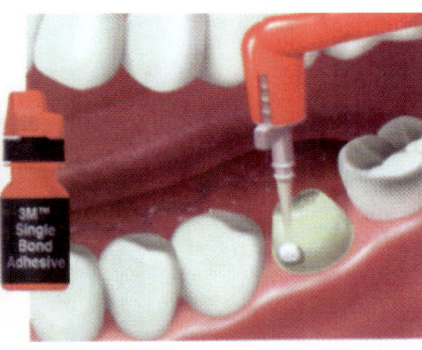

Fig. 8.4b: Application of adhesive

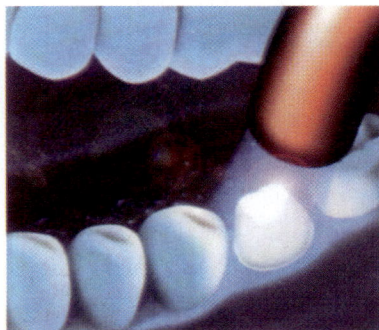

Fig. 8.4c: Curing with light

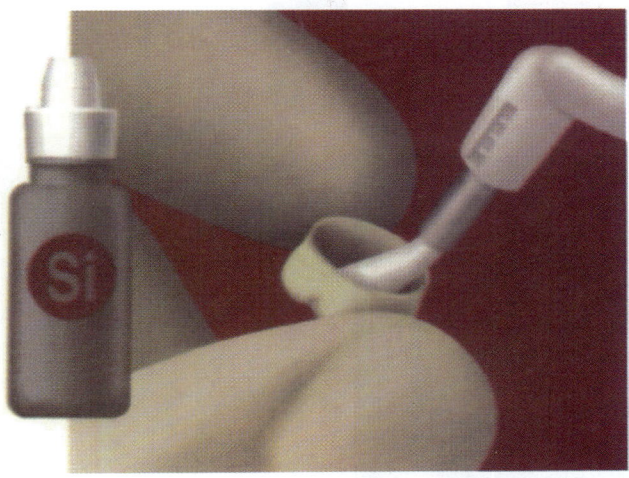

Fig. 8.4d: Preparing bonding surface, etching porcelain with ceramic primer

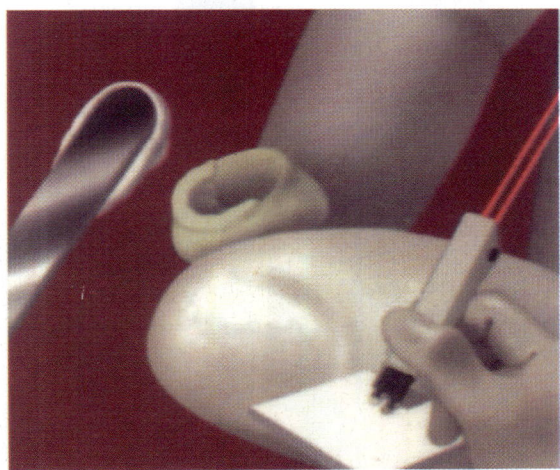

Fig. 8.4e: Mixing cement and applying thin layer

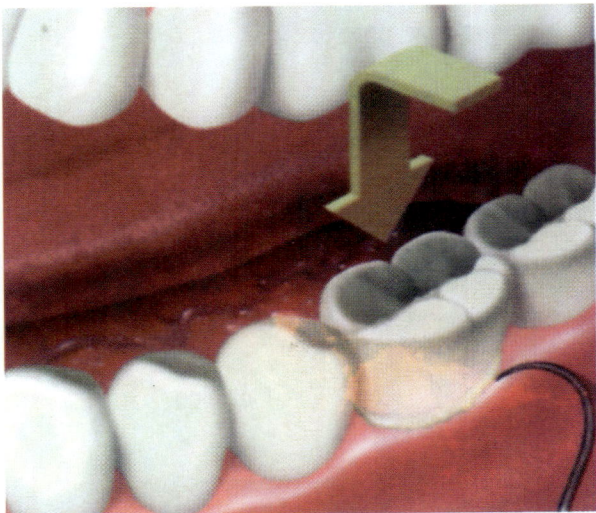

Fig. 8.4f: Seating restoration and removing excess

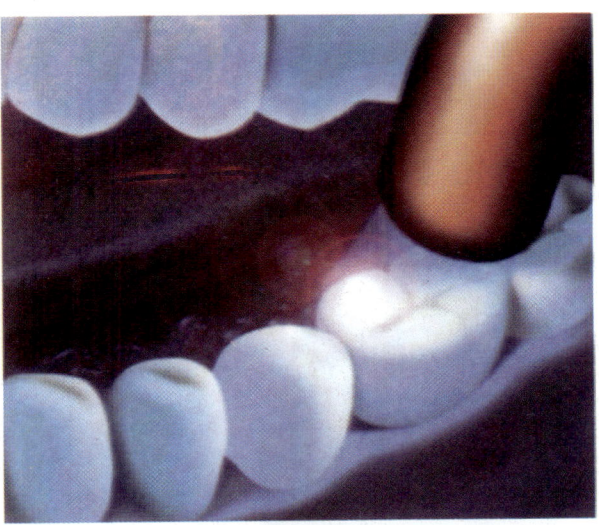

Fig. 8.4g: Light curing for 40 seconds or allowing to the self-cure

Figure 8.5: GIC restorative filling procedure cervical erosions, class III and class V

Figure 8.6: GIC core build up procedure class I and class II restorations or temporary repair

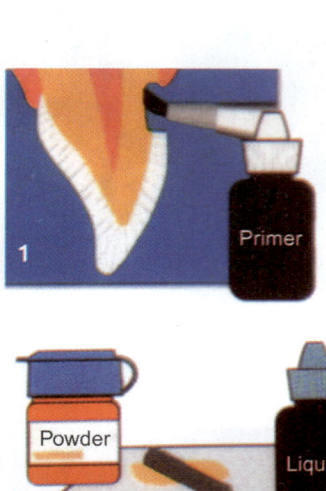

Apply primer and light cure

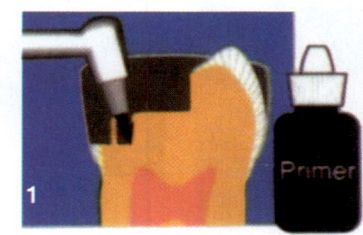

Apply primer, to enamel and dentin, pins and force, light curing

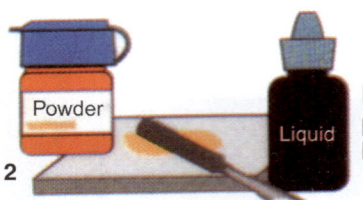

Mixing powder–liquid

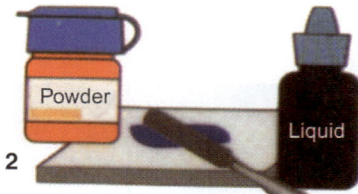

Mixing powder–liquid

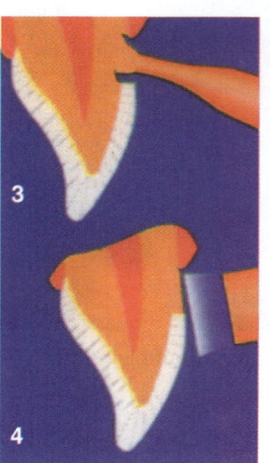

Placement of mix

Light curing

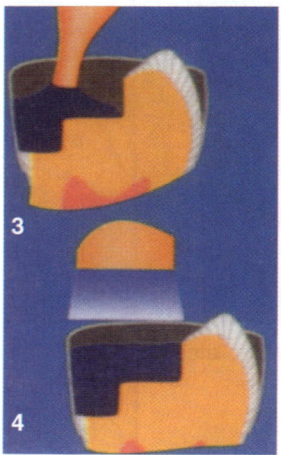

Placement in bulk, light cure, remove matrix

Light cure

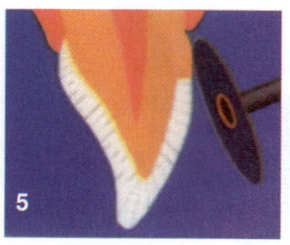

Finishing

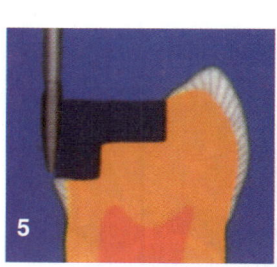

Preparing for crown

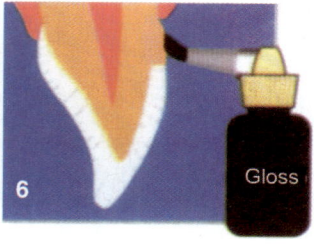

Gloss application and light curing

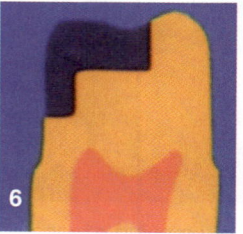

Finishing

Figures 8.7a to f: Cementation of metal-ceramics or precured composite inlays and onlays

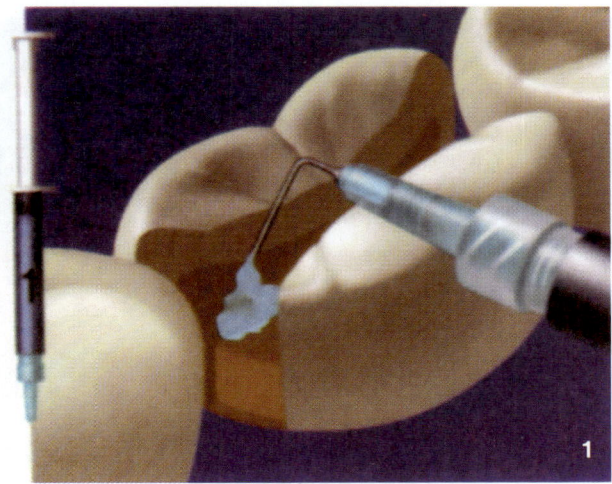

Fig. 8.7a: Apply scotch-bond etchant

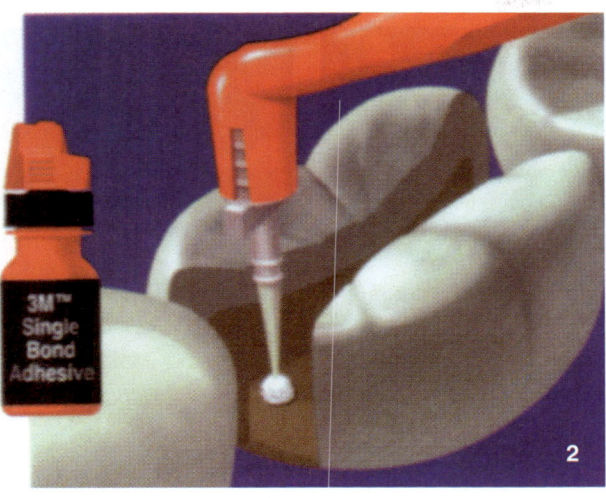

Fig. 8.7b: Apply single bond adhesive

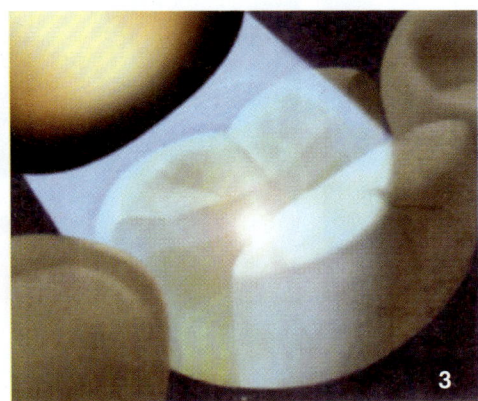

Fig. 8.7c: Light curing and roughening bonding surface

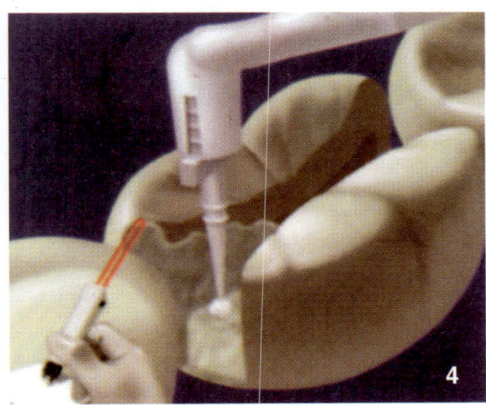

Fig. 8.7d: Apply cement mix

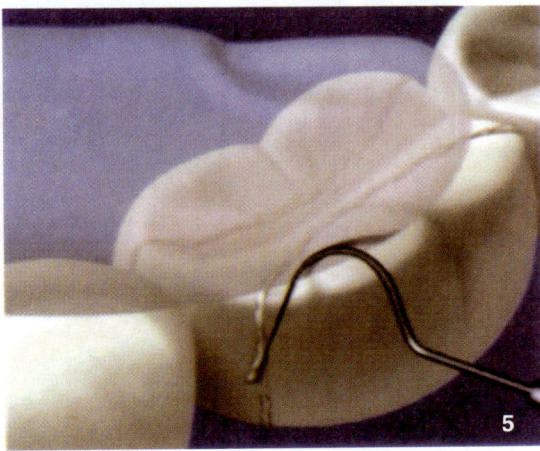

Fig. 8.7e: Seating inlay or onlay

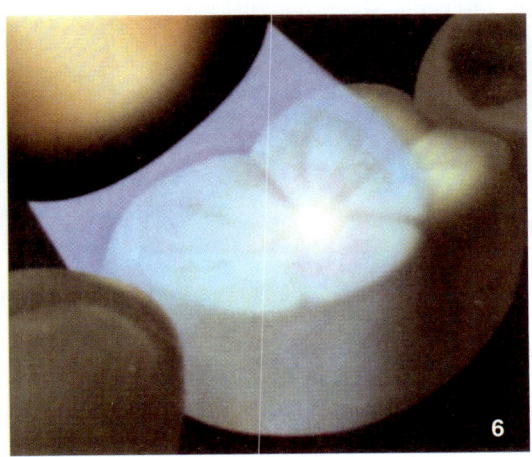

Fig. 8.7f: Final light curing of margins

Figure 8.8: Compomer restorations of primary molar class I or class II cavities

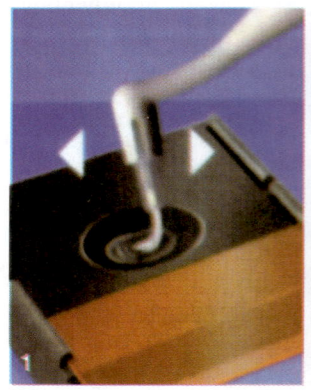
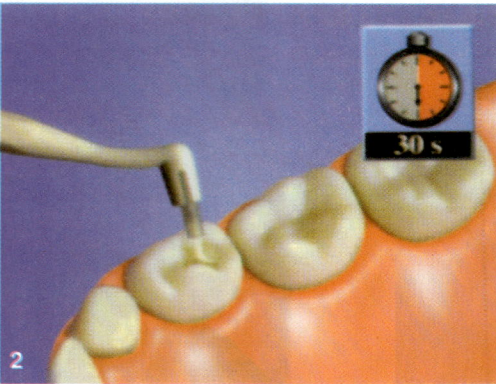
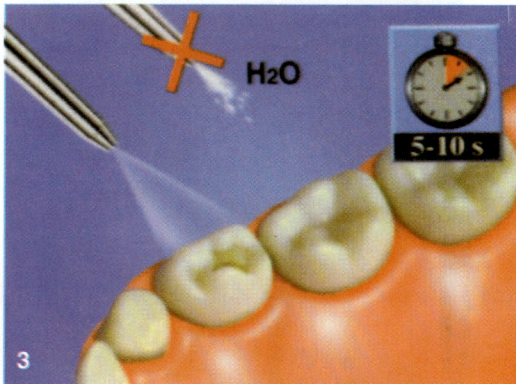

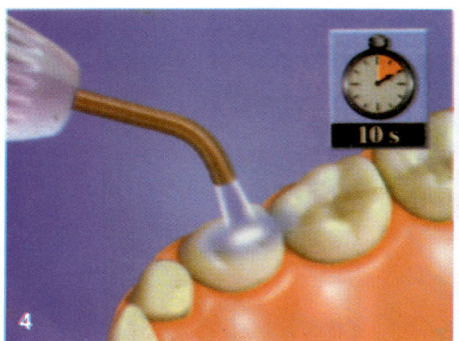
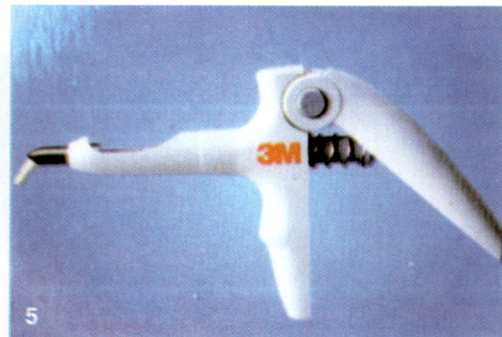
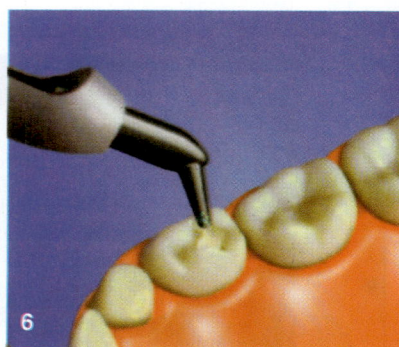

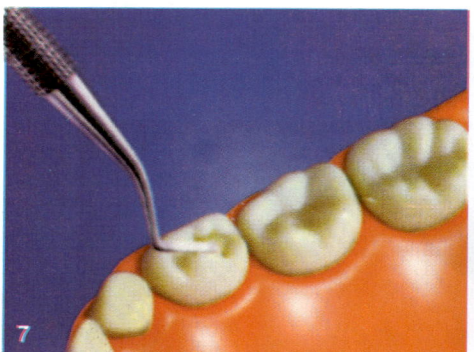
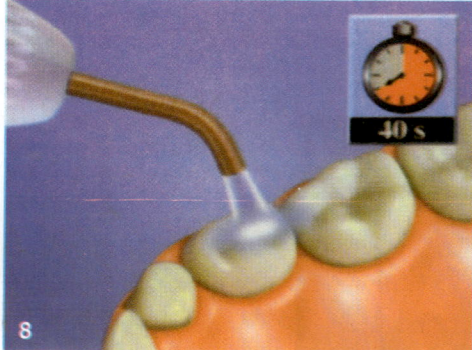
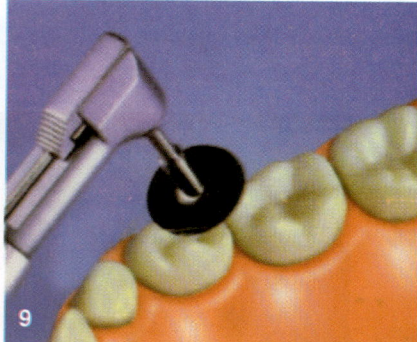

Fig. 8.8: Compomer restorations class I and II

Figure 8.9: Compomer restorations of class V

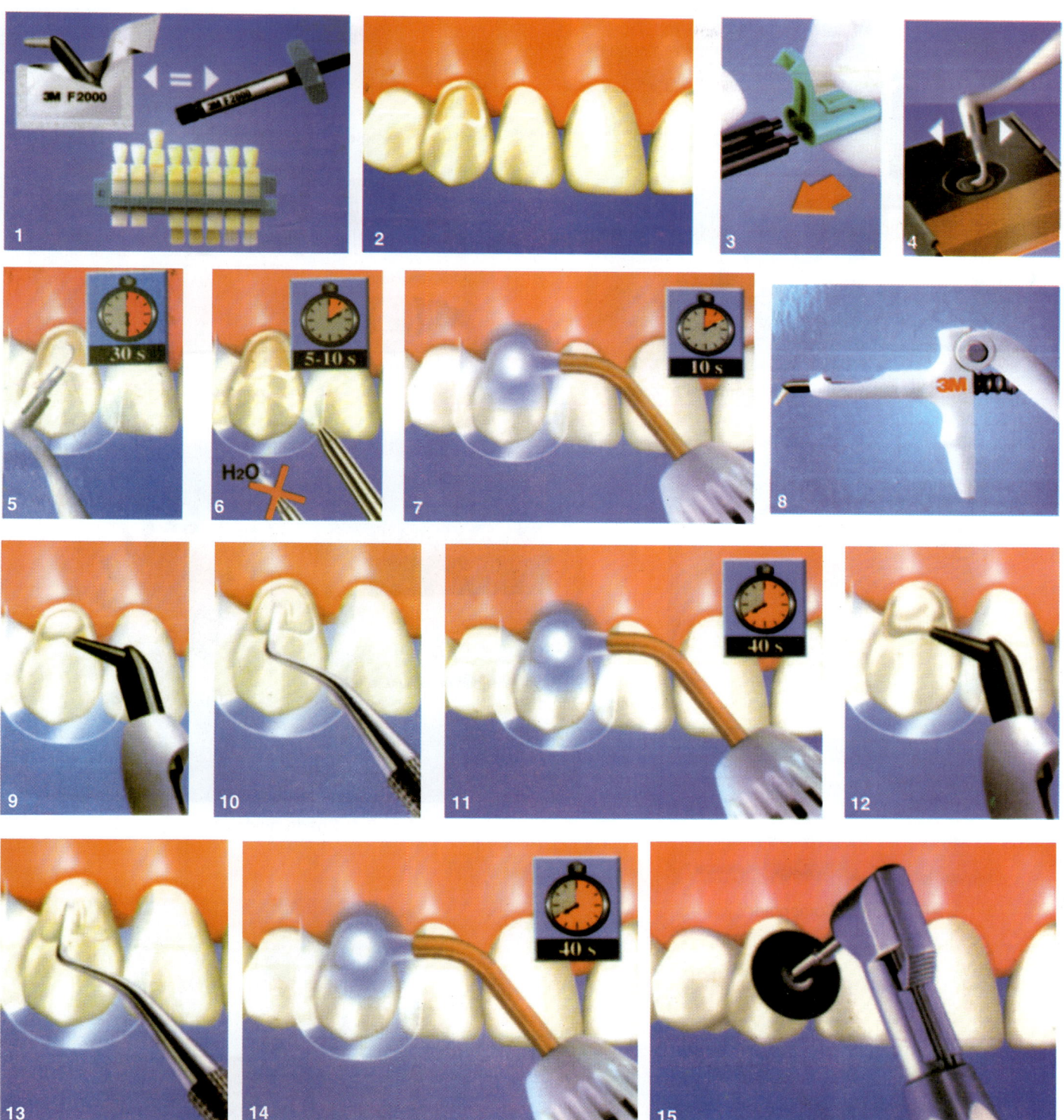

Fig. 8.9: Compomer restorations class V

CHAPTER 9: COMPOSITE RESTORATIVE RESINS

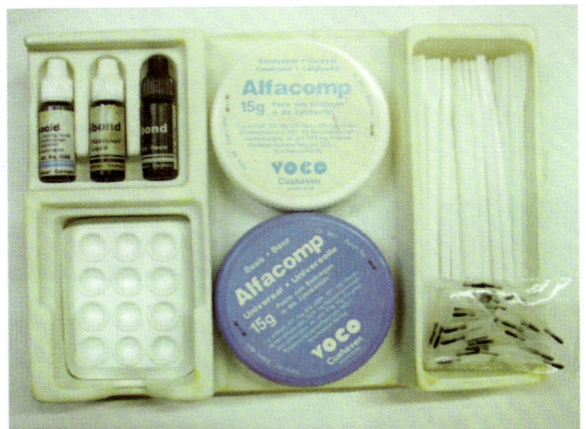

Fig. 9.1: Chemically cured composite resin

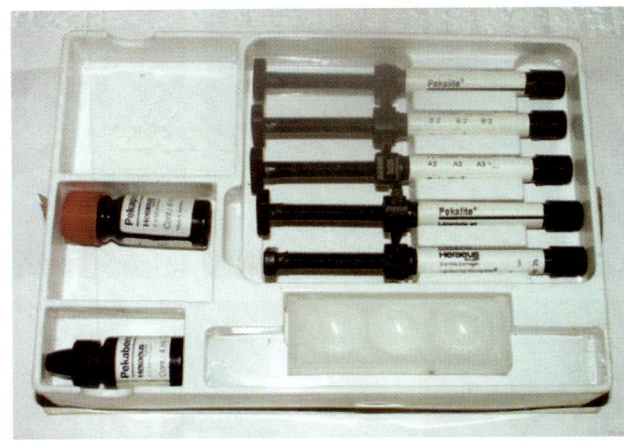

Fig. 9.2: VLC composite resin

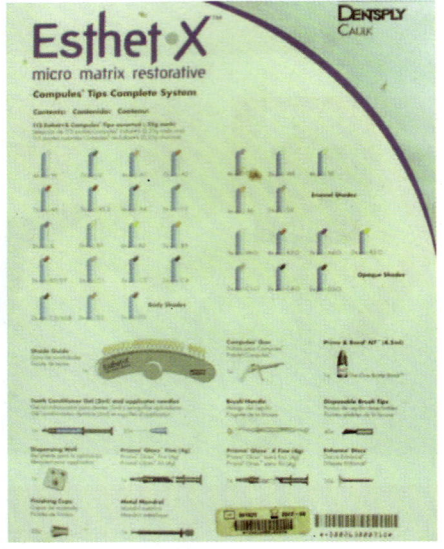

Fig. 9.3: Compomer

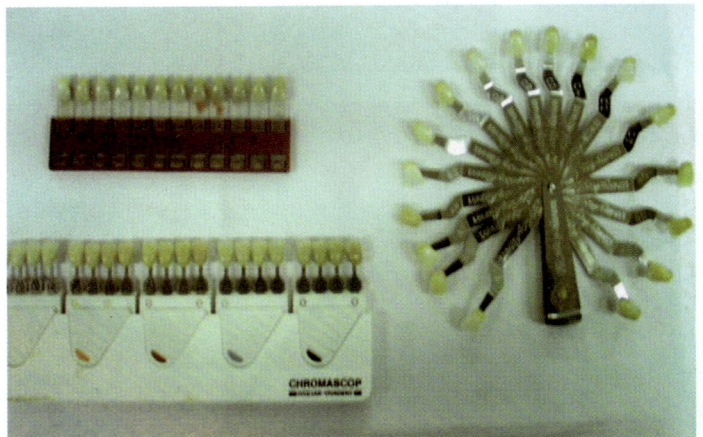

Fig. 9.4: Shade guides

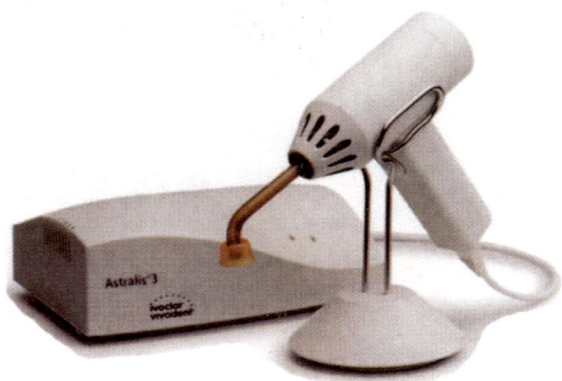

Fig. 9.5: Visible light curing unit

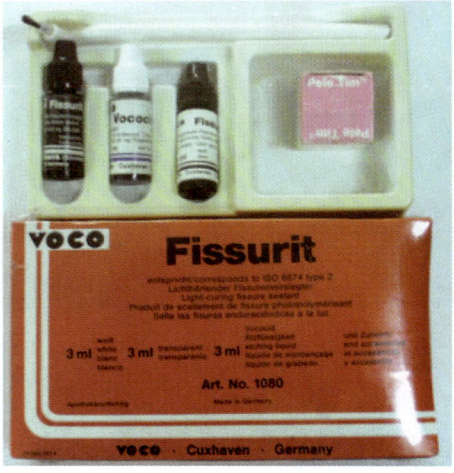

Fig. 9.6: Fissure sealant

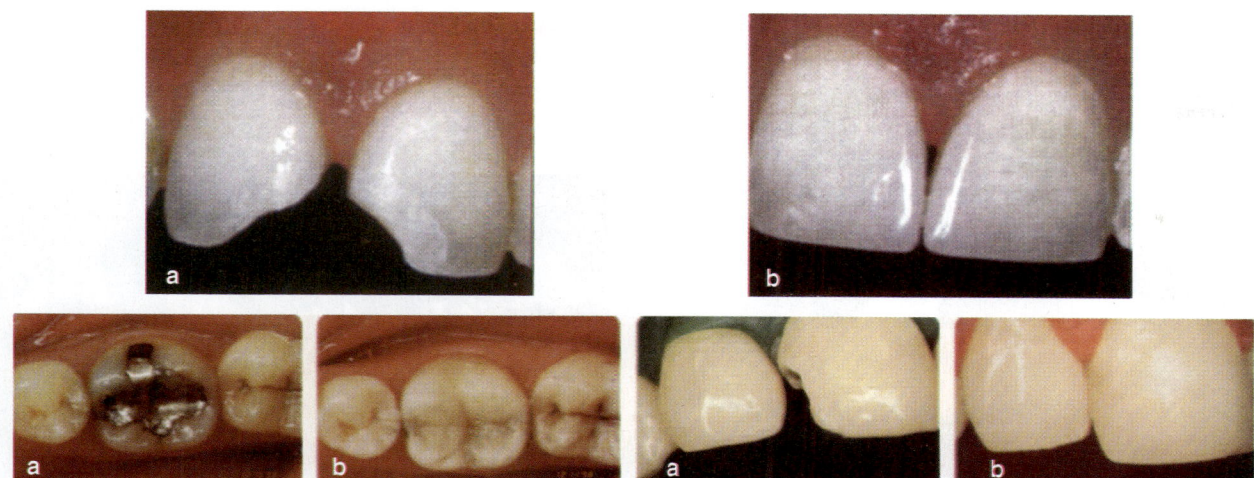

Fig. 9.7: Aesthetic composite restorations: (a) Before and (b) after

CHAPTER 10: BONDING OF RESTORATIONS

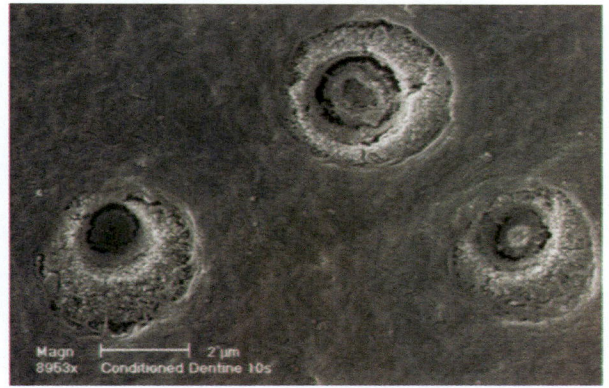

Fig. 10.1a: Conditioned dentin surfaces for ten seconds

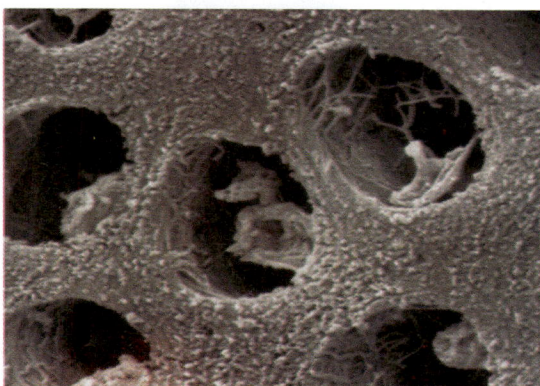

Fig. 10.1b: Dentin surface acid etched for 15 seconds (different magnification)

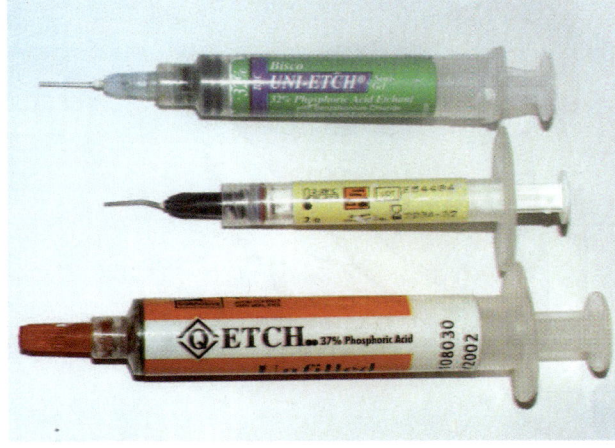

Fig. 10.2: Acid etching solution

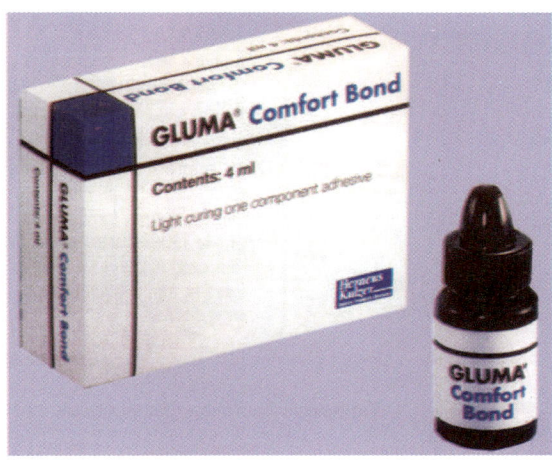

Fig. 10.3: Bonding agent

CHAPTER 11: DIRECT FILLING GOLD

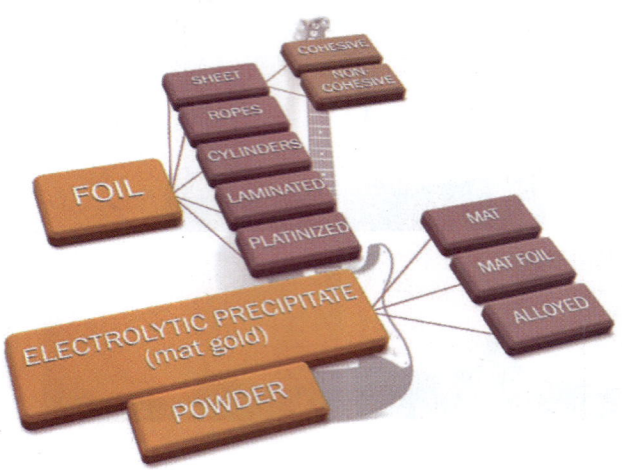

Fig. 11.1: Classification of direct filling gold

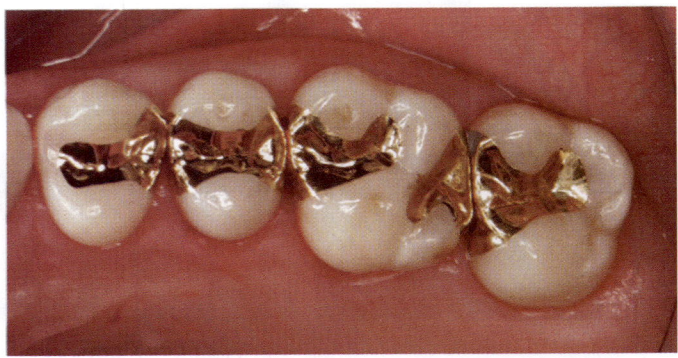

Fig. 11.2: Direct filling gold restorations

CHAPTER 13: DENTAL CERAMICS

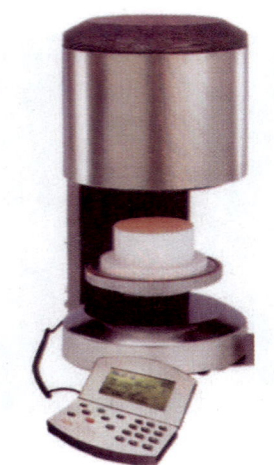

Fig. 13.1: Porcelain firing unit

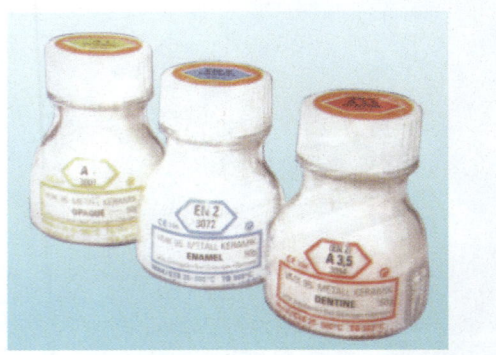

Figs 13.2a to c: Porcelain powder. (a) Opaque; (b) enamel; (c) dentin

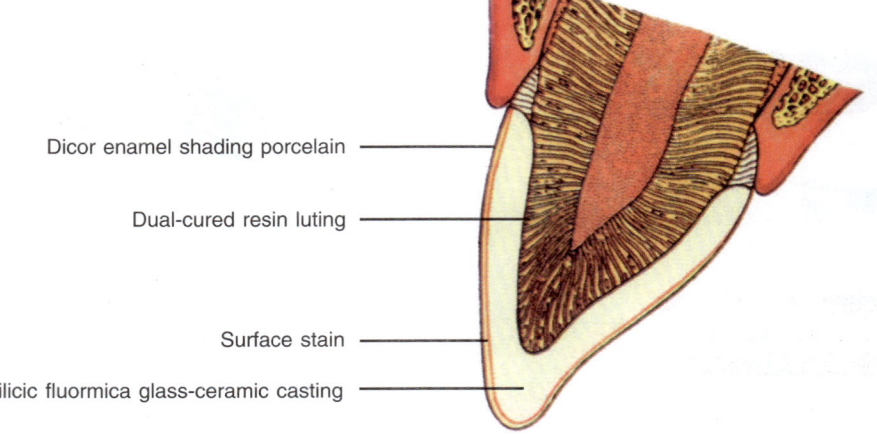

Dicor enamel shading porcelain

Dual-cured resin luting

Surface stain

Tetrasilicic fluormica glass-ceramic casting

Fig. 13.3: Cross-section of cemented dicor glass crown

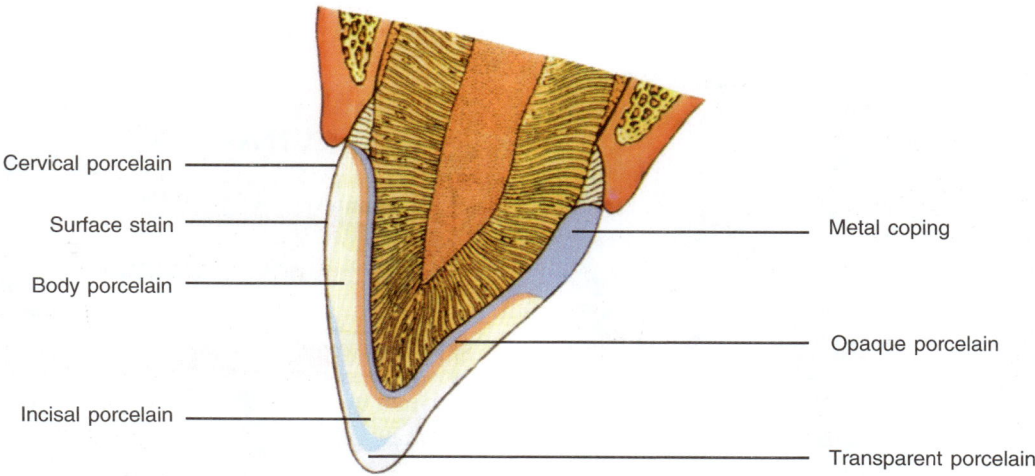

Cervical porcelain

Surface stain

Body porcelain

Incisal porcelain

Metal coping

Opaque porcelain

Transparent porcelain

Fig. 13.4: Cross-section of metal-ceramic crown

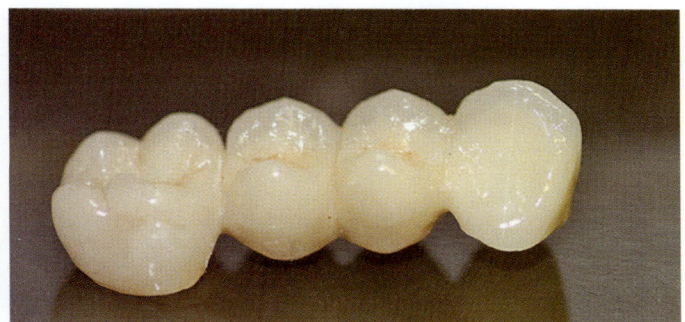

Fig. 13.5: Metal-ceramic bridge

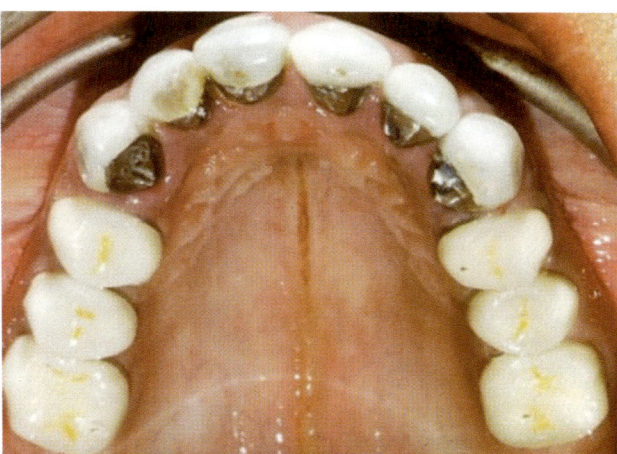

Fig. 13.6: Metal-ceramic restoration

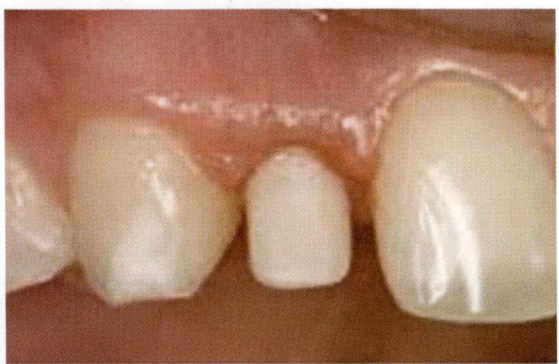

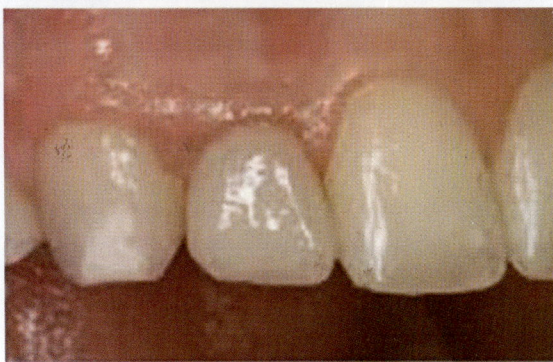

Fig. 13.7: All-ceramic crown before and after

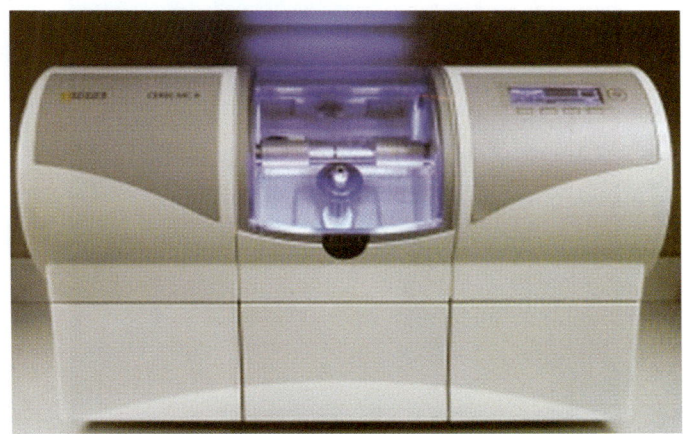

Fig. 13.8: CAD-CAM CERAC

CHAPTER 14: DENTAL WAXES (AUXILIARY MATERIALS)

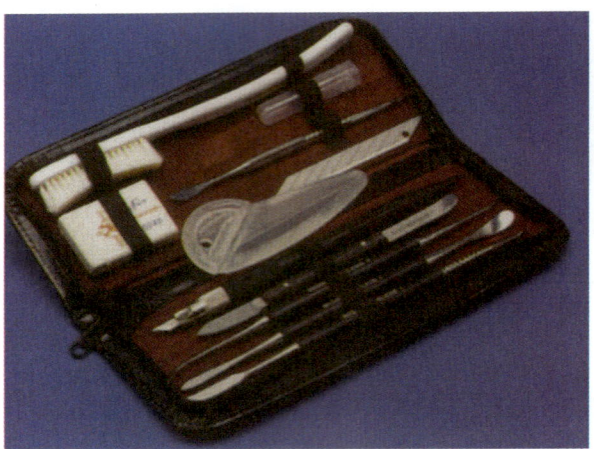

Fig. 14.1: Modelling wax instrument set

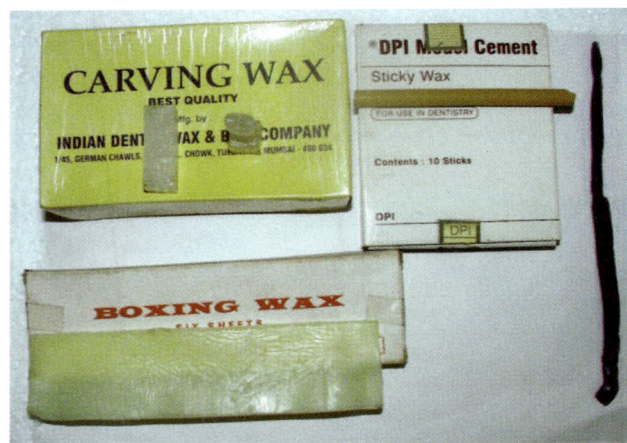

Fig. 14.2: Carving, boxing, beading waxes

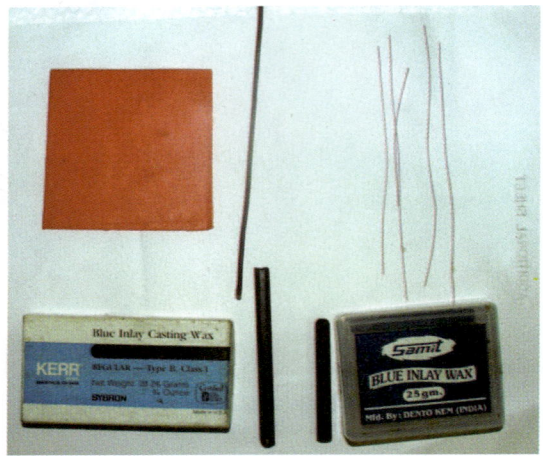

Fig. 14.3: Casting, sprue, inlay waxes

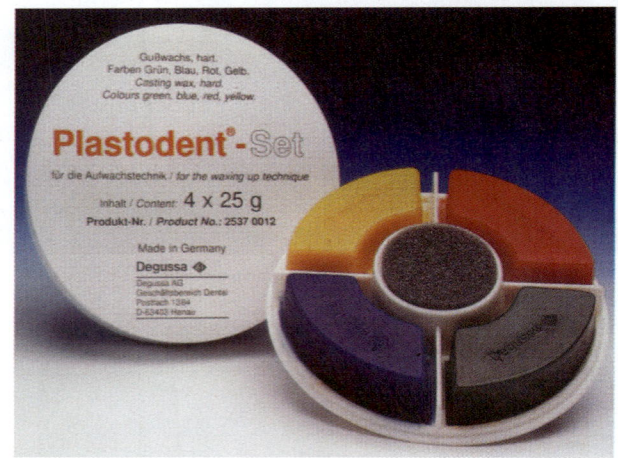

Fig. 14.4: Waxing technique wax

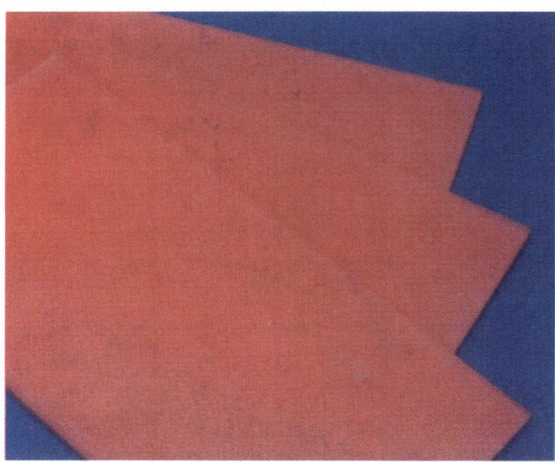

Fig. 14.5: Modelling wax

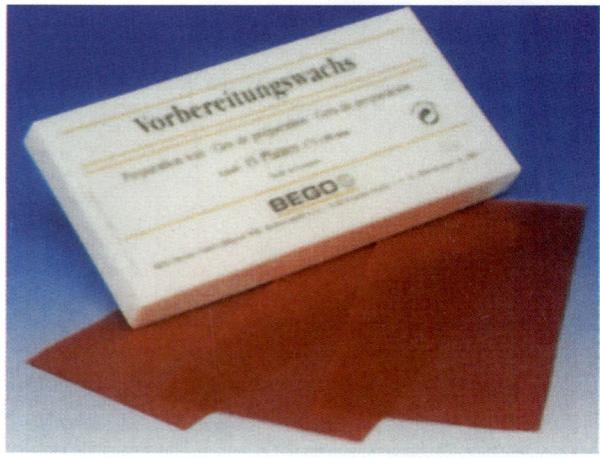

Fig. 14.6: Preparation wax for partial denture technique

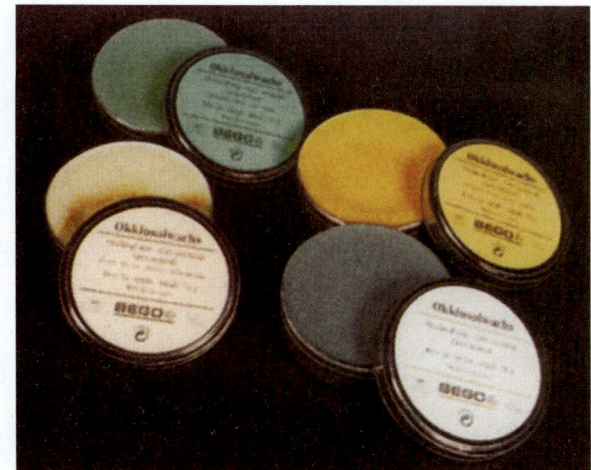

Fig. 14.7: Occlusal wax

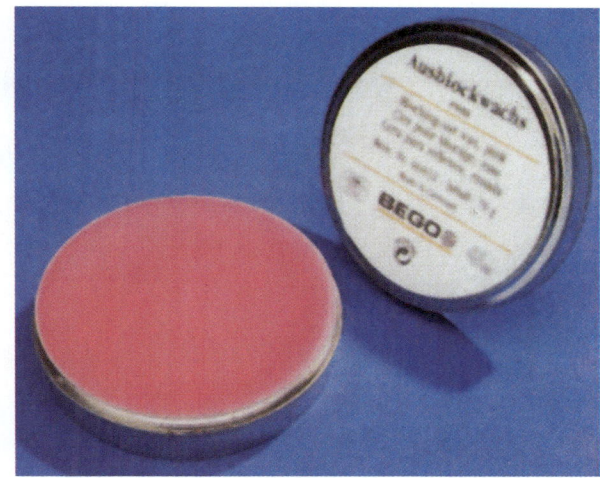

Fig. 14.8: Blocking-out wax

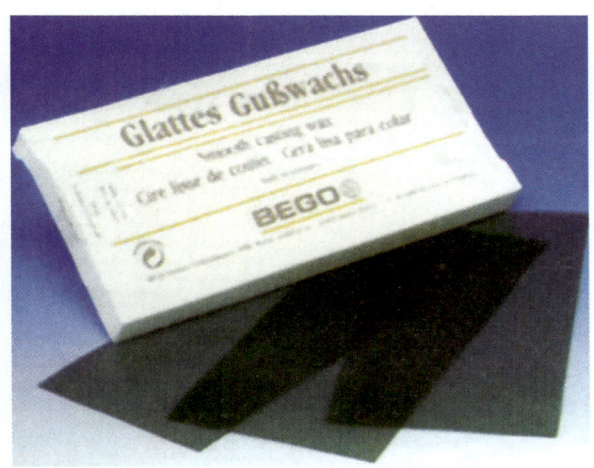

Fig. 14.9: Smooth casting wax

Fig. 14.10: Stippled casting wax

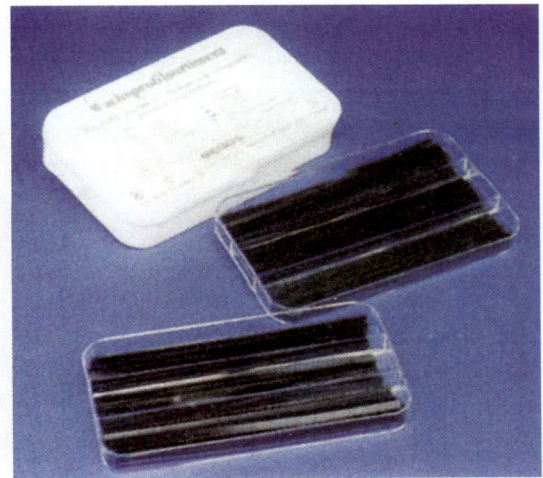

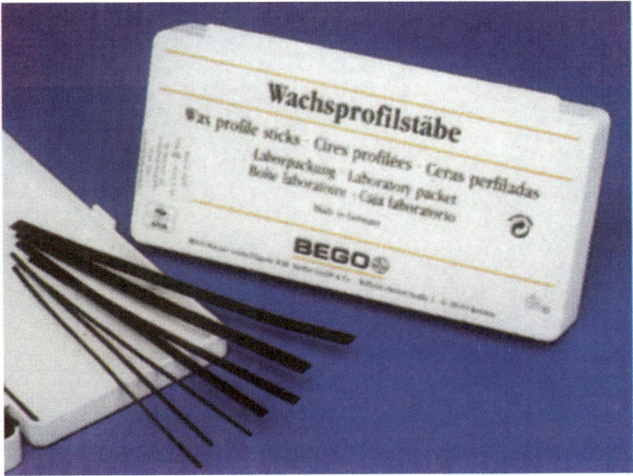

Fig. 14.11: Wax profiles assorted

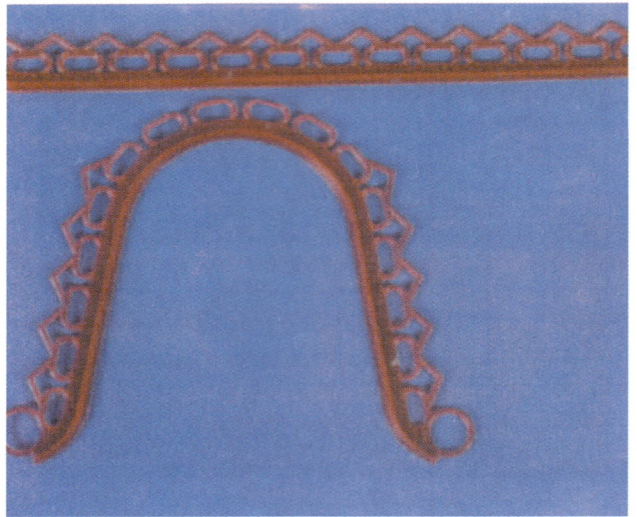

Fig. 14.12: Wax edge strips and border

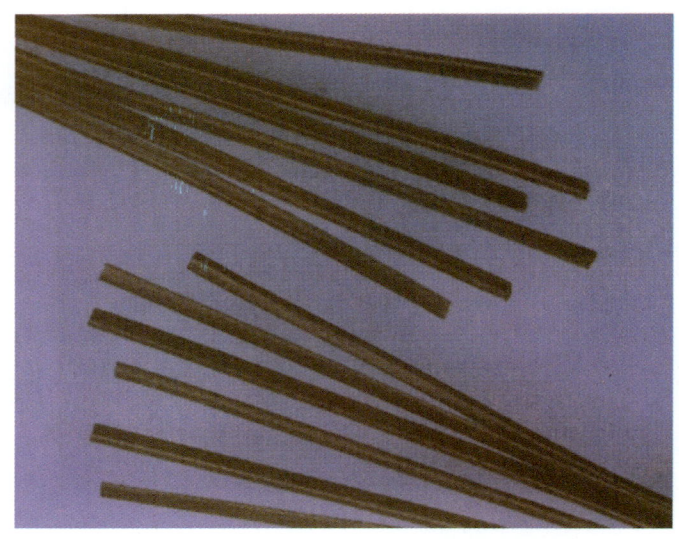

Fig. 14.13: Anatomical wax bars

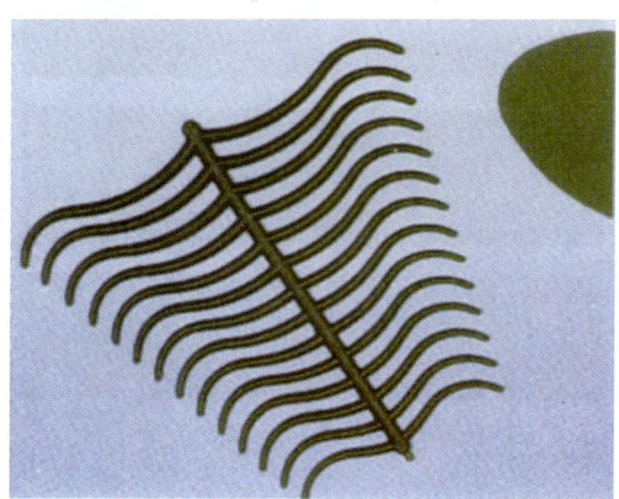

Fig. 14.14: Wax clasp

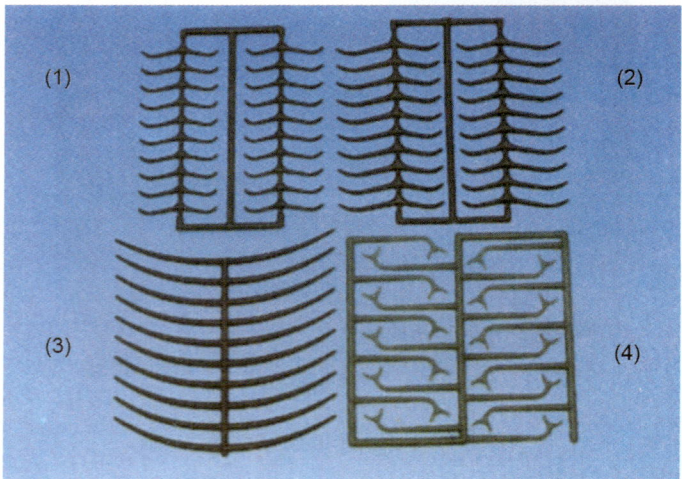

Fig. 14.15: Wax patterns for (1) premolar, (2) molars, (3) ring clasp, (4) bonyhard clasps

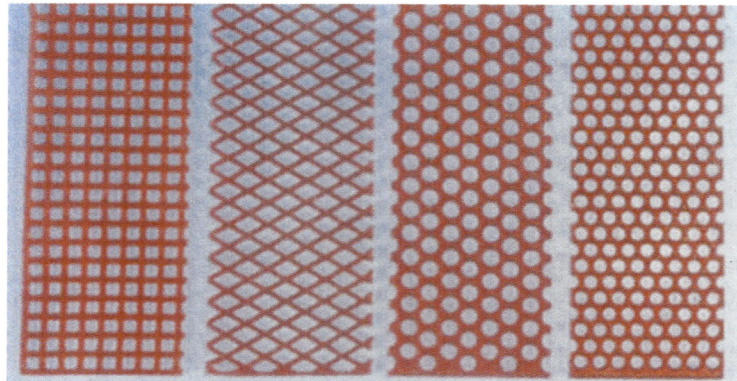

Fig. 14.16: Wax grid retentions

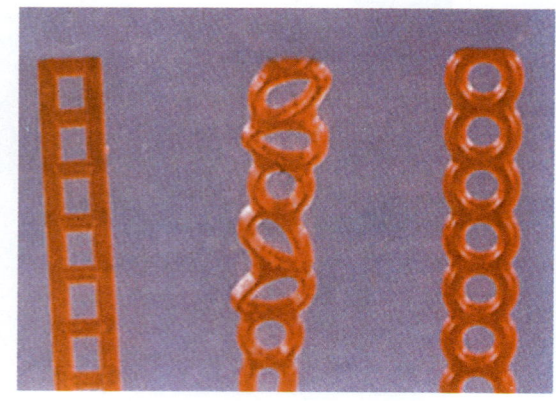

Fig. 14.17: Wax retentions

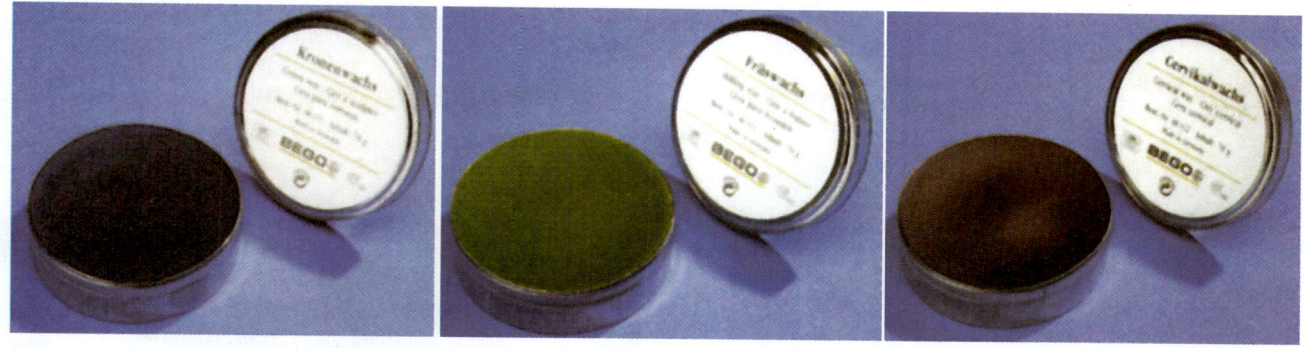

Fig. 14.18: Crown wax, milling wax and cervical wax

CHAPTER 15: CASTING INVESTMENT MATERIALS (AUXILIARY MATERIALS)

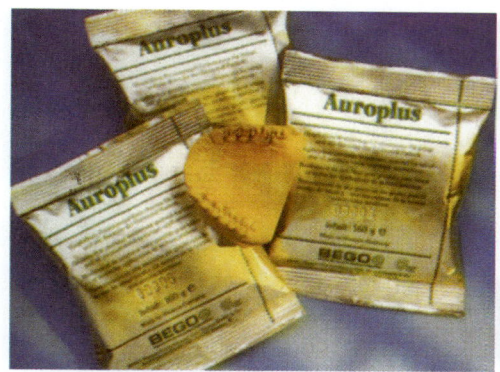

Fig. 15.1: Phosphate-bonded investment

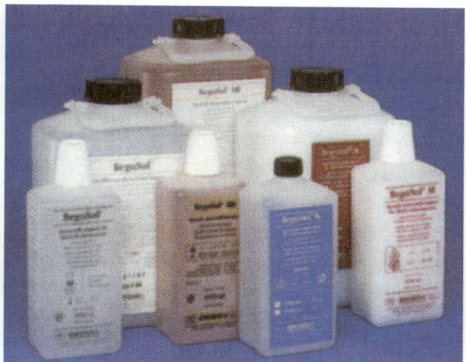

Fig. 15.2: Phosphate-bonded investment with colloidal silica liquid

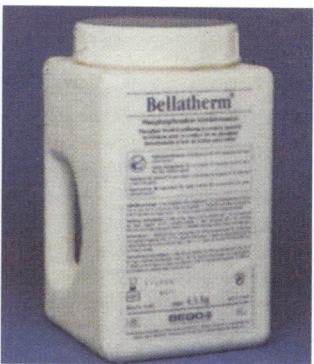

Fig. 15.3: Phosphate-bonded investment for soldering

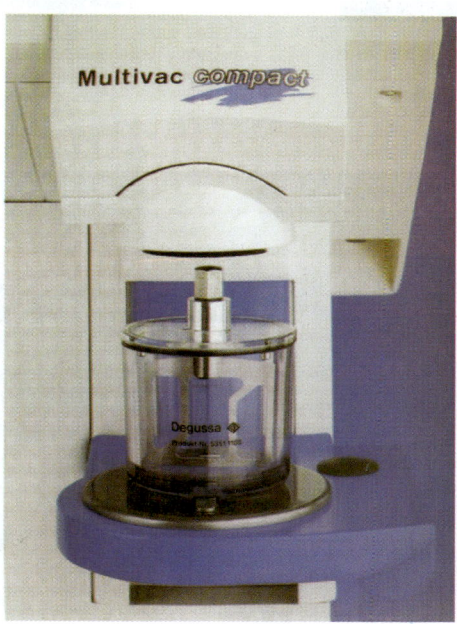

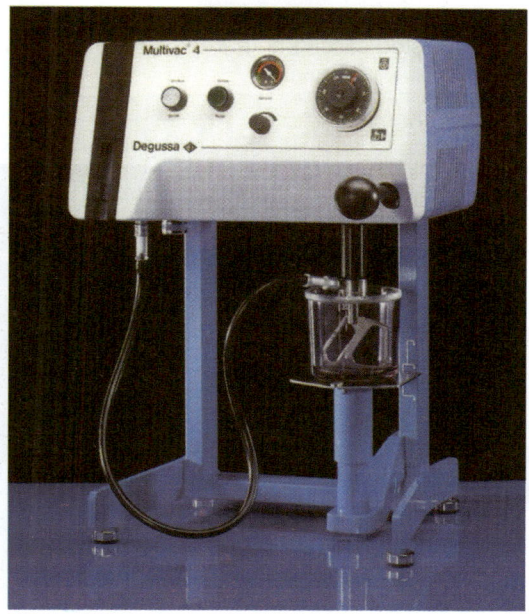

Fig. 15.4: Vacuum mixing, investing equipment with timers and speed controls

CHAPTER 19: OUTLINE OF DENTAL ALLOY CASTING PROCEDURES

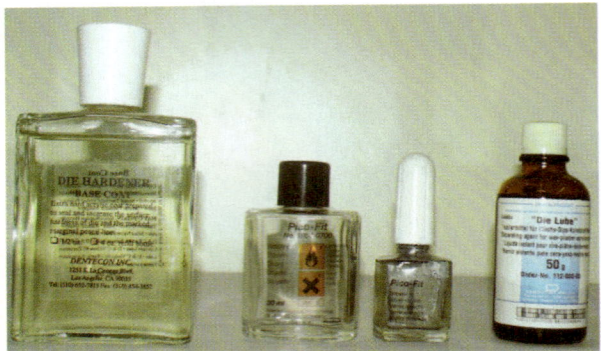

Fig. 19.1: Die-hardener, spacers, lubricant

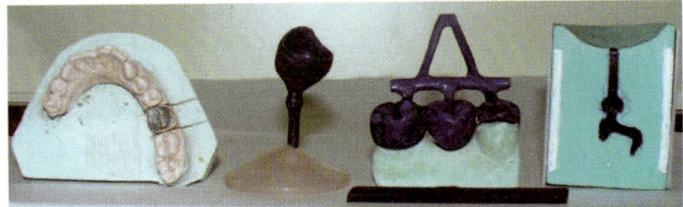

Fig. 19.2: Die, wax crown—direct spruing, crown and bridge, indirect spruing, cross-section of invested casting ring

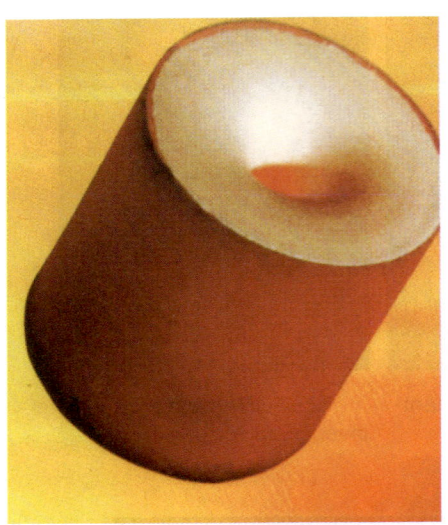

Fig. 19.3: Invested casting ring

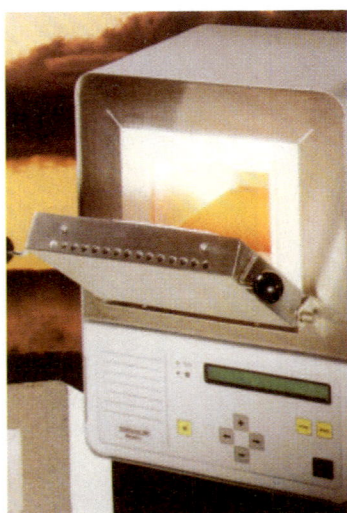

Fig. 19.4: Wax burn out furnace

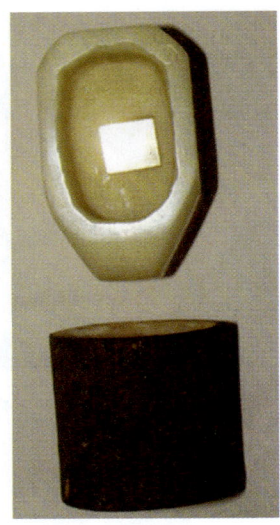

Fig. 19.5: Crucible, alloy pellet and casting ring

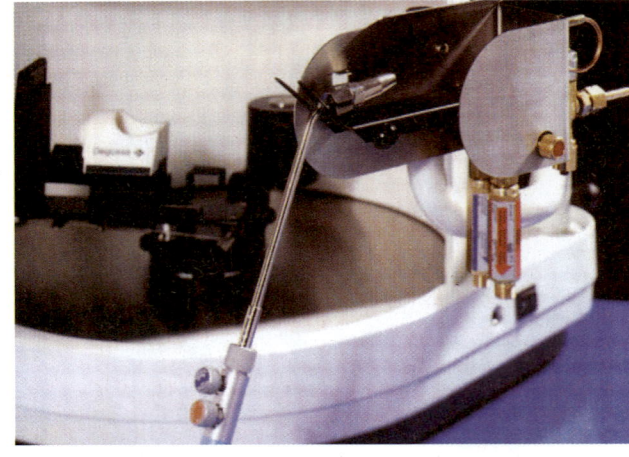

Fig. 19.6: Gas melting, motor driven centrifugal casting machine

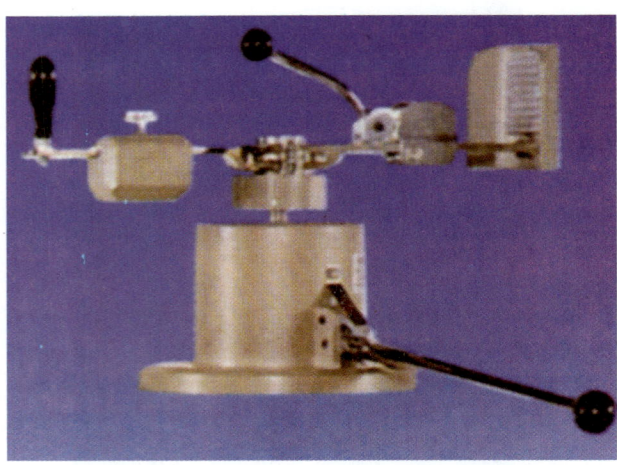

Fig. 19.7: Gas melting, spring wound centrifugal casting machine

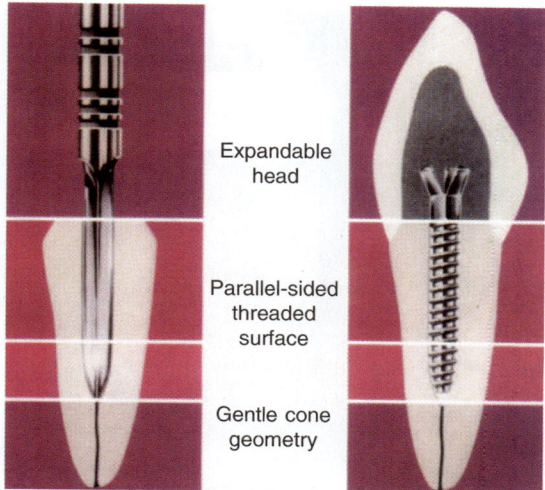

Expandable head

Parallel-sided threaded surface

Gentle cone geometry

Fig. 19.8: Post-core restoration

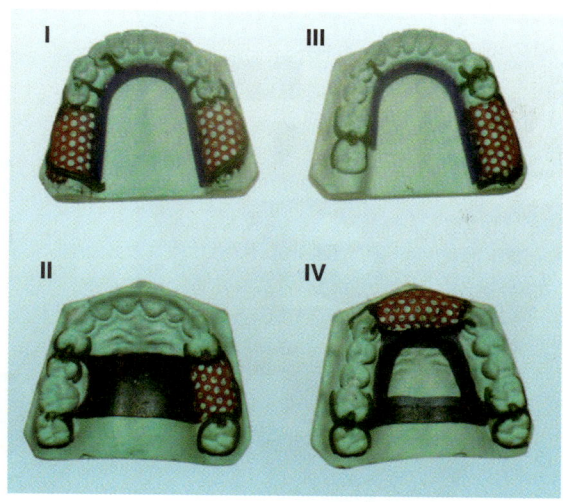

Fig. 19.9: RPD wax patterns classes I, II, III, IV

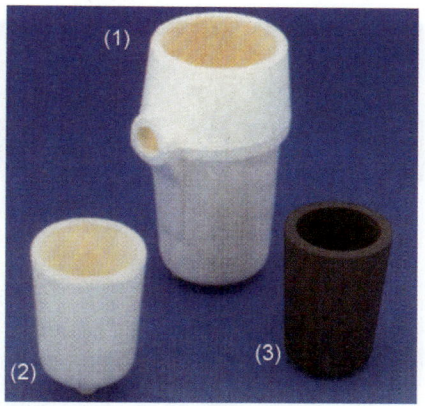

Fig. 19.10: Ceramic. (1) Crucible, (2) insert, (3) graphite crucible insert

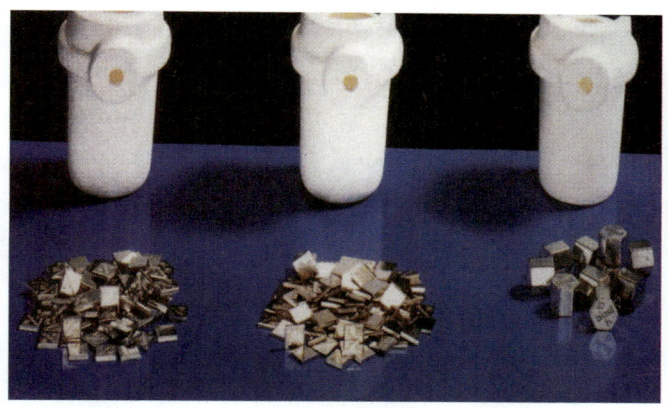

Fig. 19.11: Crucibles, alloy pallets

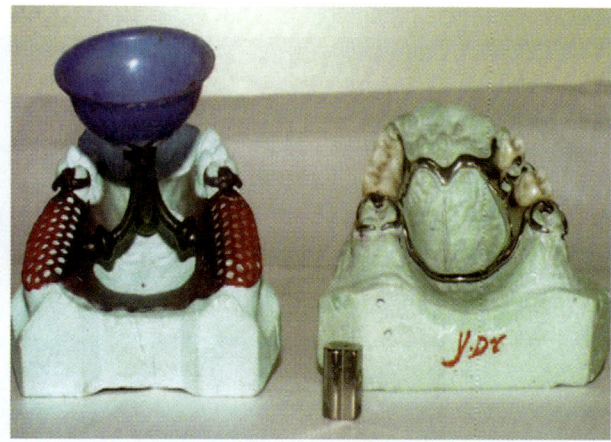

Fig. 19.12: RPD wax pattern, finished RPD

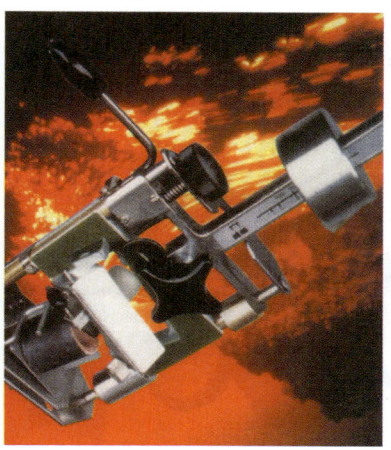

Fig. 19.13: High frequency centrifugal induction casting machine

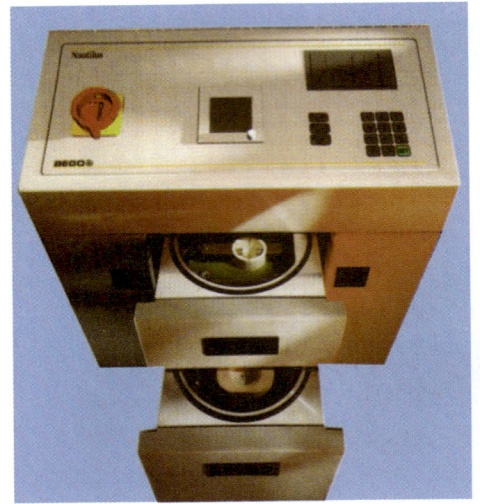

Fig. 19.14: Vacuum pressure casting machine

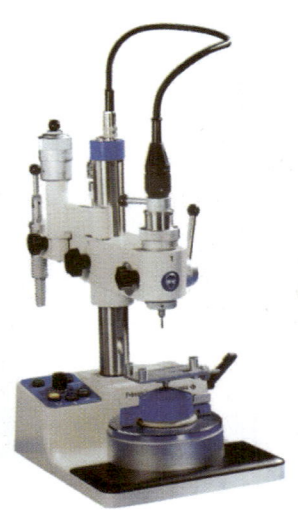

Fig. 19.15: Milling unit for surveying, drilling, scraping

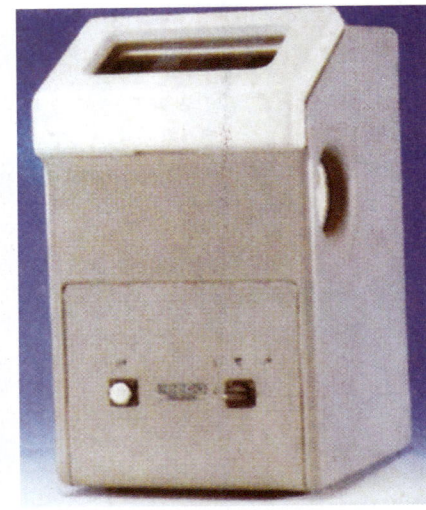

Fig. 19.16: Wet sand blasting unit

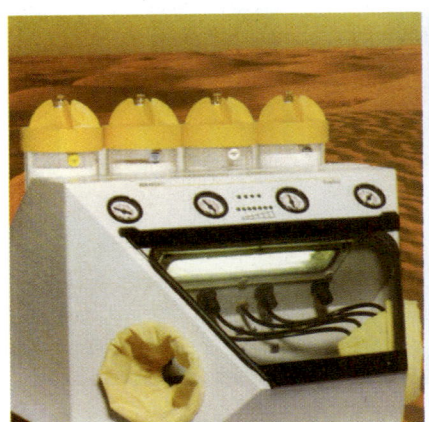

Fig. 19.17: Sand blasting—4 units

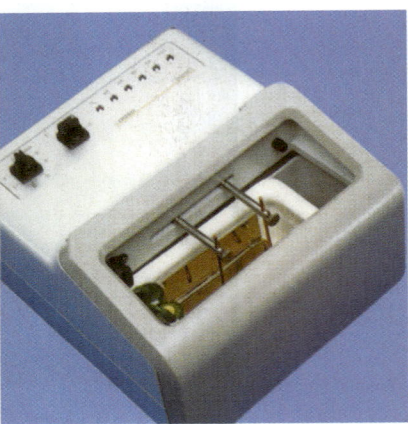

Fig. 19.18: Electropolishing unit

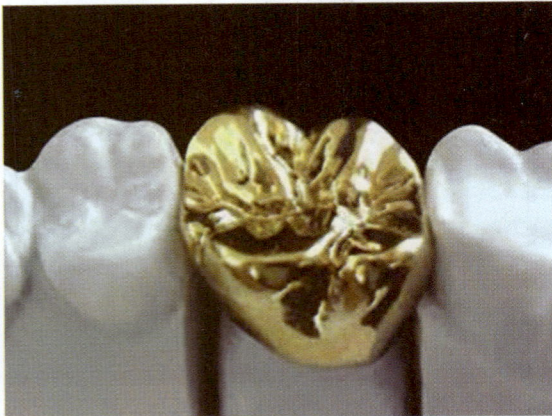

Fig. 19.19: Gold-alloy cast crown

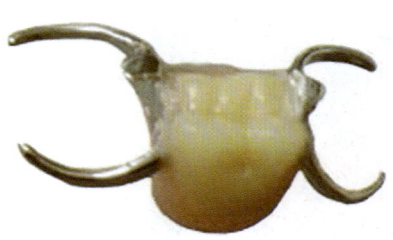

Fig. 19.20: PBM alloy cast clasp

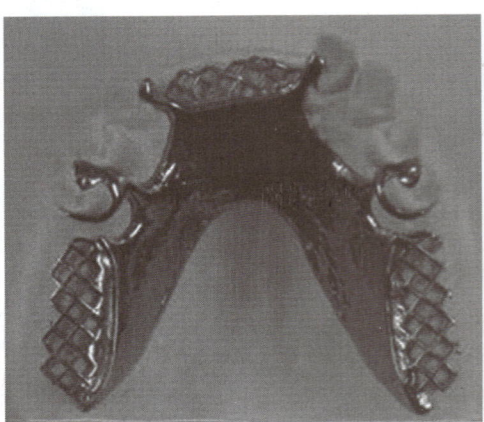

Fig. 19.21: PBM-RPD frame

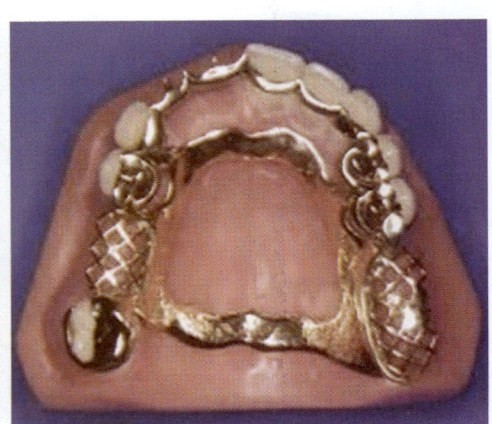

Fig. 19.22: PBM cast RPD

CHAPTER 22: MATERIALS USED IN ORTHODONTIA

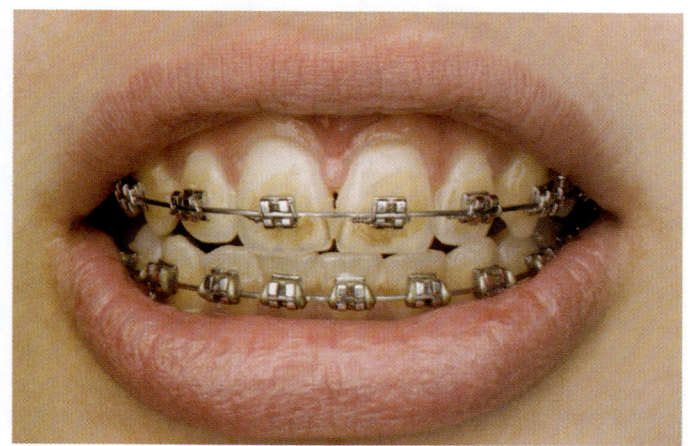

Fig. 22.1: *Ortho*-fixed appliance

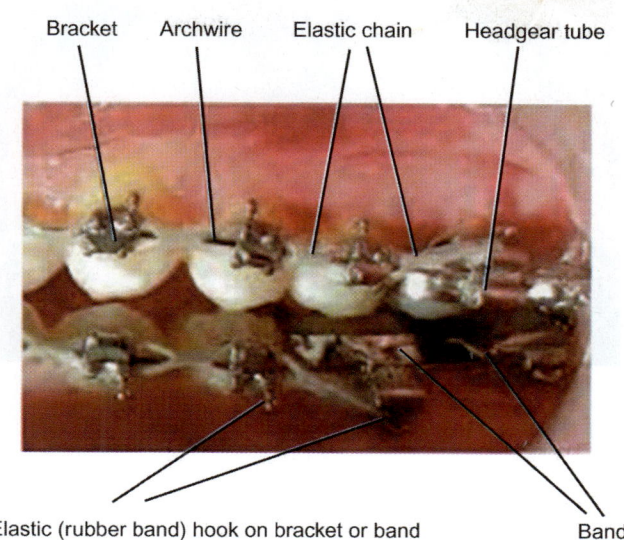

Bracket   Archwire   Elastic chain   Headgear tube

Elastic (rubber band) hook on bracket or band   Band

Fig. 22.2: Activation

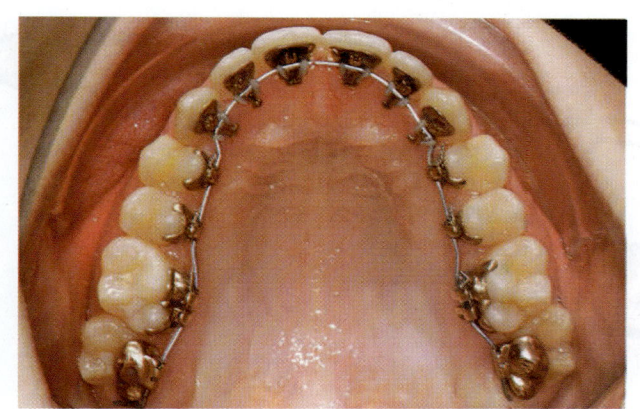

Fig. 22.3: Activation lingual orthodontics

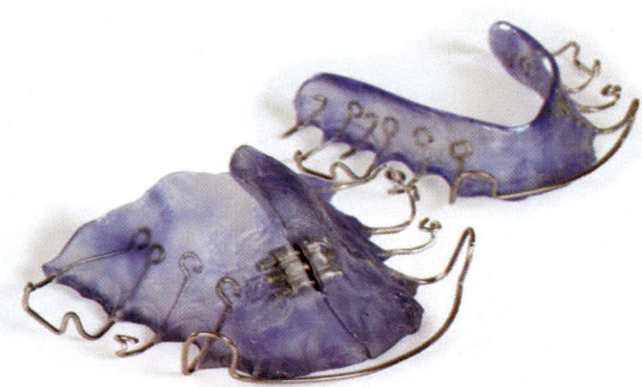

Fig. 22.4: *Ortho*-retainer

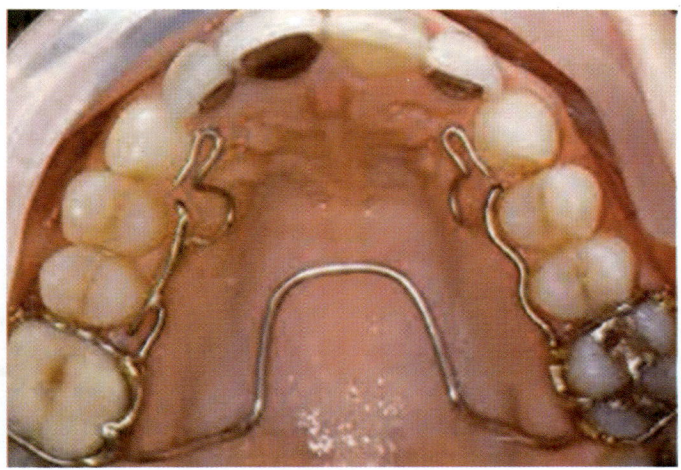

Fig. 22.5: Dentoalveolar expansion

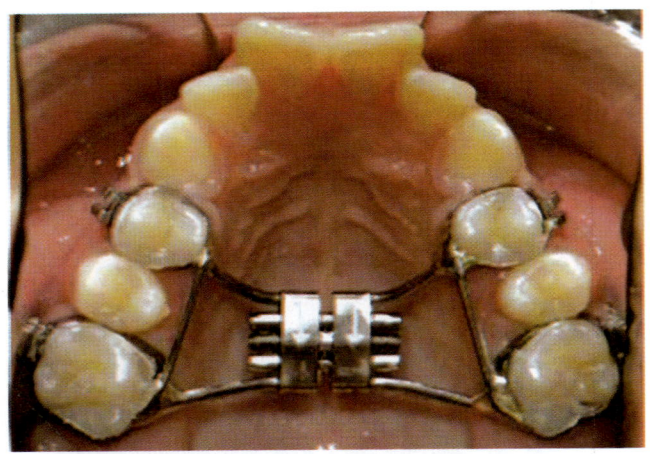

Fig. 22.6: Rapid pallatal expansion

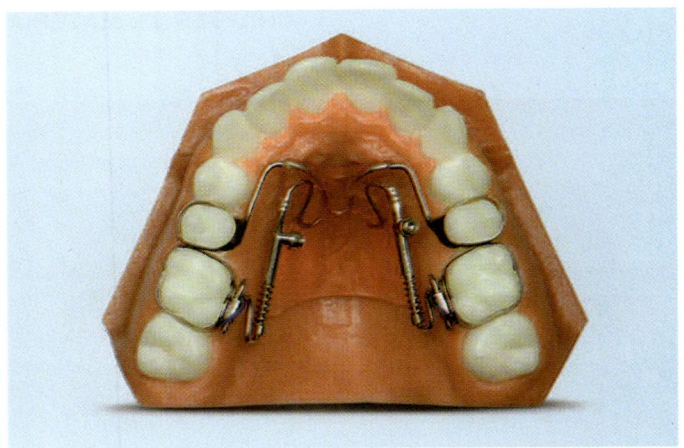

Fig. 22.7: Molar distalization appliance

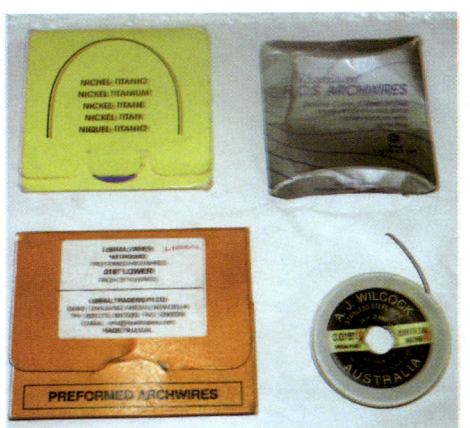

Fig. 22.8: NiTi archwire, 18-8 stainless steel wire

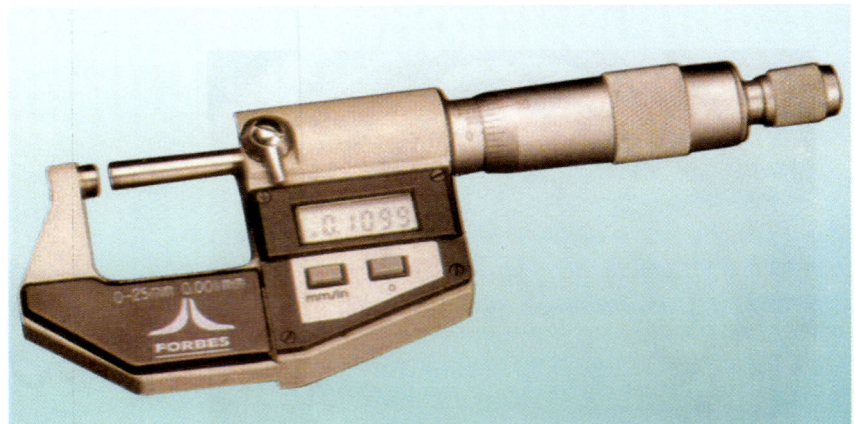

Fig. 22.9: Digital micrometer screw gauge

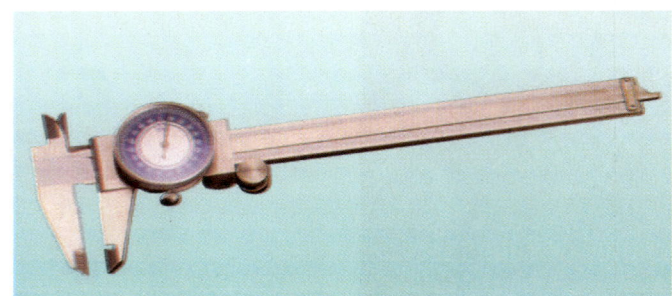

Fig. 22.10: Dial Vernier calipers

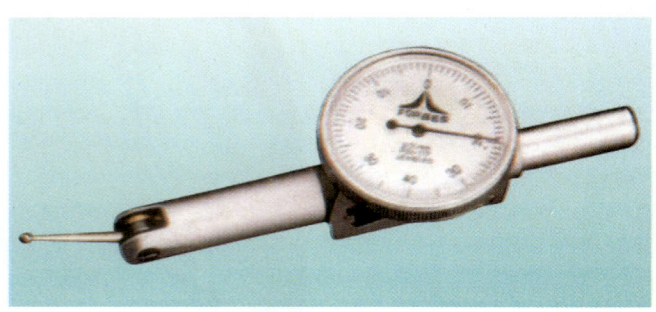

Fig. 22.11: Dial gauge

CHAPTER 23: BRAZING AND WELDING

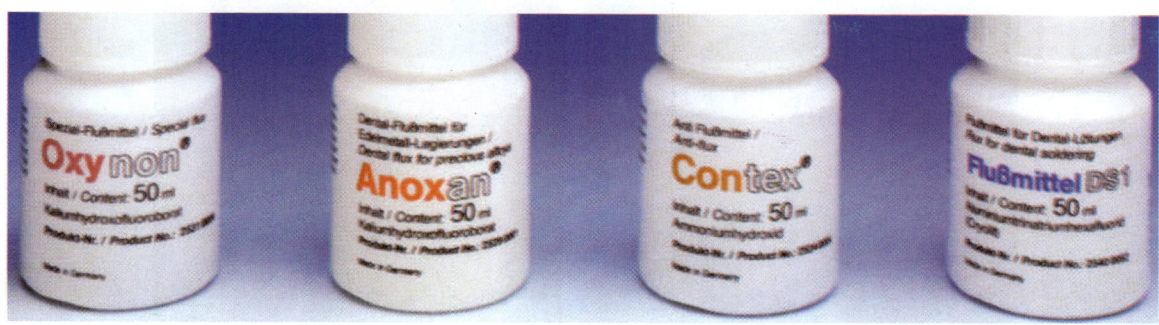

Fig. 23.1: Brazing fluxes

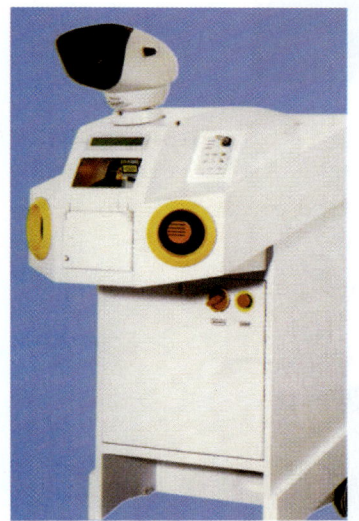

Fig. 23.2: Laser welding unit with stereomicroscope

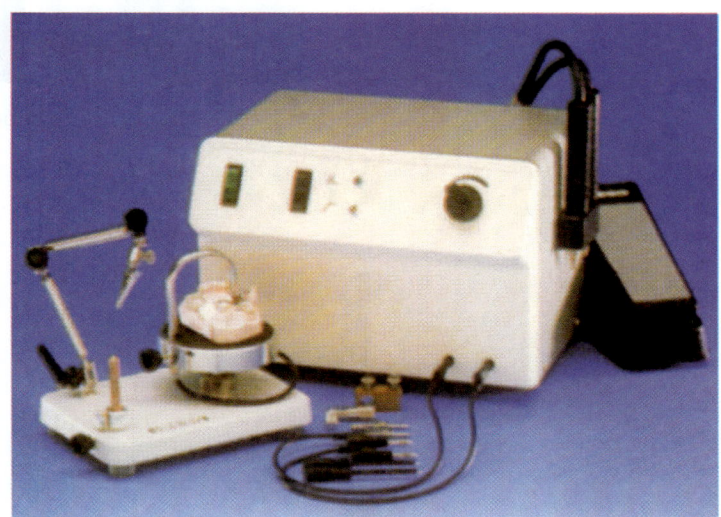

Fig. 23.3: Spot welding and soldering unit

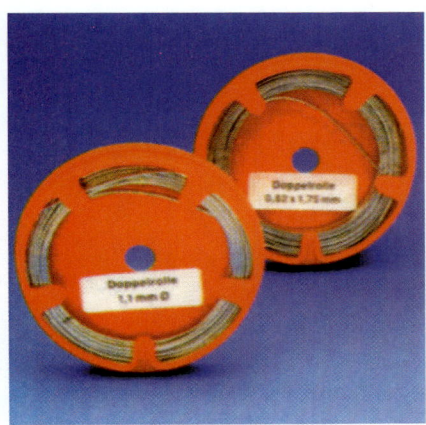

Fig. 23.4: Cobalt chromium clasp wire

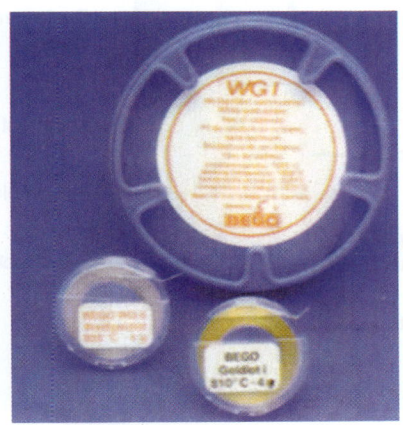

Fig. 23.5: Soldering wire

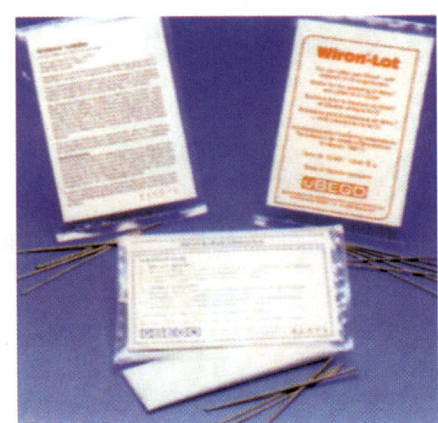

Fig. 23.6: Fluxed solders

CHAPTER 25: DENTAL IMPLANT MATERIALS

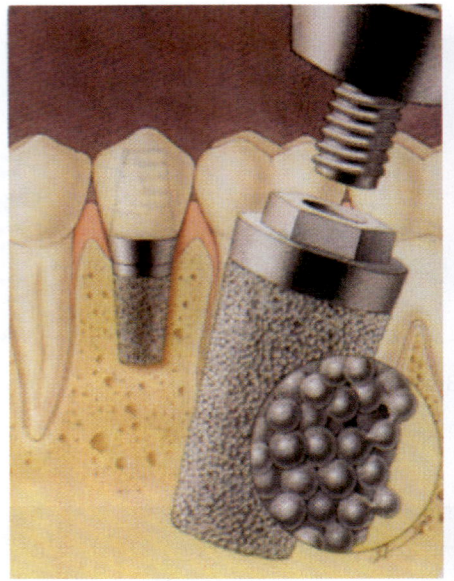 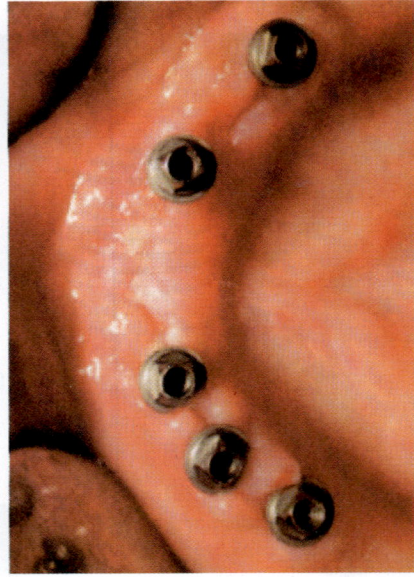

Fig. 25.1: Endopore implant

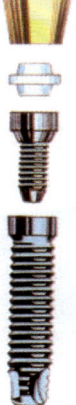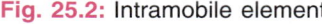

Fig. 25.2: Intramobile element

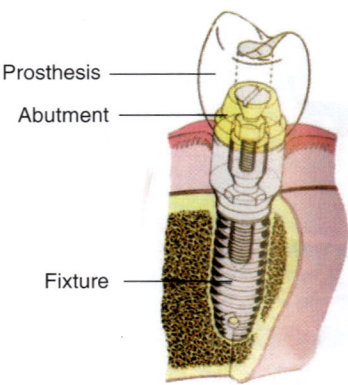

Prosthesis

Abutment

Fixture

Fig. 25.3: Implant components

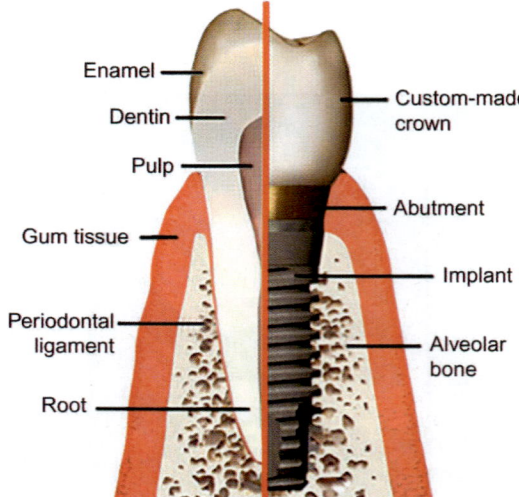

Enamel

Dentin

Pulp

Gum tissue

Periodontal ligament

Root

Custom-made crown

Abutment

Implant

Alveolar bone

Fig. 25.4: Implant anatomy

CHAPTER 26: CUTTING AND FINISHING MECHANICS: TOOLS AND MATERIALS USED

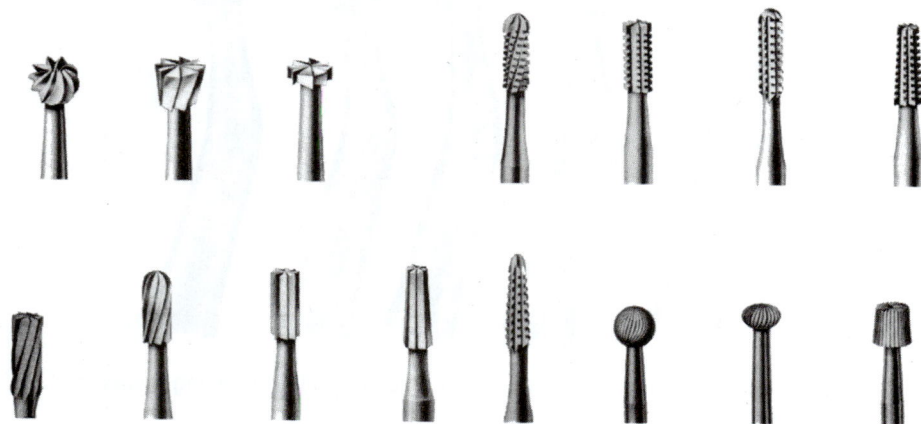

Fig. 26.1a: Steel burs—varities

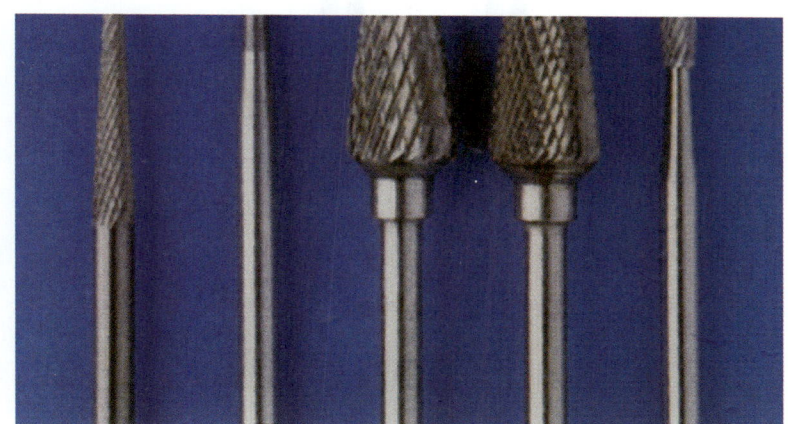

26.1b: Carbide burs

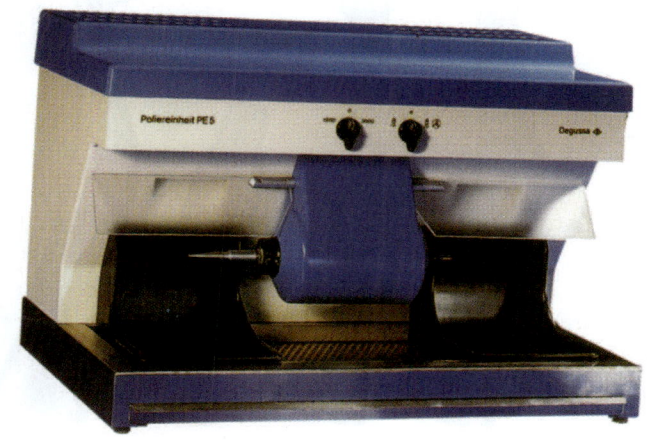

Fig. 26.2: Polishing unit with vacuum suction

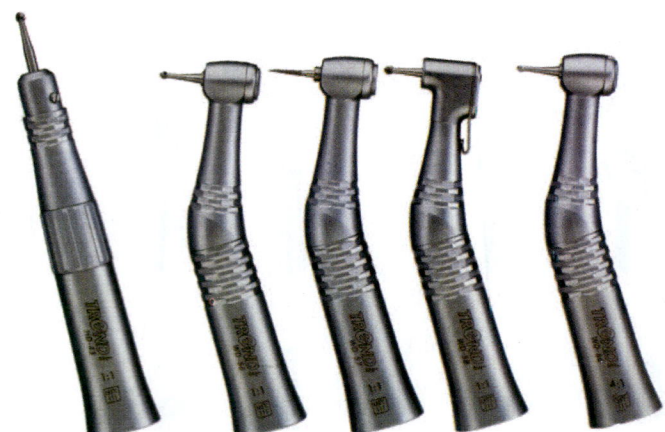

Fig. 26.3: Straight and contrangle hand pieces of different fitting systems

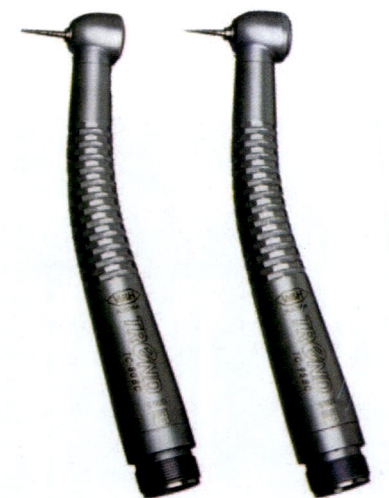

Fig. 26.4: Diamond burs—handpieces

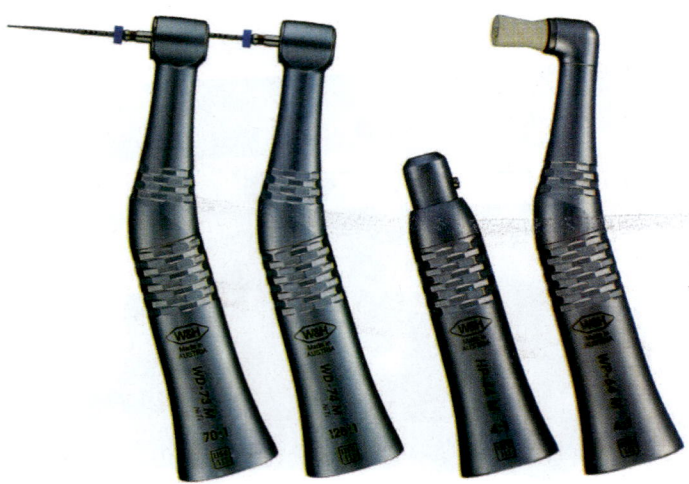

Fig. 26.5: NiTi files in contrangle handpieces (endo), and prophy brushes

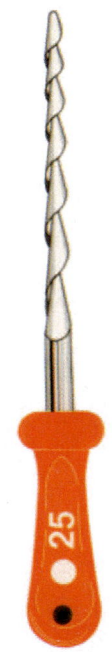

Fig. 26.6: NiTi flexible files (endo)

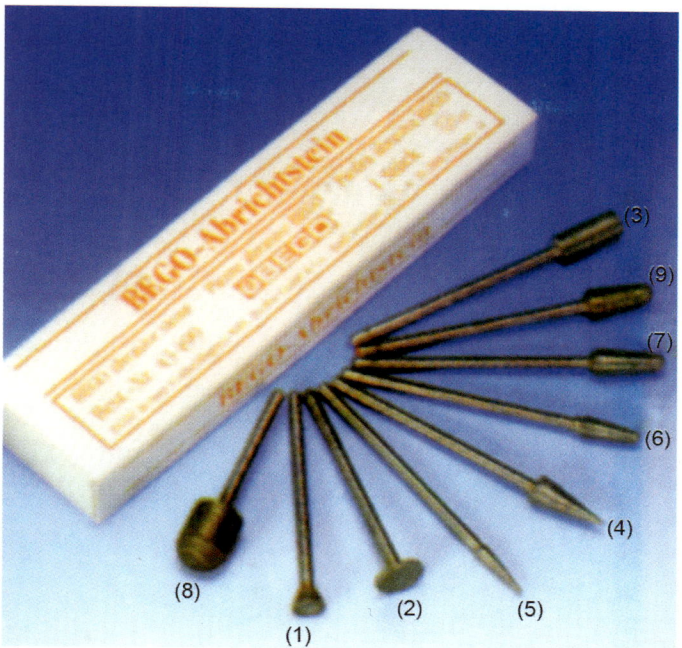

Fig. 26.7: Sintered diamond dressing stones and grinding stones

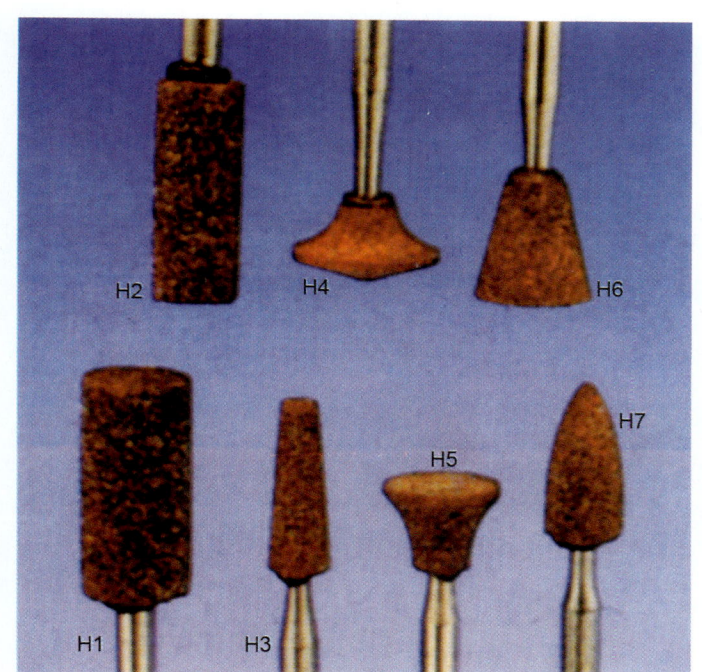

Fig. 26.8: Fine grain grinding stones

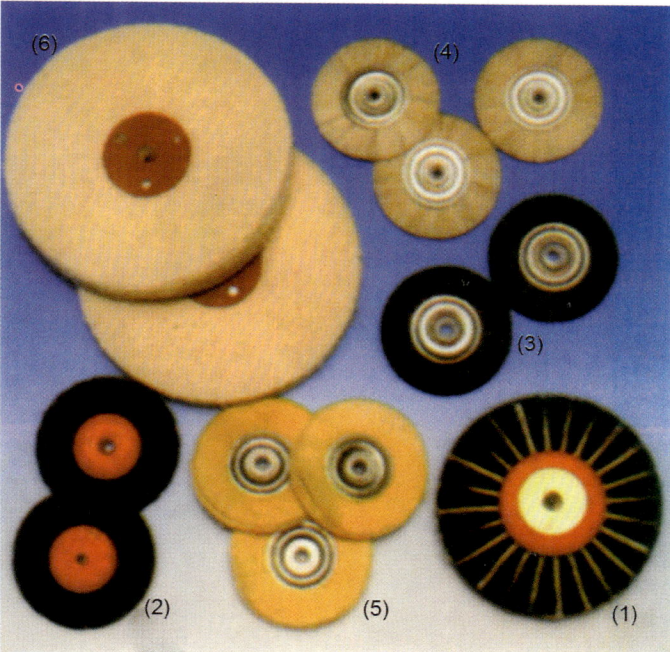

Fig. 26.9: Polishing brushes and mops

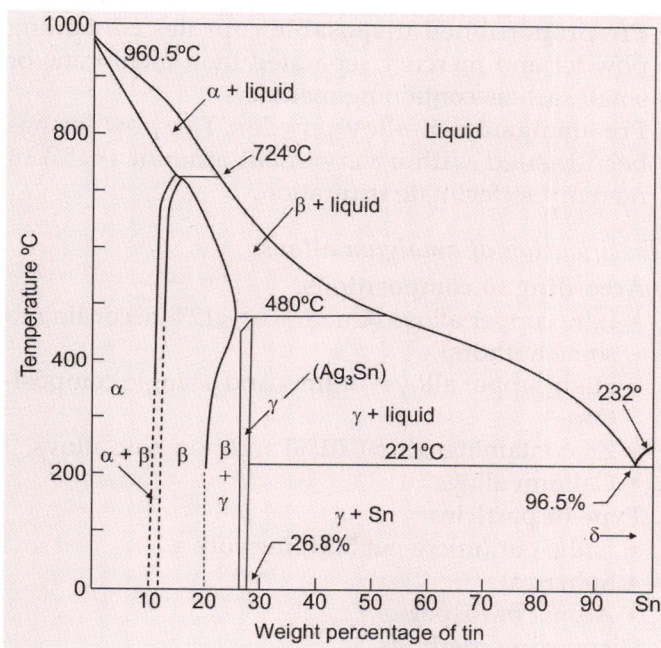

Fig. 12.1: Equilibrium phase diagram of silver–tin system

Compositions

Mainly three varieties of materials according to the particle shapes lathe-cut, spherical and admix or disperse (or a mixture of two) are prepared with different compositions, silver, tin, copper and few trace elements, Zn, In, Pd, etc. This alloy is triturated with a **triple distilled, arsenic-free mercury, for amalgamation.**

Functions of Ingredients

Silver   Has fcc structure, density 10.5 gm/cc, MP = 961°C.
Increases strength, hardness, corrosion resistance, setting expansion
Decreases creep

Tin   Has bct structure, density 7.32 gm/cc, MP = 232°C.
Decreases (controls) the rate of reaction, strength, hardness, setting expansion corrosion resistance due to the formation of β, γ, γ_2 and η phases.
Increases creep.

Copper   Has fcc structure density 8.3 gm/cc, MP = 1083°C.
Increases strength, hardness (forming eutectic phase) and setting expansions.
Decreases creep due to η crystals inter-meshing γ_1 phases.

Zinc   Has hcp structure, density = 7.1 gm/cc MP = 420°C.
(*Increases* brittleness of any HN, N metal alloys, if added).

Small amounts 1–2% are added as reducing agent (**scavenger**).
Causes delayed expansion, by moisture contamination.

Indium   Small amounts can act as scavenger and reduce mercury content.

Platinum/   In small amounts, increase hardness and
Palladium corrosion resistance

Mercury   Has density 13.5 gm/cc, BP = 357°C
Triple distilled, arsenic-free mercury is used.
Free mercury is toxic, cause many health hazards to clinicians and assistants or patients.

Manufacturing Methods

1. **Lathe-cut alloys:** The constituents either of low copper or high copper-single compositions are melted and solidified as an ingot of suitable dimensions. This has an **inhomogeneous cored** structure. It is then heated at about 420–450°C (slightly below its solidus temperature 480°C) in an **electric oven** for about **20–24 hours,** for **homogenizing.** If it is suddenly cooled the Ag-Sn, i.e. β phase remains with small amount of Ag$_3$Sn, i.e., γ phase. If it is cooled very slowly, more γ phase is formed to reach equilibrium. By controlling this rate of cooling the proportions of β and γ phases are adjusted, which influence the amalgamation reactions. This ingot is then cut in **a lathe** by bladed instruments into fine scraps and also powdered in a **milling machine** into small particles of suitable size distributions, **about 15 to 30 μm.** Very fine particles of size about **2–3 μm** also may be present. Smaller particles have a greater surface area and require more Hg, but condensing carving becomes easier for smaller particles.

   Aging heat treatment is required for **relieving the internal stresses,** induced during lathe-cutting procedure (Fig. 12.2). For this, the alloy powder is kept at about **100°C for 24 hours.** Some manufacturers, perform some surface treatments, i.e. **acid washing** to improve the reactivity with mercury.

2. **Spherical atomized particles:** The liquid alloy is atomized (sprayed) into a chamber either evacuated or filled with inert gases. Fine liquid drops solidify into small spherical particles. This is subjected to homogenising heat-treatment, controlled cooling to adjust β and γ phases and acid washing as earlier. Low copper and a high copper single composition alloys can be prepared by this method. Particle size distribution can also be done as required (due to large surface tension, alloy-liquid drops become spherical) (Fig. 12.3).

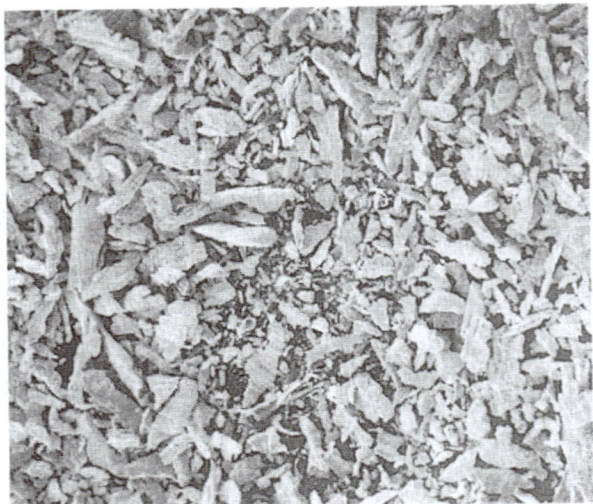

Fig. 12.2: Lathe-cut alloy powder

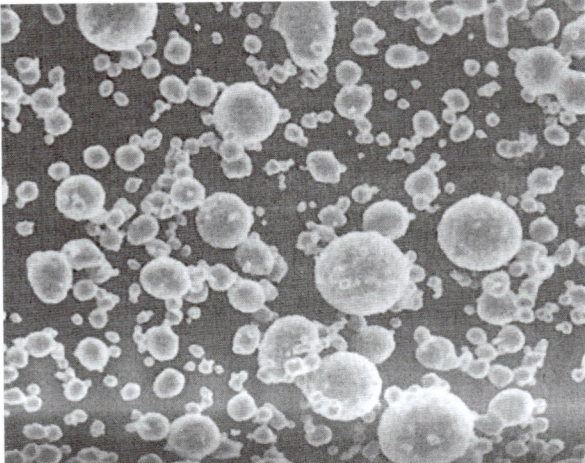

Fig. 12.3: Spherical-atomized particles

3. **Disperse or admixed alloys:** This is a physical mixture of low copper lathe-cut alloys and 30 to 55% of silver–copper (72:28 by weight) eutectic-atomized powder. Sometimes one part of spherical eutectic alloy is mixed with two parts of lathe-cut low copper alloys. Even though small spherical alloy requires less mercury and hence should have slightly higher strength, the **lathe-cut** alloys or their mixtures are **preferred** as these have better condensing properties, i.e. good resistance to condensation. It is easier to polish spherical alloy amalgams.

Dispensing methods

1. **Powder (30 gm or 100 gm)** in plastic or glass bottles and **triple distilled, arsenic-free mercury** in a dropper bottle.
2. **Pellets** of definite size, formed by heating the powder and pressing to form a loose skin.

3. **Pre-proportioned disposable** capsules containing powder and mercury separated by a membrane or small sachets containing mercury.
4. **Pre-amalgamated** alloy powder: The powder has been treated with a very small amount (<1%) of mercury to facilitate trituration.

Classification of amalgam alloys

1. **According to compositions**
   - Low copper alloys (Cu <6% or <12% according to some authors)
   - High copper alloys—admix and a single composition
   - Zn containing (Zn >0.01%) and non-zinc alloys
   - Gallium alloys
2. **Type of particles**
   - Lathe-cut (micro cut and fine cut)
   - Spherical
   - Admix or disperse
3. **Dispensing methods**
   - Powder–liquid (mercury)
   - Powder pellets + mercury
   - Preproportioned capsules (powder + mercury)
4. **Special treatments**
   - Aged alloys
   - Acid washed alloys
   - Pre-amalgamated alloys

Compositions, Amalgamation Reactions and Microstructure

1. Low copper–silver amalgam alloys

The first composition was given by GV Black (1980) and slightly modified by manufacturers.

Composition

Powder	Wt%	Liquid
Silver	= 67–70%	Mercury: Triple distilled arsenic free
Tin	= 26–29%	
Copper	= 2–5%, <6%	
Zinc	= 1–2%	
Indium, palladium/ or rarely gold	= traces	

Liquid: Pure, triple distilled arsenic free, measuring

Amalgamation Reaction and Microstructure

The alloy particles have β phase (Ag-Sn) surrounded by γ phases (Ag₃Sn). On mixing with mercury,

$$\beta(Ag\text{-}Sn) + \gamma\,(Ag_3Sn) + Hg \longrightarrow \gamma_1(Ag_2Hg_3) + \gamma_2\,(Sn_{7\text{-}8}Hg) + \text{unreacted}\,(\beta + \gamma + Hg)$$

Solubilities of Ag and Sn are about **0.035% and 0.6%** respectively. Hence, the silver–mercury γ_1 phase first precipitates and the **bcc γ_1** crystals grow. Later, the γ_2 phase—crystals formed also grow. These surround and bind the unreacted ($\beta + \gamma$) phase particles to form a composite structure (Fig. 12.4a). The properties of the set rigid mass depends on the proportions of various phases formed or present, as the **different phases have different properties:**

- Unreacted γ phase has the highest strength.
- γ_1 phase has lower strength, about $1/_{10}$th of γ phase, but has better corrosion resistance.
- γ_2 phase has still lower strength about $1/_{10}$th of γ_1 phase, has the least corrosion resistance and causes dimensional changes (creep).
- **Voids** left behind are the **weakest regions.**

Hence, to obtain better properties, i.e. higher strength and corrosion resistance and lower creep, all the following principles are used.

- **A minimum amount of mercury** (lowest Hg/alloy ratio) is used to reduce the amounts of weaker reaction products formed.
- **Elimination of the weakest** (tin–mercury) phase which is done by adding more copper.
- **A suitable modification of manipulation techniques:** Selection, proportioning, trituration, condensation, finishing, etc. to reduce the formation of weaker γ_1 and γ_2 phases, and voids.

2. High copper–silver amalgam alloys

(a) Admix (disperse) alloy (Table 12.1)

Ag-Cu eutectic (72:28) spherical alloy of small particle sizes are added by about one part to two parts (i.e. about 30 to 55%) of lathe-cut low copper alloys (**1963, Innes and Youdelis**). This hard Ag-Cu eutectic alloys were expected to increase the strength by a large value, by acting as fillers.

Composition

Powder	
Silver	50–60%
Tin	20–25%
Copper	13–30%
Zinc	1–2%

Liquid: Pure, triple distilled arsenic free, mercury.

The alloy particles have, the lamellar, Ag_3Cu_2, eutectic phase (α- and β-solid solutions) and the $\beta + \gamma$ silver–tin phases. On mixing with mercury the γ_2 phase produced react with eutectic phase and get almost eliminated.

Amalgamation Reaction and Microstructure

Ag_3Sn (γ) + Ag_3Cu_2 (ε) + Hg $\longrightarrow$ Ag_3Hg_2 (γ_1) + Cu_6Sn_5 (η) + unreacted ($\gamma + \varepsilon + Hg$)

Microstructure

The γ_1 and η phases formed crystallize **separately** binding the unreacted particles and form a harder mass. Set mass has the unreacted $\beta + \gamma$ phases and Ag_3Cu_2 eutectic ε phases bound by Ag_3Hg_2(γ_1), Cu_6Sn_5(η) and negligible amount of $Sn_{7-8}Hg$ (γ_2) phases (Fig. 12.4b).

(b) Single composition high-copper alloys

The alloy ingredients are melted together, and fine lathe cut or spherical powder particles obtained are subjected to aging heat treatment (at 100°C for 24 hours for stress relief), before dispensing.

The alloy is available as lathe-cut (fine cut) or sometimes spherical (small particles).

Composition

Powder		
Silver	=	45–60%
Tin	=	15–25%
Copper	=	13–20%
Zinc	=	0%
Traces of In, Pt, Pd		

Liquid: Pure, triple distilled arsenic-free mercury.

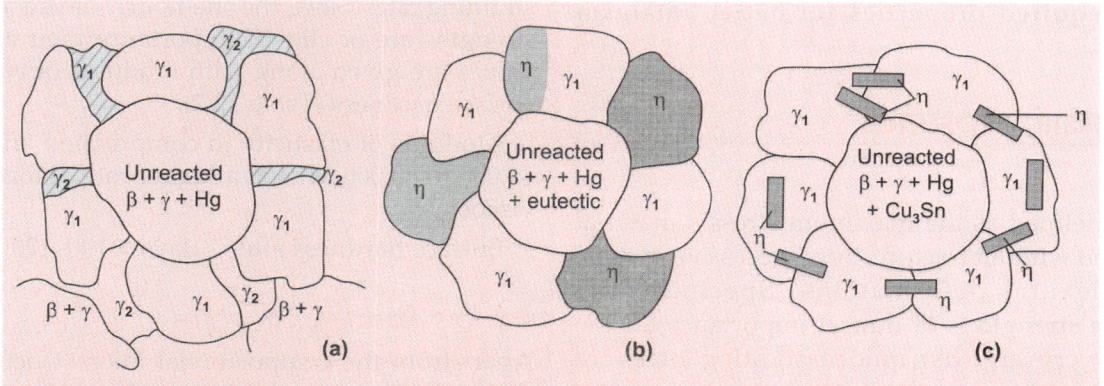

Figs 12.4a to c: Microstructure of set amalgam. (a) Low copper, (b) high copper (admix), (c) high copper single composition

Table 12.1 Composition of low copper and high copper (admix, single composition) alloys powder

Ingredients	Low copper alloys Wt%	Range Wt%	Admix alloys range Wt%	Single composition alloys (range) Wt%	Alloying properties
Silver	68.8	67–70	50–65	45–60 expansion	↑ Strength, corrosion resistance, setting ↓ Creep,
Tin	26.8	26–28	20–25	15–25	↑ Creep ↓ Strength, corrosion resistance
Copper	3.6	2–5	13–30	13–20	↑ Strength, assisting lathe cutting (comminution), corrosion resistance, setting expansion ↓ Creep
Zn	0.8	1–2	0–2	0	↑Scavenger, reducing agent ↑ Brittleness (assisting lathe cutting) and↑ setting expansion
In, Pd	Traces	Traces	Traces	Traces	↑ Strength
Micro-structure phases } Alloy	Alloy	$\beta + \gamma$	$\beta + \gamma + \varepsilon$ (Ag$_3$-Cu$_2$)	$\beta + \gamma$ + Cu$_3$Sn	
Amalgam		$\gamma_1 + \gamma_2$ + un-reacted	$\gamma_1 + \eta$ + unreacted phases	$\gamma_1 + \eta$ (rods) intermeshing with γ_1 phase + unreacted phases	

Amalgamation reaction and microstructure

Microstructure shows Ag$_3$Sn phase and Cu$_3$Sn phases are present in the alloy. On trituration with mercury finally, Ag$_3$Hg$_2$ (γ_1) and Cu$_6$Sn$_5$ phases are formed which bind the unreacted particles.

Ag$_3$Sn (γ) + Cu$_3$Sn + Hg → Ag$_3$Hg$_2$ (γ_1) + Cu$_6$Sn$_5$(η) + **unreacted material** (Fig. 12.4c).

The Cu$_6$Sn$_5$ prismatic η phase—crystals grow, intermeshing with the growing—γ_1 crystals. This causes greater resistance to slip, very high one hour and maximum strengths and decrease of the creep. All these are required properties for better amalgam restorations.

CHARACTERISTIC PROPERTIES

A. Strength

Strength is defined as the maximum stress a material can withstand without fracture, by compressive, tensile, shear or flexural deformations. **Specially, the compressive strength** is of utmost importance for the clinician, as very large dynamic masticating forces are applied, several times on these posterior, permanent restorations. **Any bulk fracture leads to failure** and

marginal fractures lead to the collection of food debris, causing secondary caries, as well as marginal leakages which are again detrimental.

The compressive strength is measured as per the standard methods (given by ADA specification No. 1). Usually a cylindrical sample of height 8 mm and diameter 4 mm is prepared, keeping the variable parameters constant, and preserved at 37°C for 7 days. These are tested by universal testing machines at definite strain rates like 0.5 mm, 0.2 mm or 0.05 mm per minute. As silver amalgam is **viscoelastic material,** its properties like strength, modulus of elasticities, depend on **stressing or straining rates**. Since, the one-hour, 7 days and maximum strengths are of clinical importance their approximate values are given along with modulus of elasticity and surface hardness (Table 12.2).

Modulus of elasticity in compression after 7 days = 40,000 to 80,000 MPa at a higher rate of loading as it is viscoelastic.

Surface hardness after 7 days = 100–120 KHN.

Factors Affecting Strengths

Apart from the compositional microstructure phases, the manipulation variables affect the mechanical properties very much. The strengths of various phases

Table 12.2	Approximate mechanical properties of different silver amalgam alloys				
Silver amalgam varieties	Compressive strength MPa		Tensile strength MPa 24 hrs	Creep % ADA <3%	Method (sample)
	1 hr	7 days			
Low copper	145	343	60	1.0–2.0	
Admix	137	431	48	0.5–1.0	
Single composition	262 (260–290)	510	64	0.05–0.1	

in the decreasing **order are γ, γ_1, η, γ_2 and voids**. Manipulative variables should be controlled to produce the **maximum amount of stronger phases such as:**

1. **Time factors (setting times):** γ_1, γ_2 and η phases formed grow into crystals gradually and bond the unreacted particles to form a rigid strong mass. Hence, strength increases with respect to time. In about 20 minutes the strength reaches about 6% of its maximum strength (i.e. about 25–30 MPa). When scratched, it gives a metallic sound, **amalgam cry,** indicating that removal of excess can be initiated. One hour strength is of much clinical importance for **'finishing'** in one sitting. Strength increases to about 95% of its maximum value in about 7 days and increases very slowly even for 5 or 6 months. For the clinician, **8 hours time is considered as setting time** and the patient can use solid food after that.

2. **Compositions:** High copper single composition alloys, form amalgam of **very high one-hour** compressive strengths **(250–290 MPa),** and highest maximum strengths (up to 520 MPa) due to **interlocking of γ_1 phases by the 'η' phase rods growing into the γ_1 phases. These increase slip resistance, and decrease creep.** Lathe-cut, spherical and disperse alloys have nearly the same **lower one hour** compressive and 24 hours tensile strengths. But high copper single composition alloys have higher maximum strength due to the elimination of weaker γ_2 phase (Table 12.2) and intermeshing of γ_1 and η phase.

3. **Mercury/alloy ratio:** If more mercury enters into the reaction, greater amounts of weaker γ_1 and γ_2 phases are formed, which decreases the strength. Hence, minimum mercury is used. **All factors decreasing this Hg alloy ratio, lead to an increase of strength,** such as time of optimum trituration, condensation force, spherical particles, etc.

If the percentage of mercury is below the limits shown in Fig. 12.5, the compressive strengths fall sharply as the unwetted particles are not bonded. The spherical alloys require **smaller%** of mercury as the surface **area is less,** and hence have higher strengths (*refer* to manipulation—proportioning).

4. **Effect of particle size and shapes: Smaller the particle size, greater is the strength** and adaptability to margins. Lathe-cut irregular particles can withstand higher condensation pressure and get higher compressive strength. Spherical particles easily slip during condensation. **Small condenser tips can pierce during** condensation, and large pressure cannot be applied.

5. **Effect of trituration:** Trituration is required for facilitating amalgamation reactions. **Prolonged trituration,** increases the weaker reaction products, γ_1, γ_2, and η phases and hence **decreases strength.** Under-trituration does not produce enough γ_1, γ_2 and η phases to bind the stronger unreacted γ phase, which therefore should decrease the strength. Also the mix becomes less plastic, cannot be condensed properly and voids or porosities are left. This also decreases strength.

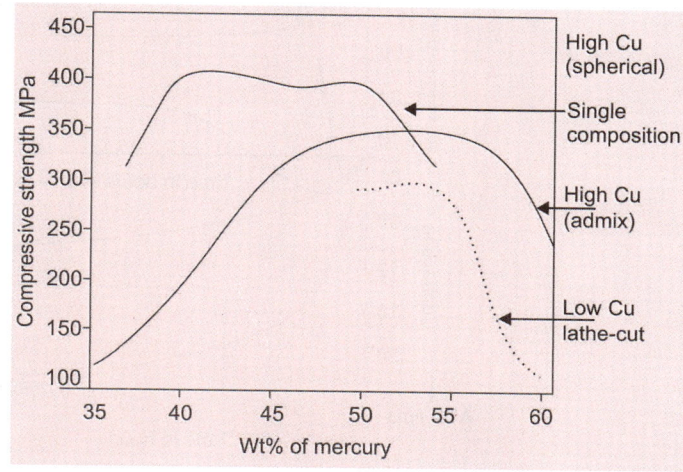

Fig. 12.5: Effect of mercury content on compressive strength

These porosities or voids become the centers of stress—concentrations and lead to fractures. During service, the porosities can cause contractions and marginal gaps.

6. **Condensation pressures:** Larger condensation forces cause better adaptation, cohesion and hence higher strength. The condensation pressure applied is about **1.5–1.7 kg.** Larger condensation forces also **express more excess of mercury,** and reduce the voids or porosities. For spherical particles lower condensation pressures are applied as condenser may pierce into the condensing mix.

Note: However, the tensile strength, shear strength, modulus of elasticity, etc. mechanical properties are not so severely affected by the above factors, except the rate of loading.

B. Dimensional Changes

1. *Setting expansion and contraction*

Theory: When the alloy powder is triturated, the molecules on the surface, react with mercury and produce γ_1 and γ_2 (or η) phases. Due to lower solubility of silver in mercury, first γ_1 phase precipitates and growth of γ_1 phase crystals take place. As there is a reduction in volume, the formation of γ_1 phase, first undergo contraction. As the crystals grow **they push each other, causing expansion until a rigid γ_1 matrix** is formed. After that, the **γ_2 crystals grow into the intergranular spaces.** Formation of γ_2 phase later may not contribute to expansion. Similarly, η phase growing as rod-like structures into the γ_1 phase also does not produce much contraction or expansions.

However, the older alloys, having a larger particle sizes and hand-mixing at lower speed, showed a **net expansion,** whereas the **modern alloys** having smaller particles and mechanical mixing **at higher speeds,** show a net contraction, as shown in Fig. 12.6.

Factors which increase setting expansion are

- Higher mercury alloy ratio
- Larger alloy particle size
- Spherical particles
- Slow mixing speed
- Prolonged trituration
- Low condensation pressures
- Moisture contamination (delayed expansions)
- A large excess of mercury left behind cause mercuroscopic expansion.

Measurement of dimensional changes

As per ADA specification, a cylindrical sample of 4 mm diameter and 8 mm height is prepared and kept at 37°C to simulate oral conditions. The expansion which is quite small is measured by using a **dial gauge or interferometer** (by measuring the changes in the bandwidths of alternate dark and bright bands, formed by interference, i.e. superimposition of monochromatic coherent lights) at various time intervals for different alloys.

ADA specification No. 1: According to this, the dimensional changes, either contraction or expansion should be <0.2%.

Clinical significances

- **Setting expansion:** Small setting expansion cause better attachment/retention to cavity walls.

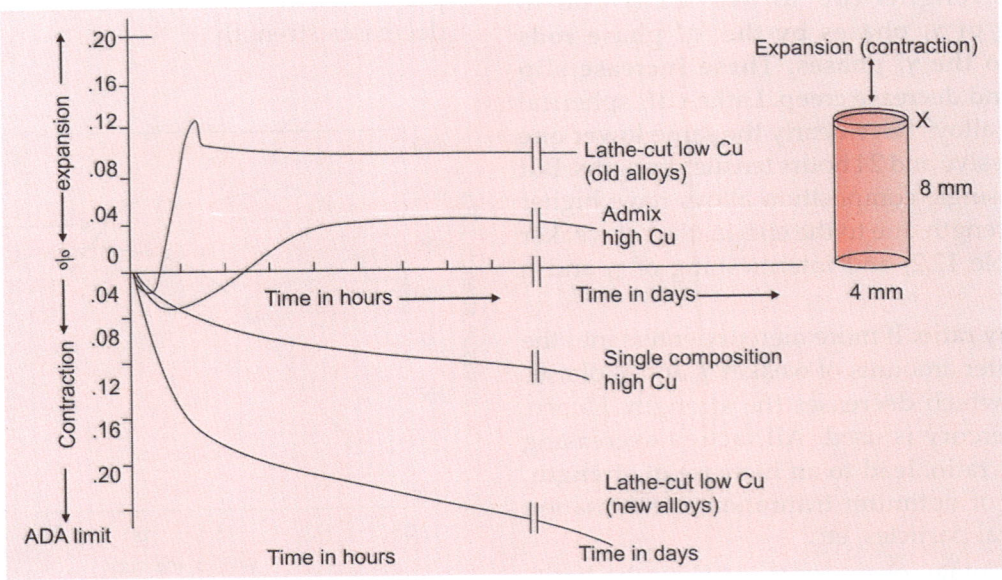

Fig. 12.6: Dimensional changes during setting of different alloys—amalgams

Excessive setting expansion causes, pulp injuries (pains), hyperocclusion that is protrusion at the occlusal surface and sometimes fracture of thin cavity walls by lateral pressures.

- **Any contraction** causes, detachment from the cavity walls, resulting in **microleakage** (or marginal leakage), a collection of food debris, leading to secondary caries. (**Microleakage** is also enhanced due to percolation. Silver amalgam has a large coefficient of thermal expansion, around 25 ppm/°C, which is double that of tooth enamel 11.4 ppm/°C. However, in due course, the small amount of **corrosion products** enter the marginal gaps and **seal it well, stopping the microleakage.**) However, cavity varnish is coated to the cavity walls before restoration.

2. *Delayed expansion—moisture contamination effect:*
Large setting expansion of about 4% (20 times of ADA specification limit) sometimes takes place, after a few days (3–7 days), in the case of zinc containing alloys, if there is moisture trapping or contamination during restoration (Fig. 12.7).

This is due to the electrolysis of trapped water into hydrogen and oxygen, by the particles of zinc and copper or silver acting as electrodes, i.e. $2H_2O \rightarrow 2H_2 + O_2$.

The H_2 and O_2 gases produced **gradually accumulate and exert a large internal pressure,** causing this expansion, after a few days.

Clinical significance of the delayed expansion
Large expansion causes **severe pains** and some time cause fracture of thin cavity walls. Only removal and replacing a fresh restoration is the remedy. Cavity restoration should be done, in dry condition using rubber dams or using non-zinc containing alloys.

3. *Mercuroscopic expansion*
Inhomogeneous condensation pressure and wrong burnishing techniques can shift the **mercury-rich thin mix to the margins of the cavity.** The portions at margins have high mercury content. This excess mercury **slowly** reacts with the alloy and produce weaker phases and large setting expansions at the margins. This is called mercuroscopic expansion. As the margins contain a higher amount of weaker phase, and form **thin ledges,** marginal breakdown or fracture takes place **causing ditched restoration.** Hence, for better restorations, proper selection, mixing, condensation, finishing, etc. are quite important.

4. *Creep*
This is the **time dependent deformation or strain, taking place in case of viscoelastic materials by static or dynamic repeating forces.** For such materials the mechanical properties are significantly affected by the **rate of loading**.

Silver amalgam restoration behaves as a **viscoelastic material.** Its modulus of elasticity ranges from about **40,000 MPa to 80,000 MPa,** when the rate of loading is increased. The restoration is subjected to large dynamic masticating forces, many times which cause creep or 'flow' of restoration on the occlusal surface, forming thin sections. These thin extensions fracture, causing marginal crevices, which collect food debris, fluids, etc. resulting in marginal leakage and secondary caries. Alloys producing **least creep value are to be selected**. ADA specification No. 1 has the creep values <2.0% for the present alloys, and for older alloys <8%.

Determination of creep
A cylindrical sample of **4 mm diameter and 8 mm height is prepared, preserved for 7 days at a temperature 37°C** and then subjected to a static load of **36 Newtons**. The percentage decrease in height x, in 3 hours ($creep = \frac{x}{8} \times 100$) in-between the ends of 1 hour and 4 hours is taken as a creep. The creep can be measured using 'dial-guage' in micrometers or optical methods (*refer* to Table 12.2 for values).

Factors minimizing creep
- *Composition*: Single composition—high copper (non-zinc, lathe-cut, small, aged particles), etc. alloys
- Minimum mercury alloy ratio
- Optimum trituration
- Large condensation pressure
- Homogeneous condensation
- Proper cavity design
- Good finishing

Accordingly, the alloys are selected and suitable precautions are followed during manipulations.

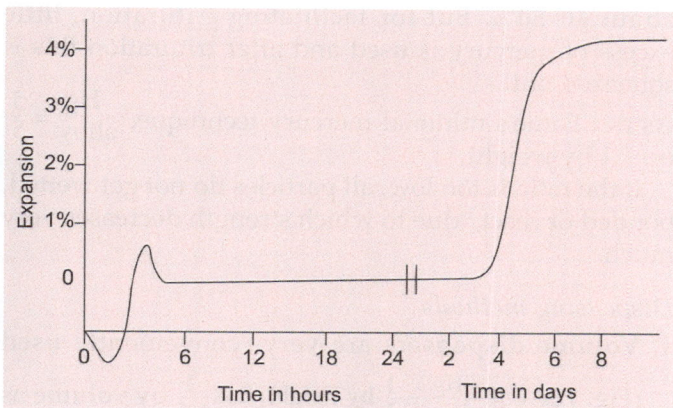

Fig. 12.7: Dimensional changes—delayed expansion

Manipulation of Silver Amalgam

The silver amalgam restoration on the average can survive for about **12 to 15 years** if proper selection and manipulative precautions are followed. The clinicians should therefore have a thorough knowledge of these, to achieve the best properties.

Criteria for Selection of Alloys

This depends upon the individual cases. The ANSI/ADA specification No. 1 should be strictly followed, to obtain

- High, one hour and maximum strengths
- Minimum dimensional changes
- Lowest creep value
- Good condensing property
- High corrosion resistance
- Good polishing and finishing abilities.

Selection is made as follows

- A high copper single composition
- Small particles
- Lathe-cut/spherical/admixed (clinical situation)
- Aged particles (to reduce distortion by relaxation of internal stresses)
- Non-zinc alloys (to avoid delayed expansion)
- Sometimes acid washed particles (for better reactivity)
- Triple distilled arsenic (and other dissolved impurities) free mercury.

Manipulation steps

1. Preliminary cavity preparations
2. Selection of instruments
3. Proportioning
4. Trituration
5. Condensation
6. Finishing

1. **Preliminary preparations:** Class I and class II cavities.
   - Should have **large volume** for bulk filling, required for greater resistance to impact forces.
   - **Large undercuts** for better mechanical retention.
   - **Proper design** for minimizing formation of thin extensions in the occlusal surface to avoid marginal fractures.
   - Suitable pulp protection by calcium hydroxide and hard insulating **bases**.
   - Cavity varnishes are applied to the cavity walls.
   - Stainless steel matrix bands are contoured with the help of band retainers, of No. 1 or No. 8.
   - Rubber dams are fixed for isolating the tooth from the damp-moist oral environment.

2. **Instruments used are**
   - Glass mortar and pestle or amalgamator
   - Amalgam carrier
   - Plastic mix carrier
   - Amalgam condenser (round)
   - Amalgam condenser (rectangular)
   - Diamond carver
   - Wartz carver
   - Hollenback carver
   - Ball burnisher
   - T-burnisher
   - Matrix band retainers
   - Polishing rubber cup

Mechanical condensers

The hand-condensation method is slightly modified. The condenser tips are attached to hand pieces of special design so that vibratory or impact mechanisms can be utilized. This saves the condensation time and reduces **the fatigue of clinician.**

3. **Proportioning**

To get the most suitable properties, such as high strength, low dimensional changes, low creep values, etc. weaker reaction products must be minimized or Hg alloy ratio should be minimum. Formerly, the ratios were expressed as:

$$\frac{Hg}{alloy} = \frac{3}{5}, \frac{4}{5}, \frac{5}{5}, \frac{6}{5}, \frac{7}{5}, \frac{8}{5}, \text{etc. } \textbf{parts by wt,}$$

e.g. $\frac{Hg}{alloy} = \frac{6}{5}$ means, it has the weight percentage of

mercury $= \frac{6}{6+5} \times 100 = 54.54\%$

For obtaining good properties for low copper lathe-cut

alloys $\frac{Hg}{Alloy}$ ratio should be in-between **50 and 54%**

(i.e. $\frac{5}{5}$ and $\frac{6}{5}$) by wt.

For high copper single composition alloys, it is about 40–50%. But for facilitating trituration, little excess of mercury is used and after trituration this is squeezed out.

As per Eame's minimal mercury technique, $\frac{Hg}{alloy} = \frac{5}{5}$ or 1:1 by weight.

If the ratio is too low, all particles do not get wetted, bonded or react, due to which strength decreases very much.

Dispensing methods

- **Volume dispensers** are very conveniently used (Fig. 12.8). If $\frac{Hg}{alloy} = \frac{1}{1}$ **by weight**, it is $\frac{1}{1.5}$ **by volume** as the density of mercury is about 1.5 times that of powder.

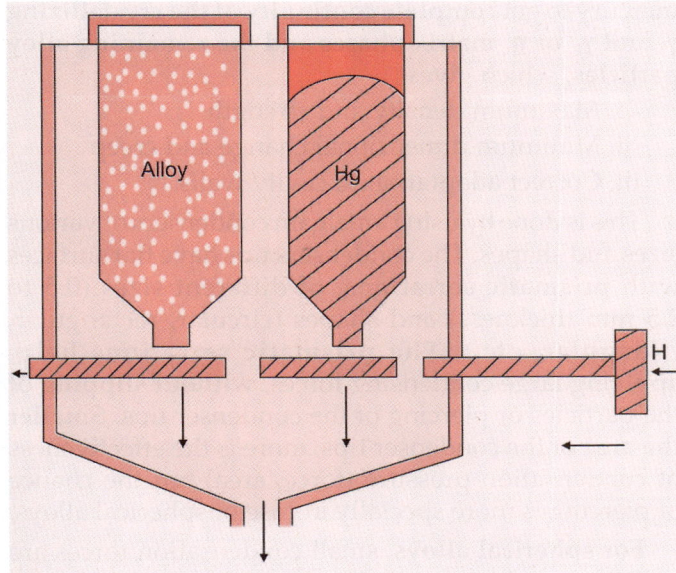

Fig. 12.8: Volume dispenser

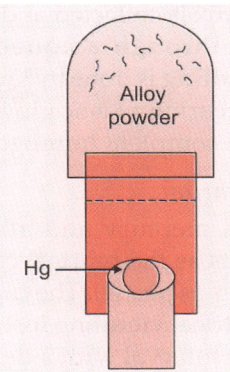

Fig. 12.9: Capsule

These volume dispensers are now incorporated in the amalgamator itself. Volume dispensers contain mercury and powder in two separate compartments. These should have more than half—full of mercury or alloy to get correct Hg/alloy ratio. When the handle H is pressed a small amount of alloy and required mercury come out and collect in the mixer. The ratio can be adjusted by controlling the orifice size. The orifices through which alloy and mercury pass out should be **kept clean.**

Small pellets of the alloy were used in some special volume dispensers. On releasing, one pellet and a drop of mercury of suitable size also comes out.

- **Preproportioned disposable capsules:** These contain, a certain amount of powder and a small sachet of mercury in two separate compartments or powder and mercury separated by a membrane, in the capsule (Fig. 12.9). The first few vibrations bring them into contact, during the mechanical trituration. **The advantages of this pre-proportioned system** are the mercury will not get spilled out, the correct mercury alloy ratio is maintained and very convenient for trituration.
  The disadvantage is that it is not possible to change the ratio by small amounts if required by the clinician.

4. Trituration

Mercury does not wet by itself or come into close contact with the alloy particles due to:

- A very thin oxide film present as an atomic layer on the surface of the alloy particles
- The large surface tension (460 dynes/cm) of mercury tending to retain the spherical shape of the drop

- The large angle of contact of mercury (130°–140°) with different phases of the alloys.
  Trituration is the mixing procedure, to remove the oxide film by friction and enhance the amalgamation reactions.

Trituration methods

- **Hand trituration** using glass (ceramic) mortar and pestle
- **Mechanical trituration** by violent vibration of the mix in special capsules.
- Amalgamators with time and Hg/alloy ratio controls.

Hand trituration

Suitable mortar and pestle of glass or ceramics are selected so that the tip of the pestle comes into close contact with the curved space at the floor of mortar. They are cleaned and roughened using **carborundum paper.** The proportioned mercury and alloy are collected, and triturated. The pestle is held by, **palm grip, thumb or fist grips,** to apply adequate force, to rub off the oxide layer on the particles and wet them with mercury. Trituration should be done **vigorously for about 45 to 60 sec** until a **homogeneous shining paste-like** mix is obtained.

Precautions

- Inadequate (or under) mixing causes noncohesive mix with a large number of dark spots.
- Low Hg/alloy ratio, i.e. too much alloy powder, cause incomplete wetting and noncohesive mix with black spots.
- High Hg/alloy ratio cause too thin, and shining mix with more fluidity.
- Overmixing (trituration) increases flow, consumes more mercury, produces a larger amount of weaker γ_1 and γ_2 phases.
- Correct trituration produces a **homogeneous plastic mass.**

The triturated mix is collected and the **extra mercury is squeezed out through a squeeze cloth** using a tweezer. **Hand mulling** is done by kneading in the palm of the left hand (wearing plastic gloves) and right hand thumb, to achieve complete **homogeneity**.

Mechanical trituration

The proportioned mercury and alloy are taken in a capsule (which acts as the mortar) containing a plastic cylinder (which acts as pestle). The capsule is vigorously vibrated in an electrical vibrating instrument (Fig. 12.10) for a definite time interval with a definite frequency of vibrations.

The present amalgamators have the volume dispensers (with facilities of changing Hg alloy ratio by small percentages), regulators of the speed of vibration and time controls. It is possible to triturate at **shorter times (20–30 sec) and get reproducible mixes.**

The capsules should not be opened immediately, as the fine particles or vapours of mercury come out and pollute the atmosphere or enter into the respiratory system of the clinical personnel. After a few seconds it is opened, the **pestle rod** is removed and again vibrated for a very short time **5–10 sec.** This **mechanical mulling** gives more homogeneous mix. (If required the excess mercury is squeezed out. But according to **EAME's minimal mercury technique" Hg/alloy ratio is adjusted to 1:1 by weight and no squeezing is to be done.**)

If the alloy is used in **pellet form**, a small metal (stainless steel) cylindrical pestle is used inside the plastic or metal capsule (mortar), as it is more difficult to break the pellets (Fig. 12.10).

The trituration time cannot be given exactly as it depends on the composition of the alloys shape and size of the particle, speed of vibrations, etc.

5. Condensation

Condensation is the procedure of compacting the **Hg + alloy mix** into the prepared cavity with sufficient

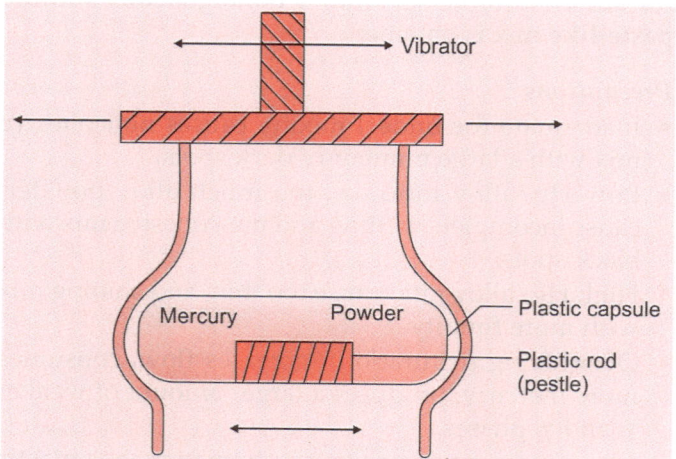

Fig. 12.10: Electrical vibrator

(labels in figure: Vibrator; Mercury; Powder; Plastic capsule; Plastic rod (pestle))

mercury to get **complete continuity of the crystallizing γ_1 and γ_2 or η matrix phases and the remaining alloy particles,** which gives

i. Maximum density and strength
ii. Minimum dimensional change and creep
iii. Correct adaptation to cavity walls.

This is done by using amalgam condensers of various sizes and shapes. The condensers tips have flat surfaces with **prismatic serrations,** of different sizes (0.5 to 2.5 mm thickness) and shapes (circular, rectangular, triangular, etc.). **The prismatic serrations help,** applying large condensing forces, **without slipping** of the particles or piercing of the condenser tips. **Smaller the area** of the condenser tips, more is the effectiveness of condensation pressure (force/area) but the chance of piercing is more specially in case of spherical alloys.

For spherical alloys, small condensation forces are sufficient, and larger condensers can be used. Also the mechanical properties are not seriously affected by condensation forces.

Methods of condensation

a. Increasing dryness technique

After mulling, the mix is carried through the amalgam carrier and ejected into the cavity. It is then condensed, first with larger condenser, thoroughly applying large **forces (1.5–1.7 kg)** for adapting properly. The excess mercury squeezed to surface is **partly removed** (the remaining parts help to bond the next increment). Then the next increment is carried, ejected, condensed homogeneously and part of excess mercury is carefully removed. This is repeated until the cavity is slightly overfilled (for carving). Smaller condensers and of different shapes are suitably selected for **marginal adaptations.** Mercury left out, after compacting each increment should be gradually decreased to nil on the final layer, i.e. "increasing dryness, technique".

b. EAME's minimal mercury technique

This is much simpler and commonly used. Mercury/alloy ratio is made 1:1 by weight. After trituration **squeezing of excess mercury is not done.** After condensing each increment, the excess mercury on the surface is left behind, to bond with the next increment.

Precautions

- Large condensation forces 1.5 to 1.7 kg are to be applied carefully and homogeneously for lathe-cut alloys.
- During condensation, **mercury rich thin mix should not be moved** or pushed to the cavity boundaries. Excess mercury continues amalgamation reaction

producing more weaker phases at margins, producing **mercuroscopic expansion** and marginal breakdown.

Restoration is to be conducted under perfect **dry conditions using rubber dams** (*refer* to delayed expansion). For large cavities, the single mix may not be sufficient. Two or three mixes should be arranged and used immediately, as the working time is only about 3–4 min.

Carving and finishing

Carving of restoration is required only to **simulate anatomy** and not to get finer details. Carving is delayed usually for about 15–20 minutes until the material shows certain resistance to the carving instrument, otherwise the restoration may be pulled away from the margins. Carving instruments need not have very sharp blades. These have different shapes and named as diamond carver, Wartz carver, Hollenback carver, etc.

Burnishing

This is the procedure for smoothening the carved surface by carefully **rubbing** with sphere-tipped-ball burnishers or T burnishers usually made up of stainless steel. Final burnishing can be done by moving **a wet cotton pellet** over the surface. **The burnishing removes small pits or scratches on the surface** (and reduces the chances of concentration cell or crevice corrosion).

Burnishing has become a **controversial subject.** Even though it gives a smooth surface and improves marginal adaptation, there is a chance for pushing or **moving mercury-rich thin mix** to the margins of restoration (where mercury reacts further, etc. mercuroscopic expansion, creep).

Final finishing is delayed for about 24 hours for low copper alloys and at least **1 hour for high copper** single composition alloys. The material should set into a sufficiently hard surface. If required contouring can be done with slow-speed handpieces using fine diamond points, brown or green rubber points. Fine pumice, zirconium silicate, tin oxide, etc. polishing powders can be finally used. These powders are made into a **thick slurry** in water/alcohol and applied with a rotary felt wheel or brush on the surface. Polishing with the **dry powders should not be done** as they can quickly **raise the temperature of restoration above 60°C** and cause some irreversible changes. Very smooth polished glossy, lustrous surface does not have much advantages, on corrosion resistance, longer life, etc. But certain polishing is required for resisting corrosion and prevent the collection of food debris.

Marginal Deteriorations (Ditched Restorations)

Marginal breakdown or failures are quite common in amalgam restorations (Fig. 12.11). These are mainly due to improper cavity preparations, wrong selections, and manipulation of the alloys. Following are the main causes.

1. **Improper cavity preparation and finishing:** The amalgam is a brittle material having a low modulus of resilience (R). The posterior restoration is frequently subjected to large dynamic masticating forces. **The ability to withstand these large dynamic, impact forces is** $= KVR$, where V is the volume, R is the modulus of resilience and K is the **geometric design factor**. The cavity of large volume V is to be designed without producing any thin extensions. The thin extensions are liable to fracture very easily, causing marginal failures. Finishing of the margins should **not cause flattening or thinning**.

2. **Mercuroscopic expansion:** Careless condensation and burnishing procedures may push the **mercury-rich thin mix to the margins** and continue to react with the alloy producing more weaker matrix for a long time. High mercury/alloy ratio also may cause these weak margins and expansions which can fracture easily.

3. **High creep of the alloy restorations** also results in a fracture. Proper selection, low mercury/alloy ratio, correct trituration, and condensation procedures, can reduce creep and the chance of fracture.

Food debris collected at these deteriorated margins, **cause crevice cell corrosion,** unhygienic condition, and secondary caries. **Ditched restoration** has poor aesthetic qualities. Suitable precautions can reduce these failures. Such marginal failures can also be repaired.

Repair of Amalgam Restoration

Small broken parts specially at the margins can be repaired. The surfaces are cleaned and a fresh amalgam mix is condensed against remaining part. However, the **old and new** restorations do not combine with good bond strength and may fracture again at this site, if it is a high stress bearing area.

If the tooth enamel is exposed, it can be acid etched. Then special dentin bonding agent (amalgam bond) can be applied. Fresh amalgam mix is **immediately condensed before the bonding agent sets.**

As the bond strengths are weak such repairs should be attempted only at the non-stress bearing areas.

Preparation of the old amalgamation restoration or its removal with diamond points, carbide burs, etc. release mercury which is health hazardous and hence the repair procedures are minimized.

Tarnish and Corrosion of Amalgam Restorations

Tarnish is the discolouration of metallic restorations in the oral environments. Sulphur, chlorine, and fluorine containing food may react with silver, copper, and tin to cause discolourations.

Corrosion is the continuation of the chemical attack or electrochemical reactions, resulting in the loss of material from the surface. **Tin has the least corrosion resistance.** Silver amalgam is a multiphase in homogeneous material and undergoes several types of corrosions. The γ_1, **i.e. Ag_2Hg_3 phase has highest, and γ_2, i.e. Sn_{7-8} Hg phase has the lowest corrosion resistance.** Different phases can be arranged according to increasing order of corrosion resistance as, Sn_{7-8} $Hg(\gamma_2)$, $Cu_6Sn_5(\eta)$, Cu_3Sn, $Ag_3Sn(\gamma)$, $Ag_3Cu_2(\epsilon)$ and Ag_2Hg_3 (γ_1).

The corrosion products are chlorides, fluorides, sulphides and sometimes mercury also get released, which again produce weaker γ_1 and γ_2 phases.

In low copper alloys due to the intermeshing of γ_2 phase, corrosion takes place throughout and is highest. High copper alloys have greater corrosion resistance. If the surface is **not well polished,** and **margins are not properly adapted, crevice corrosion** can take place. **Electrochemical corrosion** also takes place, when a **high copper amalgam** (cathodic) comes into contact with the low copper (conventional) amalgam opposing restorations. Similarly, amalgam restoration coming into contact with **base metal or noble metal alloy** restorations (in the opposing teeth), undergo galvanic corrosion.

To minimise corrosion
- Avoid dissimilar (high and low copper) amalgams in the opposing teeth.
- Avoid amalgam restoration against any other metallic restorations
- Proper condensation at the margins
- Do not use low copper alloys
- The surface should be well polished
- Mercury/alloy ratio should be minimum.

The severe corrosion at the margins can cause ditching and deteriorations. However, the corrosion products, initially collect and **seal the margins of restorations and reduce microleakage.**

Microleakage

The penetration of oral fluids, through the marginal gaps between restoration and tooth walls is known as micro (or marginal) leakage. The causes are:
- Amalgam has a higher coefficient of thermal expansions (25 ppm/°C) than tooth enamel (11.4 ppm/°C). When the patient takes hot or cold foods, the restorations and the teeth **expand differently. This causes percolation of oral fluids resulting in marginal or microleakage.**

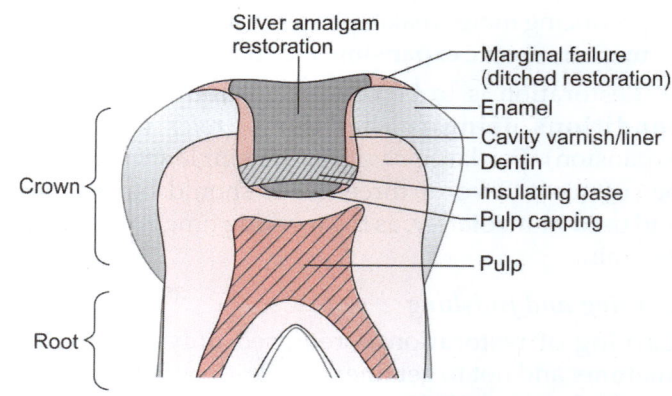

Fig. 12.11: Amalgam restoration steps

- **Contraction** of amalgam during hardening. Recent high copper alloys undergo less contraction during setting.
- Marginal breakdowns due to various factors. Microleakage causes deterioration at the cavity walls and fails the restorations (Fig. 12.11).

Remedies
- Apply cavity varnishes, to seal the exposed dentin tubules
- Use amalgam bonds (special dentin bonding agents, 4-META)
- The initial corrosion products seal the margins automatically
- Select the alloy having least dimensional changes
- Condense the amalgam carefully.

Amalgam Bond

One of the main drawbacks of the amalgam is its **inability to chemically bond** with the tooth structure. Due to this, microleakage and poor retention of thin sections, cannot be avoided.

Particular dentin bonding agent which can bond composite resins with metals and teeth 4-META (4-methacryloxyethyl trimellitate anhydride) has been tried for bonding amalgam to teeth structure successfully. The bonding agent is supplied as a powder–liquid system with adhesives, acid etching agents, etc. **Amalgam mix is to be condensed along with this material before it sets.**

However, the bonding agent **cannot bond amalgam to amalgam** in the repairing procedures.

MERCURY HEALTH HAZARDS

Silver amalgam has a long history of more than 100 years as a posterior restorative material, but since few decades it has become the most controversial dental material due to mercury toxicity. But BisGMA and other composite restorative resins, on which dentists had much hopes, as they can be a better substitute silver amalgam, have also been recently found to be estrogenic materials.

High toxicity and the resulting health hazards of mercury are well-established facts. Mercury can enter into the body through respiratory and circulatory systems, by ingestion, through the skin or as vapours into the respiratory system and through food diet into the circulatory systems. **Mercury is present as pure metal (Hg^{++}), as metal ions (Hg^{2+}) or organic forms methyl or N-ethyl mercury. (This most toxic form is released by bacterial activities on food debris.)** In dentistry, mercury is released, during abrasion of amalgam restorations, or trapped in the restoration, which can migrate easily to body systems.

Also, mercury vapours are inhaled during use in the clinics by clinical personnel and also by workers in mercury processing factories. The only minimal amount of mercury is excreted, through urine and feces, and large parts accumulate in the body system.

Symptoms of mercury toxicity depend on the form and amount of mercury in the body system. The mercury levels are found to rise in the blood, liver, bile, kidneys, spleen, lungs, renal cortex, etc. Some of the symptoms of mercury toxicities are fatigue, weakness, headache, dizziness, tingling sensations at the extremities (paraesthesia), eyelids, fingers, renal disorders, etc. depending on the accumulated mercury. For example, paraesthesia if mercury content is ≥ 0.5 mg/kg, ataxia if ≥ 1.0 mg/kg, joint pains if >2 mg/kg and death if ≥ 4 mg/kg, weight of person.

The occupational safety and health administration (OSHA) and ADA have prescribed threshold level values (TLV) for the amount of mercury vapours in atmosphere as <50 mg/m^3, in blood <3 mg/liter and <7 mg/liter in urine.

People working in mercury processing factories inhale more mercury vapour and have a TLV about 350–500 mg per day.

Large dosages of mercury enter into our body system, through the seafood (fish, etc.), other dietary foods, even water, atmosphere, etc.

However, a lot of dental researches, have shown, that the amount of mercury released by wearing or trapped in the amalgam restoration even if there are 10 or 20 amalgam restorations in the amalgam restoration in the patients mouth are **very negligible** and perhaps the patients have no grounds to complain regarding the health hazards of the amalgam restoration.

But the dentists and clinical personnel have to take it up very seriously, as they are constantly exposed to mercury in the clinics, directly or to vapours. Mercury is a highly volatile substance, with a saturated vapour pressure (20 mg/m^3) which is about **400 times the TLV**. Hence, the following precautions should be followed very strictly.

- Keep the mercury always in air-tight bottles. Open the bottles only for short times when needed.
- Do not touch mercury directly and hence wear plastic hand gloves and masks.
- Do not spill mercury on the floor or carpets (better not to use carpets as they are difficult to clean).
- Do not open the capsules immediately after trituration.
- Do not throw the waste excess mix into the wash basins, dustbin or on the floor.
- Collect all the waste underwater or **sodium thiosulphate** solution.
- This waste should be disposed by burying at large depth.
- Wash the clinics everyday with special detergents.
- Keep the clinics well-ventilated.
- Check the mercury vapour content in the clinics periodically.
- Conduct the mercury level determination tests in blood, urine, nails, etc. of the clinical personnel frequently. They can wear the special mercury indicator badges.

SPHERICAL SILVER AMALGAM ALLOYS

The high copper single composition amalgam alloys are sometimes manufactured and supplied as small spherical or spheroidal particles to have better properties. The molten alloy liquid is atomized or sprayed into a chamber evacuated or filled with inert argon gas. Fine spherical or spheroidal liquid drops solidify as such. Particles of sizes 15 to 75 μm are selected, heat treated for forming enough γ phase and then acid washed.

The spherical particles have the least surface area and hence require less mercury for wetting and reactions. Accordingly the advantages over lathe-cut alloys are:

- Shorter setting time
- Easier trituration
- Lower condensation pressure
- Higher one hour and final strengths
- Lower creep values
- Less mercuroscopic expansion
- Better surface finish and easy to finish
- No delayed expansion as no zinc is used.

Disadvantages

- Too short working time
- Larger dimensional changes during setting
- The triturated mix is more plastic and difficult to condense. As the spherical particles easily slip during condensation, the **wedged matrix** is required for establishing proximal contour.

Advantages and disadvantages of silver amalgam restorations

Silver amalgam posterior restorations became very popular during the last century due to its superior mechanical properties and simple restoration techniques compared to other metallic restorations.

Advantages

- Adequate mechanical properties like high compressive strength, modulus of elasticity, abrasive resistance, etc.
- The direct filling restoration method is quite simple compared to other alternatives, like castings.
- Sufficient long service time, about 5 to 15 years if the manipulation is done carefully.
- Can retain the anatomic forms.
- Microleakage stops after a few months by the collection of corrosion products, in the margins.
- Not expensive like metal castings.

Disadvantages

- Mercury contamination, health hazards to dental personnel
- Poor corrosion resistance
- Allergic, and toxic to a few patients
- Brittle material undergoes bulk fracture or marginal failures (ditched restorations).
- Low impact strength. Hence, the cavity should be designed with large volume, that is more healthy tooth material is to be removed.
- Large dimensional changes during setting, delayed expansions, creep, etc.
- Large thermal expansion, $\alpha = 25$ ppm/°C which is double that of tooth structure, 11.4 ppm/°C, and causes microleakage.
- Not a good insulator of heat or electricity. Thermal shock, galvanic shock, etc. should be prevented using insulating bases.
- Poor aesthetic quality.
- No chemical bonding. Hence, a large undercut is needed for mechanical, retention. **Amalgam bond (using 4-META) has been tried.**
- Proper precautions are to be followed in every step of manipulation for achieving best results.

Applications

- Permanent posterior restorative materials for class I and class II cavities and also for class V cavities, when aesthetic is not important
- Sometimes retrograde root canal fillings
- Silver retentive pins are used for reinforcement
- Sometimes as die materials, for rigid impressions.

OTHER DIRECT FILLING ALLOYS
Gallium Alloys

Gallium is a greyish metal of low density, 5.9 gm/cc and **low melting temperature 29.8°C** which can be used as an alternative to mercury. The melting temperature of gallium is **depressed by adding tin and indium,** and makes it remain as liquid at room temperatures. This can be triturated with the Ag-Sn-Cu alloys like mercury.

One such gallium alloy has the following composition

Powder	Liquid
Silver = 50%	Gallium = 65%
Tin = 25%	Indium = 18.5% }
Copper = 15%	Tin = 16% } depress MP of Ga
Palladium = 9.0%	Trace elements 0.5%
Trace elements = 0.35	

Trituration and Microstructure

On trituration the new phases formed are $CuGa_2$, $PdGa_5$, Ag_9Ga_3 and beta-tin. These surround and bind the unreacted particles.

Properties

Compressive strength is quite high at one hour = 343 MPa and at 24 hours = 383 MPa. Tensile strength = 57 MPa, low creep = 0.17%. The setting expansion is more. The greater corrosion takes place like conventional amalgams as the powder have the same components.

Biocompatibility

Initial researches have shown that **biocompatibility is not good** but there is no mercury health hazard.

Advantages

- No mercury health hazards.
- Less microleakages as the **paste** has better marginal adaptations.
- Mechanical properties are adequate.

Disadvantages

- The mix is like **a paste and difficult to fill**
- Very dry field is required for filling
- Lower corrosion resistance
- Cause adverse effects on the pulp
- More cytotoxic than traditional alloys

Manipulation (trituration) with alcohol improves the handling properties.

Copper Amalgam

The antibacterial effect of copper initiated the use of copper amalgam for deciduous teeth in case of rampant caries. This is supplied in the form of pellets of amalgamated copper. This has about **30–40% copper and 60–70% mercury.** The **pellets are heated in steel spatula until the mercury droplets come to the surface,** and then triturated and condensed into the cavity-like conventional silver amalgam. This is not used nowadays due to:

- Low corrosion resistance
- Large excess mercury, i.e. poor mercury hygiene
- Lower mechanical properties.

Indium Containing Amalgam Alloys

A quaternary alloy with Ag = 59%, Cu = 13%, tin = 24% and indium = 4% has been developed and supplied in spheroidal form. The **indium content** in mercury has been increased up to about **30%** in some of experimental alloys. The properties of this alloy are almost similar to high copper single composition alloys. This has low static creep value, 0.06 to 0.1% and high mechanical properties—compressive strength, at one hour = 210–240 MPa, and after complete setting = 430 to 480 MPa. **Indium has a low melting point of 157°C** and replaces some mercury. Hence, mercury vapour pollution is reduced.

Properties

- Low static creep value, 0.06–0.11%
- Sufficient compressive strength at 1 hour = 210–240 MPa at 24 hours = 430–480 MPa
- Indium has a low MP (157°C) and replaces some mercury, i.e. less mercury vapour pollution
- Metallic lustre

Further research is needed regarding the toxicity, marginal leakage, failures, etc. However, instead of this, more research is concentrated **on hybrid composite resins for posterior restorations** due to its aesthetic properties and bonding to tooth structures through bonding agents.

MODEL QUESTIONS

I. Long Essays   (20 minutes each)

1. Describe the compositions, manufacturing method, amalgamation reactions, and microstructures of various silver amalgam alloys and set masses.
2. Describe the high copper silver amalgam alloys, their amalgamation, microstructure, and their advantages.
3. Describe, in detail, manipulation of silver amalgam.
4. Describe the various causes for dimensional changes of silver amalgam. Add a note on creep.

II. Short Essays   (10 minutes each)

1. Manufacturing of lathe-cut alloys
2. High copper amalgam alloys
3. Amalgamation reactions and microstructures
4. Trituration
5. Strength of silver amalgam
6. Dimensional changes on the setting of silver amalgam
7. Microleakage
8. Delayed expansion
9. Creep of silver amalgam
10. Clinical significance of dimensional changes (ditching)
11. Mercury health hazards and precautions in clinical practices.

III. Brief Answers   (5 minutes each)

1. Spherical alloys alternate to lathe-cut silver amalgam alloys
2. Microstructures of high copper amalgam
3. Disperse alloys
4. Mercuroscopic expansion
5. Criteria for selection of silver amalgam alloys
6. Properties of silver amalgam
7. Silver amalgam condensers
8. Condensation of silver amalgam
9. Eame's technique
10. "Increasing dryness" technique
11. Burnishing
12. Finishing of amalgam restoration
13. Amalgam bond
14. Repairing of amalgam restorations
15. Copper amalgam
16. Gallium amalgam
17. Indium amalgam

Dental Ceramics

Search for aesthetically suitable, ideal restorative materials, lead to the research and development of many varieties of ceramics. In dentistry, there are mainly **four varieties of materials**, with different characteristic properties. These are **metals (alloys)**, **polymers, composites,** and **ceramics.** Dental alloys have high tensile strength, toughness, hardness, fracture resistance, abrasive resistance, elasticity, ductility malleability, fatigue resistance, etc. Polymers have **inferior mechanical properties**, whereas composites have superior aesthetic qualities even though, they may undergo brittle fractures like polymers.

Ceramics are nonmetallic inorganic structures of simple compounds of oxygen with one or more metallic or semimetallic materials (like Si, Al, Ca, Li, Na, K, Mg, P, Ti, Zr, etc.). Many dental ceramics have amorphous glass, crystalline or semicrystalline phases.

There can be four varieties of ceramics

1. **Amorphous silicate ceramics** (SiO_2 with small amounts of glass formers, i.e. Al_2O_3, MgO, ZrO_2, etc.
2. **Crystalline oxide ceramics** ($MgO + Al_2O_3$, $3Al_2O_3 + SiO_2$ $Al_2O_3 + TiO_2$ etc., used as refractory materials of modern investments for titanium castings).

3. **Partially crystalline glass ceramics** (like DICOR, glass matrix with tetrasilicic fluormica crystals.
4. **Non-oxide ceramics** (borides, carbides, nitrides, selenides, silicides, etc.) which are not used for dental restorations, but only as abrasives.

Structure and Characteristic Properties

Glass Formers

The tetrahedral structure of SiO_2, $-O-\overset{\displaystyle O}{\underset{\displaystyle O}{\mathrm{Si}}}-O-$ has the Si^{4+} cations at the center, and the anions at each of the corners. This structure due to short range oxygen valency bonding is amorphous and very rigid. Similarly, Al_2O_3, MgO, ZrO_2, etc. also act as glass formers. These have very high fusion temperatures, very low thermal expansions and are perfect insulators. That is why, during solidification, these form **vitreous** (liquid) structure.

Glass Interruptors

By adding the metallic ions (K^+, Na^+, Al^{+++}, Ca^{++}), it is possible to break the oxygen bonding, which causes certain amount of crystallization, or devitrifications, and an increase of COTE (as required for metal ceramic bondings.) These are known as **glass interrupters**.

Following are the characteristic properties of most ceramics

- Chemically inert, biocompatible
- Insoluble in oral fluids, but absorb water, etc. and undergo slight degradation.
- **No free electrons, but only oxygen bonding and hence**,
  - Brittle, nonductile, nonmalleable
  - High compressive strength and hardness
  - Low tensile, shear and flexure strengths
  - Low COTE (6–12 ppm/°C)
  - **Perfect insulators**, due to lack of conducting electrons. Solidifies as amorphous vitreous structure with a very large number of **microcracks.** Glazing improves surface integrity and flexure strengths.
  - **Transparent or translucent** colour pigments or frits added, give permanent excellent desired aesthetics.

Porcelains are a class of ceramics which contain glass matrix with one or more crystalline phases, but crystal formation does not take place by controlled nucleation or crystal growth (as in alloys).

Enormous research is taking place in this field of dental ceramics. Recently many varieties of ceramics have been developed, and fabrication of restorations is done by utilizing the sophisticated modern technologies. Many of the drawbacks of ceramics have been overcome by new technologies, such as metal ceramics, glass infiltration, CAD-CAM, copy milling, etc.

CLASSIFICATION OF DENTAL CERAMICS

1. **According to compositions**
   - Feldspathic (K, Na or Ca aluminosilicates)
   - Leucite based
   - Lithia based
   - Aluminous
   - Pure alumina, silica, zirconia.
2. **According to processing**
   - Condensation and sintering or firing in the air, in diffusible gases, or in vacuum
   - Partial sintering and glass infiltration
   - Hot pressing, casting, slip casting
   - Computer-aided designing and computer-aided machining (CAD-CAM)
   - Copy milling and machining.
3. **Varieties used**
   - Core porcelain
   - Opaque porcelain
   - Body (dentin) porcelain
   - Gingival, neck or cervical porcelain
   - Enamel (incisal) porcelain
   - Colour frits (pigments)
   - Glaze porcelains
4. **According to fusion temperatures**
   - High fusing (>1300°C) used for artificial teeth
   - Medium fusing (1100°–1300°C) used for artificial teeth
   - Low fusing (850°–1100°C), crown and bridges, veneers, metal ceramics
   - Ultra low fusing (<850°C), metal ceramics and casting.

Note: Since medium and high fusing porcelains are used only for fabrication of porcelain teeth, others are sometimes classified as, high fusing (850°–1100°C) and low fusing <850°C.

5. **According to microstructure**
   - Amorphous glass
   - Crystal-containing glass
   - Crystalline porcelain
   - Partially crystallized porcelain.
6. **According to transparency**
   Opaque, translucent, transparent.
7. **According to applications**
   - Porcelain or ceramic jacket crowns and veneers
   - Post and cores
   - Fixed partial dentures
   - Stains and colour frits glazes
   - Metal ceramics (PFM—porcelain fused to metal)
   - Anterior and posterior restoratives.

Dispensing methods

The ceramic compositions are melted fritted (quenched to produce microcracks), and powdered into small particles of different sizes. This mixture helps better close packing during condensation to reduce firing volume shrinkages. Opacifiers, shades, colour frits are also incorporated before melting. Sometimes shades and colour frits are provided separately. The powders of various shades transparencies like opaquers, dentin, enamel, incisal and colour frits, are provided in different varieties in large numbers for selection (*see* Colour Plate 24, Fig. 13.2).

Special binder liquids are sometimes provided for use, instead of distilled water.

Feldspathic Porcelains

These ceramics are called porcelains. These contain SiO_2 (52–62%), Al_2O_3 (11–16%), K_2O (9–11%), Na_2O (5–7%), small amounts of lithium, boron, etc. oxides and colour frits. These have an amorphous glass matrix with one or two crystalline phases. All porcelains are not ceramics as the crystal formation is not formed by nucleation and crystal growth. The feldspathic porcelains have low and ultra low fusion temperatures due to the presence of devitrifiers. Glazes and stains are included in this. Composition of dental is ceramics shown in Table 13.1.

Table 13.1	The compositions of dental ceramics	
Ingredients	**wt%**	**Functions**
1. Feldspar	60–80	Basic glass former
2. Alumina	8–20	Strengthener, glass former, opacifier
3. Kaolin	3–5	Binder during firing
4. Quartz	15–20	Filler
5. Boric oxide	2–7	Glass former, flux
6. Oxides of Na, K, Ca	9–15	Glass modifiers, interrupter, fluxes
7. Metallic pigments	<1	Colour matching (oxides of Zn, Sn, Ti)
8. Many other oxides of	Trace	As colour pigments and ZrO_2, SnO_2, BaO, TiO_2, shade B_2O_3

VARIETIES OF FELDSPARS

These are obtained as mineral ores of three varieties, of aluminosilicates as:

- Potash feldspar: $K_2O. Al_2O_3. 6SiO_2$
- Soda feldspar: $Na_2O. Al_2O_3. 6SiO_2$
- Lime feldspar: $CaO. Al_2O_3. 6SiO_2$

These form clear, colourless glasses, which require suitable colour pigments to be added.

Silica: SiO_2 exists in four varieties, i.e. crystalline quartz, tridymite, cristobalite and amorphous fused quartz. On melting at very high temperatures, they form transparent glasses with **three-dimensional SiO_4 networks.**

GLASS MODIFIERS

By adding metallic ions of K^+, Na^+, Ca^{++}, as their oxides, the silica covalent oxygen bonding can be **interrupted** and many linear chains are formed. These can rather more easily slip one over the other. This **reduces the slip resistance, Tg, fusion temperatures, COTE and cause devitrification or partial crystallization.**

Absorption or addition of water also act as glass modifier by **hydronium ion H_3O^+** replacing the metal ions and cause slow deterioration of the mechanical properties. Addition of too much devitrifiers cause **degradation** of ceramics.

Kaolin is purified clay, used as a binder during fabrication. This is **hydrated aluminosilicate Al_2O_3.**

$2SiO_2. 2H_2O$. When mixed with water, it becomes sticky and holds the ceramic powder particles together. **It increases opacity and shrinkage** during firing (some manufacturers add starch instead of kaolin).

Colour pigments metallic oxides are added in small amounts to impart different colours, e.g. **Cr_2O_3, CuO (green), Fe_2O_3 (brown), CoO (blue), TiO_2 (yellowish brown), MnO (lavender),** etc. Uranium oxide and lanthanides are used to provide fluorescence, ZrO_2, TiO_2, SnO, CeO, etc. act as opacifiers. These are prepared as fine powders, by grinding along with the glasses, and supplied in different opacities, shades, fusion temperatures, etc. varieties.

Properties of Feldspathic Porcelain (Table 13.2)

1. **Excellent** biocompatibility, chemical inertness in oral conditions.
2. **Inadequate** mechanical properties, the disadvantage
   - High brittleness
   - Low shear and diametral tensile strengths
   - Low compressive strength
   - Low impact strength or fracture resistance
   - Greater surface hardness (460 KHN) than tooth enamel. (This causes the abrasion and wearing of the opposing natural tooth.)
   - Structural degradation (porcelain absorbs slowly small amount of water and ionic solutions which cause **degradation due to interruption of silica network,** and decrease the mechanical properties further).
3. Low COTE, nearly same as tooth enamel
4. Good thermal insulator
5. **Excellent aesthetic properties.** Suitable colour pigments, stains or shades can be applied on the finished article, and then glazing is to be done. This gives **natural lifelike appearance.** The decalcified check lines on the natural tooth surface can easily be reproduced. **The colour parameters (i.e. hue, chroma and values) are permanent (Table 13.2).**

Table 13.2	Some properties of feldspathic porcelain	
1.	Compressive strength	170 MPa
2.	Ultimate tensile strength	25 MPa
3.	Shear strength	110 MPa
4.	Transverse strength (unglazed)	70 MPa
5.	Transverse strength (glazed)	140 MPa
6.	Diametral tensile strength	35 MPa
7.	Elastic modulus	70,000 MPa
8.	Hardness (KHN)	460 kg/mm^2
9.	Fracture toughness	0.7–0.8 MPa $\sqrt{m}$
10.	Refractive index	1.504
11.	Coefficient of thermal expansion	9–12 ppm/°C

Leucite

When feldspathic porcelain is heated to a high temperature (1150°–1530°C), it undergoes incongruent melting, forming a glossy liquid and leucite crystals. It begins to flow and coalesce the particles, i.e. liquid phase sintering. This incongruent melting is represented as

$$\text{Feldspar (solid)} \xrightarrow{\text{(1150°–1530°C)}} \text{liquid + leucite crystals}$$

Leucite is a potassium aluminosilicate **$K_2O.Al_2O_3.4SiO_2$ and has higher COTE = 20–25 ppm/°C,** compared to feldspar 7–10 ppm/°C. This is an advantage for bonding metal ceramics as the COTE can be raised to mismatch slightly with COTE metal castings.

Recrystallized alumina Al_2O_3, is used as core porcelain. It is added as glass modifier, and also as hardener due to **interruption of crack propagation.** But the addition of Al_2O_3 **increases opacity.**

TOUGHENING OF PORCELAIN

During solidification, first, the outermost layer of the liquid solidifies forming a **skin,** which contracts exerting large compressive forces on the liquid inside. The liquid inside solidifies slowly as there are no conducting free electrons. It forms a **vitreous (liquid) solid.** The reaction exerted inside against the compressions due to thermal shrinkage of the outer solid layer causes a large number of microcracks. These decrease the mechanical properties due to **crack propagation,** as a very large concentration of stresses takes place at the tips of the cracks. **These brittleness and poor strength due to crack propagation is remedied by the following methods:**

1. Introduction of residual compressive stresses.
2. Interruption of crack propagation.
3. Proper design of articles reducing the stress raisers.

1. Introduction of Residual Compressive Surface Stresses

Principle: Ceramics are brittle materials having high compressive strengths and low tensile strengths. Let 100 MPa be the tensile strength of a ceramic article having a stress-free structure (or surface). Let a residual compressive stress of say 80 MPa, has been introduced. In such case, as the tensile stress is gradually increased, initially the induced compressive stress of 80 MPa get released and then the tensile stress can be further increased by 100 MPa. In other words, a total of 100 + 80 = 180 MPa, tensile stress can be applied to fracture the material, or the UTS becomes 180 MPa.

Methods

- **Ion exchange or chemical tempering**
  If a **soda feldspathic porcelain** article is kept immersed in **molten KNO_3** solution at about 450°C for few (20–30) minutes, the **smaller Na^+** ions are exchanged (or replaced) by the **K^+ions** which are about **30% bigger** in size. This replacement by ion exchange introduces large residual compressive surface stresses and increases tensile strengths. But this **chemical tempering** cannot be applied if ceramics do not have Na^+ ions (Fig. 13.1a).

- **Thermal tempering**
  If the ceramic article is **suddenly cooled** the outer surface solidifies first **forming a thicker skin** surround the softer molten core. The **rapid cooling** causes contraction, introducing residual compressive stresses. This method is used to **toughen, the automobile window shields, glass windows, etc. by sudden cooling** the surface, with a jet of cold air. If the glass windows are examined with polarized light, many concentric circular patches (made by the colliding air jet) can be observed.

- **Thermal compatibility or mismatching thermal expansions**
  The residual compressive stresses can be introduced in the surface, by choosing two or more layered, and bonded, ceramic compositions which have slightly different coefficient of thermal expansions. The veneering ceramics with two or more layers, **metal ceramic appliances, incerams, etc.** have residual compressive stresses due to, one layer contracting slightly more than the other adjacent layers, e.g. if the metal has slightly greater COTE (α_m = 13.5–14.00 ppm/°C) than the ceramics (α_c = 13.0–13.5 ppm/°C), the greater contraction of the metal introduces higher compressive stresses on the veneer surface.

2. Interruption of Crack Propagations

When a deforming force acts, it is most effective at the tips of chisel-like cracks, and separate the atoms, propagating the crack. If a harder particle (p) (Fig. 13.1) is introduced, cracks cannot easily propagate, i.e. strength increases. This is done by two methods.

- **Dispersion strengthening:** This is by introducing very hard crystalline phases, before fusing the porcelain, e.g. we have
  - Alumina-core porcelain with 90–95% alumina
  - Aluminous porcelain with 40–50% alumina (This is also used as core material. But an addition of higher percent of alumina **increases opacity**).
  - By introducing crystalline **leucite** ($K_2O.Al_2O_3.4SiO_2$), **lithia disilicate** ($Li_2O.2SiO_2$), **magnesia alumina spinel, zirconia,** etc.

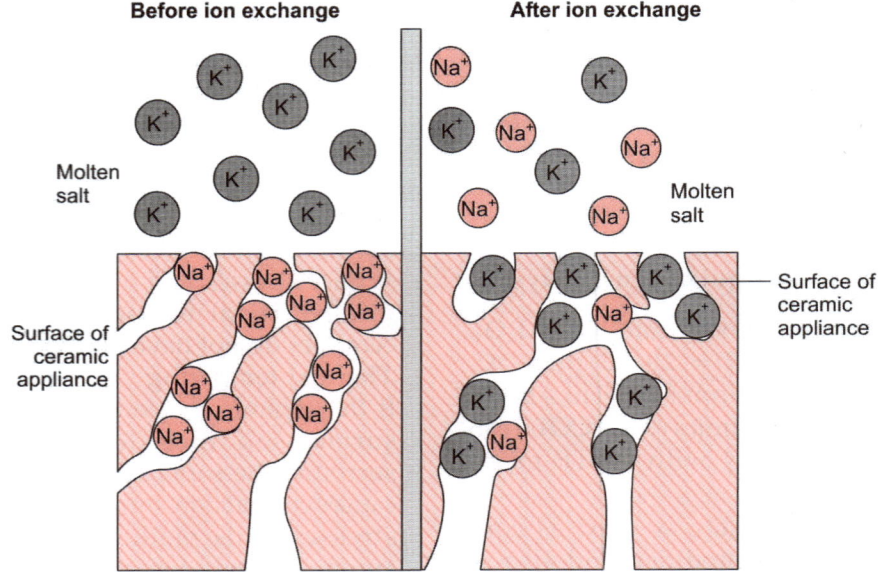

Fig. 13.1a: Strengthening of porcelain surface by replacing sodium ions with larger potassium ions

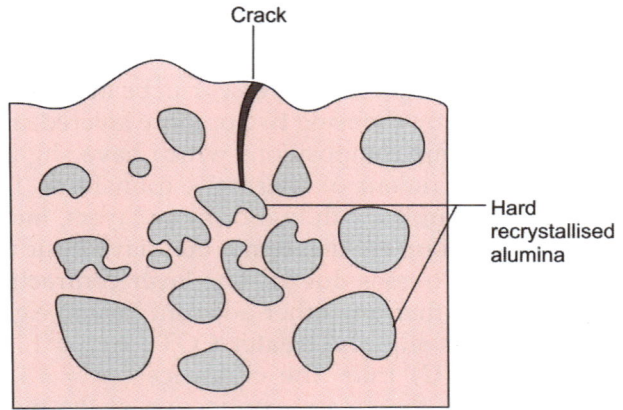

Fig. 13.1b: Dispersion strengthening

– By forming a crystalline phase by **devitrification as in ceramming.**

• **Transformation toughening:** Partially stabilized zirconia (metastable tetragonal) is introduced into ceramics at high temperatures. At a lower temperature, it transforms into more **stable monoclinic phase with 3% an increase in volume.** This transformation also takes place when the high stresses act at the crack tips. The monoclinic form is much harder and interrupts the crack propagation. **These are several mechanisms of the crack shielding principle (Fig. 13.1c).**

3. Design of the Article Avoiding Stress-raisers

Any **abrupt changes** in the thickness of the article, **sharp corners, wrinkles** in swagged metal copings,

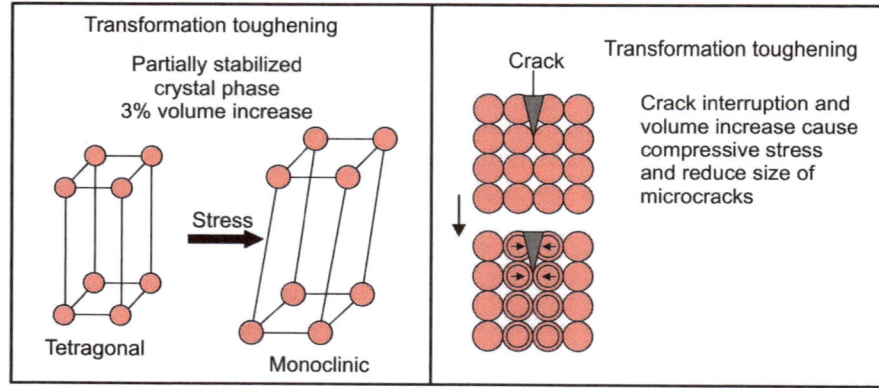

Fig. 13.1c: Toughening of ceramics by transformation toughening

etc. are the areas of large stress concentrations. These areas are known as **stress-raisers,** where the fracture failure takes place easily. Such weak points or areas of stress raisers should be avoided while designing the articles.

The various steps involved are

1. **Preliminaries**
   After recording the impression, a hard die of prepared tooth is made in a refractory material which is then closely adapted with a thin, **platinum foil (matrix) of 1/40 mm** without wrinkles. The matrix supports unfired porcelain and will not allow porcelain to flow during firing. The porcelain powders of suitable shades are chosen. A suitable amount of powder is mixed with water or a special liquid to form a **thick slurry** which is then applied over the platinum foil adapted on the die (Fig. 13.2).

2. **Condensation**
   The porcelain powder particles within the mass are closely packed to reduce the volume shrinkage of porcelain and minimize the porosity in the fired porcelain. **The process of closely packing the powder particles together and removing excess water is known as condensation.** There are 4 methods, which also can be combined.

   a. **Spatulation:** Surface of the article is carefully smoothened with a spatula when extra water from inside comes to the surface by capillary action which is removed by blotting paper or linen cloth.

   b. **Brush technique:** A small amount of dry powder is sprinkled over the article and carefully tapped with the brush. The powder absorbs the water from inside which can be removed.

   c. **Vibration method:** The article is carefully vibrated and the excess water coming out is removed.

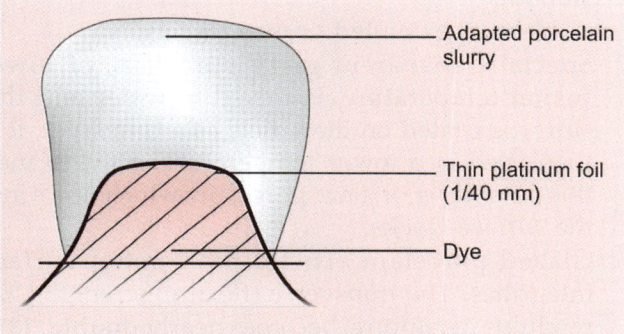

Fig. 13.2: Condensation of porcelain slurry

d. **Ultrasonic method:** The ultrasonic vibrations are transmitted and water coming out is removed, using blotting paper or linen cloth.

Even with these methods void or air trapping cannot be removed entirely.

3. **Firing (sintering) procedure**
   Porcelain firing unit (muffle chamber) is preheated to 650°C. The article to be fired is placed in a fire clay tray and then placed on the platform of the instrument and held **near the door** of the muffle chamber for 5 minutes (Fig. 13.3). The article slowly dries up (sudden heating may disintegrate). The platform is then raised and the article is held inside the muffle chamber for 5 minutes. The remaining water is converted into steam and comes out. The door of the muffle chamber is then closed.

   It is **evacuated** by connecting it to a vacuum pump, immediately in the case of vacuum firing technique. The temperature is gradually raised to about 950°C, i.e. firing temperature of porcelain, **in about 5 minutes, at the rate of 1°C per second.** The article is held under that temperature for a short time until the completion of the firing stages.

Stages of firing (sintering)

- **Low bisque stage/low biscuit stage:** As the temperature gradually rises, the surface particles soften and just begin to join. There is **no volume shrinkage or cohesion.**

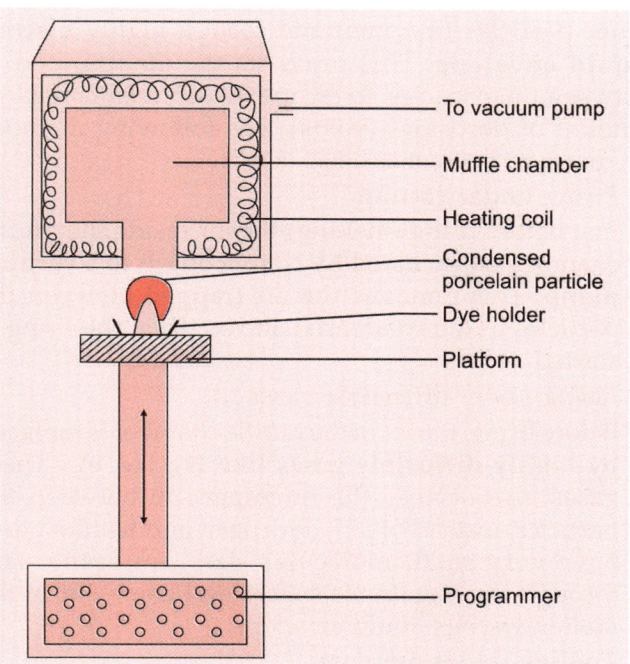

Fig.13.3: Porcelain firing equipment with muffle chamber, computerised programmer (*see* Colour Plate 24, Fig. 13.1)

Firing can be stopped at any stage. If the firing is stopped at this low bisque stage, the particles only just join together forming a porous mass as a core. This partially sintered material is used as a core in glass infiltrated ceramics: **incerams**.

- **Medium bisque stage**
  On further heating more softening of particles takes place and those on the surface begin to melt and join. There is better cohesion and slight volume shrinkage.
- **High bisque stage**
  Further heating causes **melting of all particles** producing complete cohesion and maximum volume contraction. As the liquid is **highly viscous**, the shape is retained for a short time. If this heating is prolonged, the liquid gradually flows under gravity, i.e. **pyroplastic flow** and the article loses sharp corners and shape.

4. **Cooling of the fired article**
   Firing or heating is discontinued, usually at the high bisque stage on complete melting. The muffle chamber is **gradually cooled** according to the manufacturers instructions. This is to minimize the formation of **microcracks.** Then the platform is brought down and the article is removed.

   In the modern equipment the entire firing operation is controlled by computer programming, namely the pre-firing temperatures, times, evacuation, the rate of temperature rise, cooling, etc.

Methods to minimize internal porosities

During firing in the low and medium bisque stages, the outer particles first melt and form a highly **viscous liquid envelope.** This prevents the air, trapped in between the particles, to escape, which results in large amount of porosities (voids). The following methods are used, to overcome this.

- **Firing under vacuum**
  Just before firing (melting) the air inside the muffle chamber is **evacuated by connecting it to a vacuum pump.** This **removes the air trapped** between the particles in the condensed slurry. Then the firing is started.
- **Firing under diffusible gases**
  Before firing, the air in the muffle chamber is **replaced by highly diffusible gases like H_2, He, etc.** These gases also occupy the interspace in-between the particles, instead of air. Hydrogen and helium gases have very small molecular size, can easily pass through the ineratomic spaces and come out of the molten viscous liquid envelope.
- **Cooling under pressure**
  Immediately, after firing is discontinued, air is let inside the evacuated muffle chamber and then the controlled cooling is done. If the low pressure created, by evacuation is say about 1/20 atmospheres, the pressure, when the air is let inside, becomes one atmosphere, i.e. increase by **20 times,** which reduces the size of voids to 1/20th of previous size.

Methods to minimise volume shrinkage

With all skill and methods used in condensation and firing, still, a **volume shrinkage of about 30–40%** takes place when all the particles melt. Hence, the fired article becomes quite small. To compensate this large shrinkage, the following methods are used:

- The powder is made to contain particles of varied sizes to achieve closer packing.
- The porcelain mix or slurry is again applied over the article and refired. This may require 3–4 times repetitions. But repeated firing **decreases** the mechanical properties.
- A skilled technician, initially prepares, an **oversized article by 13–14%** linear. On firing, the required size is obtained by contraction.
- But in most cases, **firing is done in increments of 0.5–2.0 mm thickness,** like core porcelain dentin (body) porcelain, enamel porcelain, glazes, etc. This automatically **compensates** the shrinkage.

5. **The glazing of fired porcelain articles**
   As the porcelain is very hard and brittle material, it cannot be polished. Diamond points, discs, carbide burs, etc. can be used to remove the unwanted excess parts. There are a large number of microcracks on the surface, which cannot be removed. Because of these microcracks, porcelain has very low tensile, flexure or fatigue strengths. The flexure strength is only about 75–80 MPa. **To remove the surface cracks and improve the flexure strength, following glazing methods are used.**

- **Autoglazing or self-glazing**
  The finished article is kept in the furnace and the temperature is quickly raised (or fired), only to melt the surface particles, which flow and fill all the microcracks. The surface becomes glossy and smooth.
- **Add-on or extended or overglazing**
  Special transparent glaze porcelain, of **lower fusion temperature,** is mixed in water and this slurry is coated on the article as a thin layer. It is then fired at a lower temperature, only, to melt this outer layer or glaze porcelain, which flows into the surface cracks.

  Glazed porcelain articles have better surface integrities. The transverse (flexure) strengths, i.e. modulus of rupture, becomes nearly **double, 135–140 MPa.**

6. Shading of ceramics

To get permanent shade and **imitate the check lines** (formed by decalcification on the tooth surface), the shades, **colour frits or stains are applied before the overglazing** (add-on glazing). **This gives a more natural life-like appearance.**

METAL CERAMICS

To overcome the mechanical deficiencies and retain the aesthetic excellence, the ceramic appliances are strengthened by bonding to metallic structures. This **combination** is known as metal ceramic restoration. This is fabricated by selecting suitable materials and sophisticated techniques, with expensive equipment and auxiliary materials. For metal-ceramic bonding different techniques are applied.

Ideal requirements of materials used for metal ceramics or porcelain fused to metal (PFM) techniques.

1. **For selection of metals (alloys), they should have**
   - Adequate biocompatibility, nontoxicity, non-carcinogenic properties.
   - High corrosion resistance, and chemical stability
   - Chemically bond with ceramics, through oxygen bonding.
   - High proportional limit, yield strength, compressive, tensile, shear and fatigue strengths.
   - **High modulus of elasticity to get enough sag resistance** at the high temperature of bonding.
   - Low creep value
   - High fusion temperature, more than porcelain, and **low COTE (13.5–14.0 ppm/°C),** close to that of porcelain which should slightly mismatch by 0.5 ppm/°C, by using more platinium (Pt) or palladium (Pd).
   - Should not cause discolouration of porcelains **(Cu and Ag are to be avoided).**

2. **For the selection of porcelains, they should have**
   - High biocompatibility
   - Good mechanical properties (if possible)
   - High COTE, close to that of metal. COTE is raised to **13.0–13.5 ppm/°C** by **devitrification or using leucite porcelains** for mismatching and thermal bonding.
   - Ability to **wet and bond** with the metal surface.
   - Fusion temperature should be **lower than that of the metal (alloys).** Ultra low fusing ceramics are used now.
   - Good colour stability.

Alloys used for Metal Ceramics

These alloys should have their fusion temperatures, (or solidus temperatures), more than that of ceramics and slightly mismatching COTE. High noble (HN) and predominantly base metal (PBM) alloys of various compositions are used.

- **HN alloys used are** pure gold (99.7%), Au-Pd-Ag, Au-Pt-Pd or Au-Pd. Pt and Pd are specially added to increase the fusion temperature and decrease COTE nearer to that of ceramics. These alloys have melting temperatures, 1000°–1150°C.
- **N alloys used are mainly palladium alloys,** with Au-Ag-Cu, i.e. Pd-Au, Pd-Au-Ag, Pd-Ag, Pd-Cu-Ga, Pd-Ga-Ag. In the presence of Pd, the tarnishing effect of Ag and also Cu are reduced. These alloys have melting points around 1000°–1250°C.
- **PBM alloys are mainly** chromium containing or titanium containing alloys. These have very high temperatures of fusion, 1300°C or above.
  These are Ni-Cr-Mo-Be, Ni-Cr-Mo, Co-Cr-Mo, Co-Cr-W, CpTi, Ti-AI-V, etc. These have superior mechanical properties and high melting temperatures 1250°–1400°C.

METAL-CERAMIC BONDING

Ceramics used have fusion temperatures about 900°–1000°C. On melting it becomes a highly viscous liquid, having **large surface tension (about 365 dynes/cm) and angle of contact (about 130°)** with alloy surface. That is why ceramic liquid does not wet and bond with the metal surface. The following principles are used:

1. **Mechanical bonding:** The bonding surface of the cast metal is made **rough** by using diamond and carbide burs, or sandblasting (with pure alumina). This creates an **increased surface area** to improve wetting and mechanical bonding.

2. **Thermal bonding:** COTE of alloys is **decreased** (by adding Pt or Pd to HN or N alloys) to about 13.5–14.0 ppm/°C. Similarly, COTE of ceramics is **increased** by adding Na^{++}, K^+ or Ca^{++} ions or forming more leucite, to about 13.0–13.5 ppm/°C, the small amount of mismatching, 0.5 ppm/°C helps to bond by mechanical interlocking, sometimes known as **thermal bonding.**

3. **Chemical bonding:** This is achieved by the bonding of ceramics through oxygen of the thin oxide layer formed on the metal surface. In the case of HN or N alloy cast copings, electrodeposition of pure gold layer is formed by electrolysis. This improves aesthetics. **Then "flash" electrodeposition of tin** is formed as an atomic layer. Before fusing the ceramics, the cast coping is placed in the furnace at about 950°C for a few minutes for **"degassing".** But during this process, **a thin tin oxide layer** is formed on the surface. This tin oxide bonds with silica of ceramics. The PBM alloys used, contain a small amount of Sn,

In, and Fe (about <1%). After sand blasting to get rough surface, the cast coping is kept in the furnace at about 950°C for a few minutes for **"degassing,"** which forms a thin tin oxide layer to chemically bond with ceramics.

Metal-ceramic Bond Failures

As the molten ceramic liquid has a high surface tension (365 dynes/cm) and a large angle of contact (130°), it will not wet the metal surface, which has oxide coating or other impurities. **Mechanical interlocking, thermal mismatching and chemical or electrodeposition techniques** are used for good adhesion. The bond failure can be caused in the following manners mainly due to the tensile or shearing forces (*see* Fig. 2.25b).

1. Ceramic failure due to low tensile strength and porosities of ceramics.
2. Ceramic-metal oxide bond failure due to inadequate oxide formation.
3. Metal oxide failure due to too thick or poor strength of metal oxide layer.
4. Metal oxide-metal bond failure.
5. Metal failure due to low tensile strength or porous defects of metal copings.

To minimize these failures, selection of materials and proper techniques of manipulations for better bonding are to be used, by the technician. The patient also should be instructed to minimize the applications of specially tensile and shearing forces.

Outline of Metal-ceramic or Porcelain Fused to Metal (PFM) Fabrication

1. After preparing the tooth, an accurate elastomeric impression is obtained and a ceramic refractory material die is prepared. Suitable metal coping is formed to fit the die exactly by any one of the following methods:
   - Casting a pure metal CpTi, or alloys of HN, N, or PBM, by the usual lost wax casting procedure.
   - CAD-CAM technique from a cast alloy ingot.
   - Electrodeposition of gold or other metals on the duplicate die.
   - Burnishing metal foils on the die and then heat treating.
2. In case of HN or N metal alloys first, **electrodeposition of pure gold, and then 'flash' electrodeposition of tin are done.** In the case of PBM alloys the presence of small amounts of Sn, In or Fe, results in a thin atomic oxide layer.
3. The articles are then kept in a furnace at about 950°–1030°C for some time for "degassing". That is to drive away gases or air trapped inside while casting. But actually, this forms a **thin atomic layer** of oxides of tin, indium or iron on the surface. This helps chemical bonding with ceramics. The surface of bonding should be **perfectly clean**.
4. Then a thin layer of about 0.3 thickness of **opaque porcelain** (opaquer) is applied to this and fired. This is to prevent reflection from white-coloured PBM alloys. In the case of yellow-coloured alloys this opaque layer is not given, as the yellow-coloured surface reflecting light makes it more **lifelike (vital).**
5. Over this, the **translucent, body (or dentin) porcelain** slurry is applied to build the tooth form and condensed. Gingival porcelain with **slight red tint is** also applied near the gingiva and fired together.
6. Then more **transparent enamel** porcelain of thin layer is applied and fired. The article is finished with diamond points, discs or carbide burs.
7. Next, apply the **colour shades and stains. Over this glaze porcelain thin coating is applied and then fired.** This finished article is finally cemented to the tooth structure with GIC (type I) or zinc silicophosphate, or resin cements.
   Note: **The fusion temperatures of these different varieties should be successively in the decreasing order from the metal coping to the glaze layer** (Fig. 13.5). Mechanical properties become higher due to thermal tempering by layered structures (*see* Colour Plate 25, Figs 13.4 to 13.7).

Advantages of metal ceramics
- Higher strength and durability
- Higher fracture resistance
- Adequate marginal fit
- Permanent aesthetics

Disadvantages
- Flexure strains produced in long-span bridges may fracture ceramics

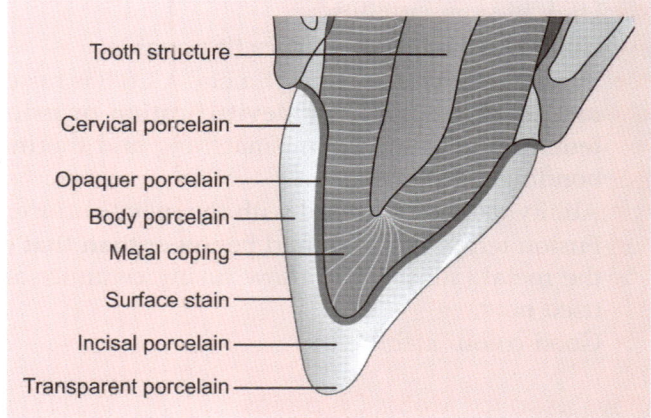

Fig. 13.4: Cross-section of metal ceramic crown (*see* Colour Plate 25, Fig. 13.4)

- Slightly poor aesthetics (than all-ceramics or aluminous core ceramics) due to metallic colour reflections
- Darker margins near the gingiva
- **More healthy tooth material is to be removed** to accommodate the thicker article (but, all ceramic crowns are more thinner). This disadvantage can be overcome by preparing a thinner coping.
- More expensive due to complicated procedures.

Further improvements

For better aesthetics, the thickness of ceramics should be increased without sacrificing the healthy tooth material. That is, the thickness of metal coping should be reduced. Since, this is quite difficult by casting procedure, the other following methods are:

1. **Swagged gold foil metal ceramics:** Laminated gold alloy foils supplied by manufacturers in fluted form are closely adapted on the die, by **burnishing or swagging.** It is then sintered by heating. Over this, the various ceramics are applied successively and fired.

2. **Bonded platinum foil:** Two thin platinum foils are adapted on the die. The outer surface is electro-deposited with tin, which is oxidized by **degassing.** Ceramic fabrication is done over this by applying the various types and firing successively. The outer foil chemically bonds with ceramics, giving more strength. It is cemented to the tooth after removing the inner foil.

3. **Electrodeposition techniques:** Various alloy copings of HN or N alloys, can be electrodeposited first with pure gold (to give better aesthetics) and **then "flash" deposition of tin.** During **degassing** the tin oxide layer formed on the coping cause chemical bonding with ceramics. Sometimes even the base metal alloys, cobalt chromium, Ti alloys, etc. are subjected to this type of electrodeposition of tin for better bonding.

ALL-CERAMIC RESTORATIONS

These are developed after 1980 as newer ceramics of better strength, toughness and aesthetics and sophisticated techniques such as casting, ceramming, etc. were introduced.

1. CASTABLE GLASSES

These castable glasses were developed and manufac-tured by the famous **Corning** Glass Works and supplied by Dentsply International; hence known as **Dicor.** This is used for fabrication of inlays crowns and veneers, **by lost wax casting** procedures and then **cerammed.** The following steps are used:

- Prepare a hard ceramic die and form the wax pattern of inlay or veneer or crown, with inlay wax. To avail adequate strength and aesthetics, **thicker patterns** are prepared. **Thick short sprues** are attached to allow the viscous ceramic liquid to enter the mould.
- Invest the patterns with the die, in phosphate bonded investment material.
- After the wax burn out, melt the casting glass ceramic pellets in the crucible in the centrifugal casting machine and perform casting.
- After casting, slowly cool it down (overnight), recover the article, finish with diamond points or discs, and then staining and glazings are done.
- **Ceramming:** The finished **casting is 'embedded', in a protective material** like gypsum or phosphate bonded investments and subjected to heat treatment, **at about 800°C for about 10–12 hours** in a furnace below its fusion temperature. **Devitrification** takes place in the **middle of the** article forming **mica crystals,** well inside. **This improves the strength as it interrupts crack propagation and also aesthetics** (Fig. 13.5a to c). Due to this the inside layers reflect light incident on them.

This nucleation and crystal growth is known as **'ceramming'.** The crystal layers formed have a higher refractive index or optical density. Due to this, the inside denser layers reflect light incident on them. Surprisingly, this shows the excellent aesthetic property as light reflected from neighboring teeth enters into this and get reflected and refracted out, with almost the same colour or hue. This is known as the **chameleon effect.** Cast glass restorations are suggested to anterior restorations, at very low-stress acting areas.

However, this Dicor is not used nowadays as

- The tensile strength is very low and fractures easily when used for stress acting areas.
- Thick crowns are required. Hence, more healthy tooth material is to be removed.

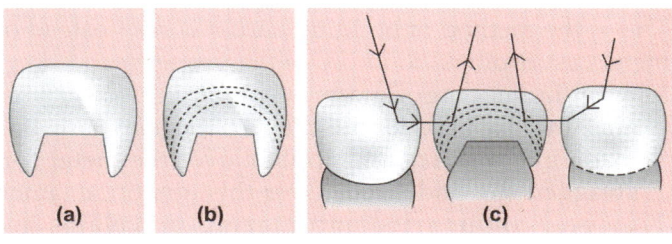

Figs 13.5a to c: (a) Cast glass crown, (b) micacrystals formed on ceramming, (c) chameleon effect

2. OUTLINE OF INJECTION MOULDING GLASS CERAMIC TECHNIQUE

The suitable wax pattern is prepared on the die, with short thick sprue and invested in phosphate bonded investment. Wax burn out is done by the usual method. High **leucite content glass ceramic** supplied as small cylinders, is softened or fused at high temperature (about 1080°C). It is then **injected into the mould at high pressure,** maintained at high temperature for some time and then cooled. Colour frits are then applied and glazed.

In another technique, **the ceramic powder is blended with a resin.** It is softened at about 200°C and injected into the mould at high air pressure. This **core article** is taken out and then fired at a lower temperature for several hours. Then staining and glazing are done.

Advantages
- Higher flexure strength (100–400 MPa)
- Better fit due to the lower firing temperature
- Better aesthetics than metal ceramics.

Disadvantages
- Lower shear strength and higher brittleness cause fracture of posterior restorations.
- Complicated procedure and expensive equipment.

3. HOT PRESSABLE GLASS CERAMICS

This procedure is similar to casting ceramic crowns. The ceramic ingots are heated to high temperature, to soften and then forced into the mould prepared, by applying high pressure. Hot pressing procedure requires about 45 minutes at high temperature. The crown form, undergoes ceramming, that is forming **leucite crystals, as needles, plates or mica, during the devitrification.** These increase the strength as interrupters of crack propagation and improve the aesthetics by **chameleon effect.**

Advantages and disadvantages are similar to castable ceramics or injection moulded ceramics.

Core Ceramics (Porcelain)

This is the method of building harder cores (instead of metal cast copings) to improve the properties.

1. **Aluminous core:** Ceramics containing **40–50% of alumina,** are used for building up the hard core. It is made into a slurry and applied over the **metal foil swagged die and fired.** Over this, dentin, enamel, incisal, colour frits, and glazing porcelains are successively fired. It gives **better strength** and aesthetics to the ceramic jacket crowns or articles.

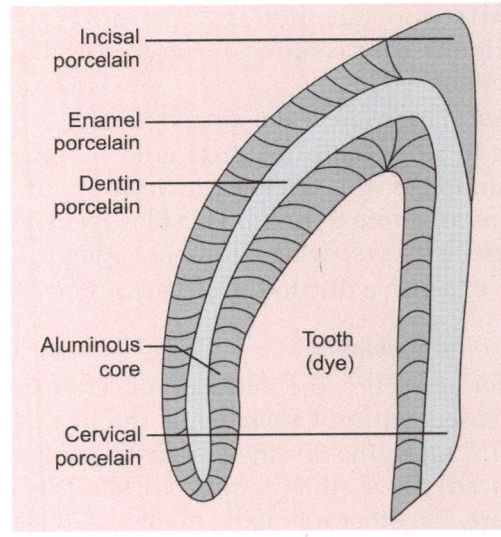

Fig. 13.6: Cross-section of core porcelain jacket crown

(This is sometimes known as aluminous porcelain crown) (Fig. 13.6).

2. **Alumina core porcelain:** This contains about 90% of alumina. The fabrication is done in a similar manner. The first fired alumina core has much **higher strength and acts as an alloy coping.** But **aesthetic** property becomes inferior due to the opacity created, by alumina.

3. **Glass infiltrated core ceramics: Inceram** (Fig. 13.7) Three varieties of inceram-core materials are:
   - **Inceram spinnel** (ICS—has $MgO.Al_2O_3$ as core)
   - **Inceram alumina** (ICA—has Al_2O_3 core)
   - **Inceram zirconia** (ICZ—has Al_2O_3 = 70% + ZrO_2 = 30% as core).

The core ceramic powder is made into a thick slurry, applied on the die, to a certain thickness by **slip casting**

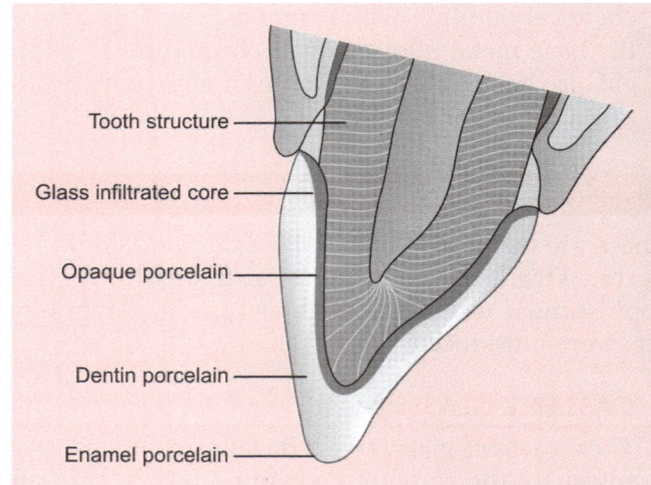

Fig. 13.7: Cross-section of an inceram crown (*see* Colour Plate 24, Fig. 13.3)

method. (The mix is applied on the porous die which absorbs the excess water by capillary action and densifies the porcelain, to a certain thickness.) It is removed, placed in the furnace and fired only **up to the low bisque stage.**

The particles just soften and join together forming a **porous mass, with very small shrinkage.** This **partially sintered** core is then applied with the glass-ceramic mix of lower fusion temperature and then fired again at **1100°C for about 4 hours.** The molten glass liquid **enters or infiltrates into the pores of the core** by capillary action and then solidifies. **Usually, sodium lanthanum glass is used.** This is a low shrinkage core. Over this core, the opaque, dentin, enamel, stains and glazes are successively applied and fired.

The main advantage of this inceram technique is its **large flexure strength of about 350–430 MPa** compared to castable glasses (100–350 MPa) or the high leucite porcelains. This method can be used for fabrications of **posterior restorations.**

The inceram spinnel (ICS) is a ceramic of $Al_2O_3.MgO$. This is also used as core porcelain. But this has a lower flexure strength than Al_2O_3 core (ICA).

Applications

- **ICS:** More translucent, flexure strength = 400 MPa is used for anterior crowns, veneers, inlays, onlays.
- **ICA:** More opaque, higher flexure strength = 500 MPa is used for posterior crowns, anterior 3 unit FPDs, onlays, inlays, etc.
- **ICZ: Highest flexure strength, 700 MPa,** and opacity is used for the posterior crown, bridges, etc.

CAD-CAM MACHINABLE–CHAIRSIDE RESTORATION TECHNIQUES

This is a new technique **alternative to metal casting** developed in 1985 (in Switzerland). The metal casting procedures for HN, N, PBM, and titanium alloys are time-consuming and require high technical skill for availing accuracy of fit. This also requires sophisticated laboratories. In spite of this, **it is quite difficult, to avoid distortion, internal porosities, and the casting defects.** Similarly, in the case of ceramics fabrications and casting procedure, internal cracks, porosities, and volume shrinkages cannot be easily eliminated. Composite resin restorations also have internal voids, shrinkages, etc. To solve these problems the **Computer-Aided Design-Computer Aided Machining** has been envisaged.

The CAD-CAM system has the following main components (see Colour Plate 25, Fig. 13.8)

- Optical camera
- Scanner or digitor

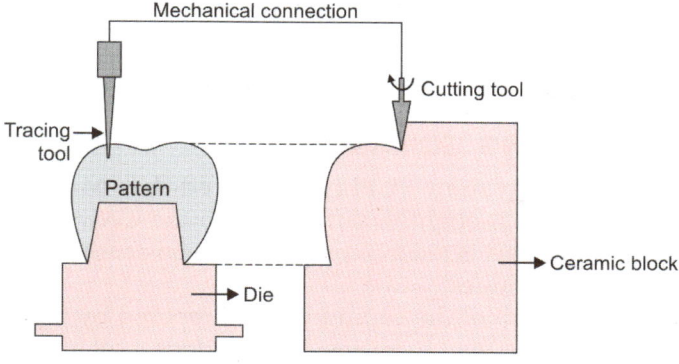

Fig. 13.8: Copy milling principle

- Computer connections
- Milling machines

Steps

- Selection of blocks of suitable sizes, of **dense ceramics** (leucite, feldspathic, Dicor-MGC, etc.) or **metal castings** without any defects such as internal cracks, porosities, voids, etc. is done by checking the internal faults.
- Cavity preparation is done as required.
- The opaque powder is sprayed over the prepared tooth cavity to reduce the optical property of the tooth.
- The optical impression is recorded by using, three-dimensional miniature video camera.
- Camera forms **a three-dimensional optical impression or image.**
- Computer designs the restorations, according to the optical impression.
- Milling machine receives these signals and grinds the outer and inner surfaces of the block with diamond or carbide tools and finishing is done.

  In the case of ceramics appliances, glazing and ceramming can be done. Metal casting or composite resin appliances can be directly cemented.

Advantages

- **Defectless, best, toughest variety** of materials can be selected.
- **Time-saving,** the whole procedure can be completed in one appointment.
- **Chairside** procedure
- Laborious procedures like impression recording, temporary prosthesis, die forming, wax pattern preparation, casting procedure, etc. are not required.
- Better fit to the cavity.

Disadvantages

- Very expensive equipment
- Sophisticated techniques require good skill and training

- Optical impression recording procedure is technique sensitive
- Finishing, glazing is required.

COPY MILLING TECHNIQUE

This new system **(Celay, evolved by Mikron Technology)** is slightly, different than the CAD-CAM technique. This is used to prepare the substructure for crowns or bridges.

The pattern of the coping is first prepared by using a special blue wax or resins. This pattern is placed in the machine. A stylus or tracing tool, passing over the pattern, guides the milling tool which grinds the ceramic block accordingly (Fig. 13.8).

This coping is then glass infiltrated and applied with the opaque, dentin, enamel, colour frits, etc. porcelain mixes, fired each time and finally glazed.

The CAD-CAM and copy milling techniques are also applicable for **preparation of metal alloy crowns or FPDs** using the alloy blanks. This helps to **overcome many of the casting defects and the complicated casting procedures.**

3D printing in dentistry: CAD-CAM milling processes are wasteful as the material is milled from a whole block and accuracy is limited. 3D printing is used for the accurate fabrication of complex structures in a variety of materials with properties that are highly desirable in dentistry and surgery. These are used for drilling and cutting guides, crown copings and partial denture frameworks, artificial teeth fabrication, dental model for restorative dentistry, digital orthodontics, dental implants and product design, instrument manufacturing, etc.

CEMENTATION OF CERAMIC FABRICATIONS

The cement used should be **translucent** and should not affect the aesthetics of the restorations. Dual cure composite resin luting agent is used for all ceramic restorations. For better bonding of ceramic restorations to the tooth structure. Following steps are used:

- The inner cementing surface of restoration is **sand blasted** with pure alumina
- **Etching** of this surface is done **with hydrofluoric** acid gel (taking all precautions required while handling HF acid)
- A **silane-coupling** agent is then applied
- The cementing surface of the tooth also can be **acid etched with phosphoric acid**
- Apply the dual-cure composite resin for cementations.

The metal ceramic crown or bridge may be cemented by the same methods used for metal crowns.

ARTIFICIAL PORCELAIN TEETH

Porcelain teeth are manufactured by using **split metal moulds** with 2 or 3 parts. The moulds are of different sizes, and shapes and are slightly bigger, to compensate the firing shrinkages. High fusing ceramics are used. More opaque porcelain mix is packed on the lingual portion of the mould. One or more mixes of increasing transparencies are packed in the other portion of the mould, according to the individual teeth requirements. The parts of the mold are closed, and dried. The moulded teeth are placed in fire clay trays and fired in the furnace. Colour frits and shade porcelains are applied and glazed.

Certain provisions are made for mechanical interlocking (bonding) of the teeth to acrylic dentures. The anterior teeth are fitted with gold plated pins. The posterior teeth are provided with **rhetoric or diatoric holes. During packing the acrylic dough will surround the pins or enter into the holes and cause mechanical retention** (Figs 13.9a to c).

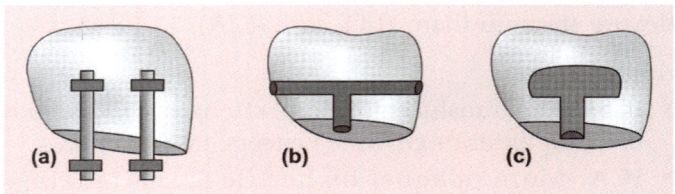

Figs 13.9a to c: Porcelain teeth—mechanical retentions. (a) Anterior with metal pins, (b) posterior with a diatoric hole, (c) posterior with a rhetoric hole

Even though porcelain teeth have an excellent aesthetic quality and high abrasion resistance, the acrylic teeth are commonly used for other reasons. (*Refer* to Table 6.5 for comparison of acrylic and porcelain teeth.)

CRITERIA FOR SELECTION AND USE OF DENTAL CERAMICS

The following are the considerations for selection and use of dental ceramic restorative materials, for availing excellent aesthetic properties and minimizing clinical failures:

1. The dentist should not select ceramic crowns for patients having extreme **bruxism, clenching or malocclusions.**
2. The **skill of the dentist** in preparation of tooth without any undercuts, obtaining accurate impressions with well-defined margins.
3. **Patients should be** informed about the benefits, risks, alternatives to the proposed treatments and also the approximate cost before commencing the treatment.

4. If the aesthetic consideration is not of prime importance, then prepare metal-ceramic restorations.

5. The laboratory technician's part is perhaps more important. He should not accept inaccurate impressions or impressions of incomplete margins, or of wrong cavity preparations.

6. **Use the toughest ceramic core material** for fabrication of posterior restorations for high stress acting areas.

7. Use all-ceramic crowns, when the adjacent anterior teeth have high translucency. All-ceramic restorations can be colour matched better for young patients or others having **high-degree** of translucency.

DENTAL APPLICATIONS OF CERAMICS

1. Porcelains jacket crowns for anterior teeth
2. Porcelain veneers
3. Metal ceramic posterior restorations (crowns, bridges, inlays, onlays)
4. All ceramic crowns and bridges
5. Ceramic inlays and onlays
6. Ceramic brackets in orthodontia
7. Artificial teeth
8. Implants, bio-glasses

MODEL QUESTIONS

I. Long Essays   (20 minutes each)

1. Classify the various dental porcelains. Give the structure and general properties.
2. Give the composition of feldspathic porcelain. Describe the methods of condensation, firing, and glazing of PJC crown.
3. Give the requirements of metals and ceramics used in metal-ceramic restorations. Outline the fabrication method for a metal ceramic crown.

II. Short Essays   (10 minutes each)

1. Classification of dental porcelains
2. Firing of porcelain jacket crowns
3. Glazing
4. Toughening methods of porcelains
5. Methods to minimise, volume shrinkage and voids
6. Requirements of metal ceramic materials
7. Metal ceramics (PFM)
8. All ceramic restorations
9. Castable glass (Dicor)
10. Core ceramics
11. Incerams
12. Porcelain artificial teeth
13. Criteria for selection of porcelain restoratives

III. Brief Answers   (5 minutes each)

1. Structure of porcelain
2. Glass formers and interrupters
3. Leucite
4. Ion-exchange toughening
5. Dispersion toughening
6. Metal ceramic bonding by thermal mismatching
7. Cast coping
8. Swagged gold foil technique
9. Bonded platinum foil technique
10. Alumina core porcelain
11. Spinnel ceramics
12. Ceramming
13. Injection moulding of porcelain
14. CAD-CAM
15. Cementation of porcelain restorations

Dental Waxes (Auxiliary Materials)

Many varieties of waxes are used in dentistry as important auxiliary materials in clinical and laboratory procedures for processing and pattern making, during fabrication of oral appliances.

Waxes are thermoplastic organic polymers containing hydrocarbons of **low molecular weight 400–4000, carbon atoms 14–52 per molecule** and their derivatives of esters, alcohols and sometimes free acids. These are obtained by various natural origins or synthetic methods.

NATURAL WAXES

Natural waxes are obtained from nature from different origins.

Mineral waxes

These are mainly straight chain hydrocarbons of general formula $CH_3\text{-}(CH_2)_n\text{-}CH_3$. Where n = 12–50. These are obtained as **byproducts in petroleum refineries.** These are paraffin, microcrystalline, barnsdahl, ceresin, etc. and mixtures of these saturated and unsaturated hydrocarbons. Their properties depend on the molecular weight and compositions. When these are heated, **the transition from platelet to needle-like crystalline structure takes place at about 5–8°C below their melting point ranges, due to which these remain soft and mouldable, in these ranges.**

Plant origin waxes

Several types of plants produce waxes which contain hydrocarbons, esters and free acids like stearic, palmitic, oleic, etc. Carnauba, Candelilla, Ouricury, Japanese wax, Cocoa butter, etc. belong to these classes. The hydrocarbons are saturated alkanes with **19–31 carbon atoms per molecule.** The properties, again depend on molecular weight and composition.

Insect origin waxes

Beeswax is a brittle material having a melting temperature ranges **63–70°C.** It is a mixture of saturated and unsaturated hydrocarbons, organic acids and **myricyl palmitate.**

Animal origin wax

Spermaceti wax (obtained from sperm-whale) is not used much in dentistry. These are mainly esters, sometimes used for coating the dental floss.

SYNTHETIC WAXES

Synthetic waxes are produced by combination of various chemicals or by chemical action on natural waxes, in the laboratory. Many of them are, byproducts in petroleum refining and other industries.

Synthetic waxes are **complex organic compounds** of varied chemical compositions, but they differ chemically from natural waxes. The physical properties such as melting temperature, flow and hardness are almost similar to those of natural waxes. Synthetic waxes have a **high degree of refinement** when compared with natural waxes which are usually contaminated with natural sources.

For example, polyethylene waxes, polyoxyethylene glycol waxes, halogenated hydrocarbon waxes, hydrogenated waxes, wax esters from the reaction of fatty acids, alcohols and acids, are used often.

ADDITIVES (RESINS, GUMS AND FATS)

Resins

Trees and other plants of many different species, produce **exudates** of natural resins, such as **dammer, rosin, sandarac,** etc.

Resins are generally complex, amorphous mixtures of organic substances that are characterized by specific physical behaviour rather than by any definite chemical composition. Natural resins are obtained from trees and plants, except **shellac** which is produced by **insects.** Most of the **natural resins are blended** with waxes to get the desirable properties for dental applications.

Natural resins such as dammer and Kauri are mixed with natural waxes to produce harder products.

Synthetic resins such as polyethylene and vinyl resins of various types are added to paraffin waxes to improve their toughness, **film forming** characteristics, resistance to flaking and chipping etc.

Natural resins and synthetic resins also may be used in organic solvents to produce film forming materials that may be used as a **cavity liner.**

Gums

Gums are the viscous substances from plant or animal sources that harden in air. Gums combine with water to form sticky, viscous liquids, e.g. gum arabic.

Fats

These are substances similar to waxes but characterized as being **soft and greasy to touch,** e.g. for fats used in dentistry are stearic acid, palmitic acid, oleic acid, etc.

CLASSIFICATION OF DENTAL WAXES

1. **According to applications**
   - **Pattern waxes**
     - Inlay: Type I, type II
     - Casting
     - Baseplate: Type I, type II and type III
   - **Processing waxes**
     - Boxing and beading
     - Sticky   – Block out
     - White   – Utility
     - Carving

   - **Impression waxes**
     - Corrective impression
     - Bite registration

2. **According to the origin (now not in use)**
   - Natural: Mineral, plant, insect, animal origins
   - Synthetic waxes

CHARACTERISTIC PROPERTIES OF WAXES (Fig. 14.1)

1. **Thermal properties**
   - **Melting range:** Waxes are amorphous materials consisting of several types of molecules with different molecular weights, so that they have melting ranges rather than a single melting point. For example, the melting range of paraffin wax is about 44–62°C. Melting range of carnauba wax is about 50–90°C.

     By varying the compositions or by mixing other varieties, it is **possible to change** these ranges, suitably according to the requirements.
   - **Thermal expansion:** When the waxes are heated their **crystal structures changes from plate to needle-shaped below their melting ranges.** Due to this, **large volume expansion and sudden increase of softness (flow)** take place, and wax becomes **mouldable.** Waxes have very large COTE, 150–400 ppm/°C and COTE increases with temperature. Due to this large COTE, contraction of wax patterns takes place by, about 0.3 to 0.8%, when cooled from oral temperature 37°C to room temperature.
   - **Thermal conductivity:** All waxes are **poor conductors** of heat. Hence, **suitable kneading** or uniform softening is required while preparing wax patterns otherwise **distortion takes place, due to relaxation of internal stresses.**

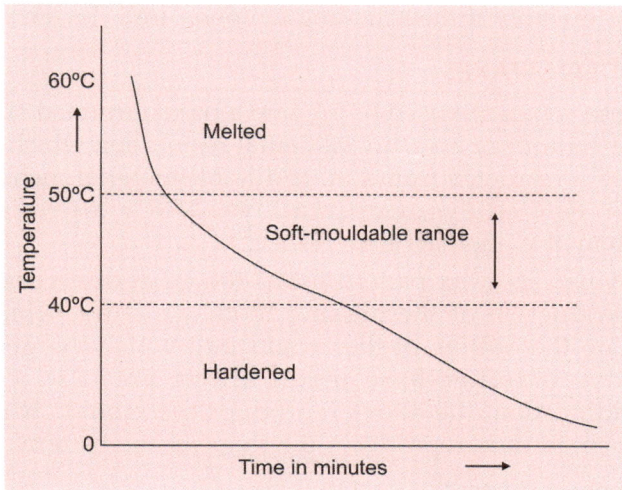

Fig. 14.1: Cooling curve for waxes

2. **Mechanical properties**
   - **Flexibility and modulus of elasticity.** These related properties change again with the rise of temperature and compositions. For waxes when the temperature is raised from 23 to 37°C the proportional limit **decreases** from 11.0 to 5.5 MPa, and **MOE decreases** from 1790 to 760 MPa. When inlay wax is heated from 23 to 40°C its compressive strength decreases from 83 to 0.5 MPa and MOE decreases from 760 to 48 MPa.
   - **Flow properties:** Flow is a very important property for **carving and preparations** of different types of (direct, indirect) wax patterns. This is determined by the percentage decrease in the height of a standard cylindrical sample, maintained at different temperatures (refer impression compound) as per ADA specification No. 4. The flow also depends on the compositions and increases with temperatures.
   - **Residual stresses:** During the preparation of the wax pattern, waxes should be melted or softened homogeneously and then moulded or shaped and finally cooled down to room temperature. The patterns are stressed and strained if the softening, moulding or cooling is not done properly. These wax patterns gradually undergo **distortion by relaxation of internal stresses**. For example, if a modeling wax sheet is slightly rolled and left, it recovers its original shape and this is known as **wax memory.** If the temperature is higher, the recovery of original shape takes place faster. That is why, the inlay wax pattern should be prepared by uniform softening, cooling under pressure, and invested immediately or stored at low temperatures.
   - **Ductility:** Like other properties, ductility also increases with temperature. Waxes have higher ductility if their melting temperature is lower.

PATTERN WAXES

These waxes are used to prepare a predetermined size and contour of an artificial dental restoration which is to be constructed from a more durable material such as cast gold alloys, Co-Cr alloys, Ni-Cr alloys or polymethyl methacrylate resins.

Note: The wax pattern forms the exact or accurate reproduction of the missing tooth structure, which create the outline of the mould into which the gold alloys or other base metal alloys are cast. On solidification, the alloys reproduce the mould shape which, in turn, reproduces the shape of the pattern.

There are 3 types of pattern waxes
1. Inlay waxes (type I and type II)
2. Casting waxes
3. Base plate waxes (type I, type II and type III).

Inlay Waxes

Inlay waxes are used to prepare the wax patterns of inlays, crowns, bridges and pontic replicas in the lost wax casting technique.

Dispensing

These are supplied as deep blue or purple rods or sticks of about 7.5 cm long and 3 mm in diameter. These are also supplied in the form of small pellets and cones.

Classification

According to ADA specification No. 4, there are 2 types of inlay waxes:

1. **Type I:** Medium wax is used for direct wax pattern technique
2. **Type II:** Soft wax is used for indirect wax pattern technique.

The Composition of Inlay Waxes (Table 14.1)

Ideal requirements for inlay waxes
1. There should be no **flakiness** or **roughening** of the surface when the wax is moulded after softening.
2. The wax should not pull out with the carving instrument or **chip out** as it is carved.
3. The wax pattern should be completely rigid and dimensionally stable at all times until it is eliminated.
4. In case of direct wax pattern technique, it should be sufficiently plastic at a temperature slightly above mouth temperature and become rigid at mouth temperature.
5. When softened, the wax should become uniformly soft, and there should be no graininess or hard spots on the surface.
6. After the mould has been formed, the wax should completely vapourize at 500°C and should have no residue.
7. It should have a flow of **more than 70% at 45°C and more than 1% at 37°C.**
8. The colour should be such that it will have contrast with die material. A definite contrast in colour facilitates proper finishing of margins.

Properties
1. **Flow property:** Type I inlay wax exhibits a marked plasticity or flow at a temperature slightly above the mouth temperature and the wax begins to harden at approximately 50°C and it solidifies approximately at 40°C, when it cools at a constant rate.

Table 14.1 The composition of inlay wax (ADA specification No. 4)

	Ingredients	Weight%	Functions
1.	Paraffin wax	60%	Provides desirable mouldability. It is used to establish a melting point. It is likely to flake when it is trimmed, and it does not give a glossy surface, so other modifiers are added
2.	Carnauba wax	20%	Increases the melting range, decreases the flow at mouth temperature and contributes to the glossiness of the wax surface
3.	Ceresin wax	5%	Improves the carving characteristics of the wax and also modifies the toughness
4.	Gum dammer	3%	Improves smoothness of the surface gives more resistance to flaking or chipping and increases toughness
5.	Beeswax	5%	Reduces the flow at mouth temperature and reduces the brittleness of the wax at mouth temperature
6.	Synthetic resins	2%	Gives stable flow properties to the wax

The maximum flow for type I waxes at **37°C is 1%**. The less flow at this temperature allows carving and removal of the pattern from the oral cavity at mouth temperature without distortion. **Both types I and II waxes** must have flow between **70% and 90% at 45°C**, i.e. when the waxes are inserted into the prepared cavity.

2. **Thermal conductivity:** Inlay waxes are softened with the heat, forced into the prepared cavity in tooth/die and cooled. The thermal conductivity of waxes is low and sufficient time is required to heat wax uniformly and cool them to body or room temperature.

3. **Co-efficient of thermal expansion (COTE):** Inlay waxes have a **high COTE 300–700 ppm/°C**. The waxes may have a linear contraction of about **0.3–0.4% when cooled from 37°C to room temperature.** If the waxes are allowed to cool under pressure, its thermal properties are **changed when reheated, and** the linear expansion also increases.

4. **Causes for distortion:** Distortion is due to any method of manipulation that creates inhomogeneity in wax involving the intermolecular distances. Distortion of wax can occur due to **relaxation of internal stresses**, caused by large thermal contraction and low thermal conduction,

   - if the wax is not heated to uniform temperature when inserted into the cavity some parts of the wax pattern may thermally contract more than the others when stresses are introduced.
   - if the wax is not held under uniform pressure during cooling.
   - if the wax is melted and added in an area of deficiency, the added wax will introduce stresses during cooling.
   - during carving, some molecules of wax will be disturbed and stresses induced, cause distortion.

Manipulation (by Dry-heat Technique Inlay Waxes are Softened)

Direct technique (type I—medium wax)

The wax is softened by heating over a flame and rotated rapidly until it becomes soft. The wax is then kneaded and shaped approximately to the form of the prepared cavity. It is then inserted into the prepared cavity and held **under pressure until it hardens**. Pressure may be applied either with the finger or by the patient biting on the wax. The wax should be allowed to cool gradually to the mouth temperature to minimize internal stresses. Cold carving instrument should be used for the direct wax pattern. Withdraw the wax pattern carefully along the long axis of the preparation. The pattern should be touched as little as possible with the hands to avoid temperature changes. **Invest the wax pattern as early as possible** to minimize distortion. Thermal contraction is about 0.3–0.5%.

Indirect technique (type II—soft wax)

- The impression of the prepared cavity is first taken with a rubber base impression material
- Die is made from the impression
- Die is coated with a **lubricant** to minimize the sticking of the wax to the stone die
- The melted, **type II** wax may then be added in layers with the wax spatula
- The prepared cavity is overfilled and the wax is carved to the proper contour
- The wax pattern is removed and **invested as early as possible.**

Methods to minimize wax distortion
- Select the proper type of waxes (type I for direct and Type II for indirect techniques) as specified by ADA.
- Soften the wax uniformly.
- Place the softened or molten increments quickly to bond with previous increment.
- After the overfilled pattern hardens, carefully do the carving without pulling from the margins.
- Remove the pattern very carefully. (A drop of oil or lubricant applied on the prepared cavity or die).
- Invest the pattern immediately without delay, or it can be stored in cold water (in a refrigerator) for a short time delay.

CASTING WAXES

Casting wax is also one of the pattern waxes used to prepare wax patterns for the metallic framework of removable partial dentures and other similar structures. These waxes are highly ductile. They should not leave any residue during wax burnout (around 500°C).

Table 14.2	The composition of casting wax
Ingredients	**Functions**
1. Paraffin wax	Establishes a melting point
2. Ceresin wax	Improves carving characteristics
3. Beeswax	Reduces flow at mouth temperature and brittleness of the wax
4. Natural resins	Give suitable flow properties to wax

Mode of supply
It is available in the form of:
- **Sheets of 0.4 mm thickness**
- **Readymade shapes** in a wide variety of ranges such as round rods that are 10 cm long, half round rods, half pear-shaped rods, etc.
- It is also provided in bulk form roles for **sprues and vent sprues**
- **Preformed wax** patterns for cast RPD frameworks, with different designs.

Uses
- To make metallic framework patterns for removable cast partial dentures
- To give uniform minimum thickness in certain areas of partial denture frameworks.

BASEPLATE OR MODELLING WAXES (Table 14.3)

These are also pattern waxes, mainly used to make **occlusal rims** in the preparation of complete dentures and partial dentures.

Table 14.3	The composition of baseplate waxes	
Ingredients	**Weight%**	**Functions**
1. Ceresin wax	80%	Improves carving characteristics
2. Beeswax	12%	Reduces brittleness and reduces flow at mouth temperature and gives a glossy surface
4. Natural or synthetic resin	3%	Give stable flow properties
5. Microcrystalline wax	25%	Establishes required melting point

According to ADA specification No. 24, they are classified as:

Type I: Soft wax used for building veneers

Type II: Medium wax tried in the mouth, used in normal climatic conditions

Type III: Hard wax used in hot (temperate) conditions.

Dispensing
Available in the form of sheets of pink/red colour.

Dimension
8 cm in breadth, 15 cm long and 1.5 mm thick.

Uses
- To make **occlusal rims** which are used on the baseplate to establish the vertical dimensions, the plane of occlusion and initial arch form in the technique for complete denture fabrications. This wax may also be used to form all or a portion of the tray itself.
- To produce the desired contour of the denture after teeth are set in position.
- To make patterns for orthodontic appliances and prosthesis other than complete dentures.
- To check various articulating relations in the mouth and to transfer them to mechanical articulators.

PROCESSING WAXES

These waxes are used mainly as **accessory aids** in construction of a variety of restorations and appliances either in the clinics, or in the laboratory. The important processing waxes (Figs 14.2 a to e) are:
- Boxing and beading waxes
- Utility wax
- Sticky wax
- Carding wax
- White wax
- Blockout wax
- Carving wax

All these processing waxes have similar ingredients of which the relative amounts are adjusted to obtain

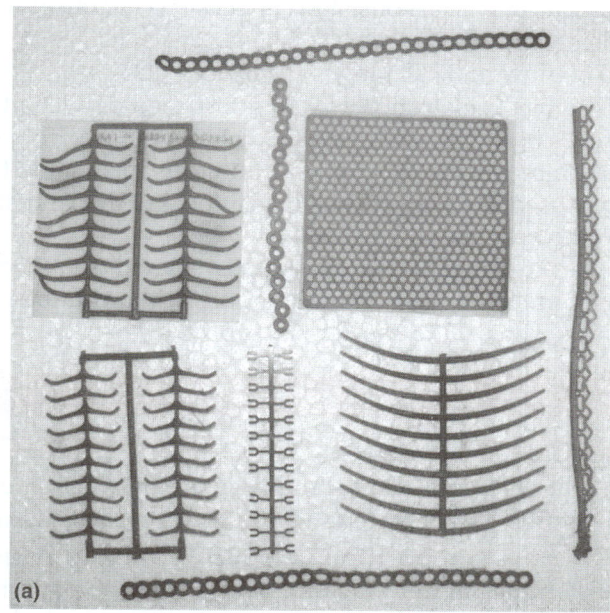

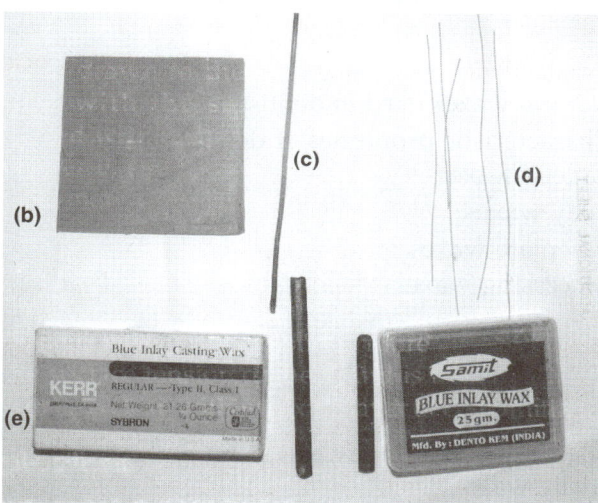

Figs 14.2a to e: Varieties of waxes. (a) Preformed waxes, (b) casting wax, (c) sprue wax, (d) vent sprue, (e) inlay wax

the required properties like ranges of melting temperatures flow properties at the working conditions, resistance to flaking and chipping, ductilities and other mechanical properties.

BOXING AND BEADING WAXES

These are mainly used to bead and box the impressions to get the casts with the required size and shapes.

Dispensing

- Boxing waxes are available as sheets of **3 cm width, 15–30 cm in length and 3 mm thickness.**
- Beading waxes are available in the form of **ropes of about 3–4 mm diameter.**

Properties of boxing and beading waxes. These are

- It preserves the extensions
- It controls the form and thickness of the base of the cast
- It conserves the artificial stone
- These are pliable and can be adapted easily
- Its **stickiness** allows it to attach to the impression.

Uses

- To build up vertical sides around the impression
- To produce the desired size and form of the base of the cast
- To preserve certain landmarks of the impressions.

Adaption of beading and boxing waxes

- Beading wax is adapted around the periphery of the impression
- Beading wax should be approximately 4 mm wide and 3–4 mm below the borders of the impression
- The height is adjusted until a boxing wax strip extends approximately 13 mm above the highest point on the impression.

UTILITY WAX

It consists mainly of beeswax, mineral wax and other soft waxes in various proportions. It is supplied in the form of **cakes, sticks and sheets**. It is used for giving a more **desirable contour** to the **perforated tray** to be used for the hydrocolloids. It is also used to **build up flange of the tray and raise a palatal portion** of the tray posteriorly in recording deep palate patients' impressions. It is pliable and can be moulded at room temperature. It has **adhesive** nature and it can easily stick to the tray.

STICKY WAX (MODELLING CEMENT)

It consists of **yellow beeswax,** rosin and natural resins such as **gum dammer.** It is sticky when melted and adheres strictly to the surface upon which it is applied. At room temperature, it is free from tackiness and is brittle. It is used for **joining metal parts** before soldering procedure and for joining fragments of a **broken denture** before repair procedure.

CARDING WAX

It is used for attaching broken parts of the denture before the **denture repair procedure** and it can also be used to join the metal pieces in **soldering procedures.**

WHITE WAX

It is used for making patterns to **simulate a veneer facing.**

BLOCKOUT WAX

This is used to **fill voids and undercuts** during fabrication of removable partial dentures.

CARVING WAX

It is used for tooth carving procedures in dental anatomy, laboratory procedures.

IMPRESSION WAXES

These are used to record zero-undercut edentulous portions of the mouth and are generally used in combination with other impression materials such as polysulfides, ZnOE impression paste or dental impression compound. The important impression waxes are:

1. Corrective impression waxes
2. Bite registration waxes.

Corrective Impression Waxes

It is used as a wax veneer over an original impression to contact and register the details of the soft tissues. It consists of paraffin, ceresin, and beeswax. The flow at 37°C is 100%. Because of this reason they **can get distorted** while removing from the mouth.

Uses

- A **functional impression** in case of partial dentures
- To record posterior palatal seal in dentures
- Functional impression for obturators (device is given for cleft palate patients).

Bite Registration Waxes

These waxes are used to record the **occlusal relationship** of the opposite quadrants (i.e. maxillary and mandibular arches). It is used to articulate an accurately certain model of opposing quadrants. Bite registration waxes consisting of beeswax, paraffin wax and ceresin wax.

The flow at 37°C ranges from 2.5 to 22%.

The bite registration wax is interposed between the 2 arches of the patient and asked to bite the wax for jaw relation recording. The indentation thus formed on the wax is used to place the cast in position and then transfer it to the articulator.

The bite waxes are supplied as U-shaped thin sheets, **which are sometimes metalized or foil laminated** (*see* Colour Plates 26 to 29, Figs 14.1 to 14.18).

MODEL QUESTIONS

I. Long Essays   (20 minutes each)

1. What are dental waxes and how are they classified? Describe the characteristic properties of these waxes.
2. Give the composition, properties, manipulation techniques of inlay casting waxes. Also, explain the various causes for wax distortions and the remedies.

II. Short Essays   (10 minutes each)

1. Natural waxes used in dentistry
2. Characteristic properties of dental waxes
3. Pattern waxes
4. Inlay waxes
5. Baseplate waxes
6. Processing waxes

III. Brief Answers   (5 minutes each)

1. Thermal expansion of waxes
2. Casting wax
3. Boxing and beading waxes
4. Sticky wax
5. Impression wax
6. Bite wax

CHAPTER **15**

Casting Investment Materials (Auxiliary Materials)

CHAPTER SURVEY

- Casting shrinkages = wax shrinkages + alloy shrinkages
- Mold expansion = Setting expansion + thermal expansions
- Compensations, by high and low heat techniques
- Classification of investment materials
- Requirements
- Refractory materials
- Gypsum bonded investment (GBI) materials

- Controlling setting and thermal expansions
- Phosphate bonded investments (PBIs)
- Ethyl-silicate bonded investments
- Divestments
- Soldering investments
- Ceramic-casting investments
- Investments for casting titanium alloys

CASTING SHRINKAGES AND METHODS OF COMPENSATIONS

Lost wax casting procedure is adopted for fabrication of metal alloy appliances like inlays, crowns, bridges, cast RPD frameworks, etc. outside the mouth. An accurate wax pattern prepared, is invested in **refractory mould** materials. After wax burns out, the mould is filled with alloy liquid, which solidifies and cools down. The final article should exactly fit the prepared teeth. During this procedure, the possible dimensional changes taking place, are to be suitably compensated.

Casting shrinkage arises due to shrinkage of wax pattern and shrinkage of alloys

1. **Wax shrinkage:** Wax patterns are prepared by direct and indirect techniques.
   - **Direct technique:** Type I, hard (or medium) inlay wax is softened by dry heat, i.e. waving carefully over a flame, directly adapted on the prepared teeth, and then carved. It is then taken out and invested. Inlay waxes have large COTE of about 300–400 ppm/°C, and undergo large thermal contractions of about 0.3%–0.4% when cooled from 37°C to room temperature. **This causes a discrepancy.**
   - **Indirect technique:** As it is inconvenient to carve the wax pattern, in the mouth, it is prepared outside the mouth.

A very accurate **impression** of the prepared tooth is obtained by the double-mix technique with elastomers and a **hard die** is made with type IV die stone or sometimes with type V die stone (for enlarged dies). Elastomers have also large COTE, of about 150 ppm/°C–225 ppm/°C, causing the **thermal shrinkage, in addition to polymerization shrinkage and incomplete elastic recoveries.** Slight setting expansion of die material, cannot compensate, these. Over this smaller die, the wax pattern is prepared with **type II soft inlay wax, by melting, applying layer by layer** and then carving. Die becomes smaller by 0.3 to 0.4%. Hence, approximately the wax pattern shrinkages in both cases are about 0.3–0.4%.

2. **Alloy-shrinkage:** Alloy liquid when poured into the mould, first cools down to the liquidus temperature and then solidifies in the mould. However, these thermal contractions of the liquid and solidification shrinkages are automatically compensated by the extra liquid present. But the **thermal shrinkage of solidified casting**, while cooling from the solidus temperature to 37°C (or room temperature) is quite large, even though, it is slightly inhibited by the first formed solid layer attached to mold walls. For low fusing (900–1000°C) HN and N alloys, these shrinkages are about **1.3–1.6%**, and for high fusing

(1,200–1450°C) **PBM alloys,** it is about **2.0–2.3%.** This also reduces the size of casting in addition to that of wax shrinkage.

Total casting shrinkage = wax shrinkage + alloy shrinkage. For low fusing HN and N alloys, it is about **1.6–1.8%** and for high fusing PBM alloys it is about **2.3–2.5%.**

These result in **misfit of castings** and need compensation. Earlier for compensation, wax patterns were expanded, by placing in warm water before investing. But this method caused, distortion of pattern and hence not practiced now.

COMPENSATION OF CASTING SHRINKAGE

Compensation of casting shrinkages is done by carefully controlling the mould expansions, by availing large **setting expansions** and adjusting the **thermal expansions** of the investment materials. Investment materials have **refractory materials (allotropic forms of silica) and a binder** (gypsum product—dental stone, $MgO + NH_4H_2PO_4$, or ethyl silicate). These powders are mixed with water (or sometimes added with colloidal silica gel), and wax patterns are invested in metal or plastic casting rings.

1. Setting Expansions of Gypsum-bonded Investment Materials

Normal setting expansion (NSE) can be increased to about 0.3 to 0.5% by:
- Decreasing water–powder ratio
- Decreasing chemical impurities
- Increasing mixing time
- Using fresh stock

Hygroscopic setting expansion (HSE) can be increased by large values (1.0–2.0%) by
- Decreasing water/powder ratio
- Decreasing chemical impurities
- Increasing mixing time
- Using fresh stock
- **Immersing** the invested casting ring in water for longer time after initial setting or by adding more extra water—**controlled water added technique after the initial setting.**

2. Thermal Expansion

This depends upon the composition and the temperature rise of the refractory material quartz, tridymite, cristobalite or amorphous quartz. Inversion from low α-form to high β-form, at higher temperatures also produce expansion which adds up to thermal expansion. When heated to about 600°C temperature, the **thermal expansions are about, for cristobalite = 1.7%, for quartz = 1.4%, for tridymite = 0.9% and for fused quartz = 0.05% (least).**

Choosing more cristobalite allotropic form, higher thermal expansion is obtained.

By adding colloidal silica (0–100%) to the mixing water for phosphate bonded investment, higher setting as well as thermal expansions are obtained. These are needed to compensate the larger casting shrinkages of PBM alloys.

Ringless casting: Flexible plastic casting ring is used instead of ceramic paper lined metal casting ring for allowing greater expansions, specially for PBI. The plastic ring is removed after investment sets, as PBI has high strength, to withstand casting force.

HIGH HEAT AND LOW HEAT CASTING TECHNIQUES

The setting expansions obtained by NSE is much smaller than that obtained by HSE method. That is why the mould invested casting ring is to be heated to higher temperatures of about 600°C for NSE method and lower temperatures of about 400°C is sufficient for HSE method. These are known as **high heat and low heat techniques.**

Under compensations or over compensations cause misfit of the cast appliances. In the case of **PBM alloys,** the melting temperatures are about 1300°C, and thermal contractions are larger, about 2.0 to 2.3%. Hence, larger compensation is obtained by greater thermal expansion obtained by heating investment to about **800°C** (Chart 15.1).

INVESTMENT MATERIALS (ADA SPECIFICATION NO. 2)

In the lost-wax casting procedure, the wax patterns are attached with sprue former and embedded (invested)

Chart 15.1: Casting shrinkage and methods of compensation can be summarized

Wax shrinkage	+	Alloy shrinkage	=	Total shrinkage	=	Setting expansion	+	Thermal expansion
0.3%		+ 1.4%		= 1.7%	=	▶ NSE = 0.4% + 1.3%, at 600°C (high heat technique		
						▶ HSE = 1.0% + 0.7%, at 400°C (low heat technique		

in a fluid mix of refractory mold material in a metallic or plastic casting ring. After setting, wax is eliminated by heating. Molten alloy liquid is forced into this **mould space to fill completely by** pressure, centrifugal force or vacuum suction or combined methods and allowed to solidify. Suitable mould expansions are obtained to compensate for casting shrinkages.

Investment material can be defined as refractory mould material used for embedding the wax pattern and obtaining the corresponding mould for casting.

REQUIREMENTS OF INVESTMENT MATERIALS

1. Should not react with inlay waxes and alloys.
2. Should not undergo chemical degradation at high casting temperatures, producing corrosive gases (like SO_2) discolouring the alloy.
3. Very fine particles to reproduce, finer details of the wax pattern and smooth surfaces.
4. Should be in fluid condition with the good flow while investing and set into hard solid.
5. Large **porosity to vent out** trapped gases or air, i.e. to avoid back pressure-incomplete casting.
6. Adequate strength to resist fracture, from casting forces. According to **ADA specification No. 2, the compressive strengths in two hours should be >2.4 MPa for GBI and >4.8 MPa for PBI.** The fracture cracks may produce **fins** on the castings.
7. **Large,** controlled **setting expansions** to compensate casting shrinkages.
8. **Large,** controlled **thermal expansions** to compensate casting shrinkages (i.e. large COTE).
9. Ability to withstand high casting temperatures that is thermal stability.
10. Readily available, long storage life, inexpensive.
11. Simple manipulation techniques.

Classification of investment materials, according to
1. **Refractory materials**
   - Quartz
   - Cristobalite
   - Tridymite
   - A mixture of quartz, cristobalite, and tridymite
   - A mixture of alumina, magnesia, and zirconia.
2. **Binder materials**
   - Gypsum product—type III
   - Magnesium oxide + ammonium phosphate
   - Ethyl silicate
3. **Principles of setting expansion techniques**
   - Type I: For small castings, with NSE
   - Type II: For small castings, with HSE
   - Type III: For large (RPD) castings, with NSE
4. **Applications for**
   - Low fusing alloys
   - High fusing (HN, N, and PBM) alloys
   - Soldering techniques
   - Ceramming techniques
   - Divestment techniques
   - Titanium and its alloys

Ceramic Refractory Materials

These ceramic refractory materials are used in investment materials for providing

- Thermal resistance to disintegration
- Higher strength to withstand casting forces
- Large controlled thermal expansions to compensate casting shrinkages
- Large porosity to vent out trapped air.

Material used is the allotropic forms of quartz (Chart 15.2)

Quartz exists in four different allotropic forms, at higher temperatures which can be retained at room temperature by quenching.

- Quartz has a **rhombic** lattice structure. When it is heated above 575°C, the **low α-form** undergoes inversion into **high β-form** with an **increase in volume**, i.e. an expansion which is added up to its thermal expansion.

Chart 15.2: Allotropic transformations of quartz

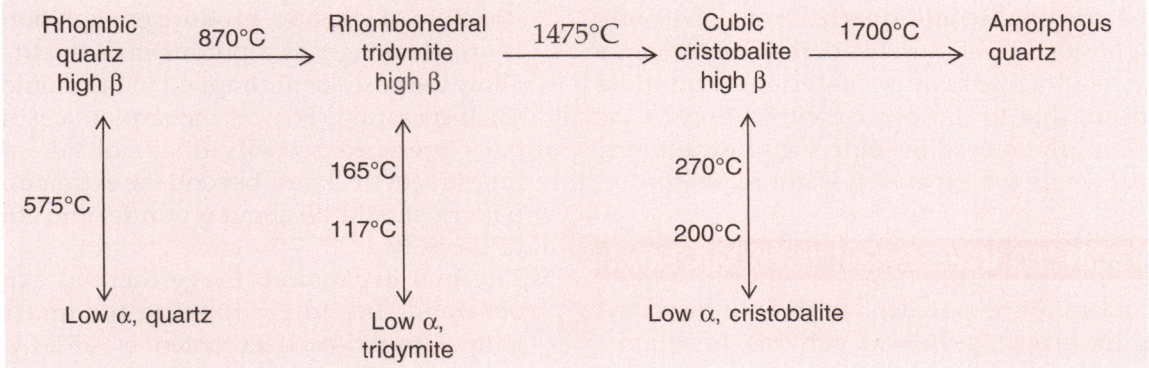

- **Above 870°C,** it transforms into its allotropic form, **tridymite,** which has **rhombohedral** lattice structure and get **low α-form** by quenching. When the **low α-**form is heated above **117°–165°C** it undergoes inversion into **high β-form** with expansion.

- When heated **above 1475°C,** it transforms into the next allotropic form—**cristobalite** which has a **cubic** structure. On quenching, the cubic structure is retained at room temperatures as **low α–**form. It also inverts to its **high β**-form above **200°–270°C.**

- On further heating, it melts **above 1700°C.** On solidification, it forms a noncrystalline **amorphous** glass which has very low COTE.

These transformations can be represented as

The different allotropic forms have different COTE and thermal **expansions are added with inversion expansions.** When these are heated to about 600°C, the expansion curves give the total expansions which are approximately (Fig. 15.1).

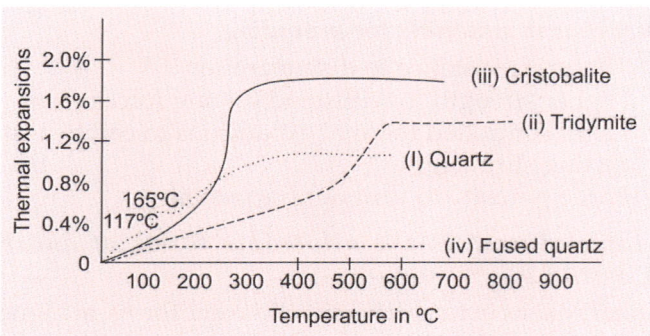

Fig. 15.1: Thermal and inversion expansions of refractory materials

Quartz	= 1.4%
Tridymite	= 1.0%
Cristobalite	= 1.8%
Fused quartz =	Negligible

Since the **cristobalite and quartz** forms, give large thermal expansions, these varieties or their mixtures are commonly used as refractory materials. Tridymite is rarely used, due to its lower contribution to the expansion but can be used in soldering or ceramming investments, where the expansion is not required.

GYPSUM-BONDED INVESTMENT (GBI) MATERIAL

It is supplied as a fine powder which is to be mixed with water for investing the wax patterns, to obtain a casting mould.

COMPOSITION (Table 15.1)

Setting action: When mixed with the recommended water/powder ratio, the calcium sulphate hemihydrate is converted into its dihydrate form, binding the refractory material particles to form a **hard, porous solid mould material, i.e.**

$$2CaSO_4 . \frac{1}{2} H_2O + 3H_2O \rightarrow 2CaSO_4.2H_2O + heat$$

Properties

1. **Setting time:** It is adjusted by manufacturer to about 8–18 min (ADA specification No. 2, is between 5 and 25 min). If required this can be varied slightly.

2. **Setting expansion:** The normal setting expansion **NSE can be increased** by lowering water powder ratio, increasing spatulation time and using fresh stock. For large hygroscopic setting expansion, **after initial set,** the invested casting ring is either immersed in water for a longer time or added with more extra water (controlled water added technique). HSE is decreased by rigid confinement of metal casting ring. For higher HSE, aluminosilicate liners are used, and plastic/rubber casting rings or split casting rings are used which later can be pulled out in PBI for PBM alloy casting procedure. Dental stone binder gives higher HSE than type II plaster. Greater the amount of refractory quartz or cristobalite, higher HSE is found to take place. Extra water added can easily diffuse between the refractory particles into their interspace and produce more expansion. If more than 75% cristobalite is used, it can compensate for the shrinkage caused by loss of water, during wax burn out heating.

3. **Strength:** According to ADA specification No. 2, **the compressive strength for GBI at 2 hours should be >2.4 MPa (and for PBI at 2 hours >4.8 MPA).** This GBI has adequate strength to withstand fracture from large casting forces. If the investment is made weak by adding too much water, etc. it may **fracture** when the hot alloy enters the mould and produce **fins.** If it contains too much silica also, the strength decreases.

4. **Porosity:** A large amount of silica and spherulitic structure of gypsum, produce enough porosity. This is an advantage, as a porous investment can easily allow the gases or air trapped in the mould to escape during casting. Hence, incomplete casting due to back pressure porosity does not take place. The investment thickness beyond the extreme end of wax pattern should be about 6 mm for the effectiveness of porosity.

5. **Thermal expansion:** Large thermal expansion is obtained due to cristobalite (or quartz) as the temperature rises. If its content is >75% by wt., it can counteract the initial contraction of the gypsum

Table 15.1	Composition of gypsum-bonded investment powder		
Ingredients		Weight%	Functions
1. Refractory material, cristobalite, quartz or their mixture		60–80%	Contributes strength, porosity, thermal expansion and thermal stability
2. Binder: Type III dental stone $CaSO_4 . \frac{1}{2} H_2O$ (α-type)		15–30%	Binds refractory material, and while setting it increases strength, porosity setting and thermal expansions
3. Modifiers: K, Li or Na chlorides or boric acid		3–10%	Prevents shrinkage due to loss of water
4. Reducing agents: Fine powders of copper, graphite		2–3%	Prevents oxidation and tarnishing of gold alloy castings
5. Small amount of colour			

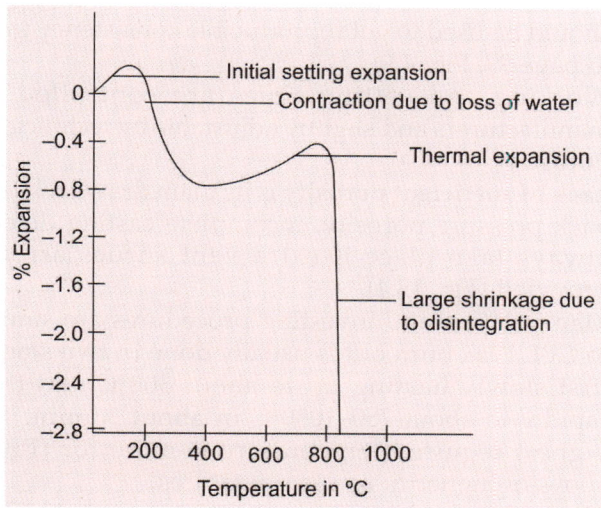

Fig. 15.2: Dimensional changes of dental stone (binder) when heated

binder (between 200°C and 400°C) (Fig. 15.2). But a larger amount of silica may decrease the strength. The total thermal expansion can even be as much as 1.2% at 800°C. According to ADA specification No. 2, the thermal expansions of type I, NSE method can be up to 0.6% at 500°C and for type II HSE method it can be 1.2 to 2.2%.

Thermal expansion becomes greater, if
- Temperature rise is higher
- Cristobalite is more
- Water/powder ratio is lower
- More modifiers (Na, Li, K chlorides or borates) are added.

However, rapid heating, prolonged heating, and over heating during wax burn out may fracture the investment. Alloy liquid may enter into these cracks, solidify and produce fins.

A disintegration of GBI takes place if heated above 600°C.
Manipulation (*refer* to casting procedure)

Advantages of GBI
- Adequate strength
- Adequate porosity
- Controlled large setting and thermal expansions
- Simple methods of manipulation and casting procedure
- Not very expensive

Disadvantages of GBI
1. The bonding agent, gypsum undergoes the following changes, when heated
   - Above 600°C, $CaSO_4 + C \longrightarrow CaO + SO_2 + CO\uparrow$ reduction by carbon.
   - Above 1000°C; $CaSO_4 \longrightarrow CaO + SO_2\uparrow + O_2\uparrow$ sulphur dioxide gas produced due to disintegration at the walls of the mould, causes tarnishing or discoloration of gold alloys. **Disintegration causes large contraction.**
   Hence, this is **not suitable** for casting of high fusing HN, N and PBM alloys and phosphate bonded investment material is preferred.
2. Too high casting force and careless wax burn out methods (prolonged, rapid or overheating) fractures and produce cracks in the investment which results: fins.
3. The GBI powder is hygroscopic and has a short storage time. Hence, large quantity should not be purchased. It should be stored carefully in air-tight containers.
4. Cannot be used for casting of titanium alloys.

PHOSPHATE-BONDED INVESTMENT (PBI)

The recent trend in casting procedure is, to use high fusing noble metals and cheaper PBM alloys for metal-ceramics, FPD and RPD frameworks. The PBI has become more popular due to its many advantages. This is supplied in sealed sachets, weighing 200 or 500 gm. It is mixed with distilled water, or water added with **freeze free silica gel** (liquid) **with a definite proportion to get a larger setting and thermal expansions,** required for compensating higher casting shrinkages of these high fusing alloys (*see* Colour Plate 20, Fig. 8.8 1 to 3) and composition of PBI is given in Table 15.2.

Setting reaction

When the powder is mixed with the prescribed amount of water (and added with colloidal silica liquid) it undergoes following **acid–base reaction.**

$NH_4H_2PO_4 + MgO + 5H_2O \rightarrow NH_4Mg(PO_4).6H_2O + heat$, or its colloidal multimolecular form $[NH_4 MgPO_4 6H_2O]_n$, around the unreacted excess MgO and binds the refractory materials.

Properties

1. **Setting expansion**
   The setting expansion can be increased by adding more colloidal silica suspension (*refer* to Fig. 15.3b). The expansion can be NSE or HSE also.

2. **Thermal changes**
   - On heating, it gets dehydrated partially at around 160°C,

     i.e. $NH_4MgPO_4 6H_2O \xrightarrow{160°C} NH_4MgPO_4 H_2O + 5H_2O$

   - On heating further to **300–650°C**,

     $(NH_4MgPO_4 H_2O)_n \rightarrow (Mg_2P_2O_7)_n + NH_3 \uparrow$

     The NH_3 gas smell produced in the wax burn out furnace can be felt around the laboratory.

   - This becomes a noncrystalline polymeric phase and finally becomes $Mg_3(P_2O_5)_2$ above 1040°C.

Thermal expansion

Contraction of investment at the temperature range 300–400°C is overcompensated by the large thermal expansion of the PBI.

It is possible to get maximum of 1.1% setting expansion and 1.3% thermal expansion by heating investment to about 800°C. The total expansion, i.e. about 2.4% is sufficient to compensate large shrinkages of high fusing 'N' and PBM alloy (Fig. 15.3a). Thermal expansion also increases with a greater amount of colloidal silica (Fig. 15.3b).

3. **Working and setting times**
   The setting takes place faster as the mixing is done rapidly, the reaction is exothermic.
   Mechanical mixing device with an electric motor, controlling speed and mixing time under vacuum should be used to get reproducible consistency (*refer* to page 97, Fig. 4.9).
   Working and setting times are controlled by manufacturers and slightly adjustable by technicians.

4. **Porosity**
   Lack of sufficient porosity is its main drawback. The back pressure porosity, incomplete casting defects always take place if extra vent sprues are not provided (Fig. 15.4).

5. Manipulation and investing procedures are similar to GBI. Wax burn out is usually done **in two stages,** first slowly heating up to about 300°C and then rapidly to about 750–1030°C **in about 30 min.** The highest required temperature is more for (PBM) alloys of higher fusion temperatures.

Advantages

- Ability to withstand high casting temperatures of HN or N, or PBM alloys and metal ceramic alloys.
- **Higher strength >4.8 MPA in 2 hours**. The more flexible casting ring can be pulled out after PBI sets.
- Sufficient controllable setting and thermal expansions.

Table 15.2	Composition of phosphate-bonded investment powder + liquid		
	Ingredients	Weight%	Functions
1.	Refractory material: Quartz or cristobalite or their mixture	80%	Withstand high temperatures, gives large setting (NSE, HSE) expansions
2.	Binder: Mixture of basic MgO and acidic ($NH_4H_2PO_4$)	20%	Increases strength, setting and thermal expansions
3.	Small amounts of carbon		Sometimes, act as a reducing agent
	Carbon or graphite crucibles should not be used for high fusing HN and N alloys, containing Pd as Pd reacts with carbon above 1500°C. The carbides and other trace metals in PBM alloys embrittle the alloys		
4.	**Liquid: Colloidal silica** suspension or freeze stable products, mixed with water, with various proportions 0–100% (but usually about 1/3 of water) to provide enough setting and thermal expansions (*refer* to Figs 15.3a and b).		

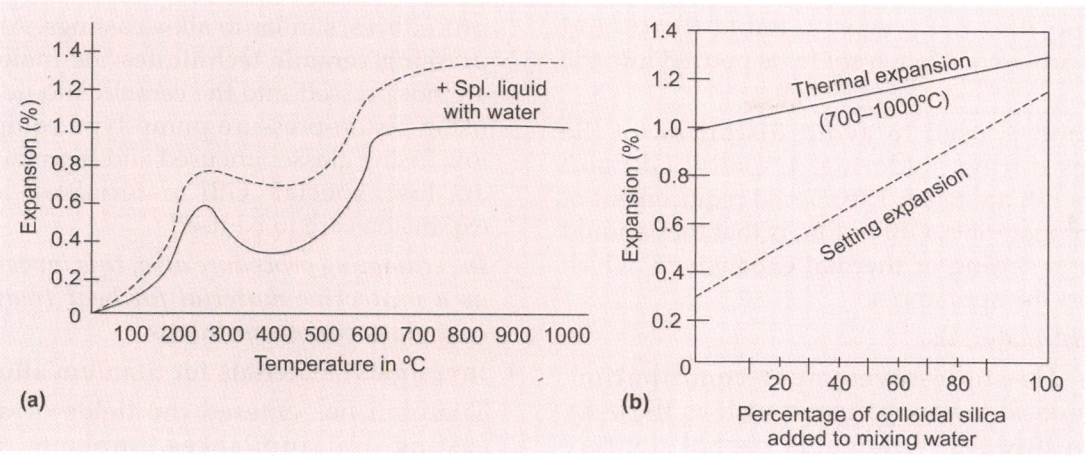

Figs 15.3a and b: (a) Dimensional changes of PBI during heating; (b) the percentage of colloidal silica net setting and thermal expansions of PBI, w.r.t.

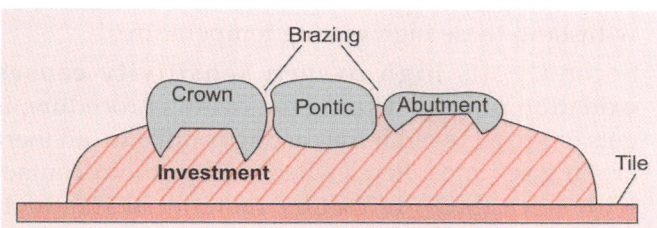

Fig. 15.4: Investment—soldering of crown and bridge parts

Disadvantages

- Insufficient **porosity cause air trapping in the mould resulting in** back pressure porosity—incomplete castings (remedy: **use thin vent sprues**).
- Strong adhesion to alloy casting: Diamond or carbide discs and then **sand-blasting** methods are required.
- **The surface finish is poor** compared to GBI castings.

ETHYL SILICATE-BONDED INVESTMENTS (ESBIS)

This has been developed to meet the refractory requirements of high fusing PBM alloys. It is supplied as a **powder of quartz or cristobalite, having selected particles distribution of different sizes and two liquids or one liquid amine system.** Setting and bonding mechanisms are more complex. In principle, the ethyl silicate is first hydrolyzed into **silicic acid** which is made to undergo gelation in the presence of HCl and MgO or certain amines. When the gel is heated to about 170°C, alcohol and water vapours escape and a **hard solid mass of cristobalite refractory nonporous material is formed**. **Large green shrinkage** occurs when water and alcohols escape.

$$Si(OC_2H_5)_4 + 4H_2O \rightarrow Si(OH)_4 + 4\ C_2H_5OH \uparrow$$

$$nSi(OH)_4 \xrightarrow{heat >168°C} [-Si-O-Si-O-]\ Cristobalite + n\ H_2O \uparrow$$

Advantages

1. The final set mass is **entirely cristobalite** (a three-dimensional-O-Si-O-network) which can withstand very high temperatures even beyond 1150°C. Hence, this can be used for high fusing PBM alloys.
2. Large thermal expansion compensates green shrinkage and also casting shrinkages.

Disadvantages

1. **Nonporous** material requires suitable vent sprues.
2. The complicated manipulation-investing procedure with vibration, tamping, setting, etc.
3. Inflammable alcohol vapours in the laboratory.
4. Cannot be used for titanium and its alloys as silica (SiO_2) can oxidize titanium or its alloys at high temperatures during casting.
5. Due to the complicated investing procedure, it is rarely used.

OTHER INVESTMENT MATERIALS

1. **Soldering investments**
RPD frameworks and long span FPDs are cast sometimes in separate parts and then soldered or brazed. The parts are assembled on the master casts, joined with molten sticky wax, and then invested in special investment materials on a tile. After

eliminating the sticky wax, suitable fluxes and antifluxes are used. Molten solder is poured into the gap.

This method is used **to avoid distortion** of the appliances during soldering. Usually, GBI and sometimes PBI are used. The special requirement of investment materials, GBI or PBI, is that they should not **undergo setting or thermal expansions**, which may distort the appliances.

2. **Divestment materials**

This is a **die-stone-investment combination**. Distortion of large wax patterns, such as those for long-span bridges, removable partial denture frameworks, etc. take place during removal from the die and investing procedures. To avoid this and get a better fit, die-stone investment technique is used.

Special GBI (with type V die stone binder) or PBI investment materials are used (Fig. 15.5). These are mixed with **colloidal silica liquid** and used to prepare a duplicate of the master cast or die. The wax pattern is prepared on this duplicate cast and **invested along with the cast in the same investment material**. The setting expansion is about 0.9% and thermal expansion is about 0.6% at about 650°C (suitable for N-metal-**high heat technique**) and about 1.2% at about 850°C (suitable for high fusing PBM alloys). The total expansion is sufficient to compensate respective casting shrinkages.

3. **Investment material for ceramics**

The casting of ceramic crowns using **castable glasses** is done in the refractory moulds, by lost wax

procedures, similar to alloy castings. Also in the **hot pressing ceramic techniques** the molten ceramics, are hot pressed into the ceramic mould by pressure using piston-pressure pump-type equipment. Since low fusing glasses are used and thermal contractions are low, special GBI materials of low thermal expansions are to be used.

In ceramming procedure also, this investment is used as a protective material for heat treatment of the cast glass crowns or inlays.

4. **Investment materials for titanium alloys**

Titanium has entered the fields of dentistry for casting oral appliances, implants (and also as orthodontic wires), etc. and is a material of choice. However, many problems are faced in the casting procedures.

CpTi has a very high melting point (1668°C) and hence requires special investment materials to withstand these high casting temperatures.

Secondly, its **high oxygen sensitivity causes oxidation quickly**. During the casting procedure, it gets oxidized (even if the casting is done in an inert argon gas atmosphere) when it comes into contact with silica (SiO_2) refractory material at this high casting temperatures.

Phosphate bonded or aluminous cement bonded investments with different refractory materials have been recently developed in Japan. These refractory materials contain,

$Al_2O_3 + Z_rO_2$, $Al_2O_3 + SiO_2$, $Al_2O_3 + Li\,Al\,SiO_2$, $MgO + Al_2O_3$, $MgO + Al_2O_3 + Z_rO$, etc. combinations.

In addition, the casting temperatures of the moulds also have to be reduced. The refractory material contains ethyl-silicate bonding agent and the mould casting temperature (after wax burn out) is lowered or reduced to room temperature to avoid oxidation, as the setting expansions can be increased to an adequate percentage (*see* Colour Plate 29, Figs 15.1 to 15.4).

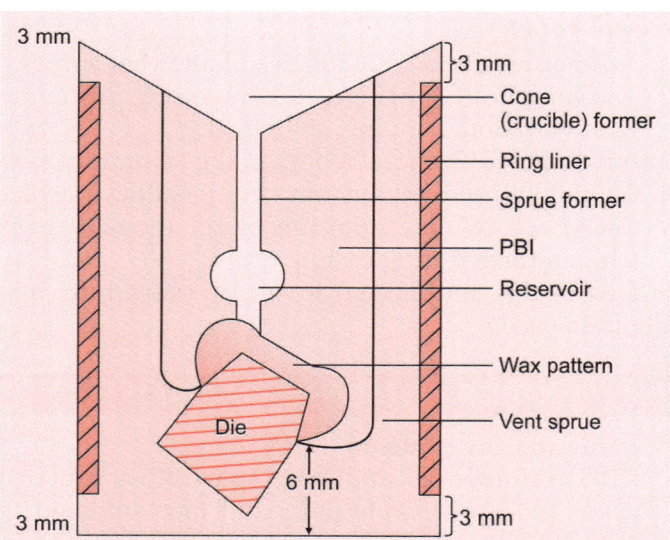

Fig. 15.5: Longitudinal cross-section of divested casting ring, with vent sprue and die

3 mm

3 mm — Cone (crucible) former
— Ring liner
— Sprue former
— PBI
— Reservoir
— Wax pattern
— Vent sprue

Die

6 mm

3 mm

3 mm

MODEL QUESTIONS

I. Long Essays (20 minutes each)

1. Explain in detail, the various causes for casting shrinkages and methods of their compensations.

2. Define the term "investment materials". Explain their ideal requirements and classify the available materials. Add a note on phosphate-bonded casting investments.

3. Describe the composition, setting action, properties, and uses of gypsum-bonded investments. What are their advantages and disadvantages?

II. Short Essays (10 minutes each)

1. Ideal requirements of investment materials
2. Gypsum-bonded investments
3. Phosphate bonded investments
4. Thermal changes and expansions of phosphate bonded investments.
5. Silica refractory materials
6. High and low heat techniques of casting
7. Investment materials for the casting of titanium.

III. Brief Answers (5 minutes each)

1. Wax shrinkage
2. Alloy casting shrinkage
3. Ethyl-silicate bonded investments
4. Soldering investments
5. Divestments
6. Colloidal silica for PBI
7. Cristobalite refractory material
8. Compositions of gypsum-bonded investment
9. Porosities in investments
10. Green shrinkage

CHAPTER 16

Metals: Solidification and Microstructure

CHAPTER SURVEY

- Metals: Noble, base, metalloids, non-metals
- Metallic bonding
- Characteristic properties of metals
- Newton's law of cooling
- Supercooled state

- Homogeneous nucleation
- Heterogeneous nucleation
- Dendrites, grain boundaries
- Grain size refinement
- Microstructures: Cast and wrought alloys

Search for biocompatible, permanent, strong, aesthetic, dental restorative materials has to lead to the use of four groups of materials, namely **metals, polymers, composites** and **ceramics**. Knowledge of metals, alloys and their microstructures is essential for the selection of materials and techniques of fabrication of the strong, permanent prosthesis. However, a recent trend is to give more importance to **biocompatibility and aesthetics, rather than strength and service time.** The metal ceramic restorations, coupled with strength and aesthetics, are recently gaining popularity.

Out of about 115 elements identified and studied, about 81 are considered as metals, few as metalloids and others as nonmetals. Metals are vaguely defined as **opaque, lustrous, chemical substances which are good conductors of heat and electricity and polishable to reflect light.**

Metals can be classified according to

1. **Noble metals:** These have high resistance to oxidation, corrosion, and dissolution in organic acids and are eight in numbers, Au_{197}, Pt_{195}, Ir_{192}, Os_{190}, Ag_{108}, Pd_{106}, Rh_{103}, Ru_{101}. Out of these, silver has low corrosion resistance in oral conditions and is not considered as noble metal in dentistry. However, alloys of silver and palladium have excellent corrosion resistance and are sometimes known as **semiprecious metals. Other seven are known as precious metals**. These terms are nowadays not used. When these are alloyed with few base metals,

their strength increases, corrosion resistance is retained as required, and melting temperatures are changed.

2. **Base metals:** A large number of metals, which occur more abundantly and undergo oxidation and corrosion easily, are base metals, e.g. Fe, Co, Ni (magnetic), Al. Ti, Cr (passivating), Cu, Sn, Zn, Na, K, Mn, Mg, Mo, etc. Some of these, can alloy with noble metals and get corrosion resistance. Cr, Ti and Al, rapidly combines with atmospheric oxygen, forming a **thin impervious** oxide layer, firmly adhering to parent metals. **This passivation** prevents further oxidation and imparts good corrosion resistance.

3. **Metalloids:** Few elements carbon, boron, germanium, silicon, sometimes behave like metals (conductors of heat and electricity) and sometimes nonmetals (do not form positive ions in solution). These and their alloys have found their immense use in semiconducting devices, communication, and industries due to their ability to conduct electricity in selective directions.

Metals also can be classified according to their physical properties

1. Ductile or brittle
2. Heavy or light
3. High fusing or low fusing, etc.

Pure metals are rarely used in industries but have limited use in dentistry, e.g. gold (direct filling gold foils and strips), platinum (foils), titanium, mercury, silver points, copper-electroformed dies, etc. The metals are alloyed with other metals or sometimes with nonmetals, and used abundantly in all fields (*refer* to Appendix: Periodic table).

CHARACTERISTIC PROPERTIES OF METALS

1. **Metallic bonding:** Metals have crystalline structure due to long-range electrostatic attractive forces between atoms which form metallic bonds. The valence electrons in the outermost shells get easily debonded at all temperatures by thermal energies, leaving behind, the atoms as positive ions in their lattice positions. These **free electrons** are moving at random in-between the positive ion—lattices **as electron gas,** form very strong attractive forces, holding the positive ions at their positions. This **strong metallic bonding** is responsible for all the following properties.

2. **Form positive ions in solution,** e.g. H^+ (in HCl), Na^+ (in NaCl), K^+ (in KCl or K_2SO_4), etc. in solutions.

3. **Good conductors of heat and electricity:** Free electron gas density is responsible for this conduction. Gold, silver, platinum, copper, etc. are very good conductors due to their **high electron gas densities**. Ceramics, polymer resins, etc. **lack free electrons** and therefore are **insulators.**

4. **Very ductile and malleable,** e.g. gold, platinum, silver, copper, tin, etc.

5. **Opaque** due to absorption of electromagnetic radiations by the free electrons. Well-polished metallic surfaces are very good **reflectors of light**, as the electrons re-emit the absorbed or incident light.

6. Most of the metal surfaces appear **white,** except few, like gold, copper, etc. as the free electrons can re-emit light of all wavelengths.

7. Most of them are solids (except few, like hydrogen, mercury, etc.) at room temperatures.

8. Have **definite melting and boiling temperatures.**

9. **High fracture toughness**—resistance to crack propagation (25–60 MPa/$\sqrt{m}$ as compared to ceramics, i.e. 0.75 to 5.0 MPa/$\sqrt{m}$, m = meter

   Fracture toughness is the energy required to produce a fine crack of unit length in the material measured by Vicker's indentation, Charpy impact testing, 3-point bending testing methods.

10. Most of them produce metallic **ringing sounds** when suddenly struck.

11. Most of them have high densities.

Newton's Law of Cooling

According to this law, the quantity of heat lost per second from a hot body, i.e. rate of cooling dQ/dt, is directly proportional to the mean excess of its temperature above the cooler surrounding. If a body of mass m, specific heat s cools from $\theta_2°$ to $\theta_1°C$ in t seconds at outside temperature $\theta_0°C$.

$$\frac{dQ}{dt} \propto \theta - \theta_0 \quad \text{or m.s.} \left[\frac{\theta_2 - \theta_1}{t}\right] \propto \frac{\theta_2 + \theta_1}{2} - \theta_0$$

$$\text{or } \frac{dQ}{dt} \propto \frac{\theta_2 + \theta_1}{2} - \theta_0$$

According to Newton's law

Temperature against the time, graph, i.e. the **cooling curve is exponential**, indicating, infinite time required for cooling of the hot body to reach the external temperature, if not disturbed (Fig. 16.1).

Temperature falls quickly in the beginning and then slowly, the difference of temperature between the body and its surroundings goes on decreasing, i.e. the rate of cooling of a hot body is directly proportional to the temperature difference between the body and its surroundings.

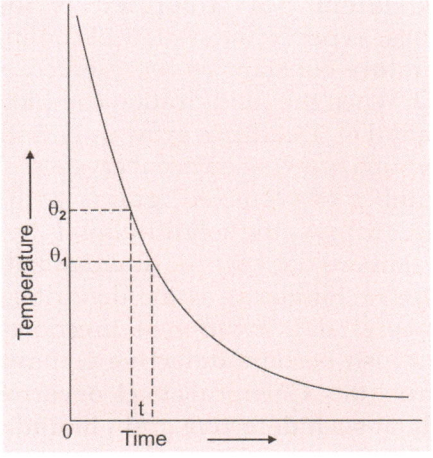

Fig. 16.1: Cooling curve

Solidification of Metals

Homogeneous Nucleation

When a liquid is gradually cooled, the kinetic energy of atoms decreases. Due to the attraction between the atoms, they begin to **cluster** together. However, many other atoms collide and destroy these clusters. If the pure liquid is carefully cooled in an inert, clean container, the temperature can **decrease slightly** below the actual solidification temperature (T°C) as represented by the part AB (Fig. 16.2). This **supercooled**

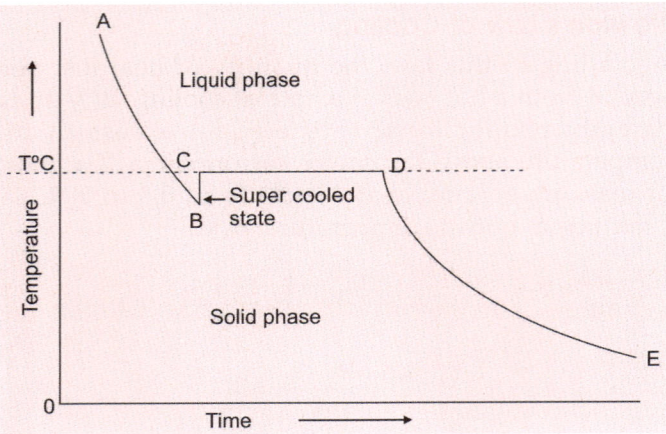

Fig.16.2: Super-cooling, solidification

condition at B is very unstable and is suitable to form stable clusters or **embryo** of crystals (as the KE of atoms is insufficient to destroy them). Such stable nuclei of crystallization are formed in very large numbers, throughout the liquid **homogeneously**. The diffusion of atoms towards the nuclei, makes them grow, forming **tree-like structures**, known as **"dendrites."** Loss of kinetic energy of atoms appears as **latent heat**, causing an immediate rise of temperature from B to C, which is the normal solidification temperature, T°C. This process continues, latent heat liberated is lost to the surroundings, as per Newton's law of cooling, keeping the **temperature constant** as represented by plateau portion CD. When the solidification completes, it cools exponentially DE. Dendrites grow only until they are stopped by such growing adjacent crystals. These form a large number of equiaxed, grains with nuclei as centers (Fig. 16.3). As the solidification is by diffusion, perfect crystals are not formed. **Interdendritic space is quite defective.** Similarly, as the dendritic growth in the adjacent crystals is in different directions, the **grain boundaries** also become **defective** or have inhomogeneous structures. **Chemical attack or corrosion takes place easily at such defective grain boundaries**.

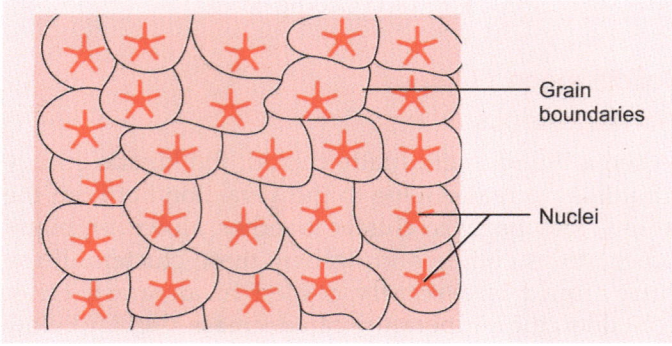

Fig. 16.3: Crystal grain boundaries

Grain Refinement

If such grains are finer (i.e. smaller) the grain boundaries become larger and produce higher resistance to slip and deformations. In other words, to have **better mechanical properties, grain size must be smaller** or the number of nuclei of crystallization should be increased. It is found that **yield strength is inversely proportional to the square root of grain size (Hall-Petch equations)**. Grain refinement can be done by the following methods:

1. **Greater super-cooling** in case of only pure metals, causes solidification to take place with more numbers of nuclei of crystallization.

2. **Faster rate of cooling,** i.e. cooling at colder environment produces smaller grains.

3. **Addition of impurities:** Grain refining trace elements, of high melting points like iridium or ruthenium (of platinum group) when added in small amounts of **0.005 to 0.1%, can increase the number of nuclei of crystallization by 100 or 150 times.**

4. **Heterogeneous nucleation:** Small amounts of very **fine dust** of the corresponding metals (silver dust to silver liquid, gold dust to gold liquid), when sifted to the liquid just at the solidification temperature, can **seed** a very large number of nuclei of crystallization, inhomogeneously. The dust particles become the nuclei of crystallization.

Microstructure

The metal surface is very well polished using a series of fine abrasives and polishing agents and then **etched** by a suitable acid. The acid reacts or corrodes at the inhomogeneous grain boundaries. It is washed and observed through a **metallurgical optical microscope** or photographed. Light scattered at the grain boundaries make them appear, dark lines—**grain boundaries.** By **linear intercept** method, an average number of grains per unit length, or unit area or unit volume x, can be found out. Grain size becomes reciprocal of these numbers, i.e. 1/x. Electron microscopes, or high magnification and resolution microscopes, can be used to study the dendrites and microstructure of grains.

Microstructure reveals the interspaces within and in-between the grains. These defects decrease the mechanical properties. Due to stress concentrations, they cause microcracks (not tears) at higher temperatures. In the casting procedures, the mould walls are at lower temperatures. Hence, the first nuclei are formed on the mould walls and the **protuberances grow as dendrites** towards the hotter portion. Thus, if the mould is cylindrical or rectangular, the growing dendrites get interfered and form radial or columnar grains respectively (Fig. 16.4).

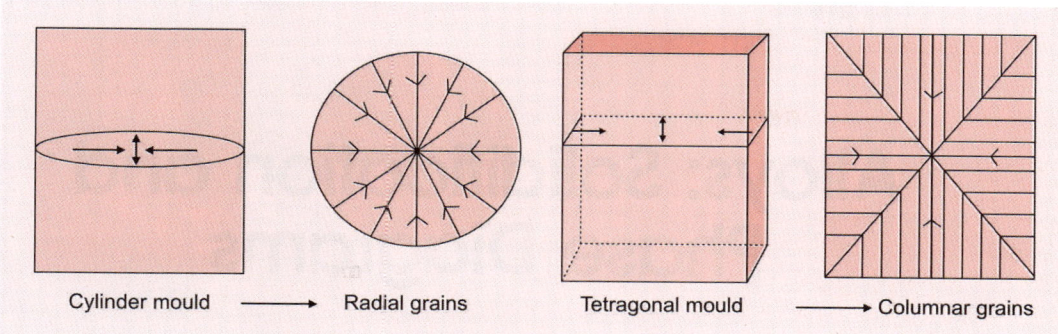

Fig. 16.4: Shapes of grains

If a large volume undergoes simultaneous nucleation, **equiaxed, spherical** crystals are formed. In small dental alloy castings, the **dendrites grow from the walls** of the small moulds towards the bulkiest part, forming **dendritic irregular grains**. Planes of interference of grains and grain boundaries are weaker parts which fail during deformations.

Alloys undergo solidification by **constitutional super-cooling,** forming grains with **cored** structures (compositions of components varying). Different phases also may solidify at a different range of temperatures. In such cases, the **phase of lowest solidification temperature, solidifies last at the interdendritic or intergranular spaces,** increasing the hardness by large value refer in carbides, in metallography—microstructure of base metal alloys.

Microstructure of Cold-worked (Wrought) Metals

Cold working operations are done to shape the cast metals into required forms by deforming, such as wire-drawing, forging or compressing into thin sheets. The grains are deformed into different shapes—**fibrous in wires, flattened in sheets,** etc. The **lattice defects move** to the interdendritic spaces and grain boundaries and increase their strength, brittleness, and decrease ductility, malleability and corrosion resistance. Annealing heat treatments, can cause recovery and recrystallisation. (*Refer* to wrought alloys—**work hardening and annealing.**)

MODEL QUESTIONS

I. Short Essays   (10 minutes each)

1. Characteristic properties of metals
2. Solidification of metals
3. Grain size and grain shapes of cast alloys
4. Microstructures of as-cast and wrought alloys

II. Brief Answers   (5 minutes each)

1. Metallic bonding
2. Metalloids
3. Supercooled state
4. Dendrites
5. Homogeneous nucleation
6. Heterogeneous nucleation

Alloys: Solidification and Phase Diagrams

CONSTITUTION—EQUILIBRIUM PHASE DIAGRAMS

An alloy can be defined as an intimate arrangement (or composition) of the atoms of two or more elements of which at least one is a metal. Since pure metals have its own characteristic properties, they can hardly be used directly in dentistry (or industries), except few, like gold, platinum, mercury, silver, commercially pure titanium, etc.

The main purpose of alloying is to get desired, corrosion resistance, mechanical and thermal properties

- **High corrosion resistance** can be achieved by alloying with noble metals like gold, platinum, etc. or passivating metals like chromium, titanium or aluminum.
- **Adequate mechanical properties can be obtained by solution hardening:** Examples—gold–copper, silver–copper, gold–platinum–palladium, chromium–cobalt or nickel, carbon–steel, etc. Mechanical properties also can be changed by **heat treatments** like tempering, annealing, precipitations of phases, etc.
- **Suitable thermal properties:** Melting temperature range can be increased by adding platinum, palladium, etc. or can be lowered by adding silver, zinc, copper or indium, etc. The coefficient of thermal expansion also can be increased or decreased (*refer to metal-ceramics thermal bonding*).

Alloys are prepared by melting the ingredients with required proportions and solidifying by casting into suitably prepared moulds. The components are carefully selected to minimize toxic materials like mercury, beryllium, nickel, etc. Compositions are usually expressed by **weight percentage.** But it is more useful to express in **atomic percentage** as this gives a better picture of the phase structures.

For example $AuCu_3$ phase has Au and Cu in 1:3 or 25 and 75 atomic percentages, whereas 45:55 weight percentage. Similarly, $AuCu$ phase has 50:50 atomic percentage and 70:30 weight percentage if gold and copper are alloyed respectively. In this book, all compositions are given by **weight%** unless otherwise stated.

The properties of alloys change according to the compositions. Hence, various properties of the alloys of different compositions are studied from 0 to 100%. The **solidification temperature ranges** determined from cooling curves are represented graphically against the compositions. This is known as the **constitution or equilibrium phase diagrams.**

Definitions

- **Alloy system:** It is an aggregate of two or more metals forming the alloy, at all possible proportions, 0–100%, e.g. Pd-Ag, Au-Cu, Ag-Cu, Ag-Sn, Fe-C, etc. alloy systems are studied in dentistry.

- **Phase:** A phase is a region of space, through which all physical properties of a material are essentially uniform. It is the **physically distinct, mechanically separable, homogeneous portion** of the alloy. These are formed by diffusion of atoms during solidification, to attain certain equilibrium phases, e.g. $AuCu_3$, $AuCu$, Ag_3Sn, Cu_3Sn, Cu_6Sn_5, NiTi, Ag-Cu eutectic, etc. Such equilibrium **phases can be identified** by their microstructure with the help of metallurgical microscope, SEM, etc.

CLASSIFICATION OF DENTAL CASTING ALLOYS

Alloys are used for casting permanent oral appliances, like all metal inlays, crowns, and bridges, metal-ceramics prosthesis, removable and fixed cast partial dentures, implants, etc. As a large number of varieties of alloys are used, their classifications are made **for identification, selection** (according to compositions and properties) and also to **estimate the cost.**

These alloys are broadly classified according to

1. **Nobility:** Noble metals are Au, Pt, Ir, Os, Pd, Rh, Ru and Ag
   - *High noble (HN) metal alloys:* Contain gold $\geq 40\%$, noble metals $\geq 60\%$, e.g. Au-Cu, Au-Cu-Ag, Pd-Au-Pt, etc.
   - *Noble (N) metal alloys:* Contain noble metals $\geq 25\%$, e.g. Pd-Ag, Pd-Ag-Au
   - *Predominantly base metal (PBM) alloys:* Noble metals $\leq 25\%$ or 0–25%
     Ex: Cr-Co, Cr-Ni, Cr-Co-Ni, Cr-Co-W, or Ni-Ti, Ti-Al-V, FeC, Fe-Cr-Ni-Co, Fe-Cr-Ni-C (stainless steel).
2. **Compositions:** Mentioned according to decreasing order of weight percentages
   - Single major elements: Gold alloys, palladium alloys, silver alloys, titanium alloys ....
   - Two major elements: Au-Cu, Au-Ag, Pd-Ag, Ag-Pd, Ni-Ti, Co-Cr, Ni-Cr,..........
   - Three major elements: Au-Cu-Ag, Pd-Ag-Cu, Co-Cr-W, Ni-Cr-Be, Ti-Al-V,.........
3. **Dominant phases**
   - Single isomorphic solid solution; Au-Cu, Pd-Ag, etc.
   - Eutectic: Silver–copper, eutectoid pearlite
   - Peritectic change; Pt-Ag, Ag-Sn, etc.
   - Intermetallic: Au-Cu, Au-Cu$_3$, Cu$_3$Sn, Cu$_6$Sn$_5$, Ag$_3$Sn, etc.
4. **Applications**
   - All metal inlays, crowns, bridges
   - Metal-ceramic prosthesis
   - Removable and fixed cast partial dentures
   - Implants, post, and cores

5. **Mechanical properties**
   Type I: Soft—burnishable, YS <80 MPa
   Type II: Medium—burnishable, YS = 80–180 MPa
   Type III: Hard—heat hardenable, YS = 180–240 MPa
   Type IV: Extra hard—heat hardenable, YS >300 MPa
   Note 1: If the alloys contain only two, three, four metals they are called **binary, ternary, quaternary,** etc. alloys.

   Note 2: More details of classifications according to compositions and applications are given in the next chapter, Dental Casting Alloys (Tables 18.2 and 18.3).

SOLID SOLUTIONS

Preliminary idea: By dissolving a solute, like sugar or common salt in a solvent like water, a homogeneously dispersed solution is obtained. The maximum amount of solute that can dissolve in 100 ml of solvent can be called as the solubility percentage at that temperature. This solubility usually increases with the rise of temperatures. If this single phase saturated solution, is cooled, it becomes supersaturated, and the **excess solute** gets precipitated or separated from the solvent.

A solid solution is formed when a mixture of liquids of two or more metals, is cooled and solidified. Then, atoms of one metal substitute atoms of other solvent metal at its lattice, or remain in the lattices space (crystal structure unchanged).

The solute is that metal whose atoms are a minority in number in solution (in the solvent lattice).

The solvent is that metal retaining its own lattice structure and has a majority number of atoms in solution lattice, e.g. copper, when added in small amounts to silver or gold, forms copper in silver or copper in gold solid solution. Copper is solute, silver or gold are solvents, whose atoms are substituted or replaced by copper atoms. Similarly, we have silver in copper (max solubility, 8.0% or copper in silver (max solubility 8.8%), i.e. β and α solid solutions. But copper in gold and silver in palladium are completely soluble in each other at all proportions. As the solid polycrystalline structure is formed it hinders the diffusion of solute atoms. Hence, to reach equilibrium conditions, infinite time is required. In metallurgy, more than two elements are usually present and different phases are mostly formed.

Hume–Rothery Conditions for Substitutional Solid Solution

- They should intimately mix with each other when liquefied.
- **Atomic size** between alloying element and host metal should be **nearly the same** and should not differ by more than 15% (within ~15%) (Table 17.1).

Table 17.1	Crystal lattices and atomic diameters of common elements in gold and palladium alloys	
Metal	Crystal lattice	Atomic diameters in AU
Gold	FCC	2.882
Platinum	FCC	2.775
Palladium	FCC	2.750
Silver	FCC	2.888
Copper	FCC	2.556
Tin	**BCT**	**3.016**
Zinc	**HCP**	**2.665**
Silicon	**Diamond cubic**	**2.351**

- **Valencies** of solute and solvent atoms must be **same** to have high solubility, otherwise solubility becomes very small.
- **Crystal lattice structure:** Should be **same** to form a complete series of solid solutions.
- **Chemical affinity,** should **not be present** to form a solid solution. Otherwise, they form, ordered **intermetallic alloys** specially when the alloy is cooled below certain lower temperatures (*refer to* gold–copper system.)
- For interstitial solid solution, the Hume–Rothery rule is: Solute atoms should have a radius no longer than 59% of the radius of solvent atoms. (Other rules are similar to substitutional solid solution.)

The most common gold alloying metal, copper, has a larger atomic size difference. **It causes greater localized lattice distortion, increases slip resistance and strength.** Small amounts zinc in gold alloys embrittles it. Tin, silicon, and zinc, harden the alloy very much but decrease ductility and malleability, as their lattice structures are different.

Types of Solid Solutions

- **Disordered substitutional alloys:** The solute particles substitute the solvent atoms at random in the crystal lattices, increasing hardness. The lattice structure of solvent or solution remains unaltered, e.g. Cu in Ag (α), Ag in Cu (β), Cu in Au, Pd in Ag, etc. (*refer to* Fig. 20.3a, page 290).
- **Ordered substitutional alloys:** Due to slightly greater **chemical affinities, at lower temperatures**, new ordered phases are formed by diffusion of atoms, which precipitate as a **superlattice**, e.g. copper in gold alloys form and precipitate AuCu and $AuCu_3$ phases around 375°C.
- **Interstitial alloys:** If the atomic size of solute is very small, compared to solvent atoms, like carbon and iron, solute atoms instead of substituting solvent atoms, directly enter into space in the lattice. This

interstitial alloy, like carbon in iron, has very low solubility of carbon, but introduces **enormous lattice distortion** and increases strength (carbon steel).

Properties of Solid Solutions

- **Corrosion resistance** of noble metal alloys changes according to noble metal contents (carat or fineness).
- **Density** and hence cost of alloy, changes.
- **Mechanical properties (solution hardening):** The small difference in atomic sizes (say gold 2.882 and copper 2.556 AU) causes **localized lattice distortion increasing slip resistance and strength.** Hence, **hardening is more, if atomic size difference and solute concentrations are higher.** Strength becomes maximum, when solute has **50% atomic percentage.** In the case of partially soluble solid solutions lowering the temperature, cause, **supersaturation** and precipitation of solute particles in the lattice space. This also increases hardness. (Copper in silver—**precipitation hardening**.)

At lower temperatures, new ordered intermetallic alloys, phases can be formed. These precipitate as **superlattices** which increase the hardness (copper–gold system, Au-Cu FCT phase in FCC solid solution. This is **precipitation hardening.** Suitable types of heat treatments of solid solutions can change the mechanical properties conveniently (e.g. hardening and softening heat treatments of gold–copper alloys, tempering of stainless steel, or Elgilloy wires, etc.). Ductility and malleability, always are lower for a solution hardened alloys.

Thermal Properties

- Alloys have **ranges of melting** temperatures which depend on the compositions. Solid solutions of different compositions have different ranges. These ranges can be raised or lowered suitably by adding suitable elements, like Pd or Cu to gold respectively.
- A coefficient of thermal expansion also can be changed lowered by adding Pt or Pd to gold alloys or raised by adding copper or silver (*refer to* metal-ceramics bonding).
- Thermal conductivity also changes.

All these changes can be tested by several methods, sometimes using sophisticated pieces of equipment like, universal testing machines, tensiometers, etc. The thermal properties, solidification temperatures with respect to the compositions can be studied with phase or constitution diagrams of the alloy systems.

Solidification of Alloys

Alloys do not have single solidification temperatures (except eutectic compositions), but small ranges of temperatures. That is, when an alloy liquid is cooled, it begins to solidify forming nuclei of crystallization at certain temperature $T_2°C$, and completes solidification at a lower temperature $T_1°C$ (Fig. 17.1).

As the temperature decreases the dendrites are formed by the growth of crystals. These growing dendrites have different compositions as the temperature falls. For equilibrium, **the alloy should be held, at the particular temperature** for a long time, for the diffusion of atoms to take place, and to attain that composition. In other words, during solidification, it should be cooled very slowly. **Otherwise, the compositions of each layer formed have different values.** This is known as a **cored structure**. Last liquid alloy of different composition, remaining at the lowest temperature, $T_1°C$, solidifies **en masse** in the interdendritic space and grain boundaries.

This cored structure is **quite brittle** as the atomic distributions are inhomogeneous. The ranges of solidification temperatures (T_1, T_2) continuously vary with the variations of composition (*refer* to Ag-Pd system phase diagram).

For examples: Silver–palladium, gold–copper, silver–copper systems.

Equilibrium Phase—Constitution Diagrams

For studying the properties of an alloy with different compositions, its phase diagrams or cooling curves should be drawn, for the entire compositions or **system.** The ranges of solidification temperatures $T_2°C$ and $T_1°C$ are determined for various compositions (0 to 100%) and plotted against their compositions, as shown in Fig. 17.2. The line connecting all $T_2°C$, is **liquidus**, and the line connecting all $T_1°C$, is **solidus.** This is known as the **constitution or equilibrium phase diagram** of the alloy system. The alloy has a **liquid phase**, above the liquidus, **solid phase** below the solidus and a mixture of liquid and solids in-between them. Theoretically, sufficient time should be allowed for diffusion of atoms, throughout solidification to attain equilibrium phase.

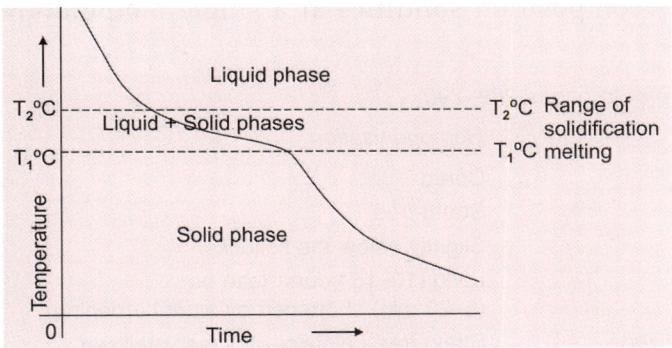

Fig. 17.1: Cooling-solidification curve for an alloy of certain composition

Silver–Palladium System (Coring and Homogenization)

For interpretation of phase diagrams and understanding the formation of cored structures, the Ag-Pd alloy system is discussed. Both silver and palladium have FCC structures, and their melting temperatures are 961°C and 1552°C respectively. They are completely soluble in each other forming solid solutions of continuous compositions (0 to 100%). By drawing cooling curves, ranges of melting (solidification) temperatures $T_2°C$ and $T_1°C$ are determined, for all compositions. A graph is drawn by plotting $T_1°C$ and $T_2°C$ against the compositions. The equilibrium phase diagram is obtained by joining all the temperatures, $T_1°C$ and $T_2°C$ separately to get solidus and liquidus as shown.

Consider an alloy of Pd = 65% by wt (i.e. Ag = 35% by wt) which is taken in liquid condition (P) and allowed to cool. When the temperature comes down to about 1400°C (Q), first nuclei of crystallization (solid) are formed. But solidification can take place at that 1400°C, only if the alloy has Pd = 78% according to **the tie line drawn through Q intersecting the solidus at M (Pd = 78%).** If sufficient time is given for diffusion of atoms, homogeneous nuclei and nucleation are formed (Fig. 17.2).

Another **tie line K, L, N at 1370°C** intersects the liquidus at K, with (Pd= 56%) and solidus at N, with (Pd = 72%). This shows, at that temperature, solid formed should have Pd = 72% and liquid remaining has Pd = 56% when equilibrium is reached.

Hence, as the temperature falls below 1400°C, the dendrites grow layer by layer, with Pd% decreasing from 78 to 65%, at 1340°C. At this temperature, remaining liquid has only Pd = 54% (silver = 46%). Since there should not be any liquid, below the temperature

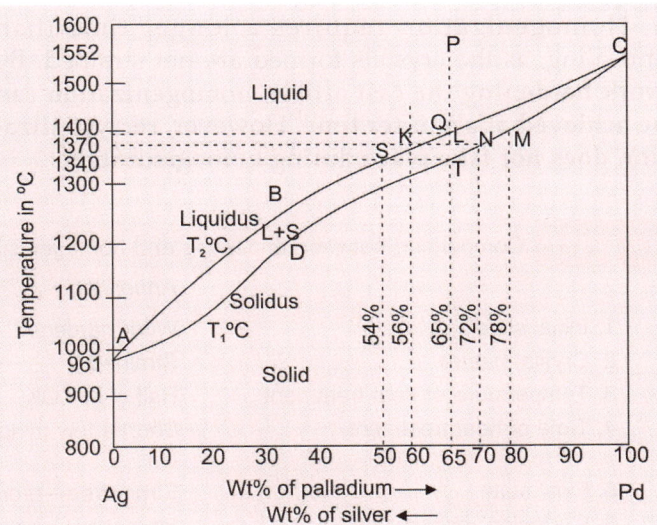

Fig. 17.2: Silver–palladium system

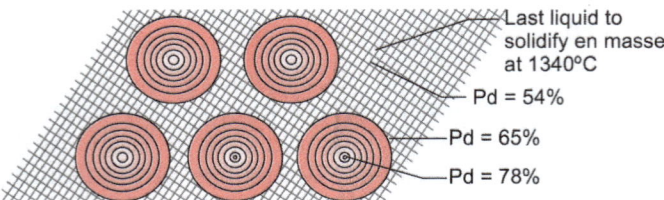

Fig. 17.3: Cored structures (Pd = 65%, Ag = 35%)

(1340°C), the entire liquid (Pd = 54%, Ag = 46%) remaining, should solidify **en masse** in the inter-dendritic space and in-between the grains, at that temperature, 1340°C (Fig. 17.3).

Coring and Homogenization

When an alloy liquid solidifies, it can be shown that the nuclei or first crystals formed, have certain compositions. The compositions gradually change from this core to the outer part. As solidification completes these cored crystals grow and finally get embedded in a matrix of different composition, which solidifies last.

Such inhomogeneous cored structure is very brittle and has low ductility or malleability. These are different from the expected properties of the homogeneous phase of the solid solution of that composition.

During casting procedure of noble or base metal alloys, always cored (brittle) structures are formed. To achieve the expected (soft, ductile) properties, the as-cast cored material should be homogenized.

Homogenization heat treatment

The as-cast article is heated to a high temperature, **slightly below the solidus**, and held at that temperature, for a **long time (10–15 hours).** The solute atoms can diffuse at a faster rate at this higher temperature and form homogeneous structure.

Homogenization requires a longer time than annealing, as the crystals formed are not strained. By **work hardening the cast article, homogenization can be achieved at a shorter time.** However, **recrystallization does not take place** during homogenization.

Applications of Pd-Ag Alloys

Palladium is an important noble metal used in dental casting procedures, orthodontic wires as well as metal-ceramics. Pd with Ag forms alloys in all proportions and has excellent corrosion resistance. Pd is used in smaller quantities in HN, but in larger quantities in 'N' metal alloys. Pd is also alloyed with copper, gallium and small quantities of tin, and indium.

Properties (*refer* to casting alloys).

Comparison between annealing and homogenizing (Table 17.2).

SILVER–COPPER SYSTEM

Both silver and copper belong to FCC structures and have their melting points 961°C and 1083°C respectively. They have **limited solid solubilities** in each other, and form, copper in silver (silver-rich α) and silver in copper (copper-rich β) phases, both being **disordered substitutional solid solutions.** The phase diagram shows the liquid phase above the liquidus AED and solid phases below the solidus, ABEGD (Fig. 17.4).

FEATURES OF EQUILIBRIUM PHASE DIAGRAMS

Note: These details are only for understanding

1. **Alpha phase**
   When the amount of copper is says, 5% or <8.8% (max. solubility at 779°C), solidification takes place along dotted line.........A' forming substitutional, cored α (Cu in Ag) phase in liquid (L + α) which solidifies around 860°C into the silver-rich solid terminal phase (Fig. 17.4a).

2. **Beta phase**
   When the amount of silver is says, i.e. 5% or <8.0% (max. solubility at 779°C), solidification takes place along dotted line ..... B' forming substitutional Ag in Cu, i.e. copper-rich β terminal phase (Fig. 17.4b).

3. **Liquidus and solidus meet** at E when the alloy has composition, silver 72% and copper 28%. This is the **lowest (eutectic) temperature,** below which there is only solid phase, i.e. liquid of this eutectic composition solidifies at a single temperature

Table 17.2	Comparison between annealing and homogenising (*refer* to pages 289–290)	
	Annealing	*Homogenisation*
1. Initial state	Work hardened	Cored
2. Crystal nature	Strained	Strain-free
3. Temperature of heat treatment	Half of MP OK	Slightly below the solidus
4. Time of heat treatment	Short a few minutes	Long (10–15 hours) (can be (5–20 min) shortened by work hardening)
5. Final state	Strain-free—recrystallized	Strain-free crystals—not recrystallized
6. Corrosion resistance	Increases	Increases

forming **lamellar structure α-solid and β-solid terminal phases, i.e. alternative layers** (Fig. 17.4c) **of silver-rich and copper-rich (α and β) phases** (dotted line H.)

Eutectic reaction: Liquid $\xrightarrow[779°C]{Cool}$ α solid solution + β solid solution which forms in alternate layers

4. **Hypoeutectic phase**

   When the amount of copper in the alloy is about 15% (i.e. above 8.8% up to 28%) **on cooling** (along with the line I), first crystallization begins at about 875°C with 5% copper (and 95% silver). Dendrites grow, with an increase of copper up to 8.8% at 779°C. These are α phase primary cored crystals. At this temperature 779°C liquid remaining will have 28% copper and 72% silver, that is eutectic composition and **solidifies en masse** forming alternate layers of α and β phases, i.e. the eutectic phase. This is hypoeutectic alloy, which has **α crystals embedded** in the eutectic phase (δ) (Fig. 17.4d).

5. **Hypereutectic phase**

   Similarly, when the alloy liquid having silver 8% to 72% is cooled (along with the line g), the primary cored crystals of copper-rich β phase (silver in copper) are formed. This gets embedded in the eutectic phase alternate layers of α and β phases. This is hypereutectic alloy (dotted line 'G' in Fig. 17.4e).

Note

Similar solid-to-solid transformation occurs when FCC austenitic steel is cooled, below 723°C, forming ferrite, hypoeutectoid (ferrite+pearlite), eutectoid (pearlite) and hypereutectoid (pearlite + cementite), equilibrium phases **on slow cooling**. Rapid cooling causes distorted FCT **martensite—the hardest phase** (*see* Fig. 21.1).

Precipitation (Age) Hardening

Solubilities of Cu in Ag and Ag in Cu at different temperatures are represented by the solvus lines CB and FG respectively. Maximum solubilities in the solid states are 8.8% and 8.0% respectively at the eutectic temperatures 779°C. Consider an alloy with 5% copper, 95% silver, cooling and solidifying. First solid formed at 940°C has about 2% copper and the outermost layer has more copper. Below about 860°C complete solidification of cored α structure is formed.

When this is cooled, it gets saturated by 5% copper at about 650°C. If it is further cooled below 650°C

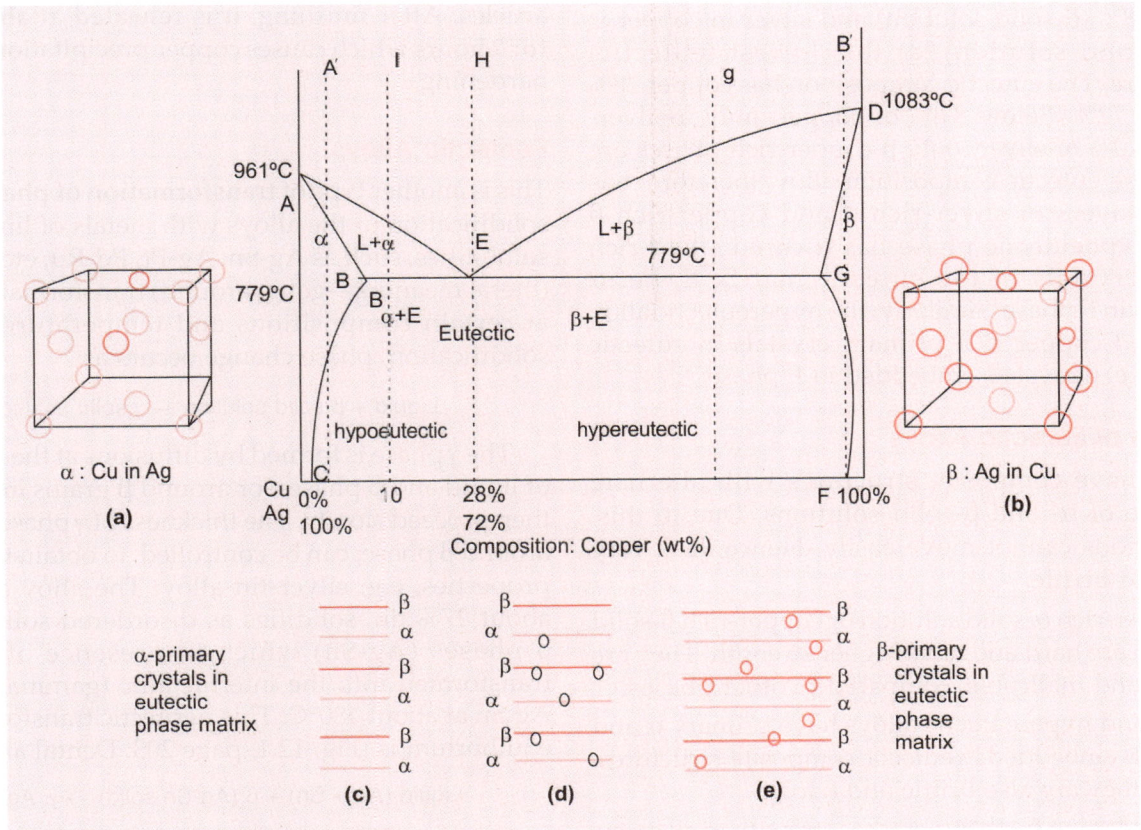

Figs 17.4a to e: Constitution diagram of silver–copper system. (a) Cu in Ag—α-solid solution, (b) Ag in Cu—β-solid solution, (c) eutectic phase, (d) hypoeutectic phase, (e) hypereutectic phase

α-solid solutions become **supersaturated**, and copper atoms **precipitate** in-between the lattices. These precipitated atoms cause **localized lattice distortions,** which increase slip resistance or hardness. When the temperature is lowered, more copper atoms should precipitate. However, in the solid state, diffusion takes place very slowly and the hardness increases gradually in a long time. Sometimes, this is known as **age-hardening**. This phenomenon is used in industries (rivetting of sheets, with certain alloys of aluminum which hardens in a few months).

This precipitation or age hardening takes place in the entire phase distributions, i.e. α and β phases, hypoeutectic, eutectic and hypereutectic phases.

Eutectic Alloys (Short Essay–Alternate Simple Answer)

Different solid solutions of limited solubilities, precipitate as alternate layers, of α and β solid solutions at the certain eutectic compositions which have a single, lowest melting point like 799°C in Ag-Cu eutectic alloy, with Ag = 72%, Cu = 28%.

In case of **partially solid soluble alloys** like copper and silver, for a definite composition, it has a single lowest melting temperature and not a range. For example, the maximum solid solubilities of copper in silver is 8.8% (α-solid solution) and silver in copper is 8.0% (β-solid solution), at this lowest (eutectic) temperature. The eutectic composition has copper 28% and silver 72%. Below 8.8% of copper, only α-silver-rich and 8.0% of silver, only β-copper-rich phases are formed. The eutectic composition alloy, therefore, has alternate layers of silver-rich α and copper-rich β phases. Hypoeutectic phase has α cored silver-rich primary crystals in the eutectic matrix E, i.e. α embedded in E phase. Similarly, the hypereutectic alloy has β cored copper rich primary crystals in eutectic matrix E, i.e. β crystals embedded in E phase.

Properties of Eutectic Alloys

- Alloys have composite structures with alternate lamellae of α- and β-solid solutions. Due to this, dislocations cannot move easily. Hence, it is **very hard and brittle.**
- The silver-rich α-solid solution or copper-rich β-solid solution are hard and have higher strength. They are ductile and malleable, compared to other phases.
- Hypo- and hypereutectic alloys have primary α and β crystals embedded in eutectic composite structures. Hence, they are also brittle and hard.
- Age-hardening further increases strength in all cases.
- Corrosion resistance: The silver-rich α phase has excellent corrosion resistance compared to other phases.

Applications

1. **In paediatric dentistry,** the silver-rich α phase, i.e. an alloy of silver with a small amount of copper (causing solution hardening) is used for temporary crowns.

2. **Disperse, or admix high copper silver amalgam alloys** The hard, brittle, silver–copper eutectic alloy (72:28 wt%) is used for strengthening low copper silver amalgam alloys: Eutectic liquid is solidified by atomizing, as fine spherical particles (spherical alloys) and **dispersed** in lathe-cut low copper alloy powder.

3. **Grain refinement of gold alloys:** Small amount of **ruthenium or iridium (0.005%) added, form** eutectic composition with gold, **depressing the melting temperature,** cause more nucleation and grain refinement.

Sterling Silver

Contains 7.5% copper, and solidifies, forming an equilibrium α phase on slow cooling. On continued heating, some copper-rich β phase also may precipitate. Silversmith uses this idea to prepare silver wares. Solution heat treatment, i.e. heating at 775°C for 30 min. and quenching makes it very soft and ductile. This is very convenient to mold by cold working into silver articles. After finishing, it is **reheated at about 325°C for 2 hours** which causes copper precipitation, and age-hardening.

Peritectic Alloys

This is another type of **transformation of phases** during solidification of the alloys with metals of limited solid solubilities, such as Ag-Sn. Ag-Pt, Pd-Ru, etc. Peritectic (literal meaning—going around) transformation occurs at certain compositions and temperatures. During solidification, phase change occurs as:

Liquid + β solid solution → γ solid solution

The γ phase is formed by diffusions at the interphase of liquid and β phases, or around β grains initially and then proceed slowly. The thickness of γ phase-envelope around β phase, can be controlled, to obtain the desired properties, e.g. silver-tin alloy: The alloy containing about 27% tin, solidifies as disordered solid solution β phases (Ag-Sn) which in presence of liquid is transformed into the intermetallic (gamma), γ phase, Ag_3Sn at about 480°C. This peritectic transformation in equilibrium is (Fig. 12.1, page 203: Dental amalgam):

Liquid (Ag + Sn) + β (Ag-Sn solid) → γ. Ag_3Sn

However, during solidification around 480°C γ phase is formed around β crystals. The relative amounts of β and γ phases influence the amalgamation reaction, dimensional changes, and corrosion resistance. This can be controlled by rate cooling.

GOLD–COPPER SYSTEM

Gold and copper have close melting points, 1063°C and 1083°C respectively and both have FCC structures. They are completely soluble in each other forming solid solution at high temperatures. These form disordered substitutional alloys, below the solidus. The equilibrium phase diagram has a narrow region in-between the liquidus and solidus (showing a small amount of coring) and meet each other at 911°C when the gold is about 80 wt% (Fig. 17.5).

Below the solidus temperature, when the atomic percentage of gold is more than 50%, disordered substitutional solid solution of Cu in Au phase is formed. When this α phase is slowly cooled, below 375°C or 410°C, the attraction between gold and gold or copper and copper atoms, cause the precipitation of two different phases as shown:

- **Au-Cu₃ FCC phase:** If the amount of copper atoms is more (gold 40 to 65 wt%) or Au:Cu = 25:75 atomic percentage solid state reaction takes place by ordering the copper atoms in the middle of the faces and gold atoms at the corners of FCC unit cell (Fig. 17.6a).

Under this arrangement, it can be shown that there are 3 copper atoms situated, nearest to each gold atoms. This AuCu₃ phase has the same FCC structure and does not contribute to the hardening of the alloy significantly (Fig. 17.6b).

- **Au-Cu, FCT phase** (Fig. 17.6c): When the percentage of gold is more (65–85 wt%), the solid state reaction takes place by forming intermetallic alloy Au-Cu equilibrium phase, with **copper atoms and gold atoms in alternate layers.** These are equiatomic 50:50%, **superlattices** (with gold 75 wt%). Due to the small difference in atomic sizes and interatomic forces, between copper atoms, the superlattice formed has one axis shorter, i.e. *face-centered tetragonal FCT structure. This phase precipitates by slow cooling, in different orientations at different sites.* At each site, it distorts of disordered FCC lattice or produce localized elastic strains. Such regions prevent the movement of dislocations when deforming forces are applied, i.e. slip resistance and hardness, increase, as more superlattice precipitates. This method of hardening is known as **precipitation hardening.**

The formation of such equilibrium superlattice phases can take place only by very **slow cooling.** However, in dental casting procedure for gold

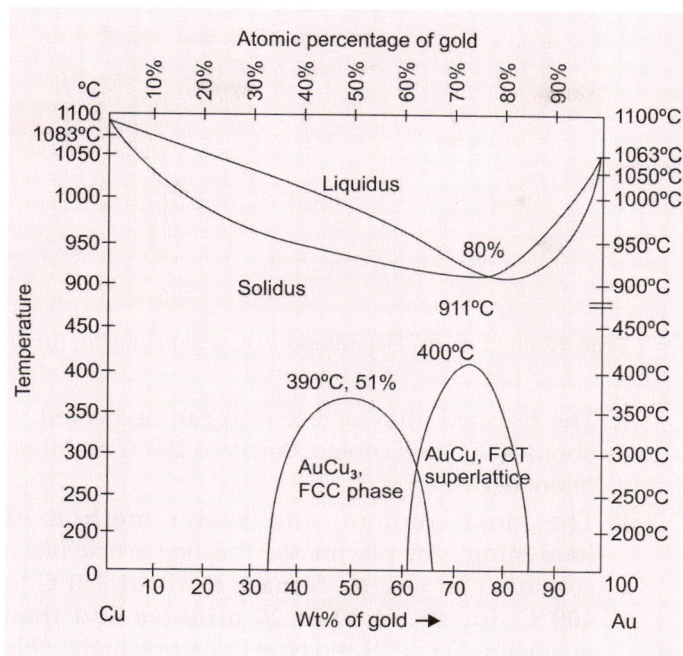

Fig. 17.5: Gold–copper equilibrium phase diagram

alloys, the casting is quickly cooled by quenching (sudden immersion in water). This does not allow sufficient time for atomic diffusion. Soft and ductile casting is obtained, and this property is **quite suitable for finishing.**

- **Order-disorder heat treatment of gold alloys**

Type III and type IV casting gold alloys fall in this composition range (gold 65–85 wt%), suitable for precipitation hardening heat treatments. The **as-cast, solution hardened,** and cored gold alloy-casting is soft and ductile and can easily be trimmed and polished (finished). During these procedures, the alloy also gets work hardened and strained.

- **Softening or solution heat treatment**

The casting is heated to a high temperature, about 700°C, just below the solidus and held at that temperature for about 10 min. for the atomic diffusion to take place. It is then quenched. The soft ductile nature is again recovered. This annealing heat treatment removes the work hardening effects and also cause homogenization of the cored structure.

- **Hardening heat treatment methods**

  i. If the above alloy is heated to 700°C and **cooled very slowly,** the equilibrium superlattice, **Au-Cu-FCT phase precipitates** when the temperature falls below 410°C. It can be quenched, when it cools below 250°C, as atomic diffusions are very slow, below this temperature and become ineffective.

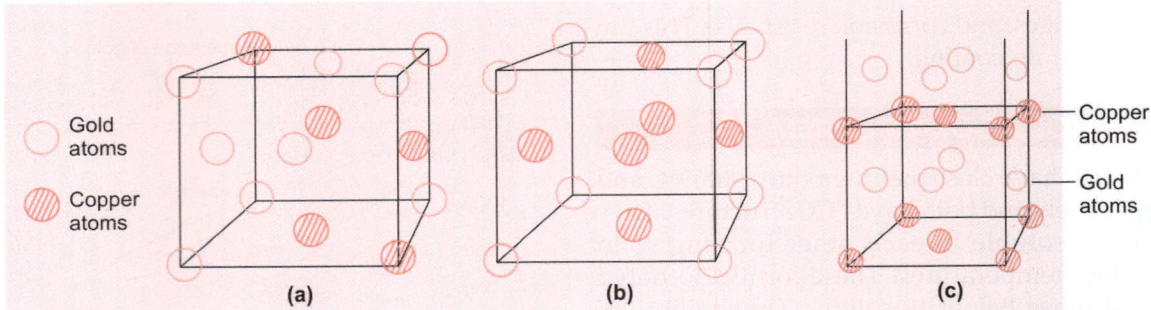

Figs 17.6a to c: (a) Disordered FCC solid solution, (b) ordered FCC AuCu$_3$ phase, (c) ordered FCT Au-Cu superlattice

ii. The finished alloy article also can be heated to about 400°C and cooled slowly to 250°C and then quenched.

iii. The most common and **easier method of hardening** is by placing the finished article like a crown, in an **electric furnace at about 350°C to 400°C**, for about **10 to 20 minutes** and then quenching. Type III and type IV casting high noble gold alloys can be subjected to this superlattice precipitation heat treatments. Their surface hardness increases approximately from 120–180 VHN and 150–250 VHN respectively. Their yield strength increases from 200 to 275 MPa for type III and from 270 to 500 MPa for type IV.

Subjecting this heat treatment for **longer times, cause excessive FCT phase precipitation and makes the casting brittle.** Hence, it is always safer to follow the manufacturers instructions for conducting heat treatments.

This precipitation or age-hardening of gold alloy crowns, bridges can also take place very slowly at oral temperature 37°C. But this requires a very long time, months or years.

Binary Alloys

The properties of the casting alloys depend upon the constituent elements and the compositions, specially those of main ingredients. The equilibrium phase diagrams help to analyze and study the properties of alloys. The constitution equilibrium phase diagrams become very complicated for analysis of ternary (3 elements), quaternary (4 elements), etc. alloys.

The binary alloys, containing mainly two elements, can be studied and their properties can be predicted by their equilibrium phase diagrams which is required for its formulation.

Noble metal binary alloys used in dentistry are, Au-Cu, Au-Ag, Au-Pd, Au-Pt, Pd-Cu, and Pd-Ag. Out of these Pd-Ag, Pd-Au and Au-Ag form continuous solid solutions at all concentrations mostly above the room temperatures. Properties of different compositions vary uniformly and can be predicted.

Au-Cu system shows complete solid solubility at high temperatures and form intermetallic—ordered phases Au-Cu and Au-Cu$_3$ below about 400°C. The **controlled precipitation of the Au-Cu superlattice,** increases the hardness of the alloy (precipitation—age heat treatment) very much. Au-Pt and Pd-Cu alloys show similar properties.

The binary alloy phase diagrams considered frequently are Ag-Cu (eutectic system), Ag-Sn (peritectic transformation) and Fe-C eutectoid transformations. These arise due to partial solid solubilities, and solid state reactions.

Ag-Cu binary alloy phase diagram shows the eutectic alloy precipitations at 780°C for Ag:Cu= 72: 28. and α and β, lamellar structure, causes an increase of hardness.

Ag-Sn binary alloy phase diagram shows a peritectic transformation for 27% Sn, from disordered (Ag-Sn) phase, to ordered (Ag$_3$Sn) phase as:

$$\text{Liquid} + \beta \text{ phase} \rightarrow \gamma \text{ phase}$$

Fe-C system shows the eutectoid transformation from Austenite γ Ferrite + Cementite phases by solid state reaction at 723°C when the alloy containing **C<2.0% is cooled slowly. If cooled suddenly or quenched, very hard martensitic** steel precipitates increasing hardness to a very high value.

For these elements, the chemical affinities become higher at the lower temperatures and form intermetallic alloys.

Intermetallic Compounds (Covalent Compound/ Intermediate Solid Solution)

Schulze (1967) defined the intermetallic compound as solid phases containing two or more metallic elements with optionally one or more non-metallic elements whose **crystal structures are different.** One of the conditions to form a substitutional type of single phase-disordered solid solutions is that the alloying metals should not have chemical affinities. However, many metals **show slight chemical affinities** during solidifications or when the solid solution is cooled below certain temperatures. In such cases, the atoms of the metals occupy certain positions in the lattice structures of alloy, forming intermetallic compounds. In disordered solid solutions, properties of alloys are changing with respect to compositions. These intermetallic compounds (like chemical compounds) have **different properties than their constituent metals.** These **superlattices** formed may have **different lattice structures** or **distorted (strained) lattices,** and **mixed bonding** (metallic and non-metallic or ionic), which makes the phase more hard and brittle.

Properties
- More hard and brittle, slightly lower toughness
- Higher melting temperatures, and respond to heat treatments
- These are in-between ceramic and alloys
- Display desirable magnetic (Alnico) superconducting, etc., properties.

Applications
- Many varieties of alloys used in dentistry (N, HN, PBM, Ti, etc.) for casting dental fabrications in prosthodontics, implants, etc.
- NiAl hardening phase in Ni-based superalloys.
- Titanium aluminides as grain refinements of Ti alloys for turbine blades.
- Intermetallics containing silicon are used in microelectronics.

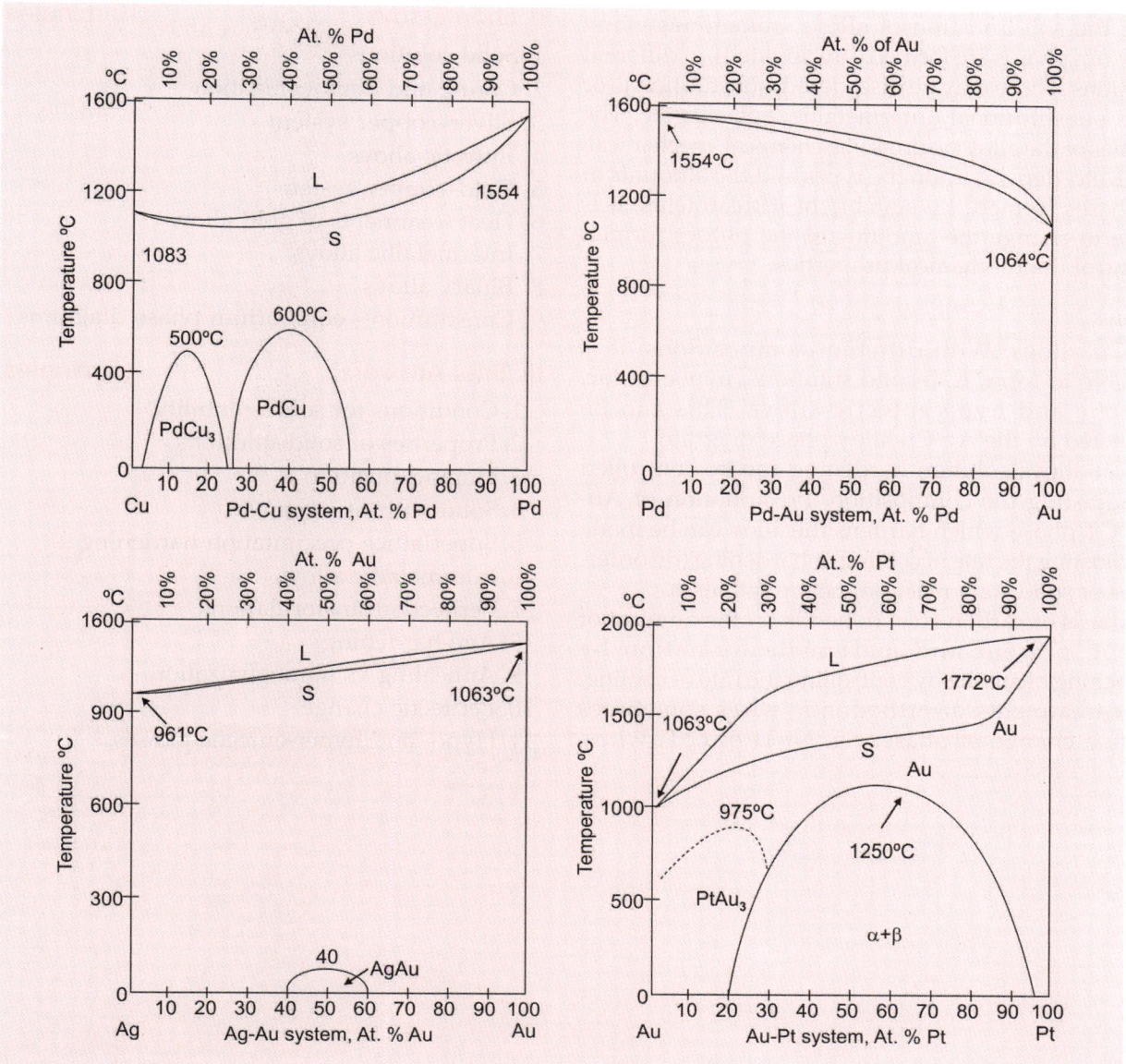

Fig. 17.7: Equilibrium phase diagrams of some binary alloys ● Palladium–Copper, ● Palladium–Gold, ● Silver–Gold, ● Gold–Platinum

Examples

- Certain critical composition in Ag-Sn alloy system with Ag = 73.2% (fcc) and Sn = 26.8% (bct), during solidification at 480°C ordered, intermetallic Ag_3Sn (orthorhombic), γ phase is formed. Similarly, during amalgamation, the intermetallic $γ_1$ (Ag_2Hg_3), $γ_2$ (Sn_7Hg) phases formed have different properties than Ag or Sn or Hg (see Fig. 12.1, page 203).
- The precipitation of many intermetallic phases like $PtAu_3$ (Pt-Au system), Ag-Au (Ag-Au system), Pd-Cu or $PdCu_3$ (in Pd-Cu system) below 600°C and 500°C respectively contributed to improving the properties. HN and N metal casting alloys by suitable heat treatments.

Applications of equilibrium phase diagrams (Fig. 17.7) During the solidification of alloys, sometimes many equilibrium phases are formed (precipitated), in different proportions. These may be disordered, substitutional or ordered substitutional, intermetallic, eutectic, etc. The properties of the alloy castings like chemical, mechanical, thermal, etc. depend upon the types and the amounts of such phases formed. By suitable heat treatments, it is possible to change the amounts of the phases formed and control the mechanical properties.

Examples

- Ag-Cu alloys: With different compositions, it is possible to form, α, β-solid solutions, hypoeutectic, eutectic and hypereutectic alloys. This can be predicted by the Ag-Cu alloy phase diagram.
- Au-Cu-alloys solution hardening can be controlled by adjusting the composition. Precipitation of Au-Cu FCT phase which hardens the alloy can be made by adjusting the rate of cooling or hardening (disorder-order or solid state reaction) heat treatments.
- Hardness of carbon steel depends on the amount of carbon present and martensite formation by quenching austenite by controlling the rate of cooling.
- Heat treatments of orthodontic wires sometimes cause a change of phase, e.g. Ni-Ti or cpTi wires.

Suitable alloying can stabilize the alpha or beta structures of cpTi. This also can be brought about by **changing the temperature or stressing** (*refer* to Ni-Ti elastic memory, superelasticity).

- Silver–amalgam alloy phases (microstructure, metallography) can be adjusted by varying the compositions and clinical procedures to avail its required the best properties.

MODEL QUESTIONS

I. Long Essay   (20 minutes)

1. Classify the dental casting alloys : Give the conditions for forming a solid solution, explain the properties of solid soutions.

II. Short Essays   (10 minutes each)

1. Solid solutions
2. Coring and homogenization
3. Silver–copper system
4. Eutectic alloys
5. Gold–copper system
6. Heat treatments of gold alloys
7. Intermetallic alloys
8. Binary alloys
9. Constitution—equilibrium phase diagrams

III. Brief Answers   (5 minutes each)

1. Conditions for solid solubility
2. Properties of solid solutions
3. Homogenization
4. Solution heat treatment
5. Superlattice precipitation hardening
6. Intermetallic alloys
7. Peritectic transformations
8. Age-hardening
9. Annealing vs homogenization
10. Peritectic change
11. Hypo- and hyper-eutectic phases.

Dental Casting Alloys

BRIEF HISTORY

Pure gold is the noblest of all metals and has excellent biocompatibility. Since many centuries, pure gold restorations have been attempted, and in 19th century, certain techniques of filling were evolved. However, it lacked strength and aesthetic qualities.

During the last century, the constant search for permanent, hard, corrosion resistant, biocompatible aesthetic materials to **replace the missing part of the tooth, and missing teeth** has lead the research scientists and engineers to develop various metal alloys, ceramics, polymers, composite resins, etc. as well as sophisticated equipment and techniques.

1907: Taggart's presentation of revolutionary **lost wax gold alloy casting** procedure was immediately accepted for fabrication of inlays, onlays, crowns, bridges, etc. To get higher mechanical properties, gold alloys, with similar compositions of gold jewellery, were tried. Soon many varieties of the gold alloys of different compositions, containing Cu, Ag, Pt, Pd, etc. were produced.

1932: American National Standard Institution/ American Dental Association **(ANSI/ADA)** found the necessities of classifying these alloys for selection, application, cost estimation, etc. According to ADA specification No. 5, the simple **classification** was according to hardness and only gold contents as types I, II, III, IV.

Also, types I and II were known as inlay casting alloys (Table 18.1). Types III and IV were called **crown** and **bridge alloys.**

Type IV was called **removable partial denture alloys**.

1933: **Base metal alloys:** As the price of gold, increased and the mechanical properties were found somewhat inadequate, base metal alloys (used in industrial castings) were tried. Soon many corrosion resistant alloys of Co-Cr, Co-Ni-Cr, etc. were introduced into the field. Accordingly, the simple casting methods had to be modified.

1950: As the polymer resins were introduced as denture base materials, and restoratives, the resin veneering of gold alloy crown and bridges were used for better aesthetics.

Table 18.1	Earlier classification according to ADA specification No. 5 for casting gold alloys			
Types	Nature	Min gold content%	Hardness VHN	Used at
I	Soft	85%	50–90	Non-stress bearing areas
II	Medium	78%	90–120	Low stress bearing areas
III	Hard	78%	120–150	High stress bearing areas
IV	Extra hard	75%	> 150	Very high stress bearing—posterior restorations

1960: **Metal-ceramic techniques** were introduced to combine the excellent aesthetic and higher strength properties of ceramics with stronger metal cast backings.

1968: **Palladium alloys:** At that time cheaper and lighter **palladium** (noble) metal alloys, having almost similar properties to gold alloys were introduced (as semiprecious—Pd-Ag casting alloys).

1970: **Nickel–chromium** base metal alloys were found to be more suitable due to better mechanical properties, for all metal castings, metal ceramics, RPDs, etc. This was also due to the very high cost of gold alloys.

1980: **All-ceramic technologies** of fabrication of dental restorations with sophisticated firing and casting equipment and several technologies to obtain tooth-coloured matching materials, were introduced.

1984: Classification of alloys according to the nobility, i.e. high noble, noble and predominantly base metal alloys.

1997: Classification according to functions (properties) and description.

1999: As the cost of palladium suddenly shot up, again the gold alloys, substituted them.

2002: Modifications suggested by ANSI/ADA for mechanical properties requirements of new alloys.

REQUIREMENTS OF DENTAL CASTING ALLOYS

The permanent restorations should be able to withstand the hostile oral environments such as corrosion, biodegradation, large dynamic masticating impact forces, thermal fluctuations, etc. **They have to restore the functioning and enhance aesthetics and maintain occlusion.** Hence, the alloys chosen should have the following properties.

1. **Biocompatibility chemical**
   - Should not be toxic or allergic, like Hg, Be, Ni, etc.
   - Chemically inert, i.e. they should not react with oral fluids and release harmful products

   - High tarnish and corrosion resistance—gold should be present >75%, and passivating Cr in predominantly base metal alloys >11%
   - Noncarcinogenic
   - Insoluble and stable (without biodegradation).

2. **Physical and mechanical**
   - High proportional limit and yield strengths to resist permanent deformations.
   - High modulus of elasticity to resist elastic deformations.
   - High modulus of resilience and impact—strengths to resist dynamic impact forces.
   - High compressive, tensile, shear and flexure strengths to withstand fracture.
   - High fatigue strength and endurance limit for long service.
   - High sag-resistance, to resist deformations at high temperatures for metal-ceramics.
   - Suitable surface hardness—low values to assist finishing and polishing, but high values to resist abrasion.
   - Excellent castability: Alloy liquid should have low viscosity to flow into the thin sections of the mould to avoid incomplete castings.
   - Ability to bond with ceramics for good (metal-ceramic bonding).
   - Low density to decrease cost and weight, i.e. to improve retention.
   - Ductile and malleable for adjustments of clasps and burnishing.
   - Should not absorb gases like H_2, N_2, O_2 in the liquid state, to avoid gas-inclusion porosities and oxidation during casting.

3. **Thermal**
   - Low coefficient of thermal expansions to reduce casting shrinkage.
   - Adjustable low thermal expansions for slight mismatching with ceramics (for bonding).
   - Low solidification contraction to reduce micro and localized shrinkage porosities.
   - Low latent heat of fusion for quicker and easier melting and solidification.

- Suitable melting temperatures—low values for all metal castings and high values for metal-ceramics.
- Minimum coring (small range of melting points) to reduce inhomogeneity and brittleness.
- Ability to control hardness by heat treatments.

4. **Aesthetics**
- Ideally, colour should perfectly match with that of patients teeth which is not possible.
- Should not contain Cu and Ag (as these discolour ceramics) in metal-ceramic restorations.

5. **Others**
- Alloy and its auxiliary materials-like investments should not be expensive, and should be readily available.
- Simpler equipment and laboratory facilities.
- No intense training or high skill for fabricating technician.

Note: However, the fabrication of precision castings of predominantly base metal alloys, like Cr-Co, Cr-Ni, titanium, requires expensive investment materials, sophisticated laboratories with costly modern equipment. Technicians should have high skill as well as intensive training, specially for fabrication of titanium castings, metal-ceramic appliances, and CAD-CAM techniques.

CLASSIFICATION OF DENTAL CASTING ALLOYS

Several hundreds of varieties of noble and base metals alloys were soon developed. These are gold alloys (Au, Cu, Ag), palladium alloys (Pd, Ag, Au), chromium alloys (Cr-Co-Ni), titanium and its alloys, etc. The cost of these alloys mainly depend on gold and noble metals contents, which mainly contribute the corrosion resistance. For the purpose of calculating the relative cost to inform the patients, billing and insurance claims, a simple classification of all these alloys was proposed by ADA in 1984, according to the **noble metal contents or nobility.**

The noble metals are Au, Pt, Pd, Rh, Ru, Ir and Os. Silver undergoes tarnish and corrosion in oral environment and hence it is not considered as noble metal in dentistry. Pd-Ag alloys have good resistance to corrosion and have slightly better mechanical properties. Pd >50 wt% alloys were named as **semiprecious and predominantly base metal alloys as nonprecious but these terms are not used now.**

1. **Classification by stress-bearing abilities or functions:** However, for the dentist to select the alloy according to their **mechanical stress-bearing properties, various functions**, and the identification of **component elements**, better classifications were suggested by ANSI/ADA specification No. 5, in 1997 modifying the earlier gold alloy classifications type I, II, III, IV. This does not involve the composition percentage but mechanical properties and functions and includes all casting alloys, in types I, II, III and IV. The minimum yield strengths prescribed for 0.2% offset values in quenched or annealed conditions are listed in Table 18.2.

Note: Types I and II are sometimes known as **inlay casting alloys.**

Table 18.2 Classification by stress bearing abilities or functions

Types	Hardnesss or strength	Yield strength in MPa ADA 1997	ADA 2002	Elongation% 1997, (2002)	Functions (applications)
I	Soft: Low strength	80	80	18, (18)	Non-stress bearing areas—inlays strength
II	Medium strength	180	180	12, (10)	Moderate stress bearing areas: Inlays, onlays, crowns
III	Hard: High strength	240	270	12, (5)	High stress bearing areas: Onlays, thin crowns, copings, saddles, etc.
IV	Extra hard: High strength	300 (>450 hardened)	360	10, (3) (>3 hardened)	Extra hard: Saddles, clasps, lingual bars, crown and bridges (FPD), RPD frameworks, abutments, post-cores, etc.

Type III and type IV are **crown and bridge alloys.** Type IV is also known as **partial denture alloy.** Metal-ceramic alloys are considered separately, but are similar to type IV alloys.

2. **The classification suggested by ADA according to nobilities** is given in Table 18.3.
   - **High noble (HN)** metal alloys contain **gold ≥40 wt%, with noble metals ≥60 wt%**
   - **Noble (N)** metal alloys contain noble metals **≥25 wt%**
   - Predominantly base metals alloys **(PBM)** contain **noble metals ≤25 wt%**, i.e. 0–25 wt%.

Note: Pd-Ag alloys with Pd ≥25 wt% is considered as noble.

IDENTIFICATION OF DENTAL CASTING ALLOYS

The dental casting alloys are identified by:
- Single most abundant metal, e.g. Au alloy, Pd alloy, Ti alloy
- Two most abundant metals in decreasing wt%, e.g. Au-Cu, Au-Ag, Pd-Ag, Ag-Pd, Ni-Ti,.....
- Three most abundant elements: Au-Cu-Ag, Au-Pd-Ag, Pd-Ag-Cu, Pd-Au-Pt, Co-Ni-Cr, Co-Cr-W, Ag-Sn-Cu, Ni-Cr-Be, Ti-Al-V, etc.

CLASSIFICATION BY APPLICATIONS AND DESCRIPTIONS

All metal prosthesis, metal-ceramic prosthesis and partial denture frameworks (Table 18.3).

Note: All alloys used for a metal-ceramics prosthesis, can also be used for all metal casting prosthesis. Partial denture frameworks, nowadays, are cast by PB metal alloys.

Carat (Karat) and Fineness

Gold is the most common major component of HN dental casting alloys, due to its excellent corrosion resistance. The amount of gold present is an indication of the corrosion resistance of the alloy. Carat and fineness are the terms used to represent this. Carat is the number of parts of gold in 24 parts of the alloy by weight. For example, 24-carat gold is 100% pure gold, 18-carat gold alloy has $18/24 \times 100 = 75\%$ pure gold and **22-carat gold has $(22/24) \times 100 = 91.6\%$ pure gold and is 916 fine gold.**

Fineness of the alloy is the parts of pure gold by weight in 1000 parts of the alloy, e.g. 750 fine gold alloy refers to $750/1000 = 75\%$ pure gold, or $75/100 \times 24 = 18$ carats gold alloy. Even though these old terms are not used nowadays, gold solders are indicated by fineness. For adequate corrosion resistance, the restorations should have more than 750 fineness and gold solders should have more than 650 fineness. At present, the **weight percentage** has become more common and explicit. 916 fine gold contains 91.6% gold or 22 carats.

The term carat is also used to indicate the weight of gems. **One carat gem has 200 mg weight.**

ALLOYING PROPERTIES OF METALS USED IN GOLD ALLOYS

Every metal has its own characteristics properties such as resistance to corrosion, biocompatibility mechanical and thermal properties, etc. which may not be suitable for use directly in dentistry. The purpose of alloying are to suitably changing their following properties:

Table 18.3 Classification of dental casting alloys by description

Metal types	Metal-ceramic alloys (MCA)	All metal casting alloys	Partial denture frameworks alloys
HN (Au >40 wt% with noble metals >60 wt%)	Pure (99.7%) Au Au-Pt-Pd Au-Pd- Ag (Ag 5–12 wt%) Au-Pd-Ag (Ag >12 wt%) Au-Pd	Au-Ag-Pd Au-Pt-Pd Au-Pt-Pd Au-Cu-Ag Au-Ag-Cu	Au-Ag-Cu-Pd +HN-MCA
N (Noble metals >25 wt%)	Pd-Au Pd-Au-Ag Pd-Ag Pd-Cu-Ga Pd-Ga-Ag	Ag-Pd-Au-Cu Ag-Pd +N-MCA	All MCA
PBM Noble metals 0–25%	CPTi Ti-Al-V Ni-Cr-Mo-Be Ni-Cr-Mo Co-Cr-Mo Co-Cr-W	Cu-Al PBM-MCA	All MCA

- Corrosion resistance and biocompatibility
- Strength, stiffness, hardness, ductility, and malleability
- The range of melting temperatures, and coefficients of thermal expansions
- Castability, density, cost, and techniques of fabrication to simple methods, etc.

For alloying, they should satisfy the Hume-Rothery conditions for solid solubility (page 253).

Few important properties of metals commonly used for alloying with gold are listed in Table 18.4. These help selection of the metals for alloying with gold.

1. GOLD

This is the major element, ≥40 wt% in high noble (HN) metal alloys used for dental casting and purest form is used for direct filling restorations.

Properties

- Noblest of metals, highest corrosion resistance, and biocompatibilities.
- FCC structure, form solid solutions of copper (and silver) at all proportions above 400°C and below 400°C ordered AuCu (FCT) and $AuCu_3$ (FCC) intermetallic phases precipitation.
- Highest ductility, malleability and high density (19.3 gm/cc).
- Very low surface hardness (about 25 KHN) and strength. On work hardening (gold compaction) the hardness increases to about 68 KHN and transverse strength increases to about 160–270 MPa.
- High melting temperature (1063°C), low COTE (14.2 ppm/°C,) very high thermal conductivity.
- **Cold-welding properties**
- Yellow colour, changes to red with Cu and white with Pd or Pt **(white gold).**
- Expensive and also appliance becomes more costly due to high density.

Applications

- Direct filling—tooth restorations, in purest form (99.99%) as foils, strips, powder, etc.
- Alloys with silver, and copper for casting inlays, crowns, bridges, partial denture frames
- Alloys with Pt and Pd orthodontic wires
- Alloys with Pt, Pd, Ag, etc. for casting metal-ceramics.
- Alloys with Ag, Cu, Zn for soldering gold alloys.

2. PLATINUM

Properties

- High corrosion resistance, biocompatibility
- High density (21.3 gm/cc), ductility and malleability
- Has FCC structure, forms a solid solution with gold, and increases its hardness
- Low COTE (8.9 ppm/°C) and high melting temperature (1769°C)
- White colour

Addition of Pt to gold

- Increases strength (by solution hardening), density, cost, melting and recrystallization temperatures.
- Decreases COTE, as required for metal-ceramics bonding and whitens gold alloys.

Applications

- Platinum foils in PJC preparation
- Metal-ceramic HN and N alloys
- Orthodontic (PGP) wires of high recrystallization temperatures.

3. PALLADIUM

Properties (similar to platinum)

- High corrosion resistance, biocompatibility.
- FCC structure, density 120 gm/cc white noble metal, form a solid solution with silver.
- The strength of Pd alloys is higher than gold alloys.
- High melting temperature (1552°C) and low COTE (11.8 ppm/°C similar to the tooth).

Table 18.4	Properties of metals in gold alloys				
Metal	Atomic wt	Crystal structure	Density gm/cc	Melting temperature°C	Coefficient of linear thermal expansion ppm/°C
Gold	197	FCC	19.3	1063	14.2
Platinum	195	FCC	21.5	1769	8.9
Iridium	192	FCC	22.5	2454	6.8
Silver	108	FCC	10.5	961	19.7
Palladium	106	FCC	12.0	1552	11.8
Copper	63.5	FCC	8.9	1083	16.5
Indium	114	FCT	7.31	156	33
Zinc	65	HCP	7.1	420	39.7

Addition of palladium to gold

- Increases corrosion resistance of silver containing alloys and strength of gold, copper, silver alloys by solution hardening and also increases melting temperature ranges.
- Decreases, COTE, and even small amounts make the **gold alloys white.**

Applications

- A major element in noble metal (N) alloys used for casting all metal (for resin veneering) crowns and bridges, and metal ceramics.
- Orthodontic PGP wires of high recrystallization temperatures.

4. SILVER

Properties

- Low corrosion resistance in the oral environment. But silver-palladium alloys have adequate corrosion resistance, for oral appliances.
- FCC structure, lower density, form a solid solution with gold and palladium.
- Has limited solid solubilities (max. 8%) in copper and form α, β solid solutions and hard eutectic phases causing **precipitation hardening.**

$$Ag : Cu = 72 : 28\%$$

- Lower melting temperature (961°C) and higher COTE.

Addition of silver to gold alloys

- Slightly lowers corrosion resistance
- Increases hardness by solution hardening
- Increases hardness if copper is also present by precipitation of α, β and eutectic phases
- Slightly lowers melting temperature ranges (gold solders) and increase COTE
- Alloying with palladium increases strength, corrosion resistance
- Alloying with copper—lowers melting point and increases hardness (eutectic alloys).

Applications

- Gold–silver–copper HN alloys for casting all metal (resin veneered oral appliances).
- Palladium–silver–copper (PSC) orthodontic wires.
- Palladium-silver noble metal casting alloys.
- Gold–silver solders and silver solders.
- Silver–copper–tin alloys for silver amalgam.
- Pure silver pins for strengthening amalgam restorations.

5. COPPER

Properties

- Low tarnish and corrosion resistance (as it forms, sulphides and carbonates in oral environments)
- FCC structure, low density (8.8 gm/cc), high ductility, malleability and reddish colour
- High melting point (1083°C), and a good conductor of heat and electricity.

Addition of copper

- Decreases tarnish and corrosion resistance of noble metal alloys.
- Increases the strength by solution hardening of gold alloys and silver alloys.
  Precipitations of ordered Au-Cu superlattice of 'FCT' structure by heat treatment (around 375°–400°C). Forming α, β and eutectic phases with silver present (at around 780°C)
- Strengthens the silver–tin amalgam alloy restorations and helps **comminution**
- Makes gold alloy more reddish
- Decreases melting temperature ranges of gold alloys to facilitate casting and soldering.

Applications

- Important hardening metal in HN gold alloys.
- Used in HN and sometimes in noble metal (N) alloys.
- Silver–copper casting alloys, sterling silver (Cu = 7.5 wt%).
- Gold solders contain copper, to decrease melting temperatures.
- Palladium–copper–gallium alloys have similar, i.e. hardened properties as base metal casting alloys.
- Palladium–silver–copper (PSC) alloy is used as orthodontic noble metal alloy wire.

6. IRIDIUM

It used as trace metal to improve the mechanical properties. It is a noble metal of the Pt group. It has a very high density (22.5 gm/cc), **very high melting temperature (2454°C)** and very low COTE (6.8 ppm/°C). A small amount (0.005%) of iridium forms a eutectic alloy with gold, causes greater nucleation and **grain refinement** of gold alloys.

7. ZINC

Properties

- It has close-packed hexagonal (HCP) lattice and hence **cannot dissolve** (or form solid solution) in FCC structured noble metals.
- High oxygen affinity

- High COTE (39.7 ppm/°C)
- Low melting point 420°C.

Addition of zinc

- **Embrittles** gold alloy
- Sweeps out oxygen absorbed by molten alloy liquid (i.e. reduces gas inclusion porosity in casting).
- Lowers the melting temperature ranges (of gold solders).

Applications

- Small amounts in gold alloys act as a **scavenger** of oxygen.
- Gold and silver solders contain zinc to lower their fusion temperatures ranges.
- A small amount in (0–1%) in silver–tin–copper amalgam alloys to act as a **scavenger and assist lathe cutting**. However, moisture contact during trituration and condensations cause **delayed expansion.** Hence, zinc free alloys are preferred.
- Experimental gold coloured—**technique alloy** is used for training in casting procedures. Japanese gold contains Cu:Zn:Al = 55:35:10 wt. percentages, approximately.

8. INDIUM

It has **tetragonal** lattice, high COTE (33 ppm/°C) and very low melting temperature (156°C). It is not tarnished by moisture or air. **It replaces zinc, for scavenger.** In certain Pd-ag alloys, indium is added up to about 30 wt% to impart strength and yellow colour. Sometimes used in Ag amalgam alloys.

9. GALLIUM

The greyish yellow metal of FCC structure, low density (5.98 gm/cc) and very low melting temperature, 31°C. Oxides of gallium formed in gold and palladium alloys help to chemically bond the cast alloys with ceramics (metal-ceramics). Experiments to replace mercury of silver amalgam alloy, have yielded some positive results.

HIGH NOBLE AND NOBLE METAL CASTING ALLOYS

According to ADA specifications for classifications, high noble metal alloys should contain gold ≥**40%** with noble metals (Au, Pt, Pd, Rh, Ir, Os) ≥**60%** by weight, to have excellent resistance to corrosion and good biocompatibility. By alloying with many base metals like copper, and noble metals, many varieties of these alloys are made. The noble metal 'N' alloys should have noble **metals ≥25%** by weight. These are mainly silver or palladium based alloys (sometimes called **semiprecious alloys**).

Approximate composition ranges of HN alloys and their varieties

Gold	= 40–80%
Silver	= 10–25%
Copper	= 6–15%
Palladium, platinum	= 1–4%
Gallium, zinc, indium, iridium	= Small amounts, trace metals

Zn and In are scavengers to sweep out metal oxides, and iridium is grain refiner.

In these varieties are Au (99%), Au-Pt-Pd, Au-Pd-Ag, Au-Pd, Au-Ag-Pd, Au-Pd-Cu-Ag, Au-Ag-Cu-Pd, etc. varieties, which are used for metal-ceramics, all metal castings, resin veneering, and RPD frameworks (Au-Ag-Cu-Pd).

Composition ranges of N alloys

Silver	=	40–70%
Palladium	=	5–60%
Gold	=	0–40%
Copper	=	8–14%
Ga, In, Zn, Ir	=	Trace metals

The **N alloy varieties** have mainly Pd and Ag and are Pd- Au, Pd-Au-Ag, Pd-Ag, Pd-Cu-Ga, Pd-Ga-Ag, Ag-Pd-Au-Cu, Ag-Pd, etc. These are **white** coloured, noble metal alloys used for metal-ceramics, all metal prosthesis and resin veneering.

GENERAL PROPERTIES OF HN AND N METAL CASTING ALLOYS

1. **High biocompatibility** and resistance to corrosion. Alloys containing small amounts of silver may have sufficient corrosion resistance. Ag in the presence of Pd shows better corrosion resistance.
2. **Mechanical properties** are mostly controlled by the compositions. Au-Cu alloys can be softened by solution heat treatments and **hardened by large values** by precipitation of Au-Cu superlattices on heating to about 375°–400°C. According to the classification, their **minimum yield strengths in softened conditions** are specified by ADA (Tables 18.5 and 18.6).

Table 18.5	Ranges of yield strengths of casting alloys in softened-quenched condition		
Types	Property	Min YS softened MPa	Softened condition range of YS MPa
I	Soft	80	80–180
II	Medium	180	180–270
III	Hard	270	270–360
IV	Extra hard	360	>360

Table 18.6 Mechanical properties of HN and N alloys in softened and heat hardened

Properties	Softened by quenching or annealing	Heat hardened
1. Yield strength at 2% offset	100–430 MPa	270–580 MPa
2. Surface hardness	80–180 VHN	180–270 VHN
3. Elongation at fracture	35%–39%	6%–20%
4. Modulus of elasticity	90,000–100,000 MPa	Same

Depending on the clinical situations, these, soft, medium, hard and extra hard varieties are selected for fabricating the desired appliances. The **soft and medium alloys are burnishable** to get better marginal fit. HN alloys have higher densities (14–16 gm/cc) and hence become more expensive compared to N metal alloys of lower densities (10–12 gm/cc).

3. **Thermal properties:** The HN alloys have ranges of melting temperatures around 920°C to 960°C and the N alloy have around 850°C to 1100°C. These can be melted by ordinary gas flames or electrical resistance heaters.

    Casting shrinkages of about 1.3 to 1.6% are caused due to their high coefficient of thermal expansions. When the solidified alloy is cooled from solidus temperature to oral temperature, the thermal contraction is inhibited to a certain extent by the first solidified layer on the mould walls.
    Type III and IV HN alloys can be age hardened effectively, if copper present is **15–35%, by** maintaining the temperature around **375–400°C** for few minutes.

4. Most of the HN alloys have a yellow colour which becomes more red with copper and N alloys have a white colour.

5. The auxiliary investment materials GBI is not very expensive and the method of casting is comparatively simpler and less technique sensitive than base-metal alloy casting procedures.
    These alloys are quite suitable for all metal castings like inlays, full crowns, crowns and bridges as well as, for resin veneering appliances. Some high fusing hard varieties can be used for metal-ceramic appliances.

Note: If required additional information like alloying properties, hardening and softening heat treatments and compensation of casting shrinkage, can be added **for a long essay.**

HN AND N METAL ALLOYS FOR METAL-CERAMICS

Metal-ceramic cast restorations are fabricated, by initially conducting alloy casting, and then, fusing or bonding, aesthetically selected ceramic materials of **lower fusion temperatures**, over it. The restoration is a combination of the strength and toughness of the metal with the aesthetically excellent ceramics. HN and N metal alloys were used earlier. Recently predominantly base metals, chromium–cobalt–nickel alloys, titanium and its alloys are used.

Requirements of metal-ceramic alloys

In addition to the general requirements for the dental casting alloys, such as biocompatibility, resistance to corrosion, adequate mechanical and thermal properties, these metals require the following:

1. Ability to bond chemically (through the metal oxide layer) with ceramics, at high temperatures.
2. High modulus of elasticity and sag resistance at high temperatures to reduce thermal deformations and **interfacial debonding shear stresses.**
3. High solidus temperature at least about 100°C above that of ceramics. This is done by adding Pt or Pd to the alloys, which raise the melting temperatures of gold alloys.

Table 18.7 General properties of HN and N metal-ceramic alloys

Properties	High noble metals	Noble metals
1. Corrosion resistance	Very high	High
2. Metal-ceramic bonding	Good	Good
3. Yield strength (annealed)	450–680 MPa	460 MPa
4. Surface hardness (softened)	180–220 VHN	190 VHN
5. Modulus of elasticity	100,000 MPa	90,000 MPa
6. Elongation at fracture	5%–20%	10–30%
7. The range of melting temperatures	1250°C–1300°C	1150°–1300°C
8. Density	14–18 gm/cc	10–12 gm/cc
9. Colour	Yellow or white	White

4. Good thermal compatibility: The COTE of metal and that of ceramics must be **nearly the same.** The COTE of metals is lowered to about 13.5 to 14.0% by adding Pt and Pd.

5. Should not contain copper whose sulphides, discolour the ceramics with a greenish tint. Silver also should not be used in a large amount for the same reason.

6. Good castability, low viscosity, for the molten alloy liquid.

METAL-CERAMIC BONDING

Due to large surface tensions (365 dynes/cm) and high angle of contact (130°), the **ceramic liquid (at 1050°C) does not wet** the metal surface and bond with it strongly. The shearing stress produced at the interface cause **bond failure** (*see* Fig. 2.25b, page 37).

Bonding of metals and ceramics is achieved by mechanical, chemical and thermal mismatching, methods (*refer* to metal-ceramics, pages 37 and 226).

1. **Mechanical bonding:** Surface of the metal casting is roughened by sand-blasting. This rough surface has a larger area to interlock with ceramics.

2. **Chemical bonding:** This is supposed to be superior to mechanical interlocking. This is achieved by two methods:
   i. Adding **passivating** metals which combine with atmospheric oxygen and form oxide layers, like chromium oxides on Co-Cr-Ni alloys, or titanium oxide on titanium or its alloys.
   ii. By **electrodeposition** on the substrate: First pure gold layer is formed by electroplating the article, and then a short flashing electrodeposition of **atomic layer of tin** is formed. During the fusion procedure, tin oxide is formed which chemically bonds with ceramics.

3. **Thermal mismatching:** By developing **residual stresses** between metal and ceramic surfaces. This is done by slightly mismatching the COTEs of metals and ceramics. COTE of the alloys can be decreased to about 13.5 to 14.0 ppm/°C by including Pt and Pd. Similarly, COTE of ceramics is raised (to about 13.0–13.5 ppm/°C) by forming more **leucite** or by adding **alkali metals** K or Na ions.

Metal-ceramic shear bond strength can be raised by using all these methods from about 20 to 110 MPa.

The composition of HN metal-ceramic alloys (approx)
- Au-Pt-Pd, Au-Pd-Pt with Ag <5%
- Au-Pt-Ag, Au-Pd-Ag with Ag = 5–12%
- Au-Pd-Ag with Ag >12%
- Au-Pd, Pd-Au

Composition of N metal-ceramic alloys
- Pd-Au with Au = 5–35%
- Pd-Ag with Ag = 5–35%
- Pd-Cu-Ga with Cu = 10%, Ga = 5–10%
- Pd-Ag-Ga with Ag = 1–5%, Ga = 5–10%

GENERAL PROPERTIES OF HN AND N METAL-CERAMIC ALLOYS

These alloys cannot be easily melted with a gas torch flames. Oxyacetylene gas torch flames, electrical resistance or **induction methods** are required for melting. More expensive **phosphate-bonded investment** is required and **centrifugal casting machines** can be used (Table 18.7).

RECENT NOBLE METAL ALLOYS

1. Pd-Cu-Ga alloys: Contains about Pd = 75%, Cu = 10% and Ga = 5–10% and trace metals.
   These alloys have superior mechanical properties, **similar to those of base metal alloys.** Discolouration of ceramics due to copper and gallium cause brownish tint. The surface oxide layer, formed can help chemical bonding along with thermal mismatching and mechanical interlocking metal-ceramic bonds.

2. Pd-Ga-Ag is another recent alloy containing, Pd = 80–85% Ga = 5–10% and Ag = 0.5–8% and trace metals. The properties, clinical study reports, etc. are not yet available.

3. High gold alloys with more than 90% gold can be used for ultra-low fusing metal ceramic appliances. The yellow colour gives a better aesthetic (vitality, lifelike) quality to ceramics.

HN AND N METAL CASTING ALLOYS FOR REMOVABLE PARTIAL DENTURE FRAMEWORKS

Few HN and N metal alloys satisfying the properties of type IV, alloys, i.e. Y.S. >360 MPa, were used for this purpose. HN alloys contain Au-Ag-Cu-Pd (Au = 70%, Ag = 13%, Cu = 10% and Pd = 4%) with a few trace elements Fe, In, Sn, Ga. The N alloys have Pd, Ag, Cu as major elements with the trace metals.

The HN alloys can be heat hardened. Similarly, palladium–silver–copper alloys are also heat hardenable. These alloys have higher melting temperatures 950–1100°C. Phosphate-bonded investments, electrical resistance or induction alloy melting methods are preferred.

Due to the advent of many base metal alloys like, Co-Cr, Ni-Cr or Ti and its alloys, which have better mechanical properties, lower cost, lower density, the **HN and N alloys are not preferred.**

Note: If required additional information can be given briefly to HN and N metal casting alloys and metal-ceramic alloys for long essays, such as

1. Alloying properties of major constituents (Au, Ag, Cu, Pt, Pd, Zn)
2. Solution—softening heat treatment and age hardening heat treatments
3. Casting shrinkage and principles of compensations.

PREDOMINANTLY BASE METAL (PBM) CASTING ALLOYS

These are mainly base metal alloys which may or may not contain any noble metals (i.e. 0–25%). The following are their characteristic properties:

- **High corrosion resistance** comparable to noble metal alloys due to the formation of strongly bonded impervious chromium or titanium oxide film **(passivation), on the surface.**
- **Superior mechanical properties** like high modulus of elasticity (stiffness), yield strength, ultimate strength and surface hardness (abrasion resistance).
- **Low density** (lighter appliances), at low cost.
- **High fusion temperatures around 1300°–1600°C**
- White in colour and shine-**like stars (stellites).**

Now these are replacing the more expensive HN and N alloys for the fabrications of:
- All metal crowns and bridges
- Metal-ceramics
- Cast removable partial denture frameworks
- Implants, etc.

CLASSIFICATION ACCORDING TO PBM CASTING ALLOYS

1. **Passivation—oxide film**
   - Chromic oxide film in Co-based or Ni-based alloys
   - Titanium oxide film in titanium and its alloys.
2. **Compositions**
   - Cobalt-based, Co-Cr-W, Co-Cr-Mo, Co-Ni-Cr
   - Nickel-based, i.e. Ni-Cr-Mo, Ni-Cr-Be, Ni-Ti
   - Titanium, Ti-Al-V, Ti-Mo-Zr-Sn, Ni-Ti
   - Aluminum–bronzes.
3. **Fusion temperatures**
   - Low fusing PBM alloys: Solidus temperature **<1300°C**
   - High fusing PBM alloys: Solidus temperatures **>1300°C**
4. **Applications**
   - All metal crown and bridges (FPD)
   - Cast removable partial denture (RPD) frameworks
   - Metal-ceramics
   - Dental implants

- Orthopaedic implants: Hip joints, bone plates, bars, screws, etc.
- Wrought alloy orthodontic wires
- Dental instruments

Note: Stainless steels, i.e. ferritic, austenitic (18-8) and martensitic, varieties are not included, as they are mostly used as wrought alloys—wires, plates, sheets, etc.

According to ADA specification No. 14, these alloys should have
- Passivating metal: Cr >20% by wt.
- Major elements: Co + Ni + Cr >85% by wt. (But other compositions complying toxicities and hypersensitivity limits are also accepted).
- Yield strength >500 MPa
- Modulus of elasticity >1,70, 000 MPa
- Elongation percentage >1.5%

Compositions (approximate weight percentage)
- Cobalt: 0–65% or
- Nickel: 0–80% or
- Cobalt + nickel = 60%–65%
- Chromium: 15–30% in cobalt-based alloys and 11–17% in nickel-based alloys
- Molybdenum or tungsten: 5–10% hardeners
- Beryllium: 1–2%, decreases the melting temperature
- Trace metals for increasing mechanical properties: Al, Fe, Cu, W, Mo
- Trace metals for grain refinements: Iridium, ruthenium
  Trace metals for scavenging: Manganese, zinc, indium, carbon 0.2–0.5% effective hardener. The types of **carbide precipitations control hardness.**

Note
- The alloys used for casting removable partial denture frameworks are Co-Cr or Co-Ni-Cr (Co + Ni about 60–65% and Cr = 15–30%) with carbon, etc.
- The alloys used for casting crown and bridges and metal-ceramic FPDs are mainly Ni-Cr alloys with nickel about 75–80%, Cr (11–17%), carbon, etc.

ALLOYING PROPERTIES

1. **Chromium:** Medium density = 7.15 gm/cc, high MP = 1875°C.
   Increases: Corrosion resistance, by forming Cr_2O_3 film, yield strength, modulus of elasticity (stiffness) by solution hardening, and MP.
   Decreases: Ductility, malleability, and elongation at fracture, **Cr >30% causes brittleness.**
2. **Cobalt** has medium density = 8.85 gm/cc, MP = 1495° C
   Increases: Hardness, YS, MOE (stiffness), MP.

Decreases: Ductility, malleability, elongation at fracture.

3. **Nickel:** Medium density = 8.9 gm/cc, MP = 1453°C
Increases: Hardness, YS, MOE and MP **to less extent**
Decreases: Ductility, malleability and percentage elongation to **less extent**.
Note: Nickel-chromium alloys have greater ductility, percentage elongation, and lower hardness, YS, MOE, and MP compared to Co-Cr alloys. **Nickel vapour inhalation causes lung cancer.**

4. **Mo or W:** *Increases* hardness, **YS,** and MOE. But Mo does not decrease ductility and percentage elongation as W.

5. **Beryllium:** *Increases* strength but decreases melting point and grain size. **Inhalation of toxic-vapour or dust in the factory, and laboratories cause health hazards, dermatitis,** etc.

6. **Sn, Al, Cu, W, Mo** are trace elements which increase hardness (Ni_3Al phase **precipitations**).

7. **Iridium, ruthenium** (in traces) are grain refiners and hardeners.

8. **Mn, Zn, Si** in traces act as scavengers.

9. **Carbon:** 0.2–0.5% **traces effective hardener, respond to heat treatments.**

GENERAL PROPERTIES OF PBM CASTING ALLOYS

1. These have high corrosion resistance due to the passivation effect of Cr_2O_3 surface film.

2. Nickel and beryllium are said to be toxic. Inhalation of vapours or dust of these metals causes health hazards. Nickel vapours inhalation is found to be **carcinogenic,** and **beryllium** vapours cause **dermatitis, chest pain** (berylliosis), etc.

3. Nickel-containing alloys have slightly lower, melting temperatures (easier to melt) stiffness or modulus of elasticity, YS, UTS, and hardness but higher elongation at fracture.

Approximate properties of a few PBM casting partial denture alloys are given in Table 18.8.

4. Many of these alloys respond to heat treatments, usually by age hardening, annealing, homogenization, etc.

5. All PBM alloys are white in colours (**stellites**).

6. Trade names:
Co-Cr alloys: Vitallium, Genesis, Novarex, Ultra 100
Ni-Cr alloys: Ticonium, Resillium III, Neptune, Litecast, etc.
Co-Ni-Cr alloys: Nobillium
Gold alloys: Orion, Deva 4, Jelenko-SMG-3, Dequdent, Cameo (for comparison).

CLINICAL ASPECTS

1. Clasp adjustments: Modulus of elasticity (stiffness) of PBM alloys (200,000 MPa) are nearly double that of HN or N alloys. The force to be applied for clasp adjustment is hence nearly double. Also since double force is required to dislodge the clasp, tooth preparation with **lesser undercuts is sufficient. The advantage is less removal of tooth material.**

2. PBM alloys undergo **work hardening more easily** which reduces its lifetime.

3. Even though the PBM alloys are cheaper, the auxiliary materials like phosphate-bonded investments, special casting equipment, skilled technicians with intensive training, time-consuming procedures, advanced laboratories (with sand-blasting, electropolishing, etc. equipment) **make the appliance quite expensive.**

MICROSTRUCTURE METALLOGRAPHY OF PBM ALLOYS

During solidification, dendritic structured grains of the various **solid solution phases** of different components are formed in different, directions forming grain boundaries. **Co-Cr-Mo** form **eutectic alloys at 1275°C**

Table 18.8	Approximate properties of casting PBM alloys						
Alloys	YS MPa	UTS MPa	Elongation%	Hardness VHN	Modulus of elasticity GPa	Melting temperature (range—middle)	Casting shrinkage %
Co-Cr (Vitallium)	700	870	1.6	430	225	1410°C	2–3%
Ni-Cr (Ticonium)	690	800	4.0	300	180	1275°C	2–3%
Co-Cr-Ni (Jelenko)	470	685	8.0	260	200	1360°C	2–3%
Fe-Cr Hardened gold	700	840	9	310	202	1260°C	2–3%
Alloy-type IV	490	775	7	265	90	960°C	1.3–1.4%
CPTi	340	345	13	210	103	1668°C	2–3%
Ti-6Al-4V	870	925	5	320	117	1400°C	2–3%

and precipitate as **lamellar** structures. All these increase slip resistance or hardness. Carbon can combine with all these component metals forming their carbides. These carbides have **fusion temperatures lower than other solid solutions. Hence the liquid carbides solidify last, in the interdendritic space and at the grain boundaries**. These carbide precipitation increases hardness and decreases ductility, depending on the nature and **sites of precipitation**, such as:

- **Continuous** thin dark layers or lines, at grain boundaries, if casting is done as soon as the solid alloy is melted. This increases **brittleness**, decreases elongation percentage, but produce a **smooth casting surface**.
- **Lamellar eutectoid type** structures of different phases are formed on **slow cooling**, which increases **brittleness**.
- **Spherical island**-like structure in between the grains, if the alloy liquid is heated to **100°C above its liquidus, before casting**. It has very **poor surface quality,** but higher ductility and is not usually used.

HEAT TREATMENTS

Several types of heat treatments are suggested by manufacturers, involving **precipitation hardening, solution hardening, etc**. For example, heating above 900°C and **cooling slowly increases ductility,** due to conversion of martensite to austenite. **Careless heat treatment** decreases, YS, **ductility, elongation at fracture, etc.** The type of precipitations of carbides at grain boundaries, get altered (i.e. island, continuous or lamellar) during the heat treatments and affect their properties.

PBM ALLOYS FOR METAL-CERAMICS

Chromium forms the corrosion resistant, Cr_2O_3 film on the surface of Co-Cr and Ni-Cr alloys, which also helps to improve metal-ceramic bondings. Earlier both varieties were used. Nowadays, Ni-Cr alloys are preferred due to its lower melting temperature and greater elongation percentage.

Compositions of PBM—metal-ceramic alloys

Varieties: Ni-Cr-Mo, Ni-Cr-Mo-Be, Co-Cr-Mo, Co-Cr-W. All these are suitable for all metal crown and bridges and removable partial denture frameworks.

Compositions

- Ni = 70–80%: Suitable mechanical and thermal properties
- Cr = 12–20%: Solution hardener, forms corrosion resisting passivation film.

- Mo or W = 1.5–5%: Hardeners and grain refiners (Mo is preferred as it does not decrease ductility as much as W).

Trace metals

- Al, Fe, Cu, Be: 0.1–1.5% act as solution hardeners, grain refiners
- Mn, Si, B: 0.1–3.0% act as scavengers, may cause brittleness.
- Small amounts of Sn for metal-ceramic bonding through the tin oxide.
- Small amounts of carbon are usually present to act as hardner only in Co-Cr alloys used for all metal crowns and bridges and RPD frameworks.

Properties

- Adequate corrosion resistance, biocompatibility, metal-ceramic bond strength, like, noble metal alloys.
- Superior mechanical properties, more suitable for metal-ceramics.
- The higher modulus of elasticities (180,000 MPa, nearly double that of HN and N alloys) and sag resistance.
- The higher yield strengths 300–800 MPa and tensile strengths 600–900 MPa, much higher than hardened type IV gold alloys.
- The higher surface hardness (320 VHN) and abrasive resistance, difficult to reduce and polish.
- Difficult to do clasp adjustments due to lower elongation percentage 5–10%, higher modulus of elasticity and yield strengths.
- The higher fusion temperatures 1200–1300°C (lower than Co-Cr alloys) (difficult to melt and cast).
- Larger thermal shrinkages after casting, 2.2–2.4%
- COTE is nearly mismatching with ceramics.
- White colour-nonvital appearance is a **disadvantage compared to the yellow colour of HN alloys** (which impart vital appearance to ceramics).

The cast coping is initially applied with **opaque ceramics** on this to reduce reflection from metal. In view of these properties, the casting methods require some **modifications:** Preformed wax patterns, phosphate-bonded investments, plastic removable casting rings, electrical resistance, induction or arc-melting instruments, diamond burs, discs, sandblasting and electropolishing equipment is to be used.

The metal-ceramic bonding is achieved by (pp. 226, 271)

1. Mechanical interlocking—making the surface of the casting rough by sand blasting.
2. Thermal compatibility—COTE of Ni-Cr alloys slightly mismatch, that of ceramic as required.
3. Chemical-oxide bonding by forming an oxide layer of Sn, In, Al and Cr. Before applying the ceramic-slurry, the article is heated in the muffle chamber, at

about 800°–900°C for a few minutes when the **oxide** layer is formed for bonding. This is **sometimes known as degassing** as it was intended to drive out gases trapped during casting procedure.

OUTLINE OF CASTING PROCEDURE OF HIGH FUSING PBM ALLOYS

As the casting procedure is more complicated and technique sensitive, it is done in specially equipped, sophisticated laboratories by well-trained technicians. Certain modifications are done in the gold-alloy-casting procedures, due to the different properties.

1. **Master cast and duplicates:** Dentist prepares the teeth, to receive the fabrication of a required design, obtains an accurate impression, prepares the dental stone master cast and sends to the laboratory. Using agar-agar duplicating material, the technician prepares an exact duplicate of the master cast in a hard die stone (type IV) or divestment material. Type V die stone is preferred to get the slightly enlarged die, for helping the compensation of larger casting shrinkages (*see* Colour Plates 31 and 32, Figs 19.9 to 19.22).

2. **Preformed-smooth casting wax patterns supplied** are used for designing the partial denture frameworks on this duplicate cast. This reduces the trimming and finishing work of the very hard PBM alloys. **Ready-made sprues of required** dimensions are attached. Fine **vent-sprue-wax** wires are also attached, for eliminating the chances of incomplete castings, due to inadequate porosity in the phosphate-bonded investment.

3. **Investment and die-investment:** As the alloys have high casting temperatures, phosphate-bonded investment is required. To minimize distortion of wax pattern, it is invested along with the die, **die investment technique**. Special investment materials and divestment materials are also available, which are gypsum-bonded for low fusing alloys or phosphate-bonded for high fusing alloys. **Colloidal silica liquid** is added in required proportions to avail **higher setting and thermal expansions** (*refer* to phosphate-bonded investments for compensation of larger casting shrinkages of about 2.2–2.3%). Flexible rubber or plastic casting ring is first used in the investing procedure and later pulled out (known as **ringless casting method**). Strong investment does not need the metal casting ring which inhibits the lateral expansions. It is allowed **to set for about 2 hours.**

4. **Wax-burn out** is done in an electric furnace by slowly raising the temperature first **up to 300°C and then quickly to about 750° to 850°C** and maintained for about **2 hours for completing the thermal expansion and wax elimination.**

5. **Melting of the alloys:** Type I low fusing PBM alloys are of nickel-chromium, having melting temperatures 1150°–1300°C and type II high fusing alloys are of Co-Cr having fusion temperature range 1300°–1450°C. These cannot be melted by gas flames. Alloys are usually melted in ceramic, clay or graphite crucibles. Electric furnaces with high fusing **Pt-Ir or silicon carbide,** resistance heating coils, or argon gas or carbon arcs are used for melting.

The **induction heating centrifugal casting machines** (*see* colour plate 31, Fig. 19.13) have become more common. The ceramic crucible is surrounded by the copper-tube coil through which high frequency AC is applied to induce **large heat, along with the axis of the coil** (and crucible), which can melt the alloy within a minute. Cold water current is also circulated through the copper tube to protect it from melting (*see* Fig. 19.4, page 281). The wax eliminated mould (investment) is mounted against the crucible, in the rotating arm of centrifugal casting machine and casting is done. It is allowed to **cool slowly by itself**.

RECOVERY AND FINISHING

Divesting is done by carefully fracturing the hard PBI investment. The unwanted sprue parts are removed by using diamond discs, diamond points or carbide burs and finished. To remove the hard investments sticking to the casting, **sandblasting method** is used. Final polishing is done by **electropolishing method** that is suspending the article, as an **anode in sulphuric acid solution bath and passing direct current for some time.**

The denture is prepared with PMMA denture base materials and acrylic/porcelain teeth, on this framework.

BRONZE: COPPER ALLOYS FOR CASTING

These copper-rich alloys are commonly known as bronze and mainly contain copper about 80–88%. Different types of bronzes are: Aluminium bronze (Cu-Al), silicon bronze (Cu-Si), beryllium bronze (Cu-Be). The traditional bronze contains copper, tin, and sometimes Zn and P, in small quantities. Small amounts of nickel (2–4%) and iron (1–4%) may also be present.

One popular dental-bronze, known as **technique alloy or Japanese gold** has Cu:Zn:Al approximately **54%, 34% and 12% by weight.**

Properties

- Due to the formation of copper sulphide, the alloys have low tarnish and corrosion resistance and very soon become dark, when exposed to the atmosphere.

- Mechanical properties are similar to type II and type III dental casting alloys.
- Low density (8.0–8.2 gm/cc) and inexpensive
- Low fusion temperature, 750–850°C, can easily be melted by ordinary gas torch flames.

These alloy-appliances (crown, bridges with acrylic facings) continue to have gold colour in the oral environment due to continuous washing of tarnish products by saliva. **Patients may get easily be duped as when polished it appear just like gold!**

These alloys are contraindicated for dental castings. However, they are quite suitable for the **technicians to get good training in casting procedures** using gypsum-bonded investments with centrifugal casting machines. Hence, these are known as **goldent, nonprecious gold or technique alloys, and supplied as small pellets.**

MODEL QUESTIONS

I. Long Essays   (20 minutes each)

1. Explain the necessity of alloying gold, for casting. Describe the ideal requirements of dental casting alloys and classify them according to their functions or descriptions.
2. Describe alloying properties of various metals used in high noble and noble metal casting alloys.
3. Give the composition of PBM casting alloys. Explain the microstructure of cast alloys and give the outline of the casting procedure.

II. Short Essays   (10 minutes each)

1. High noble casting alloys
2. Noble metal casting alloys
3. PBM casting alloys
4. HN and N alloys for metal-ceramics
5. PBM alloys for metal-ceramics
6. Requirements of metals and ceramics for metal-ceramics
7. Metal-ceramic bonding
8. Outline of casting steps of PBM alloy
9. Casting problems of titanium alloys (*see* page 286)

III. Brief Answers   (5 minutes each)

1. Alloying properties of platinum/palladium
2. Alloying properties of silver/copper
3. Scavenger in casting procedure
4. Metal-ceramic bondings
5. Sandblasting and electropolishing
6. Technique alloys
7. Microstructures of PBM cast alloys
8. Heat treatment of gold alloys
9. Carat and fineness.

Outline of Dental Alloy Casting Procedures

INTRODUCTION

The objective of casting is to prepare an exact permanent metallic duplicate of the missing tooth structure as accurately fitting as possible.

The lost-wax-casting procedure is to be carefully planned and the precautions should be meticulously followed to achieve this goal of perfect fit (Fig. 19.1). Preparation of tooth or teeth, then the wax pattern, investing the wax pattern, melting of the alloy, casting and finishing is the major steps.

For this, the **technician** also should have deep knowledge of compositions, microstructures (metallography), phase diagrams, heat treatments, etc. for selection and use of the alloys. In addition, he should have **excellent skill and scientific background** for using the sophisticated equipment and techniques of casting in the modern casting and ceramic laboratories.

Preparation or cavity cutting of the tooth or teeth to **receive the appliance is done by the dentist** after studying clinical situations and planning the design of appliances.

1. WAX PATTERN

- **Direct pattern technique:** Dentist has to select type I hard inlay wax, soften it uniformly by waving carefully over a flame and adapt it directly on the prepared teeth (coated with lubricants for easy removal without distortion) and then carve it as required. However, as it is very inconvenient to carve it in the mouth, this method is used very rarely.
- **Indirect pattern technique:** Dentist has to obtain a very accurate elastomeric impression of the prepared tooth (double mix-syringe techniques) with finer details reproduced accurately. The impression or its master-cast with type IV die stone is sent to the laboratory technician (*see* Colour Plate 30, Fig. 19.2).

The technician performs the following steps
- **The increase of surface hardness** by immersing the die in certain surface hardener solutions (like K_2SO_4, borax, cellulose-resins, etc.). The electroforming method has not become popular.
- **Die spacers:** Like nail paints, resin paints, or certain suspensions with silver and gold colours, which, on coating alternately, controls the space. This is required for obtaining suitable cementing space. This method is also made use for die enlargement for compensating large casting shrinkages (*see* Colour Plate 30, Fig. 19.1).
- **Lubricant** or thin layer of oil is then applied for easy removal of the wax pattern without distortion.

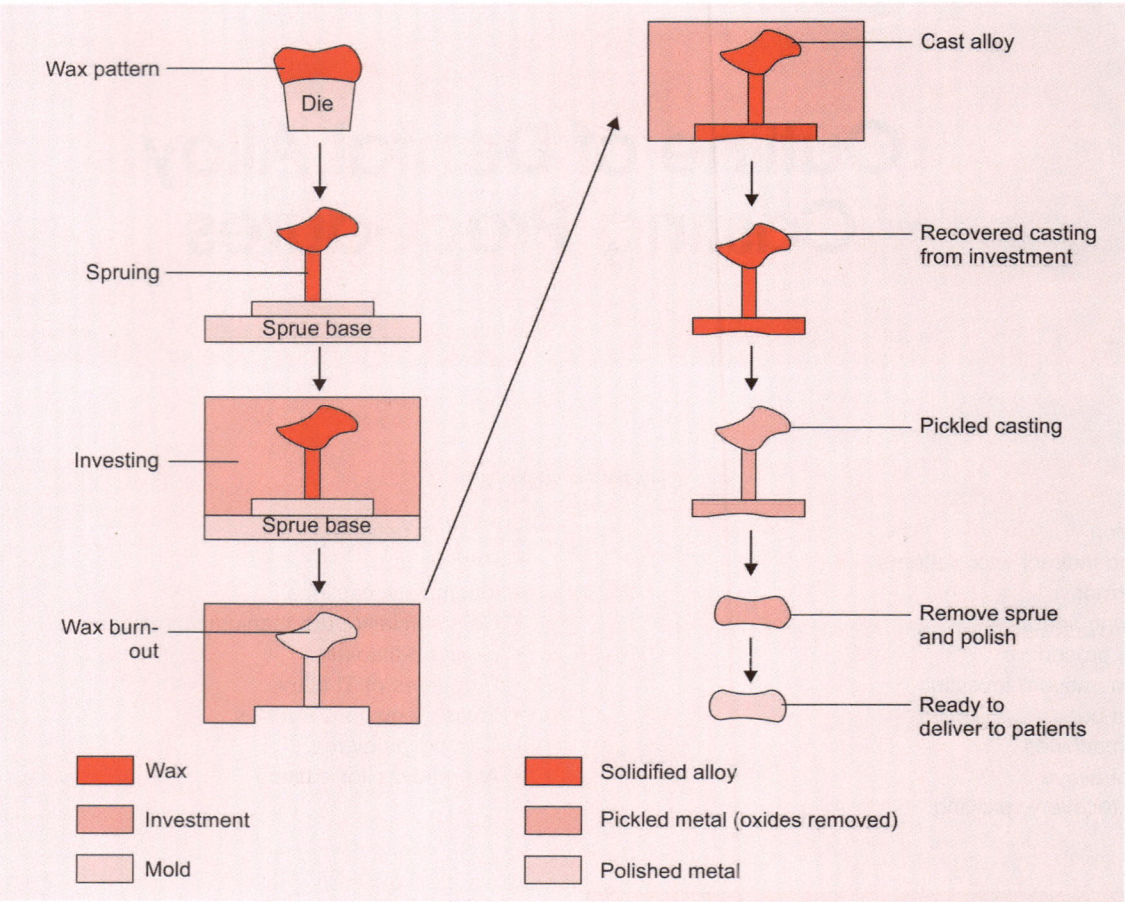

Fig. 19.1: Outline of lost-wax casting steps

- The **wax pattern** is then prepared by using the type II soft inlay wax. It is carefully melted by **dry-heat** and placed on the prepared die, **layer by layer** until some excess is formed. **Care is taken to uniformly heat, melt and bond the increments to minimize distortion** due to relaxation of internal stresses. Carving is done with sharp carvers without pulling the wax away from margins or abrading the die surface.

  Sprue is fixed to the wax pattern, and then the pattern is very carefully withdrawn from the die, to minimize distortion.

  If there is some delay in investing, the pattern is to be stored, immersing in cold water or refrigerator to minimize distortion by internal stress relaxations.

2. SPRUE FORMERS

Sprue is a channel or ingate to the mould of the wax pattern invested in the casting ring, to allow the molten wax to come out and molten alloy liquid during casting, to enter and completely fill the mould space. Sprue formers are selected and attached carefully to minimize many casting defects.

- **Materials of sprue formers or sprue**
  - Special wax supplied in rope form (rolls) of different diameters (gauges) for selection.
  - Hollow stainless steel wires of different diameters and lengths. These are to be coated with thin layer of **inlay wax** by dipping in molten wax. This is for easy removal of sprue former after setting of investment.

- **Sprue former diameter:** This should be approximately equal to the **maximum thickness** of the pattern. For bigger patterns, sprues of larger diameters are used. The diameters usually vary from **1.3 mm** (16 gauge) up to about **2.6 mm** (10 gauge) for small castings. If the **diameter is too small, pre-solidification** in the sprue and insufficient liquid entering, cause **incomplete casting.** Sprues of large diameters cause rough surface, suck back or localized shrinkage porosities, fracture or distortion of thin segments.

- **Length of the sprue:** Should be such that the wax pattern must be positioned in the **middle** of the casting ring to minimize distortion and the thickness of investment beyond the extreme end of the pattern be about **6 mm, for gypsum-bonded investment or**

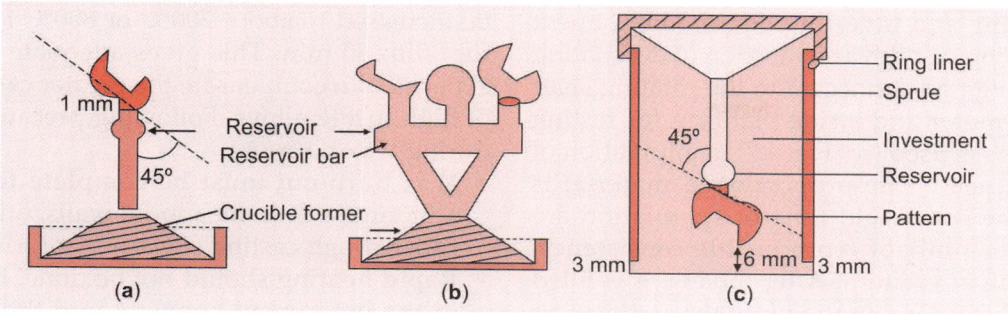

Figs 19.2a to c: Methods of spruing. (a) Direct, (b) indirect spruing, (c) positioning of wax pattern in casting ring

3–4 mm, for phosphate-bonded investments (as it has less and inadequate porosity). This consideration is necessary to have sufficient porosity to allow the trapped air to escape out

If the sprue and casting ring is **too long, or sprue former is too thin**, alloy pre-solidification in the sprue, blocks it, causing incomplete casting. Too short (or thick) sprue, causes rough surfaces, suck back porosity, as well as damage to thin sections.

- **Sprue attachment**

  Attachment of the sprue to the wax pattern is done by a **small drop** of molten wax or flaring, with the following considerations:
  - **At the bulkiest part** so that alloy liquid first enters and flows to the thinner portion with lower speed and less turbulence, i.e. without damaging. Localized shrinkage porosity will not take place as the last portion solidifying, has adequate liquid in the connected reservoir.
  - **Sprue is oriented at 45° inclination** to the proximal area to **reduce turbulent** flow to the extremities of mold. If it is at the right angle, casting forces may fracture investment.
  - **Reservoir:** In direct spruing, the reservoir (Fig. 19.2a) is made by a large drop of wax at 1–2 mm distance from the attached position. This is to minimize **localized shrinkage porosity**, by reserving a portion of the last liquid from solidifying in it.
  - **Indirect spruing:** The reservoir bar provides extra liquid to compensate solidification shrinkage (localized shrinkage porosity). In this multiple casting method (Fig. 19.2b), 3 or 4 patterns can be invested as shown, with a common bar (reservoir). This method also **saves expensive phosphate-bonded investment and also casting time.**
  - **Sprue axis** should not be oriented or directed towards the extreme thin sections of the wax pattern. The component of casting force is highest in this direction which may damage it.
  - A plastic or ceramic crucible former is attached to the other end of sprue former (Figs 19.2a to c).

3. CASTING RING LINERS

Formerly asbestos sheet liners were laid inside the casting ring leaving about 3 mm at the ends. Due to health hazards of inhaling asbestos dust or vapours which is carcinogenic, now **cellulose or alumina silicate ceramic liners are used** (Fig. 19.2c). The functions of the liners are:

- To allow enough lateral expansion of mold (investment), during setting or heating.
- Longer longitudinal expansion is reduced by adhesion of investment at the ends (3 mm space, Fig. 19.2c). This minimizes the distortion.
- If wetted, these liners provide some **extra water for the HSE** of the mould. Two or three layers give **higher HSE** of the mould laterally.
- Split casting rings or plastic casting rings are used to get adequate lateral expansions specially for high fusing alloys. In base metal alloy casting procedures ringless casting investment is done.

4. INVESTING PROCEDURE

The wax pattern is washed with a dilute detergent solution to remove greasy materials. This detergent layer left behind, reduce surface tension and cause **better wetting.** This special surfactant or wetting agents can also be applied as a thin layer, to wet the hydrophobic surface of wax pattern, which otherwise collects air bubbles from the mix and causes **nodules of casting.** Two methods of investing are:

- **Hand mixing investing method:** Required amount of distilled water (or a mixture of water and colloidal silica gel, special liquid for phosphate-bonded investments) is taken in a clean flexible bowl. A weighed amount of powder is added and mixed thoroughly. A small amount of **mix is painted** on the surface of the wax pattern for better wetting and then the remaining mix is vibrated carefully into the casting ring to fill completely. Too much **vibration causes sedimentation of larger investment** particles, leaving a thin mix close to the pattern, which may cause a rough surface.

- **Vacuum mixing and investing:** Special investment mixing closed bowl, with a connection to evacuating pump, a mixing pad connected to the rotating shaft of an electric motor and a side platform for resting the casting ring is used (*see* Fig. 4.7, manipulation of gypsum products). The proportioned material is taken in it, the speed and time of spatulation are adjusted to get a **mix of reproducible consistency.** Mixing is done in vacuum. After mixing, it is tilted to flow the mix under vibration into the casting ring on the platform (*see* Colour Plate 29, Fig. 15.4).
- **Compensation of casting shrinkages by**
  - Increasing normal setting expansion of investment
  - Increasing hygroscopic setting expansion
  - Adjusting thermal expansion by heating the invested casting ring to a required temperature
  - Adding colloidal silica liquid (for PBI).

After allowing to **set** for about 1 hour, the **crucible former is carefully removed.** If metal sprue is used, that also is easily pulled out as exothermic reaction softens the wax coating. The crucible formed is carefully cleaned by removing the loosely adhering investment particles which otherwise may fall into the sprue and block it. The invested casting ring should be dewaxed, when it is quite wet, otherwise it is to be stored in 100% humidor to prevent drying.

5. WAX BURN-OUT

It is then placed in the furnace, with the **crucible downwards,** on a ceramic mesh stand, to allow the molten wax to flow down. The temperature is slowly raised to about 400°C in the low heat (HSE) technique or 700°C in the high-heat (NSE) technique, for about half an hour, and is maintained for about **30–60 minutes for completion of the thermal expansion.** As wax is melted and evaporated, some carbon may deposit in the pores of investment and block them. But the steam produced by the water of wet investment pass out through the pores, clean them and make them effective. If the temperature is more than 700°C, the GBI get reduced by carbon, producing SO_2 gas, according to:

$$CaSO_4 + C \xrightarrow{>700°C} CaO + SO_2 + CO$$

The chemical degradation causes shrinkage of investment and SO_2 gas produced causes tarnishing of HN and N metal alloys (*refer* to pickling).

In the case of PBI, after setting, the plastic ring can be taken out (ringless casting). The temperature of the furnace is **slowly** raised first to about 300°C, to prevent cracking of investment due to large steam pressure, produced by rapid heating. Then the temperature can be increased to about 700°C or 800°C and maintained for 30 to 60 min. This gives adequate larger thermal expansion to compensate the greater casting shrinkage of high fusing alloys. Following precautions are taken during wax burn-out.

- **Wax burn-out must be complete to eliminate** all adhering wax to the mould walls, otherwise, it may cause rough casting surface.
- **Rapid heating** should not be done. Excess of water in the investment converts into the steam of high pressure which may fracture the investment and produce a crack.
- **Overheating** of investment, cause disintegration resulting tarnishing of gold alloys, rough casting surface, too much mold expansions and also cracks.
- **Prolonged heating** also may fracture the investment and produce cracks (colour plate 30, Fig. 19.4).

The molten alloy liquid enters the cracks producing thin feather-like extensions **fins.**

6. CASTING MACHINES

These are devices to force the alloy liquid into the mould formed in the investment in casting ring. In a very simple old method, the alloy pellets were kept in the crucible former, melted by gas torch flame and forced by air pressure applied from a compression pump or steam pressure. This can be coupled with **synchronized vacuum suction from the other end of casting ring.**

Centrifugal casting machines, with different alloy melting systems, are now used. The alloy is melted in a separate crucible by gas torch flames, electrical resistance or induction heating or electric arc systems.

Centrifugal casting machine is a **spring-wound or electric-motor driven** rotating shaft equipment. The rotating arm has two parts, one balancing arm A and the other, broken arm B. The broken part C is rotatable through 90°. The whole arm ABC is **initially kept wound by giving 2 to 5 complete rotations** and fixed by lever-arm, connected to a strong spring 'S'.

The part C of a broken arm carries the alloy melting crucible, against which the wax burnt out casting ring can be mounted, and it is fixed at right angles before melting the alloy (Fig. 19.3) (*see* Colour Plate 30, Figs 19.6 and 19.7; Colour Plate 31, Fig. 19.13).

7. MELTING OF ALLOYS

Crucibles used for melting of alloys are made up of:
- Clay
- Graphite
- Quartz
- Zirconia-alumina

Clay crucibles can be used for low and medium fusing HN and N alloys. For high fusing high palladium

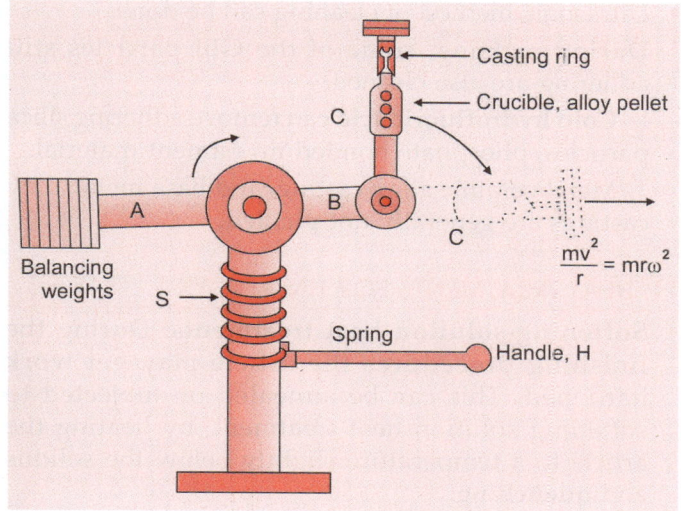

Fig. 19.3: Centrifugal casting machine

(Pd-Ag), and PBM alloys, graphite, quartz or zirconia-alumina crucibles are needed. However, to minimize carbon contamination and reactions, **graphite crucibles are not** recommended for melting high Pd and nickel containing alloys.

Methods of Melting of Alloys

- **Gas torch flames** with mixtures of natural gas and air or oxyacetylene gases are used.
  - The innermost conical portion of the gas flame has no heat content and is only gas and air (or oxygen) mixture.
  - Next outer green-coloured cone is the combustion zone (Fig. 23.3b, zones of flame).
  - Next outer, **pale blue**-coloured zone, is the **reducing flame** which is the **hottest part and should be used for alloy melting.**
  - The outermost yellow-coloured oxidizing zone also should never be used.
    The alloy pellets are placed leaning to the crucible walls and the reducing flame is carefully applied. As alloy begins to melt, it crumbles down and a large spheroidal drop is formed on the crucible floor. Small amounts of **(boric acid + borax) – flux** powder is sprinkled over it. Fluxes increase the flow and decrease melting temperatures. The brown-dark oxides of zinc (zinc-scavenger) is blown out. A **mirror-like shining surface** is formed when properly melted and if the flame is rotated or moved, its image appears moving in the opposite direction.
  - **Electrical resistance heating system:** The crucible is surrounded by a small electric resistance heater. The **advantages are: Correct adjustment of the temperature of the alloy liquid** and required delay

in the solidification in the sprue former and the mould space which rectifies localized shrinkage porosities.

- **AC electrical induction melting system:** A copper tube coil is wound loosely around the crucible. **High frequency alternating current** and cold water circulation, cause very quick rise of temperature along the axis of the coil even up to 1500°C or 1600°C, melting the high fusing PBM alloys easily. During casting, the coil is brought down and the arm (B, not broken arm) rotates by electric motor, until it is switched off. The highest temperature can be controlled, and this has become quite popular, for high fusing noble and base metal alloy castings (Fig. 19.4) (*see* Colour Plate 31, Fig. 19.13).
- **Electric arc melting system:** Electric arc is produced between the alloy and a **water cooled tungsten electrode**. Temperature shoots up to more than **4000ºC** and melts the alloy immediately. But there is no control over the highest temperature produced. Within a few seconds, the **alloy components may begin to evaporate and damage** the alloy. This method has been tried for casting cpTi and its alloys.
- **Vacuum pressure assisted casting machine:** This is designed specially for casting the high fusing **titanium and its alloys**. Titanium has a very high melting temperature 1668°C, low density (4.51 gm/cc) and **high oxygen sensitivity** at high temperatures. The centrifugal force (mv^2/r) is not sufficient to force the liquid into the mould. **Hence, the alloy is melted in a vacuum by an electric arc, and casting is done under argon gas pressure.**

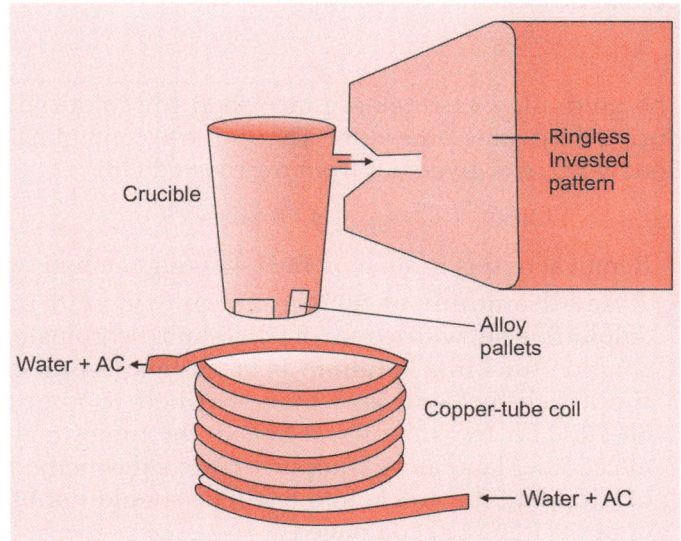

Fig. 19.4: Induction melting coil around crucible

8. CASTING OF ALLOY

The dewaxed, heated casting ring, maintained at suitable temperature in the electric furnace, is quickly transferred and fitted against the crucible, in a very short time, to prevent solidification taking place meanwhile. The gas flame can again be directed to the alloy liquid to check liquefaction, and also to the casting ring. The handle 'H' is released immediately (Fig. 19.3).

The arms begin to rotate, first with a sudden jerk when the alloy liquid enters into the mould. The broken arm turns and becomes **straight along with AB and rotates** with high speed. The centrifugal force exerted on 'm' gm of liquid = $F = mv^2/r$ or $mr\omega^2$ retains the alloy liquid to the extreme wall of the mould, and solidification takes place. When it stops rotating, liquid solidifies completely, and the excess is seen as a red hot button on the cone or crucible.

In the case of electrical resistance or induction, melting system, casting is done by switching off the heating circuit

9. DEVESTING OR RECOVERING

As soon as the rotation stops, the casting ring is **quenched in water**. The water rushes inside with a hissing sound, disintegrates investments and separates the casting. The quenching also leaves the gold alloy casting in softened (disordered alloy phase) condition which helps to cut, trimming and finishing.

For chrome cobalt or nickel alloys, the cast investment is allowed to **cool slowly by itself** overnight and then the article is recovered by carefully breaking the investment. It is then trimmed by diamond disc or carbide bur, **sandblasted** to clean the adhering phosphate-bonded investment, finished and **electro-polished.**

10. PICKLING

The gold alloy castings are tarnished (discoloured) during the casting procedure. This is due to contamination by SO_2 gas given out from overheated GBI.

$$CaSO_4 + C \xrightarrow{700°C} CaO + SO_2 + CO.$$

Removal of this is done by the following methods.

- A small amount of 50% hydrochloric acid or sulphuric acid, with a trace of potassium dichromate, solution **(pickling solution)** is taken in a test-tube, the article is kept, and then warmed to about **50–70°C** for few minutes. If boiled, the fumes may affect other laboratory equipment. Also, the method of dropping the article into test tube should not be done, as it may get damaged.
- Special pickling solutions supplied can be used.

- Ultrasonic method of cleaning can be done. During pickling, some of the GBI particles still adhering are also cleaned.

    Cold hydrofluoric acid can remove adhering silica particles, phosphate-bonded investment material.

    Metal-ceramic alloy casting, and base metal alloy castings are generally **not pickled.**

11. HEAT TREATMENTS FOR HN ALLOYS

- **Softening-solution heat treatments:** During the finishing procedures the article may get work hardened. This can be annealed or subjected to softening solution heat treatment, by heating the article to a temperature slightly below the solidus and **quenching.**
- **Precipitation-hardening heat treatment**

    After the final finishing and polishing, the article can be heated in an electric furnace (muffle chamber) **for about 10–15 min, at about 375°C. The ordered FCT superlattice** formed in HN alloys with copper 15–35% (with respect to gold), **precipitate,** causing lattice distortion which increases the hardness by a large value. Prolonged heat treatment increases brittleness.

    Dentist has to check the fitting of the article and do permanent cementation.

DEFECTIVE CASTINGS: CLASSIFICATION, CAUSES AND REMEDIES

The precision casting should have the exact shape, size, correct fitting, smooth surface and no internal or external flaws, affecting the properties. There are many chances of introduction of many casting defects in various steps, unless suitable precautions are carefully observed.

CLASSIFICATIONS OF CASTING DEFECTS

1. Distortion: Change of Shape or Size: Both Cause Misfit

Change of shape occurs by distortions of the wax pattern (Fig. 19.5) by careless removal from the die (apply lubricant), too much vibration during investment, too thick investment, delay in investing, inhomogeneous setting and thermal expansions of investment, such as too much longitudinal expansion. Too long sprue and casting ring also can cause distortion (remedy—leaving about 3 mm gap, free of ring liner, at the ends, can restrict this expansion).

Change of size occurs, due to, under- or over-compensation of casting shrinkages (which can be controlled by correct setting and thermal expansions).

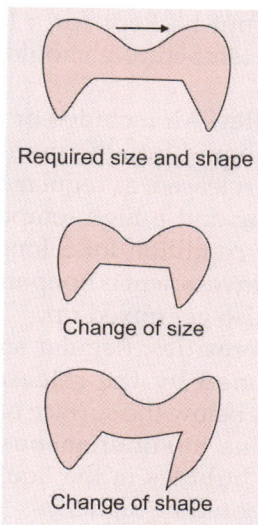

Fig. 19.5: Distortion of casting causes misfit

2. Discolouration

This is due to SO_2 gas contamination to HN and N alloys—remedied by pickling (*refer* to pickling, and disadvantages of GBI).

3. Surface Roughness, Unevenness and Nodules

The external surface defects (Fig. 19.6) can be removed by finishing procedures. Any attempt to remove the defects in tooth-tissue contact surfaces can cause misfit. Main causes of surface roughness are:

- Rough wax pattern
- Coarse investment powder particles
- High water/powder ratio of investment
- Inhomogeneous mixing of investment
- Inadequate vibrations to dislodge air trapped during investing
- Insufficient wetting of wax pattern (apply surfactant/detergent coating)
- Air bubble collection and thin water film on the surface of wax pattern cause nodules and uneven surface (apply surfactant, vibration, vacuum mixing, and investment techniques).
- Too short, too thick sprue—increase the speed of liquid entering.
- Improper methods of dewaxing, i.e. incomplete dewaxing, too rapid, prolonged and overheating during wax burn out.
- High casting force (adjust the speed of rotation, increase the length, decrease the thickness of sprue, and also, correct orientation of sprue). Liquid entering the mould **at high speed abrades** the walls and cause rough surface.

Rough surface cause, corrosion due to a collection of food debris and poor aesthetics. If the tissue surface side is smoothened, it may cause misfit.

4. Solidification Shrinkage Porosities

Almost all liquids contract during solidification as the atoms arrange in a certain order, more closely.

- **Microporosity: Small irregular voids** are formed throughout, which decrease the strength (Fig. 19.7). If the temperature of the liquid entering mould is low and close to its liquidus temperature, it solidifies simultaneously preventing diffusion of liquid properly. Contractions cause irregular microvoids throughout (remedy—the temperature of casting liquid should be higher).
- **Localized shrinkage porosity:** Large irregular void is formed close to the sprue attachment at the bulkiest part. The liquid continues to solidify from the cooler mould walls towards the bulkiest part (close to the

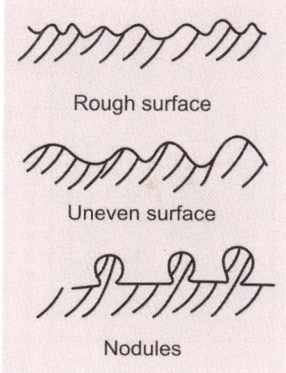

Fig. 19.6: Rough surface, uneven surface and nodules

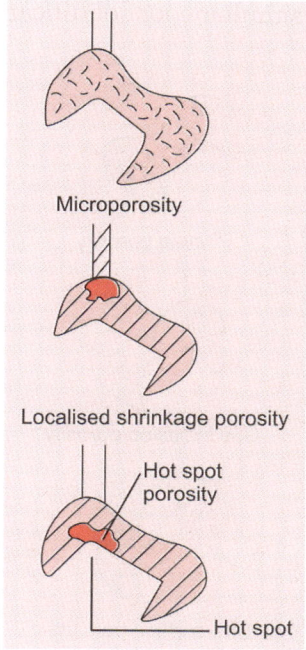

Fig. 19.7: Solidification shrinkage porosities

sprue attachment). If the sprue is blocked by pre-solidification, adequate liquid will not be available to compensate the solidification shrinkage occurred, which is localized at this bulkiest part where liquid solidifies last.

Remedies are, attaching a **large reservoir** in the sprue close to its attachment **(1 mm)** to the pattern and use a **sprue of thickness more than the thickest portion of the pattern,** such that the last portion of the liquid, solidifying is in contact with the liquid in a reservoir, which supplies **extra liquid required.**

- **Hot spot or suck back porosity:** A large irregular void is formed opposite to sprue. If the temperature of the liquid entering is very high, it raises the temperature of the mold opposite to the sprue attachment. Due to this hot spot, liquid solidifies last, near it. The other liquid is sucked back, by the solidifying liquid against it. Solidification shrinkage localizes near the hot spot.

Remedies

The temperature of liquid should not be very high and the thickness of sprue should be decreased.

5. Air Inclusion Porosities

Air can be included in the molten liquid during the casting procedure and even gases like H_2, N, etc. get absorbed during prolonged heating of the liquid, which are released during solidification as **regular voids** (Fig. 19.8).

- **Pinhole porosity:** The absorbed gases are released, throughout, as **very small spherical pinhole-like voids** due to simultaneous solidification. **Remedy** is,

liquid should not be kept for a long time before casting and its temperature should not be too close to liquidus.

- **Large air bubbles:** Air included or mixed up during rapid entry of liquid into the mould and **turbulent motion.** It gets released, as regular large voids: High speed of casting and a high temperature of liquid, keeping liquid condition for a long time should be avoided. If the investment is nonporous, the air inside the mold can also get mixed up.
- **Sub-surface porosities:** Regular small air bubble—voids are formed by the release of trapped or absorbed gases below the surface of the casting. This is said to be due to **simultaneous nucleation and release of gas bubbles** in the liquid. (Temperature of the liquid should be higher.)

All these porosities decrease strength.

6. Incomplete Castings

- These occur due to an adequate amount of liquid entering the mold (Fig. 19.9a). Reasons for these are:
  - Insufficient amount of the alloy melted
  - Incomplete melting of alloy
  - Too low casting force
  - Poor castability, i.e. high viscosity of alloy liquid
  - Blocking of sprue due to loose investment particles
  - Incomplete dewaxing
  - Blocking due to pre-solidification in the sprue, if sprue is too long, or too thin or liquid alloy temperature is too low (close to liquidus), or investment temperature is also low. (**Remedies are suggestive.**)

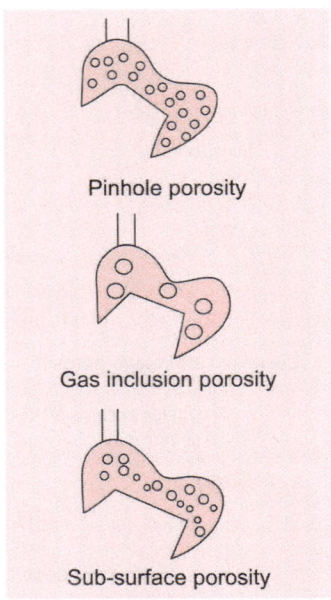

Fig. 19.8: Air inclusion porosity

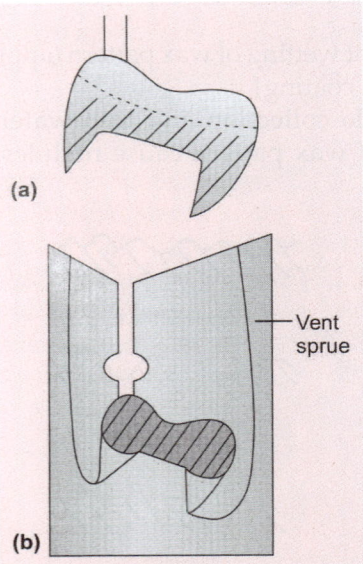

Figs 19.9a and b: (a) Incomplete castings, (b) incomplete casting (back pressure porosity)

- **Back pressure—air trapping porosity:** As the liquid enters the mould through the sprue, the air trapped in the mould is compressed at the extremities, which exert a **back pressure** preventing the alloy liquid to occupy this region. This is due to the **inadequate porosity** in the investment **to vent out trapped air.** Even though, GBI is porous, if the thickness of investment at the extremity of the pattern is more than 6 mm. the porosity becomes less effective. To increase the effectiveness of porosity **reduce the thickness** to less than 6 mm or increase water/powder ratio. The PBI has still less porosity which very frequently causes incomplete castings. **Extra vent wax sprue formers** are fitted to the extreme ends of wax pattern to make trapped air escape backward as shown in Fig. 19.9b.

7. Fins

These are feather-like thin extensions on the alloy casting surfaces, produced as the liquid enters the cracks formed in the fractured investment (Fig. 19.10). Reasons for the investment fractures are:

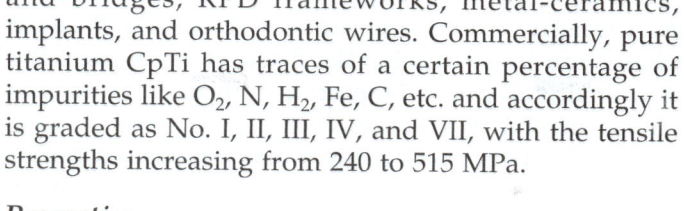

Fig. 19.10: Fins

- Weak investment
- High water/powder ratio used for investing
- Improper mixing and investing methods
- Rapid temperature rise during wax burn out
- Prolonged heating of investment
- Overheating of investment
- Too high casting forces.

Remedies

Reduce the number of turns to casting machine arms, or decrease the thickness and increase the length of the sprue, etc. Use the above precautions during wax burn-out.

Incomplete casting and fins result in misfit of cast articles.

TITANIUM

Titanium is a light, highly biocompatible material introduced into the casting appliances such as crowns and bridges, RPD frameworks, metal-ceramics, implants, and orthodontic wires. Commercially, pure titanium CpTi has traces of a certain percentage of impurities like O_2, N, H_2, Fe, C, etc. and accordingly it is graded as No. I, II, III, IV, and VII, with the tensile strengths increasing from 240 to 515 MPa.

Properties

- High biocompatibility and corrosion resistance
- High oxygen affinity forms a very thin 10 microns film of TiO_2 when exposed to the atmosphere in a very short time, 10^{-9} sec. This passivating effect is even better than chromium and TiO_2 adheres to the substrate very strongly. It gets oxidized by contact with silica of investment at high temperatures.
- Very low density, 4.51 gm/cc (centrifugal casting force becomes inadequate).
- Moderate tensile strength depending upon the allotropic—martensite and austenite (α-Ti and β-Ti) phase distributions.
- **Moderate stiffness** or modulus of elasticity, β-Ti has more flexibility (E = 71,000 MPa).
- **Fusion temperature** is very high about **1668°C** (tungsten arc or induction melting methods are to be used).
- Undergoes allotropic changes from HCP (α-Ti) martensitic form to BCC (β-Ti), complex austenitic form, when heated above 883°C or stressed.

ALLOTROPIC FORMS: MICROSTRUCTURE

At ordinary temperatures, α-Ti has a HCP structure. Above its TTR (transition temperature range) of 883°C, it is transformed into complex β-Ti of BCC structure. The change is also reversible, on cooling. The α and β forms have different mechanical properties (Table 19.1). In general, the properties of cast Ti depends on the presence of amounts of various phases, equiaxed grain structures and grain sizes, which also depends on the rate of cooling.

ALLOYS OF TITANIUM

By **adding small amounts of other metals, it is possible to control the amounts of α and β phases,** for obtaining desired properties at ordinary temperatures. **Vanadium, molybdenum and tantalum are β phase**

Table 19.1	Mechanical properties			
Properties	α-Ti	β-Ti	Ti-6Al-4V	TMA (Ti-Mo-Zr)
YS (MPa)	170–480	860–1000	975–1120	860–1200
UTS (MPa)	240–515	900–1100	1025–1152	1000–1350
E (MPa)	110,000	70,000	80,000	71,700

stabilizers and Al, C, O, N are **α** phase stabilizers. Accordingly, varieties of alloys with **α, α + β** and **β** phases can be obtained. (The **β** stabilizers depress the martensitic **α** phase formation temperature to low values, like Ni, in stainless steel.)

α + β variety has mechanical properties better suited for casting purpose. Whereas β phase varieties are more suitable for active orthodontic wires active appliances.

Ti Alloys for Casting

Ti- Pd, Ti-Cu, Ti-Cu-Ni, Ti-V, Ti-Co, etc. alloys are in the experimental stages. The titanium alloy which has been successfully used for casting dental appliances is Ti-6Al-4V (TAV) alloy.

Ti-6Al-4V Alloy

When this cast alloy is subjected to heat treatment by heating to about 700°C and quenching, equiaxed spherical grains are formed. **Slow cooling** from **β** phase produces **α + β lamellar structures. This alloy has very high fatigue strength of 860–950 MPa.**

PROBLEMS IN CASTING OF TITANIUM AND ITS ALLOYS

Titanium is becoming the material of choice for casting, all metal and metal-ceramic appliances and the various problems faced in the casting procedures have been tackled.

1. **Choice of investment materials:** Titanium has very high melting temperature and oxygen sensitivity. Titanium alloys get contaminated with oxygen, if they come into contact with SiO_2 refractory material at the high temperatures as **Ti can reduce SiO_2. Special refractory materials, Al_2O_3, ZrO_2, MgO, Zr** and their combinations developed in Japan, with phosphate bonding, are to be used.
2. **Melting of alloy:** Electric tungsten arc or induction melting methods are used in **vacuum or inert argon gas atmosphere.**
3. **Casting machine:** Due to the very low density of the alloy (about 4.5 gm/cc), the low centrifugal force ($m.V^2/R$ = volume × density × V^2/R) becomes very inadequate to force the liquid into the mould. The casting machine is modified by **adding compression as well as vacuum suction techniques, to minimize incomplete castings.**
4. The surface of titanium alloy casting becomes very hard (**formation of martensite α-case**) and special instruments and techniques are used for finishing work.

These difficulties are being tackled and the alloy becomes gradually more popular for RPD, metal ceramics and implants. Osseointegration or bioactivity of coated titanium alloys (Ti-Al-V) has resulted as one of the best implant materials.

The latest CAD-CAM technique can solve many of the above casting problems.

ALTERNATIVES TO METAL CASTING TECHNOLOGY

The casting techniques involve many stages such as preparation of wax patterns, investments, selection of alloys, casting machines, methods of melting, recovery finishing, cementation, etc. This is time-consuming and highly skilled procedure to get a **precision casting permanent restoration.** Instead various simpler technologies have been invented.

1. **CAD-CAM procedure:** Computer-aided designing and computer-aided machining has been developed in the 1980s. This is a **chairside technology** used for processing metal alloy, composite resins and the best ceramic of ideal properties, in a single sitting of short time.

   The CAD system digitally or electronically traces the surface profile of a prepared tooth or teeth and designs the fabrication of the prosthesis from **memory.** These are immediately transferred to a milling machine. Using diamond points and discs, etc. the machine prepares the prosthesis from **solid blocks or blanks, of alloy, composite resin or ceramics.** The finished article is cemented or bonded. All these can be completed in a short time of few minutes to one hour.

   Advantages
   - Various precautions to minimize casting defects are not required.
   - Work can be completed within an hour in a single sitting of the patient
   - Best varieties of ceramics can be selected and used.
   - Can be applied, to Ti alloys in preparing implants at the chair side.
   - Finishing of Ti articles are much easier, as the hard α-case is not formed
   - Limited technical skill

   Disadvantages
   - Correct knowledge of the procedure is required for a well-trained technician
   - Very very expensive equipment

2. **Copy milling:** After the preparation of the tooth or teeth, the pattern is made with certain resin-based composites. It is then traced optically or electronically and duplicated by the copy milling machine from the solid blanks and finished.

3. **Electroforming:** The master die is coated with special die spacers and a duplicate is formed. It

is first cleaned and coated with a suspension of the metallizing agent, on the required surface. This is then placed as a cathode in electrolytic bath. Electroplating is done, **for a few hours** to get an adequate thickness. The gypsum product die material is removed. The ceramic fabrication is done on this coping.

4. **Sintering of burnished foil technique:** A few layers of thin foils of gold alloys or gold platinum alloys are adapted on the die and burnished. It is then sintered by firing at about 1000°C. The thickness of this coping may be low, about 50 microns. Over this the ceramic appliance is prepared, with a ceramic layer of a small thickness of 0.3–1.0 mm for anterior, and 1–2 mm or more for posterior restorations (*refer to metal-ceramics*).

Advantages

- Very thin restorations can be prepared
- Since the coping is also very thin, **minimum removal of the tooth is required which gives better strength.**

MODEL QUESTIONS

I. Long Essays (20 minutes each)

1. Give a brief outline of a lost-wax-casting technique for low fusing alloys.
2. Classify the casting defects. Explain briefly, their causes and suggest remedies.
3. Explain the causes and remedies for solidification shrinkage porosities and incomplete castings.
4. Explain, why the surface of casting becomes rough and internal porosities occur? How can these be remedied?
5. Give the properties of commercially pure titanium and its allotropic forms. Describe the major modifications done in the casting procedure for titanium alloys.

II. Short Essays (10 minutes each)

1. Sprue former
2. Investing methods
3. Wax burn out
4. Methods of melting of casting alloys
5. Dental casting machines
6. Rough surface-casting defect
7. Solidification shrinkage porosities
8. Incomplete castings.
9. Properties of allotropic forms of CpTi and its α varieties of casting alloys
10. Modifications of casting techniques for titanium alloys
11. Alternatives to metal casting techniques

III. Brief Answers (5 minutes each)

1. Die spacers
2. Die hardeners
3. Sprue formers
4. Wetting agents
5. Direct and indirect spruing
6. Casting ring liners
7. Vacuum investment
8. Vent sprue
9. Gas-torch flames
10. Electric arc-melting of high fusing alloys
11. AC-induction melting of high fusing alloys
12. Divesting
13. Pickling/discolouration
14. Fins
15. Investments for the casting of titanium alloys
16. Titanium–aluminium–vanadium casting alloys
17. CAD-CAM technique
18. Back pressure porosity
19. Localized shrinkage porosity
20. Hot spot porosity
21. Microporosity in castings

Wrought Alloys

As-cast alloys are very rarely used directly either in dentistry or in industries. These are modified by deformations into the desired polished and finished shapes such as wires, sheets, strips, cutting instruments, etc. used in the various clinical specialities. The microstructures of the castings are also modified accordingly. These result in many changes in the properties of these **worked** or **wrought metals (alloys)**, which become brittle and fail in service, undergo corrosion and get distorted due to relaxation of internal stresses.

During casting, the alloy liquids undergo solidification by diffusion of atoms due to **thermal** or **constitutional supercooling, forming polycrystalline** structures and grains. If the cooling or solidification is done **very slowly in infinite time**, diffusions will be complete and perfect crystals are theoretically formed. Single crystals (whiskers) are formed by very slow cooling, but still all the crystal spaces will not be occupied due to the obstruction to the diffusion of atoms. In the ordinary cooling or solidification procedures, a large number of lattice imperfections or defects are caused. Due to these imperfections or defects, the material undergoes deformations easily. Such defective, as-cast polycrystalline material has low strengths compared to less defective single crystals (whiskers) or the theoretically calculated values for perfect crystal structures. The approximate ultimate shear strengths for as-cast polycrystalline, single crystal (whiskers) and the calculated values for perfect crystals of some metals are given in Table 20.1.

Table 20.1	Ultimate shear strengths of different structures		
Materials	As-cast polycrystalline USS-MPa	Single crystal whiskers USS-MPa	Theoretical perfect crystals USS-MPa
Copper	220	2,100	7,700
Iron	290	9,500	12,400
SiC	170 (Tension)	14,600	32,300

These values show the effect of lattice imperfections, on the properties of as-cast alloys.

LATTICE IMPERFECTIONS

1. **Point defects:** During fast cooling, atomic diffusions are inhibited as crystal growth is rapid, forming a rigid solid structure.

   The **unoccupied atomic sites and distortions are called point defects**. Two or more such vacancies can combine forming voids. Voids also can be due to trapping of air, during fast crystallization. Microporosities, irregular voids are also caused due to solidification shrinkages. **All these defective sites act as stress concentrations and assist fracture** (Fig. 20.1).

2. **Dislocations or line defects:** Sometimes a row of atoms may be missing. These line defects may be one or two dimensional. These defects assist the crack propagations as the wedge-shaped gap acts like a chisel, when deforming forces are applied, and separate or tear the structure.

LATTICE IMPERFECTIONS

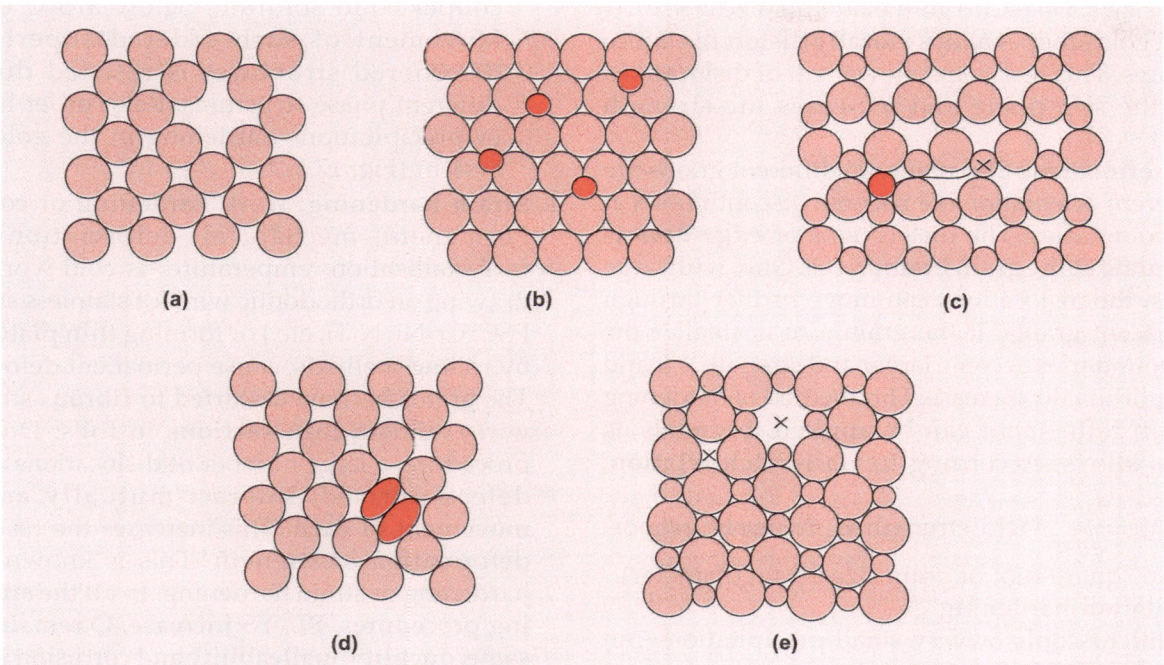

Figs 20.1a to e: Point defects in a crystal lattice. (a) Vacancy defect, (b) interstitial defect, (c) Frenkel (vacancy-interstitial pair) defect, (d) substitutional defect, (e) Schottky defect (vacancy)

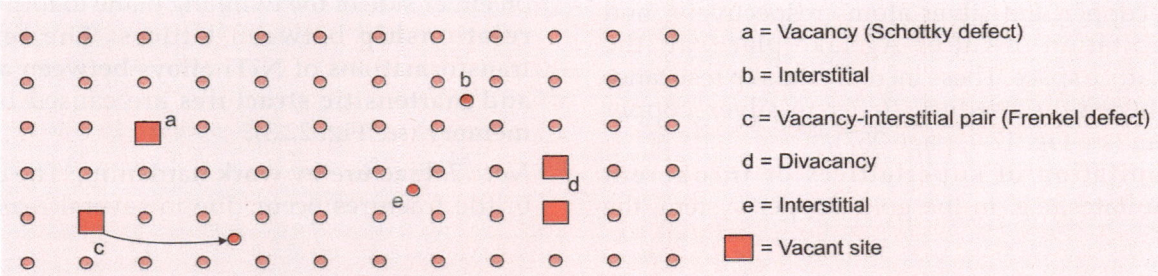

a = Vacancy (Schottky defect)
b = Interstitial
c = Vacancy-interstitial pair (Frenkel defect)
d = Divacancy
e = Interstitial
■ = Vacant site

Fig. 20.1f: Some simple defects in a lattice

SLIP RESISTANCE

The cohesive or attractive forces between the adjacent atoms resist slipping of the adjacent layers, when external shearing forces are applied. The point defects and dislocations decrease this resistance to slipping. When shearing forces are applied parallel to slip planes, the dislocations, move in the slip direction, finally reaching the grain boundaries, forming edge-dislocations (Fig. 20.2).

In **noncrystalline** (amorphous) substances, due to lack of long-range attractive forces, line defects or **dislocations cannot exist**. Since permanent deformation is only possible by the movement of dislocations, amorphous materials like ceramics, composites, polymers, certain cements, etc. are **brittle**.

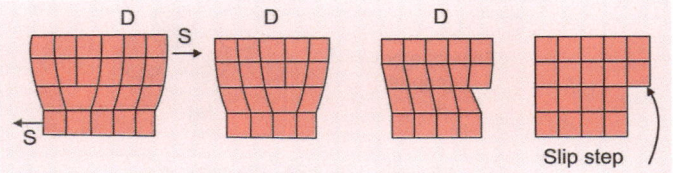

Fig. 20.2: Slip caused by the movement of edge-dislocation

Mechanisms of Strengthening Involving Lattice Defects (Increasing Slip Resistance)

The strength of materials refers to the resistance to deformation (or fracture) due to external forces that is their resistance to slip or movement of dislocations. This can be increased by several mechanisms.

1. **Solution hardening:** Presence of solute atoms of slightly different sizes (e.g. addition of copper of atomic size 2.556 AU to gold of atomic size 2.882 AU to form gold–copper alloys), **locally distort** the lattice structures. This resists the movement of dislocations along the slip plane and increases the strength (Fig. 20.3).

2. **Grain refinement:** Slip planes in different grains are in different orientations or become discontinuous at grain boundaries. The dislocations or **edge defects accumulate at the grain boundaries.** Only with large stresses, the dislocations can move further through the adjacent grains. If the grain size is smaller the grain boundaries become larger and strength, PL and YS proportionally increase. This method of hardening by grain refinement can be applied to metals as well as alloys. According to **Hall-Petch relation,**

$$\sigma_y = \sigma_0 + \frac{ky}{\sqrt{d}}$$ yield strength is inversely proportional to square root of grain size (grain diameter).

3. **Precipitation hardening**
   - **Submicroscopic** or very small precipitations can cause localized distortions in atomic arrangements in the lattice. This increases slip resistance, e.g. if alpha and beta solid solutions containing Cu <8.8% or Ag <8.0%, are cooled, they become supersaturated with copper and silver atoms respectively and precipitation of Cu or Ag take place, at the interlattice space. These increase the slip resistance and hence the hardness (*refer* to silver–copper system (*see* Fig. 17.4, page 257).
   - **Precipitation of superlattices** or **incoherent precipitates**, e.g. in the gold–copper system, the

alloy, containing 15–35% copper, form **Au-Cu, FCT. superlattice**, precipitating in the FCC gold-copper solid solution, below 375°C or 400°C. Movement of such ordered superlattice in disordered structures is resisted due to the different phase structures. Refer order hardening or precipitation hardening in the gold–copper system (Fig. 17.5).

4. **Strain hardening, work hardening or cold work:** Permanent mechanical deformations below recrystallization temperature is cold-working, e.g. drawing an orthodontic wire (of stainless steel, PGP, PSC, Cr-Ni, NiTi, etc.) or forming **thin plates or foils** by rolling methods, cause permanent deformations. The grains become **distorted to fibrous** structure in wires, and **to thin sections** in foils. During this procedure, a large number of dislocations and other defects formed, **interact mutually and resist movement of each.** This increases the resistance to deformation or strength. This is known as work hardening or strain hardening. **In all the strengthening procedures, PL, YS increase, Q remains almost same, ductility, malleability and corrosion resistance decreases.**

Note 1: **Twinning:** One method of producing deformation is by causing small atomic movements on either side of the twinning plane to form a **mirror relationship** between lattices: **The reversible transformations of NiTi alloys between austenitic and martensitic structures** are caused by **elastic memory** (*see* Fig. 22.3).

Note 2: **Fracture by work hardening:** The ductile or brittle fractures occur due to several reasons. The

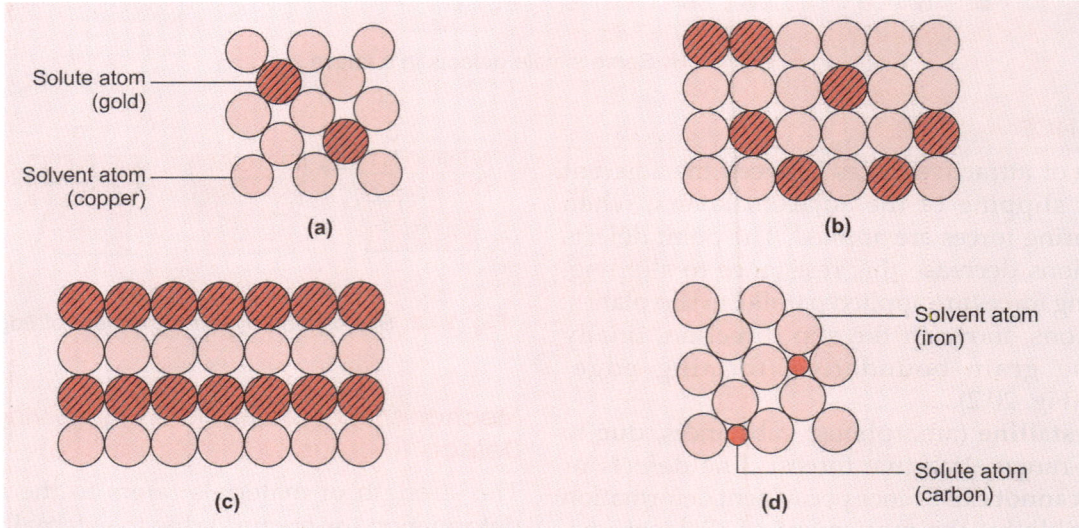

Figs 20.3a to d: Solid solution. (a) Substitutional solid solution, (b) disordered substitutional solid solution, (c) ordered substitutional solid solution (Au-Cu phase), (d) interstitial solid solution

microcracks become the stress concentrated areas, and tearing of lattices takes place. Also large numbers of dislocations at the grain boundaries, various types of phase structures (weak and strong), compositions of alloys, etc. are a few other reasons. Accumulations of dislocations at grain boundaries makes it inhomogeneous and brittle structure. The internal voids, point defects, and cracks **produce a transgranular fracture**. The grain boundaries' inhomogeneity causes an **intergranular fracture**. Stress concentrations, specially at grain boundaries also cause **greater corrosion by chemical attack.**

WORK HARDENING AND ANNEALING

One of the methods of strengthening a metal or an alloy is by work or strain hardening. When the alloy liquid solidifies, in casting procedures, many point defects, voids and dislocations are formed. When this cast structure is deformed permanently into the required shapes, such as an orthodontic wire or a foil (thin sheet), the grain structures become distorted to fibrous (in wires) or thin sections (in foils). Many more **dislocations produced during these deformations move to the grain boundaries**. However, the movements of many dislocations are complicated and are prevented by each other. **This slip resistance gradually increases** as more and more deformations take place. This **increase in hardness is known as work or strain hardening or cold work** (Fig. 20.4).

Effects of work hardening are
- Increase of PL, YS, and hardness.
- Modulus of elasticity remains almost the same.

- The decrease of ductility, malleability and corrosion resistance (specially at grain boundaries).
- Severe work hardening may slightly change the colour
- The material becomes more brittle and finally fractures.
- Distortion in service, due to relaxation of internal stresses, induced during work hardening.
  Examples
  - Pure direct filling gold foil and other varieties have low hardness, YS, and highest ductility. During compaction, it undergoes work hardening, increasing surface hardness from 25 to about 68 KHN, and transverse strength, to about 160 or even up to 350 MPa.
  - Orthodontic wires of thinner diameters have higher mechanical properties. This increases further during bending or forming repeatedly, and finally, cause a fracture.
  - Clasps of cast partial dentures, on adjusting frequently or in service, fracture.
  - **Instruments used in clinics**, cast alloy machine parts, etc. suddenly fail after long service. Fracture by work hardening (*refer* to Note 2, page 290).

ANNEALING HEAT TREATMENTS

The worsening effects of work hardening can be remedied, and the properties can be restored to the original values by annealing heat treatments. The work hardened article is heated approximately **to half of its melting temperatures in degree Kelvin (½ MP°K), for few minutes and then quenched or cooled. Time of heat treatment is shorter if work hardening is more severe or the temperature is higher**. The reversal of properties takes place successively in three stages.

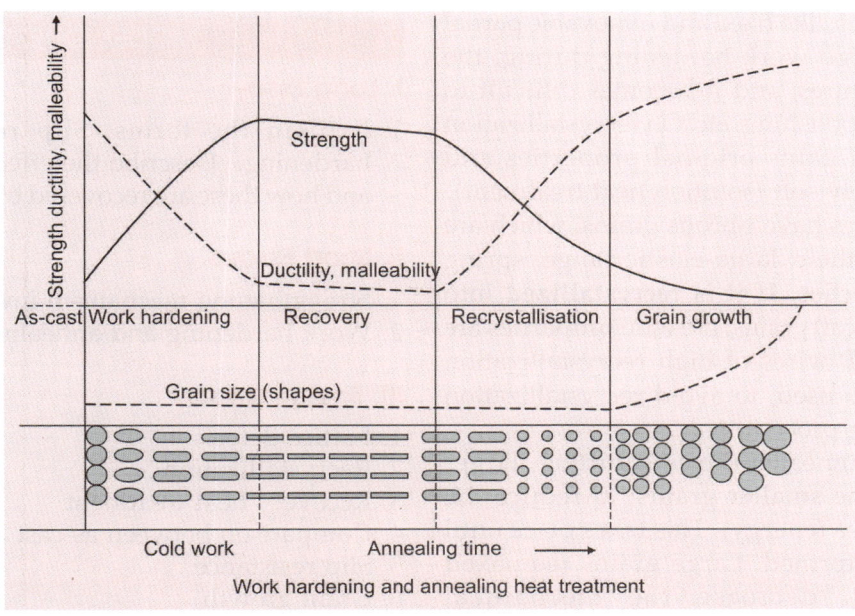

Fig. 20.4: Work hardening and annealing heat treatment

Recovery, recrystallization and grain growth: The changes in tensile, compressive, shear, flexure strengths and ductility during work hardening and annealing are represented graphically.

1. **Recovery or stress relief annealing:** The internal stresses relax initially and the effects of cold work gradually begin to disappear.

   Tensile strength, slightly decreases, corrosion resistance and electrical conductivity, increases, but ductility and microstructure do not change. The density of dislocations gradually decrease.

   Applications: Orthodontic appliances formed by bending of wires, have stress concentration at strained regions and undergo distortion in service by stress relaxation and lose their effectiveness. These **configurations are stabilized** by recovery annealing heat treatment. This annealing is done at lower temperatures and for a shorter time to avoid recrystallization and deterioration of wire properties.

2. **Recrystallization:** On further heating, changes in microstructure takes place. Atoms diffuse, deformed grains disappear, and **new grains grow from the new nuclei formed at the severely cold worked regions.** New growing grains merge with the old grain boundaries. **Fresh strain-free grains**, with dislocations are formed similarly to those formed during solidification. Equiaxed (spherical) grains are formed. However, recrystallization does not take place fast if it is not severely work hardened, and recrystallization time becomes longer. **Finer grains are formed if the work hardening is more severe.**

   Applications
   - As-cast appliances, like fixed and removable partial dentures, undergo work hardening during, the finishing procedures, and it becomes difficult to do the finishing, polishing, etc. On recrystallization anneal, it again gains original properties and becomes relatively soft (solution heat treatment).
   - Orthodontic wires have fibrous grains, which are responsible for their, large elastic range, spring back, etc. properties. **If it is recrystallized** into equiaxial (spherical) grains, the wire **properties are lost.** Hence, PGP wires of high recrystallization temperatures are used, to avoid recrystallization during soldering procedures.

3. **Grain growth:** If annealed (heated) further, **larger grains swallow** the smaller grains, to reduce the grain boundary area (energy). This takes place until coarse grains are formed. Large grains (equiaxed microstructures), decrease the mechanical properties, increase ductility (or softness) of

material which can fracture easily. **Recrystallization by careless annealing may ruin the instruments.**

Comparison of Cast (also Recrystallized Annealed) and Wrought Structures (Table 20.2)

Table 20.2	Comparison of cast and wrought structures	
Properties	As-cast	Work hardened
1. Microstructure	Many dislocations and defects, equiaxed, spherical	Dislocations shifted to grain boundaries fibrous, lamellar
2. Grain nature	Strain-free	Strained
3. Strength	Relatively soft	Higher, PL, YS
4. Ductility, malleability	Higher (tough)	Lower (brittle)
5. Corrosion resistance	Higher	Lower (stress corrosion at grain boundaries)
6. Electrical resistance	Lower	Slightly higher

Applications

Most of the dental instruments are prepared from alloy castings, by mechanically deforming—forging, drawing, beating, etc. Orthodontic wires are deformed by bending. Cast partial denture clasps are to be adjusted. Alloy castings are burnished for marginal adaptations. The clinical instruments are subjected to deforming stresses, very frequently. **All these procedures result in work hardening which finally may cause a fracture.** To save the material it is to be annealed suitably, so that strain-free fresh crystals formed, restore the original properties.

MODEL QUESTIONS

I. Long Essay (20 minutes)

1. Explain the terms: Slip resistance and work hardening. Describe the effects of work hardening and how these are recovered by annealing procedure.

II. Short Essays (10 minutes each)

1. Strengthening mechanism involving lattice defects
2. Work hardening and annealing.

III. Brief Answers (5 minutes each)

1. Lattice defects
2. Recrystallization
3. Recovery heat treatment
4. Comparison between as-cast and wrought alloys
5. Slip resistance
6. Grain growth
7. Fracture by work hardening.

Carbon Steels and Stainless Steels

CARBON STEELS

PURE SOFT IRON

Iron is one of the most abundantly available base metals and its alloys are used in industries as well as in dentistry in large amounts. **Pure iron** is soft and ductile, has density = 7.878 gm/cc and melting point = 1527°C. When exposed to moisture, it very quickly gets oxidized. The iron oxide is very **loosely bonded to substrate** and get easily lost. This **corrosion is rusting.** Iron exists in different allotropic forms at various temperatures and is ferromagnetic up to about 768°C, and above 910°C, it loses magnetic properties. The major allotropic forms are:

- Ferrite, α iron BCC up to 768°C magnetic
- Ferrite, β iron BCC up to 910°C paramagnetic
- Austenite, γ iron FCC up to 1400°C nonmagnetic
- Austenite, δ iron BCC up to 1527°C melting point.

CARBON STEELS

When alloyed with carbon, small amounts of carbon atoms can enter into the interlattice space. Since size of the carbon atoms is quite small but slightly bigger than available space, it **distorts the lattice space** and **increases slip resistance or strength by a large value.**

This interstitial alloy is carbon steel,

Soft iron + carbon (< .02%) ⟶ **Ferritic carbon steel**

The **solubility** of carbon in BCC—ferrite is very low about 0.02% at 723°C. Any excess carbon which is present forms hard iron carbide an intermetallic alloy, **cementite.** The maximum solubility of carbon in FCC—austenite structure is **2.1%.** Above 2.1% the alloy becomes very brittle and is known as **cast iron.**

Soft iron + (carbon >.02%) ⟶ **Ferritic carbon steel + cementite (Fe_3C)**

This transforms to austenite (FCC) when heated above 723°C.

Solid-state transformations: When austenitic (FCC) steel is cooled slowly it is transformed by **solid-state reaction in a range of temperature, to ferrite + cementite.** The lowest transformation temperature is **723°C,** below which there are two-phase precipitations.

Austenitic steel → Ferritic steel + Cementite (Fe_3C)

EUTECTOID STEEL

When the amount of carbon = 0.8%, there is a single–lowest transformation temperature (like eutectic change) from solid to solid and is known as eutectoid steel.

Eutectoid γ austenitic steel with C = 0.8% when cooled below 723°C → α ferritic steel + cementite in 7:1 ratio in alternate layers. This is pearlite (P).

If it is polished, softer ferritic matrix is removed easily, and the harder cementite appears under scattered light as shining pearls and is known as **pearlite.** If amounts of carbon are in-between 0.02–0.8%

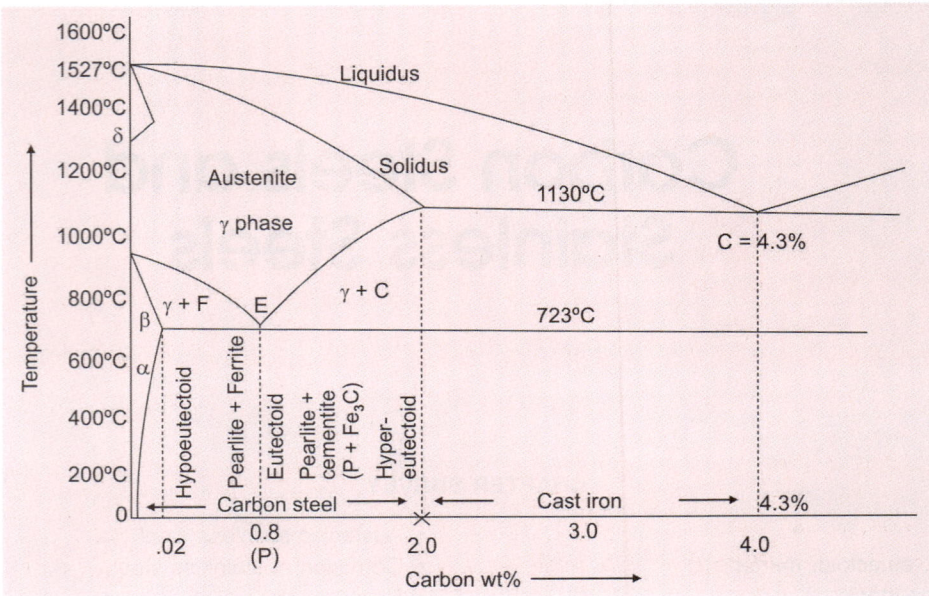

Fig. 21.1: Phase diagram of carbon steels

or 0.8–2.1%, the carbon steels are known as **hypoeutectoid** and **hypereutectoid** steels (Fig. 21.1).

Martensite or Martensitic Steel

If austenitic steel (FCC) is cooled rapidly (even the cooling in the air is not slow, but rapid), by quenching in water or oil, there is no adequate time for diffusion of atoms. The **diffusionless transformation causes distorted BCT space lattice, i.e. martensitic steel.** This is the **hardest phase** (not shown in the above phase diagram).

Thus, the hardness of carbon steels increases with, larger

- percentage of carbon added
- amount of martensitic steel precipitated, i.e. by a faster rate of cooling.

For example, pearlite with 0.8% carbon has hardness, about 300 KHN. But when completely converted into martensite, the hardness becomes **>1000 KHN.**

TEMPERING OF CARBON STEELS

This is a softening and hardening heat treatment of carbon steels by controlling the martensite precipitation. The article is to be **heated above 723°C and then cooled slowly, in a controlled manner.**

Applications

- The cutting blades of the hand cutting instruments, steel burs, saw teeth, knives, etc. are heat treated, to increase the hardness and reduce brittleness, controlling the martensitic formation by the rate of cooling.

- In austenitic stainless steel, which has very large number of applications in every field, the martensitic formation temperature of **723°C, is depressed below** room temperature by adding a **nickel** or **sometimes manganese.**

STAINLESS STEELS

Carbon steels have superior mechanical properties but the main drawback is their poor corrosion resistance. This is remedied by adding **chromium about 11 to 30% by weight.**

PASSIVATION

Chromium (like titanium and aluminum), when exposed to the atmosphere, immediately gets oxidized to form a very **thin atomic layer of Cr_2O_3 which is firmly bonded to the substrate.** This film prevents further oxidation by penetration of oxygen and thus **protects the material from corrosion.** This is known as **passivation.** If the film is removed by abrasion, immediately the protective film is again formed.

Iron + carbon + chromium → carbon steel + chromium → stainless steel

According to the lattice structure of carbon steels, there are mainly three varieties, ferritic, martensitic and austenitic stainless steels. As these have good corrosion resistances and excellent mechanical properties **(YS up to 1750 MPa, UTS = 2200 MPa, MOE = 200,000 MPa),** their uses in dentistry or industries have become **unlimited.** Thousands of varieties of, specially austenitic stainless steels have been formed with different compositions and their properties have been studied and given by the American Iron and Steel Institute (AISI) in many series.

VARIETIES OF STAINLESS STEELS AND COMPOSITIONS

- **Ferritic stainless steel:** Compositions, Cr = 11.5–27%, C = 0–0.2%, Mn = 2%, Iron = balance. This is a low-cost variety having fairly good corrosion resistance, but comparatively poor mechanical properties. This is not hardened by heat treatments. It is mostly used in industries for large sized articles like table tops, furnitures, etc.

- **Martensitic stainless steel:** This is the hardest variety. It has Cr = 11.5–17%, Ni = 0–2.5%, C= 0.15–1.2%, Fe = balance. This has **distorted BCT structure formed by diffusionless transformation** when austenitic stainless steel is suddenly cooled. Hence, it has very high slip resistance or strength. This variety has the **lowest corrosion resistance** out of the three varieties. It can be **heat hardened by quenching and tempered by slow cooling.** It has very high mechanical properties, depending on carbon content, yield strengths 500–1900 MPa and hardness 250–1100 KHN. It also has low ductility or percentage elongation <2%.

The cutting edges or the blades of hand cutting instruments, dental burs, etc. are heat treated to form suitable amount of martensite. The blades of knives, saw-teeth, sickles, etc. have been martensitic.

The AISI 200 series refer to low cost stainless steel with Mn and Ni instead of nickel and is used in industries. The AISI 300 series applies to the FCC austenitic stainless steel, and 400 series applies to ferritic and martensitic stainless steel (Table 21.1).

AUSTENITIC (18-8) STAINLESS STEELS

Many varieties of this, very useful alloys, have been developed with small differences in compositions according to the requirements for applications.

Compositions and Alloying Properties

- **Chromium:** Sixteen to twenty-six percent has a high melting point and oxygen sensitivity (like titanium) imparts strength, hardness, **and corrosion resistance by passivation.**
- **Nickel:** Seven to twenty-two percent has high melting point, imparts strength, hardness, and **depresses** martensitic formation temperature, down below the ordinary temperatures.
- **Carbon:** <0.25%. Small amounts, form an **interstitial alloy** with iron, increases strength by carbide precipitations and influence the heat treatments.
- **Manganese or molybdenum:** Two to three percent increases strength and retains ductility and malleability of iron.
- **Iron:** Balance (60–80%) is the main component to impart strength, ductility, malleability, etc.

The various varieties come under AISI 300 series and have properties slightly different according to their compositions.

Properties of Austenitic, 18-8 Stainless Steels

- **Biocompatibility**
  - High corrosion resistance below 400°C
  - Chemically stable in oral or implant environments
- **Superior mechanical properties**
  - Yield strength (YS) 1,100–1,750 MPa
  - Ultimate tensile strength up to 2200 MPa
  - Modulus of elasticity 170,000–200,000 MPa
  - Surface hardness about 250–400 KHN

Table 21.1	Varieties of stainless steels and compositions				
Varieties	**Chromium wt%**	**Nickel wt%**	**Carbon wt%**	**Others wt%**	**AISI series**
Ferritic	11.5–27	0	0–0·2	Mn = 2 Fe = balance	400 (BCC)
Martensitic	11.5–17	0–2.5	0.15–1.2	Mn = 2 Fe = balance	400 (BCT)
Austenitic	16–26	7–22	0–0.25	Mn = 2 Fe = balance	300 (FCC)
18-8 Surgical	17–19 (18) 18–20	8–10 (8) 8–12	Max .17 Max .08	Mn = 2 Fe = balance	302 (FCC) 304
Implants	16–18	10–14	Max 0.03	Mo = 2–3 Mn = 2 Fe = balance	316 L (low carbon)

- Density is 8.5 gm/cc
- Percentage elongation up to 35%
- **Undergoes work hardening by large amount. That is why, thinner wires and sheets have higher mechanical properties.**
- Fairly high formability factor, and spring back qualities = YS/Q
- **Thermal properties**
  - Melting temperature ranges = 1240–1260°C.
  - Responds to heat treatments
  - Can be welded and soldered
  - When heated above 400°C undergoes sensitization, which can be remedied to a certain extent.
- Easily available in various forms, wires, sheets, bands, etc. and not expensive.

Most of these properties are suitable for selection for reactive (passive) orthodontic appliances.

Corrosion Resistance of Austenitic Stainless Steels

Passivation

It is the formation of an **impervious**, Cr_2O_3 layer on the surface, when the base metal alloys **containing Cr (also Al, Ti)** are exposed to the atmosphere. This takes place immediately and even if it is scratched, new layer forms instantly.

Sensitizations

It is the **loss of corrosion resistanc**e when stainless steels are heated between 400 and 900°C, when the carbon atoms diffuse rapidly to the grain boundaries, combine with iron and chromium of the solid solution to form **$(CrFe)_4C$**. This reduces the corrosion resistance, due to the reduction of Cr atoms at about 650°C (which depends on the carbon content) and above this, it undergoes decomposition. The **intergranular, grain boundary corrosions and disintegrations,** reduce the strength. These temperatures are **within the range of soldering and welding** temperatures. Corrosion taking place at the soldered joints and weld-nuggets is due to the loss of passivation and localized stress in the welded, or soldered interfaces. These lead to failures known as **weld-decay.**

Stabilization

Addition of small amounts (about 6 times carbon) of **niobium or titanium with tantalum** stabilizes stainless steel. These arrest temporarily, the diffusion of carbon atoms, during brazing and welding. Stabilized steel becomes more expensive.

Sensitizations can be reduced by decreasing carbon percentage, which is not rather practicable.

During work hardening, i.e. drawing into wires, the carbon atoms are shifted to dislocation. This causes uniform distribution of carbon atoms (rather than concentrated at grain boundaries) and reduces the chance of corrosion.

Other Causes for Corrosion

1. Brazed joints have inhomogeneous compositions, and electrolytic corrosion takes place when kept in contact with electrolyte solutions. That is why hypochlorite containing solutions should not be used in cleansers.
2. Inhomogeneous surfaces also undergo such electrolytic (galvanic) corrosions. Polishing of the surface reduces this.
3. Use of carbon steel instruments like "pliers" may transfer carbon into the scratches produced during manipulation of orthodontic wires, which cause corrosion.

Remedies or Precautions to Reduce Corrosions

- Do not heat the article above 350°C for a long time
- Brazing temperature should be low and the time should be short
- Select solders of very low fusion temperatures
- Welding or brazing is performed as quickly as possible, i.e. spot welding or laser welding methods are suitable
- Do not use carbon steel instruments for manipulation of wires
- Do not use chlorine or fluorine containing cleansers.

Applications of stainless steels

- Industries: Many varieties of austenitic, ferritic and martensitic steels for machine parts
- Laboratory equipment, and facilities
- Orthopaedic surgery: Special 18-8 stainless steel for hip joints, knee joint replacements, bone plates, nuts, bolts, plates, etc.
- Dentistry: Clinical equipment, instruments and fittings
- Orthodontia: Wires, bands, brackets and instruments
- Dental implants
- Household utensils, and appliances

Note

Stainless steel denture base: It is possible to obtain sheets of stainless steel of very small thickness **about $1/20$ mm.** These can be forged or shaped into the desired form, by applying large force using a hydraulic press, between the edentulous die (of patients mouth) and its hard counter die (Fig. 21.2). Excess is trimmed off and

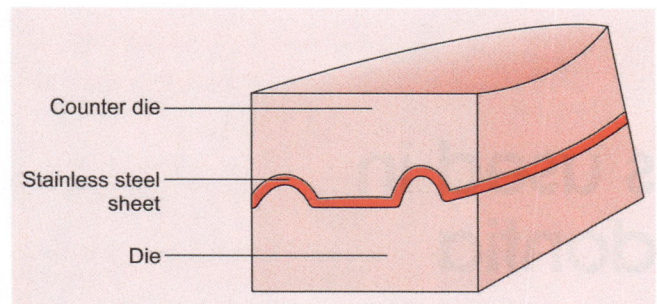

Fig. 21. 2: Stainless steel sheet is pressed in-between hard die and counter dies

denture is constructed over this denture base using same compression molding technique.

Advantages

- High fracture resistance to impact forces
- Good conductor of heat
- Lightweight (even though a density of stainless steel is about 8 times of acrylic, the thickness can be reduced to $\frac{1}{20}$ mm).

Disadvantages

- Poor fitting
- Complicated equipment and fabrication procedures.

Note 1: Brazing and welding of stainless steel: *Refer* to orthodontic 18-8 steel wires and brazing and welding chapters.

Note 2: Refer model questions in Chapter 22.

Materials used in Orthodontia

INTRODUCTION

Orthodontia is a dental speciality dealing with

- **The study of the growth of craniofacial complex or the development of occlusion and masticatory apparatus**

- **The treatments like, preventions, interceptions, corrections of malocclusions and other abnormalities, sometimes with surgeries.**

The study of the growth of the craniofacial complex, i.e. involving the positions, structures, orientations, growth occlusion of the teeth, etc. with reference to the jaws, is made with radiographs of the entire area.

A study model or diagnostic cast is prepared with dental stone. The orthodontic treatments are then carefully designed to achieve **maximum functional and aesthetic harmonies** by intercepting the deviations from the normal developments, and then stabilizing the teeth positions accordingly. These are achieved by fabricating and using various types of **force-delivery mechanisms, such as with active and passive appliances.**

Active appliances are used for translation, shifting, torquing, tripping (uprighting), intrusions and extrusions of the teeth to the desired positions and orientations. For this, **small constant forces** are to be applied through the force-delivery systems using elastically deformable appliances. That is, the materials used should have, **high modulus of resilience, flexibility, elastic ranges and low modulus of elasticities**, (e.g. Ni–Ti, β-Ti, PGP, PSC, or HN alloys) (*see* Colour Plate 33, Figs 22.1 and 22.2).

These appliances are
- Removable
- Fixed
- Semi-fixed

Passive appliances are used basically for resisting any unwanted shifting, rotation, and movements of the teeth to the undesired positions or orientations, after the initial treatments. For this, **large forces** are to be delivered through the appliances. That is, the material should have rigidity or stiffness (high modulus of elasticity) and low flexibility (e.g. elgiloy, 18-8 stainless steel, gold, and noble metal wires). These appliances are:

- **Functional appliances** to deliver the natural forces to alveolar bones in the required directions, e.g. Frankel's appliances.
- **Retention appliances** to hold the teeth in the stable positions at the end of orthodontic treatments.
- **Habit breaking appliances** to alter or correct the harmful habits, such as mouth breathing, thumb sucking, tongue thrusting, nail-biting, etc. (Fig. 22.1.)

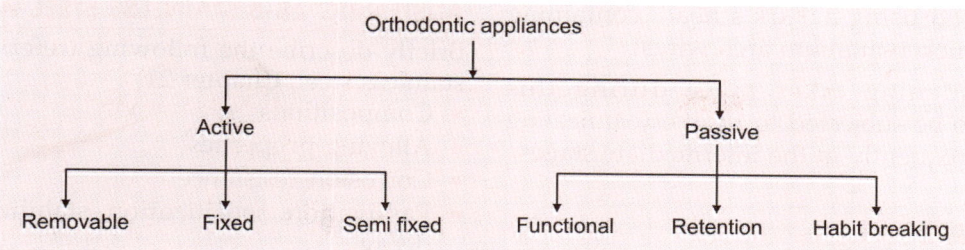

Fig. 22.1: Orthodontic appliances. Colour Plates 33, 34, Figs 22.1 to 22.7

REQUIREMENTS FOR SELECTION OF ORTHODONTIC WIRES

1. **Biocompatibility should be adequate** as the appliances are to be retained in the mouth for the desired long time. Hence, they should have high corrosion resistance, noncarcinogenic, hygienic and chemical inertness in the mouth.

2. **Mechanical properties** of suitable values are essential as the appliances are **force delivery systems,** i.e. large amount of activation energy stored should be **released at constant small rates** that is a small force delivery rates for a long time. Hence, they should have:

   - **High flexural yield strength** YS (FYS is defined as the bending moment required to produce a definite amount, say 2.9° or 0.05 radians of permanent bending strain).
   - **Large elastic activation** or working range, i.e. elastic flexibility spring-back property. For this, it should have a low modulus of elasticity, E, which gives high flexibility, i.e. large YS/E.
   - **Large modulus of resilience [(YS)²/2 E = R],** to store, large activation energy.
   - Ability to undergo large work hardening
   - Adequate hardness, or abrasive resistance
   - Able to form or shape easily and **bend through sharp corners.** The resistance to bending depends on the stiffness of the wire or elastic force delivery rate.
   - Modulus of elasticity must be **low for active appliances** (like Ni–Ti, E = 41,400 MPa, β-Ti, E = 71,700 MPa, gold wires, E = 1,00,000 MPa).
   - Modulus of elasticity must be **high for passive appliances** (like Cr-Co-wires, E = 220,000 MPa, Elgiloy, E = 200,000 MPa, 18-8 stainless steel, E = 180,000 to 200,000 MPa).

3. **Thermal properties**
   - Should not be difficult for soldering or welding.
   - **Should not undergo recrystallization** during heating for soldering or welding procedures and lose its high mechanical properties, i.e. they should have high **recrystallization and melting temperatures** (e.g. PGP wires = 1500 – 1530°C. Recrystallization temperature, **T$_R$ = 0.3** melting point in degree Kelvin).

   - Should not get annealed easily during recovery heat treatments.
   - Should not get sensitized during heating soldering or welding (*refer* to 18-8 stainless steel).

4. **Aesthetic quality** should be good. But all the metallic wires or brackets have their own colours. (Recently **polymer resin coated ceramic core wires** have been studied. These are glass fibre reinforced **aramid candidate** resins and have aesthetic qualities.)

CLASSIFICATION OF ORTHODONTIC WIRES

Classification of orthodontic wires can be done according to:

1. **Compositions**

   - HN and N alloys: Au-Cu-Ag, Au-Pd, Au-Pd-Ag, PGP, PSC, etc.
   - Base metal alloys: 18-8 stainless steel, Elgiloy, Ni-Cr-Be, Ni–Ti, cpTi, β-Ti, TMA, etc.
   - Polymer-ceramic combinations.

2. **Nature of cross sections:** Round (circular), rectangular, multistrand and braided.
3. **Heat treated conditions:** Quenched and oven cooled.
4. **Mechanical tempered conditions:** Soft, ductile, semi spring, spring, and high tempered.

Materials used for orthodontic wires

The common materials used as orthodontic wires are base metal wrought alloys

- 18-8 stainless steel
- Co-Cr-Ni-Fe (Elgiloy)
- β-Ti and TMA
- Ni–Ti alloys

(However, few HN and N metal alloys are still in use. ADA specification No. 7 for HN and N alloy has been recently withdrawn).

MANUFACTURING AND MICROSTRUCTURES

The cast ingot is subjected to successive deforming operations like

- drawing through dies of various decreasing diameters to get round wires of required diameters (stainless steel, Elgiloy, etc.)

- a rolling method using a Turk's head, containing pairs of rolls (nickel–titanium arch wires).

As work hardening takes place during this procedure, it is to be subjected to recovery annealing heat treatments frequently in the intermediate stages.

MICROSTRUCTURES

The as-cast alloys have dendritic equiaxed spherical crystals. During the wire drawing procedure, the distortions convert these into **fibrous structures** along the direction of elongations. When a well-polished wire sample is observed through an optical microscope, the microstructure appears as a **series of closely spaced lines** parallel to the direction of the wire drawing (Fig. 22.2).

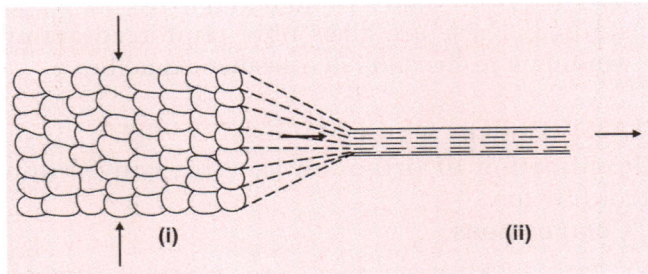

Fig. 22.2: Microstructures. (i) As-cast: Equiaxial grains with lattice defects, dislocations and voids, (ii) wrought alloy wire, fibrous grains with lesser defects

The fine fibrous microstructure is responsible for the **superior mechanical properties like YS, UTS, E, flexure strength, etc. For the same reasons, the thinner wires have still better properties.**

Hence, the mechanical properties of orthodontic wires depend on:

- Compositions
- Diameters of round wires or thinness of rectangular wires
- Recovery and tempering heat treatments.

ANSI/ADA SPECIFICATION NO. 32

Two varieties: Type I—low resilience and Type II—high resilience, base metal alloys without containing precious metals are shown in Table 22.1.

AUSTENITIC 18-8 STAINLESS STEEL WIRES

Briefly describe the following (referring to austenitic stainless steel, Chapter 21)

- Compositions
- Alloying properties
- Corrosion resistance
- Passivation, sensitization, stabilization, and weld decay
- Microstructure

1. **Mechanical properties**
   The mechanical properties depend upon the thinness of the wires and the heat treated conditions. The approximate values of as received wires are:
   - Yield strength (0.2% offset) = 1600 MPa
   - Tensile strength = 2100 MPa
   - Modulus of elasticity E = 180,000 to 200,000 MPa
   - Surface hardness = 250–600 KHN
   - Spring back = YS/E = 0.008 = 0.8%

   All these properties are **higher for thinner** wires.

2. **Heat treatment of stainless steel wire appliances**
   During the fabrication procedures, the wires are bent and unbent many times to achieve the correct shape and fit. This causes strain hardening and an increase of brittleness. To avoid distortion (misfit) due to stress - relaxation, the appliance should be subjected to careful heat treatments at low temperatures, **400–500°C, for short time intervals, say for 1 min at about 500°C.** Heating above 500°C causes:
   - Loss of corrosion resistance by sensitization
   - The decrease of mechanical properties by recrystallization and annealing.

3. **Soldering (brazing) of stainless steel**
   - **Silver solders:** Alloys of silver–copper–zinc are preferred as the temperatures of soldering. 600–650°C is lower than that for gold solders (700–750°C).
   - The soldering flux should be **fluoride fluxes, to reduce Cr_2O_3 film** for better flow of solder to improve wetting and bonding.
     - Soldering should be performed, in **a short time as possible.**

Many times, the spot welding procedure is preferred to brazing even though the weld-decay—failure at the weld joints due to sensitization is quite common. The

Table 22.1	Properties of wrought base metal alloy wires		
Properties		*Type I—low resilience*	*Type II—high resilience*
1. Flexure—YS (MPa) at 2.9 degrees or 5% radian (bending) offset		1700–2400	2400 and above
2. Number of cycles of 90° bending tests		0.3 mm wire >15 0.3–0.64 mm wire >10	0.64 mm >5

welded portion very quickly gets annealed by recrystallization during the short welding time and looses its mechanical properties.

Note: Braided and twisted (co-axial) stainless steel wires.

A large number of very thin steel wires of thickness 0.178 mm are twisted or braided to form **multistrand—**round or rectangular cross-section wires of thickness about 0.406 to 0.635 mm. These have a very **low apparent modulus of elasticity under flexure.** These highly flexible wires can sustain **very large elastic deflections with small forces.**

ELGILOY (Co-Cr-Ni-Fe)

Initially manufactured for use as watch springs (1950s) as it can be made high tempered.

Compositions

- Co = 40%
- Cr = 20%
- Ni = 15%
- Fe = 15.8%
- Mo = 7.0%
- Mn = 2.0%
- C = 0.16%
- Be = 0.04% (decreases MPa)

Properties are almost similar to 18-8 stainless steel and has higher mechanical properties

- Corrosion resistances and biocompatibilities are good.
- Yield strength, YS = 1400–1600 MPa
- Ultimate tensile strength = 2100–2540 MPa
- Modulus of elasticity = 150,000–200,000 MPa
- Hardness = 600–700 VHN

These can be soldered and welded. These wires are supplied in various tempered (cold worked) conditions, **soft, ductile, semispring and spring tempers.** Accordingly, the mechanical properties also increase as given above.

Heat treatment

Elgiloy blue is a soft tempered variety having almost similar properties as 18-8 stainless steel. This can be heat treated at **480°C for 7–12 min, to improve the mechanical properties by carbide precipitations in a furnace or by passing electric current from a soldering or welding unit.** Overheating above 800°C cause recrystallization with the deterioration of properties.

Uses

- Soft Elgiloy is used instead of steel wires even though it has slightly lower spring back properties (**0.005–0.007**) for as received and heat treatment versions.
- Thicker wires are specially used for **quad-helix** appliances.

Advantages

- Good corrosion resistance and biocompatibility
- Superior mechanical properties like 18-8 steel
- Good formability (YS/E). It can be easily bent and shaped
- Can be soldered or welded
- The heat treatment can change the soft, to different spring temper conditions.

Disadvantages

- High force delivery rate
- Lower spring back—elastic range, than 18-8 steel.

WROUGHT HN AND N METAL ALLOYS

These are nowadays, not used much, as the predominantly base metal cast and wrought alloys have occupied their place. The wrought HN and N alloys have better mechanical properties compared to the cast alloys of the same composition, by **elimination of lattice defects.** Due to their higher flexibilities, wire clasps of these alloys can be **adjusted more easily.** But now the technicians, fabricate the entire RPD castings including the clasps.

The properties of these alloys are similar to type IV alloys. The HN alloys may contain **Au-Ag-Cu, Au-Pd, Au-Pd-Ag,** etc. compositions, including small amounts of nickel. The N alloys contain **Pd-Ag, Pd-Au,** etc.

According to earlier ADA specification No. 7, two types of wires: Type—I containing Au + Pt + Pd >75% and Type—II containing Au-Pt-Pd >65% have been described and their properties are listed as follows. But now this has been withdrawn.

Two varieties of these are still used as wires, endodontic posts and clasps, to which the **RPD framework can be directly cast.** The Pd-Au-Pt (PGP) alloy has the composition as given. It has very high fusion temperatures **1500°–1530°C** so that during soldering procedures, **recrystallization does not take place and the superior mechanical properties are not lost.** As this is very expensive, cheaper variety PSC, i.e. Pd-Ag-Cu alloy is available for orthodontic uses. These have higher MOE, i.e. about 110,000 MPa compared to their cast alloys. These can be used for **active and passive since appliances** their modulus of elasticity is lower than wrought base metal alloys (Table 22.2).

These wrought noble and high noble metal alloy wires have superior corrosion resistance and biocompatibilities. Modulus of elasticity is lower than wrought base metal alloys.

β-TITANIUM AND TITANIUM ALLOY WIRES

The wires used in active appliances should have high spring back or low force delivery property. That is the

Table 22.2	Properties of wrought HN–N alloy wires					
Type of alloy wires	Compositions wt percentage	YS MPa oven cooled	UTS MPa oven cooled	Elongation% minimum quenched/oven cooled		Fusion temperatures °C
Type I	Au + Pt + Pd >75%	>860	>930	15	4	>960
Type II	Au + Pt + Pd >65%	>690	>860	15	2	>870
PGP	Pd = 25–30 Au = 40–50 Pt = 25–30	550–1030 not heat hardenable	860–1240	14–15	–	**1500–1530**
PSC	Pd = 42–44 Ag = 38–41 Cu = 16–17	690–790 heat hardenable	960–1070	16–24	8–15	1040–1080

ratio YS/E must be high. In addition, to have high resilience, i.e. $R = (YS)^2/2E$, same conditions are to be satisfied. Hence, it should have:

- High yield strength
- High flexibility and resilience
- Low modulus of elasticity.

The β-titanium allotropic form satisfies these requirements.

At the ordinary (low) temperatures cpTi exists as **α-Ti martensitic phase** that is monoclinic, triclinic or distorted **HCP** structure. When heated it transforms into **β-Ti having complex, BCC phase**, above 885°C (*refer to casting Ti alloys*).

Properties

- Good corrosion resistance and biocompatibility
- The α-Ti has YS = 430 MPa and E = 110,000 MPa. The β-Ti has higher YS = 860–1200 MPa and lower E = 71,000 MPa. These show that β-Ti has higher spring back (YS/E) property about three times more than α-Ti.
- Low force delivery property due to high flexibility.

TMA orthodontic β-Ti wire. It is possible to depress the martensite formation temperatures, from 885°C, down to ordinary temperatures. This is done by alloying with the **β-phase stabilizers**, like molybdenum **(Mo)**, vanadium **(V)**, tantalum **(Ta)**, or zirconium **(Zr)**. One such alloy TMA wire has the following compositions:

Titanium	79%
Molybdenum	11%
Zirconium	6%
Tin	4%

Properties

- This TMA wire has all the properties **similar to those of β-Ti,** i.e. high flexibility (spring back), low modulus of elasticity and large modulus of resilience.

The high elastic range (YS/E), indicates the **easiness to bend and shape.**

- Microstructure at ordinary temperatures shows β-phase.
- Can be **welded and soldered easily.** As intermediate alloy is not required for welding, the **welding is perfect, and the welded part has the same phase.**
- **High fatigue strength**

These properties are very much suitable for **active appliances.**

Uses

Wires for active appliances, heart valves, hip joint implants, orthopaedic appliances, dental implants, etc.

NICKEL-TITANIUM (Ni–Ti)—NITINOL: ORTHODONTIC WIRES

This is an equiatomic (i.e. 1:1 atomic ratio) intermetallic alloy, recently developed (1970) with many special properties like **superelasticity, elastic memory, very low modulus of elasticity, high spring back,** etc. which are very much welcomed to form active orthodontic appliances (*see* colour plate 33, Fig. 22.3).

Compositions (approx) by wt%

Nickel = 54%
Titanium = 44%

Cobalt, chromium, or copper = 2% to **depress the transition temperature slightly below 37°C or to any desired value.**

Microstructure

This has predominantly the Ni–Ti phase with small precipitates of their oxides. This has two allotropic forms.

1. **Austenite-complex BCC** (cesium chloride structure), at low stresses and high temperatures.

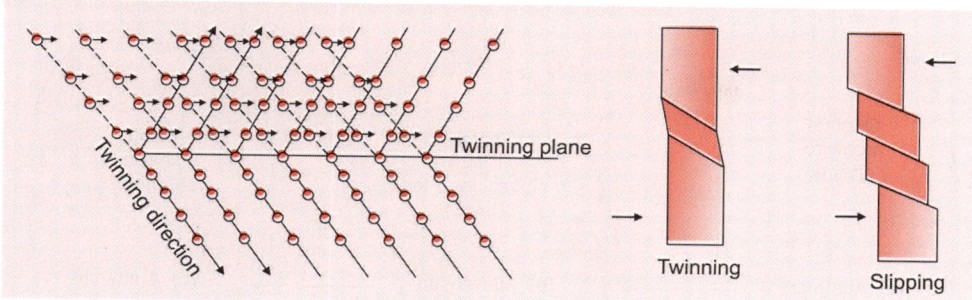

Fig. 22.3: Twinning and slipping

2. **Martensite HCP or monoclinic or triclinic** formed by high stress or cooling below the transition temperature range (TTR) (*refer* to carbon steel).

   This transformation from austenite to martensite takes place by a reversible **twinning process,** i.e. slight distortion of the lattices due to small displacements of atoms, forming a mirror image structure about the twinning plane (Fig. 22.3). During twinning **changes in volume and electrical conductivity** takes place. An intermediate rhombo-hedral R phase also is formed.

Properties

1. **Superelasticity (pseudoelasticity) (austenitic-active alloys):** When the material is **stressed (or cooled)** proportional deformations or strains are induced up to a certain value (a-b). Then the crystallographic transformation to martensite takes place with an increase in volume (or strain or angular deflection) (b-c). Further increase in stress (bending moment) increases the strain again proportionately (c-d) (Fig. 22.4).

   The total deflection or strain corresponds to the sum of all the three. Hence, it has **very large elastic deformation** which is known as **superelasticity.** On

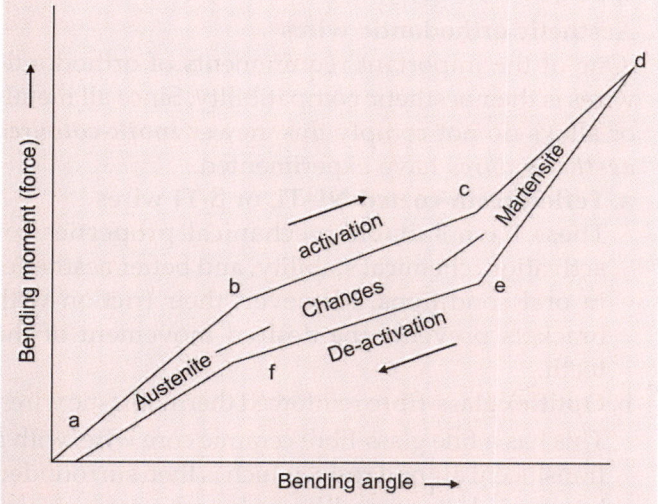

Fig. 22.4: Superelasticity of Ni–Ti wires

unloading or during **force-delivery or deactivation,** the reversal takes place with a slight loss of energy (i.e. along, d, e, f, a), given by the area, abcdefa.

2. **Shape memory (martensitic-active alloys):** This is due to the **reversal of the twinning process** on releasing the stress or heating above TTR. For example, if a straight wire (austenitic) is bent or wound like a spring and heated above TTR, it immediately unbends or uncoils and becomes straight. This is called **thermal shape memory.** Manufacturer supplies arch wires of standard shapes (a) The dentist can fix this wire through brackets to the malpositioned teeth. (b) If the TTR is about 37°C or slightly lower; the manipulated wires to different shapes (Fig. 22.5) return to the original required shape by pushing the malpositioned teeth to this ideal position. (c) The relaxation of large deactivation forces exerted quickly, by the thermal change may cause inconvenience and **pain to the patient.**

   Nickel–titanium archwires of TTR = 27°C, 35°C, 45°C are supplied.

   Mechanical properties of orthodontic wires (Table 22.3).

3. **Nonsuperelastic orthodontic wires (martensite-stabilized):** These alloys contain substantial quantities of heavily cold-worked and stable martensite and do not possess shape memory or superelasticity.

4. **Spring back property or elastic range:** Ni–Ti has moderate YS = 430 MPa and very low modulus of elasticity E = 41,400 MPa. Hence, it has **very low force delivery rate, high flexibility elastic range or spring back property**

$$\frac{\textbf{YS}}{\text{E}} = \frac{\textbf{430}}{41,400} = 0.0104 = 1.04\%$$

5. **The elastic stiffness or elastic force delivery rate depends on the length 'l' of the segment, the geometry of cross-section and modulus of elasticity.** For round wires of diameter, d,

   the elastic stiffness = $\dfrac{\textbf{Ed}^4}{\textbf{l}}$

   For a wire of rectangular cross-section of **width b and thickness t,** the elastic stiffness = $\dfrac{\textbf{E. bt}^3}{\textbf{l}}$

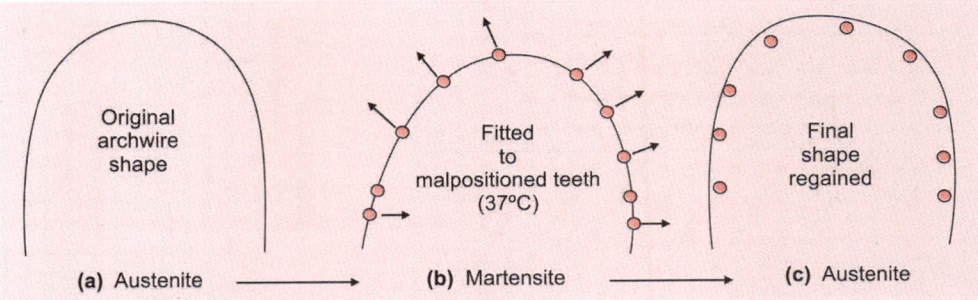

Figs 22.5a to c: Thermal elastic memory of Ni–Ti archwires

Material of wire	Yield strength	Ultimate tensile strength	Modulus of elasticity	Modulus of resilience	Elastic range spring back	Springiness
	YS MPa	UTS MPa	E MPa	R = (YS)²/2 E	YS/E	1/E × 10⁵
18-8 stainless steel	1580	2100	180,000	6.934	0.00877	0.55
Elgiloy (soft tempered)	1410	1680	184,000	5.402	0.00766	0.54
Ni–Ti	430	1400	41,400	2.233	0.0104	2.4
cpTi (beta)	930	1275	71,700	6.074	0.013	1.4
PGP	1000	1200	110,000	4.54	0.009	0.91
Coaxial 6 strand steel wire			5500	-	-	11.0
Braided 9 strand steel wire			8500	-	-	12.0
Polymer-ceramic combination	1800		-	-	55.0	

Table 22.3 Approximate properties of some orthodontic wires

Since Ni–Ti has very low E, it has the **lowest stiffness** or force delivery rate on unloading.

6. **Ni–Ti has large modulus of resilience**
$$\frac{(YS)^2}{2\,E} = 2.233 \text{ Jm}^3$$

Disadvantages
- **Cannot be soldered or welded. Hence, mechanical crimps are used for joining two wires.**
- Difficulty to bend.
- Shape memory—appliances may cause, **severe pain due to the rapid recovery and pushing of teeth by thermal change.**
- Higher archwire-bracket friction due to surface roughness.

Ni–Ti ENDODONTIC INSTRUMENTS

The superelastic property is made use in the recently developed endodontic reamers, and files. These can bend easily when used for **sharply curved root canals.** These have the austenite transformation temperature around 25°C. These can **minimize the perforations in the curved root canal and also fractures** [*see* Fig. 2.13(b)].

RECENT EXPERIMENTAL WIRES

1. Many other alloys of titanium have experimented. One alloy Ti = 76%, V= 15%, Cr = 3%, Al = 3%, Sn = 3% is found to have properties of **YS/Q, i.e. spring back, slightly better than β-titanium.**

2. **Aesthetic orthodontic wires**
   One of the important requirements of orthodontic wires is their aesthetic compatibility. Since all metals or alloys do not comply this, newer *tooth-coloured aesthetic wires* have experimented.
   a. **Teflon resin-coated Ni–Ti, or β-Ti wires**
   These have suitable mechanical properties for activation, chemical stability, and better aesthetics in oral conditions. However, their friction with brackets prevents the desired movement of the teeth.
   b. **Optiflex glass-fibre** reinforced thermoplastic wires. This has a fine glass-fibre ceramic core wire, with a translucent aramid resin, which is then surrounded by *candidate resin* like polycarbonates, polyethylene terephthalate glycol. It is also protected

Table 22.4	Comparison of common orthodontic wires		
Alloy	**Advantages**		**Disadvantages**
18-8 stainless steel	• Adequate biocompatibility and corrosion resistance. High resilience excellent formability, easy to shape for orthodontic appliances • Can be soldered and welded High rigidity—suitable for reactive appliances • Lowest cost compared to other alloys		• Low elastic range • High force delivery • Low springiness
Elgiloy	• Adequate biocompatibility • Excellent formability • High resilience (increases by heat treatment) • Can be soldered and welded • Comparatively low cost		• Lowest elastic range • Highest force delivery • Lowest springiness
Beta-titanium or cpTi, or TMA	• Excellent biocompatibility • Excellent formability • Large elastic range—spring back property • Excellent, real, weldability		• High force delivery (in-between Elgiloy and stainless steel) • High arch wire-bracket-friction, resisting tooth movement
Nickel-titanium (Ni-Ti)	• Adequate biocompatibility • **Superelasticity and shape memory** (which gives large elastic range and spring back) • Can be heat treated to adjust force delivery property • Lowest modulus of elasticity, suitable for active appliance		• Lowest *in vitro* corrosion resistance • Lowest formability • Difficult to bend wire permanently through sharp corners • **Cannot be soldered and welded** (use mechanical crimps) • **Most expensive**

by *transparent nylon,* which acts as *strain retainer.* This can be softened by warming above the Tg or glass transition temperature of the resin. This also has the same disadvantage of preventing the movement of teeth, by the friction between the wire and bracket.

MODEL QUESTIONS

I. Long Essays   (20 minutes each)

1. Give the composition, alloying properties of ingredients and microstructures of austenitic 18-8 stainless steel. Describe the properties and main causes of its corrosions. Explain briefly the remedies for corrosion.
2. Describe the composition and properties of nickel–titanium orthodontic wires. Explain their advantages and disadvantages. Write a note on TMA wires.

II. Short Essays   (10 minutes each)

1. Carbon steels
2. Ideal requirements of orthodontic wires
3. 18-8 stainless steel (austenitic steel)
4. Elgiloy
5. β-titanium (TMA) wire
6. Ni–Ti orthodontic wires
7. HN and N metal orthodontic wires
8. Heat treatment of orthodontic wires
9. Compare 18-8 stainless steel wire and Ni–Ti superelastic wire.

III. Brief Answers   (5 minutes each)

1. Ferritic stainless steel
2. Martensitic stainless steel
3. Passivation
4. Sensitization and stabilization of steels
5. Weld decay
6. Stainless steel denture base
7. Microstructure of orthodontic wires
8. Braided and twisted orthodontic wires
9. Classification of orthodontic wires
10. Active and passive orthodontic appliances
11. Superelasticity (or pseudoelasticity)
12. Elastic memory

Brazing and Welding

Metal joining techniques are frequently used in the fabrication of large, cast or wrought alloy intraoral appliances. Sometimes, large appliances are prepared by casting two or more separate parts and then carefully joining them together by soldering (brazing) or welding methods.

Solders (brazing metals)

These are low fusing alloys having their fusion (solidus) temperatures lower (by 50 to 100°C) than those of substrate metals.

Basis (substrate) metals

These are the parent metal parts which are to be joined together by soldering (brazing) or welding operations.

SOLDERING AND BRAZING

The process of joining two components of a metal appliance, by melting the solder, flowing it into the gap between the parts and solidifying it as a filler, or it is the process of building up a localized area, with a metal, or joining two or more metal parts by heating them to a temperature below their solidus temperature and filling the gap between them with a molten filler of suitable alloy having lower fusion temperatures.

The terms soldering and brazing are used when the liquidus temperature of filler is **less than 450°C and more than 450°C,** respectively. The term soldering was commonly used earlier.

IDEAL REQUIREMENTS OF SOLDERS (BRAZING FILLERS)

1. **Biological properties**
   - Biocompatible, nontoxic, and chemically inert in mouth
   - High tarnish and corrosion resistance
   - Noncarcinogenic, nonallergic.
2. **Mechanical properties**
   - High **tensile and shear strengths,** at least equal to those of basis metals
   - High **proportional limit,** to resist permanent distortions
   - High abrasive resistance
   - Solder liquid should have **low surface** tension and viscosities for **free flow**
   - Liquid should **wet** the soldering surface of the basis metal for **free flow**.
3. **Thermal**
   - Solidus temperature should be **50–100°C lower** than that of basis metals for **easy flow**
   - **Same COTE** as the basis metal, to avoid detachment during thermal cycling

- **A small range of** fusion temperatures to minimize coring and brittleness
- Components should not boil or evaporate during melting which will **cause pitting**
- Solders should melt easily and quickly. It should have a **low latent heat of fusion** and specific heats.
4. **Aesthetics:** Same colour as basis metal.
5. **Others:** The procedures should be **quite safe,** without causing accidental electric shocks and fire (by inflammable gases).

TYPES OF SOLDERS

Soft Solders

These are alloys of lead, bismuth and tin, having **low fusion** temperatures, 200°–260°C. It can be easily melted with a narrow gas flame or electric soldering irons. As the soldering procedure is **very simple and quick,** it is used for soldering parts of electronic gadgets (equipment). It is also known as **lead solder** or **tin makers' solder**.

It is not used in dentistry due to
- Very low tarnish and corrosion resistance
- Inadequate mechanical properties.

Hard Solders (Brazing Fillers)

These are alloys of gold, silver, copper, zinc, etc. and have higher
- Tarnish and corrosion resistance
- Mechanical properties, tensile strength, shear strength and abrasive resistance
- Liquidus temperature >450°C
- Fusion temperature ranges around:
  - 700–870°C for gold solders (Table 23.1)
  - 620–700°C for silver solders

Gold Solders (Brazing Fillers)

For adequate corrosion resistance, the gold alloys should have **>650 fineness,** i.e. >65% gold or >16 carats. Usually, the solder is **supplied as strips, wires, thin hollow pre-fluxed wire coils** (Table 23.1).

Properties of gold solders
- High corrosion resistance
- High mechanical properties, comparable to type IV casting gold alloys. The tensile strength is 220–300 MPa (heat hardened = 430–630 MPa) and proportional limit is 140–200 MPa (heat-hardened has 270–530 MPa)
- Fusion temperature ranges are slightly higher, i.e. about 700°–870°C
- Adequate flow properties, i.e. low viscosity for liquefied solder

Table 23.1	The composition of gold solders (brazers)	
Ingredients	wt%	Function
Gold	45–85%	↑ corrosion resistance, strength
Silver	8–30%	↑ strength, ↓ melting temperature
Copper	8–20%	↑ strength, ↓ melting temperature
Tin	2–4%	↑ strength, ↓ melting temperature
Zinc	2–4%	↑ brittleness ↓ melting temperature, scavenger
Cadmium	3–5%	Replace zinc for a clean surface

- Thermal expansion is similar to gold alloys
- Colour is usually yellow, light yellow or white.

Easy Flow and Free Flow of Gold Solders

Easy Flow

During soldering or brazing procedure, solder is melted and allowed **to flow** into the gap in between the parts of the basis metals. If the solder has lower fusion temperature it is **easier to melt** and flow. For this, the fusion temperature should be at least **55°C below** the solidus of parts of the substrate.

Free Flow

Refers to the ability of the solder liquid to **wet** the **soldering area, and flow** easily into the gap. For this free flow, the liquid alloy should have **low viscosity and surface tension.** Low gold content (fineness) and addition of tin and zinc improves this flow.

Microstructure of Soldered Joints

The brazing filler liquid wets and flows on the surfaces of basis, wrought wires or cast metals, to be joined. This forms an **intimate contact** between the interfaces. The brazing filler metal begins to solidify from the solid basis metal surfaces **forming granular crystals.** This causes **strong bonding** (Fig. 23.1).

Micrograph of perfectly brazed joints shows clear sharp boundaries in-between brazing filler and basis metals, without affecting the original fibrous structures **of wrought wires,** and **granular structure of cast metals.** However, prolonged or overheating, during the brazing procedures cause:
- Recrystallization of wrought wires.
- Grain growth in the cast basis metal parts.
- Diffusion of brazing filler into the basis metals **forming weaker new alloy phases,** to certain depths at the boundaries of the basis metals.

All these, decrease the original mechanical properties of basic metals and corrosion resistance, cause warpage, distortion of brazed joints and **failure in service.**

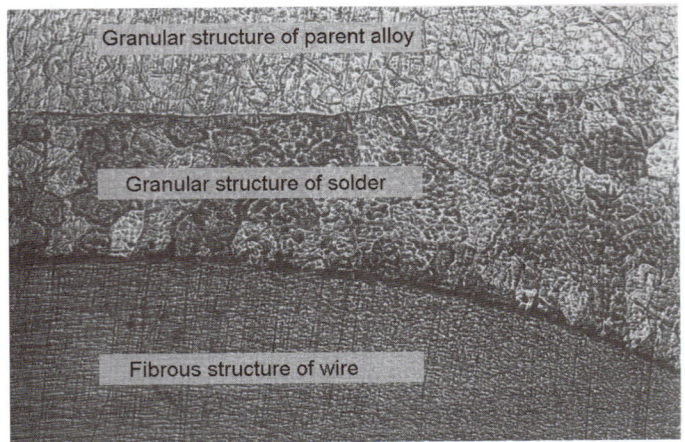

Fig. 23.1: Ideal soldered joint formed between gold based casting alloy and a gold based wire. granular microstructure of the cast alloy; bottom, fibrous microstructure of the wire. Middle, granular microstructure of the solder

Hence, suitable precautions are to be observed during brazing procedures (*refer* to technical considerations for brazing).

Pitting

If the solder liquid is maintained in the liquid state for a long time, it absorbs gases, and if overheated some elements, like Zn, Sn, Cd, boil and separates out. The gases produced, escape during the solidification, leaving small pits in the surface. The pits collect food debris and lead to **cell corrosion. Soldering must be performed quickly, by withdrawing the flame to avoid overheating and adsorption of gases.**

Silver Solders (Table 23.2)

These are hard solders of lower liquidus temperatures 620–700°C, used for brazing **base metal** alloy castings and appliances of stainless steel, Cr-Co-Ni, β-Ti, TMA, etc.

Table 23.2	The composition of silver solders	
Ingredients	wt%	Functions
Silver	10–80%	↑ strength, ↓ melting temperature
Copper	15–50%	↑ strength, ↓ melting temperature
Zinc	5–35%	↑ strength, brittleness, ↓ melting temperature
Cadmium	Small	Scavengers, ↓melting temperature, produce clean
Phosphorus	Amounts	Surface without pitting

Properties

- Tarnish and corrosion resistance is inferior to gold solders
- Mechanical properties are better
- Quick soldering of stainless steel at lower temperatures, reduces chances of sensitization
- Less pitting
- Has good flow and adhesion to base metal alloys.

Brazing Fluxes and Antifluxes

Flux (Latin word, meaning flow) is applied to the basis metal surfaces to
- Wet the surfaces of brazing and assist the flow of solder liquid
- Protect the soldering surfaces from oxidation
- Reduce the oxides on the surface
- Dissolve the oxides and impurity layers.

Three types of fluxes can be distinguished
Type I—protective flux: When applied on the surface and heated, the borax present melts forming a thin protective low fusing glass layer, covering the surface, which protects it from oxidation.
Type II—reducing flux: Sodium tetraborate or its dehydrated form borax reduces the oxides, like CuO in HN, N, metal alloy surfaces.
Type III—dissolving (solvent) flux: Fluorides (like KF) can dissolve the oxides of Cr, Co, Ni, etc. formed on the surface of base metal alloys, and causes wetting.
Purpose: Presence of an oxide film or impurities on the surface prevents wetting of the basis metal surfaces. That is why, flux is applied before brazing, on the gold alloys or base metal alloys.

Accordingly, there are gold or silver fluxes.
1. **The composition of brazing borax flux for gold alloys**
   - Borax ($Na_2B_4O_710H_2O$) = 55 parts
   - Boric acid (H_3BO_3) = 35 parts
   - Silica (SiO_2) = 10 parts

   This is a protective and reducing flux.
2. **The composition of fluoride, fluxes for base metal alloys**
   Potassium (or sodium) fluoride = 50–60%
   Boric acid = 25–35%
   Borax = 6–8%
   Potassium or sodium carbonates = 8–10%
   This is reducing and dissolving flux.

Both are supplied as
- Powder
- Paste in glycerine or petroleum jelly
- Liquid suspensions
- **Pre-fluxed or fused** to brazing fillers, i.e. fluxes are placed inside hollow cylindrical brazing fillers supplied as coiled wires.

The fluxes are applied as a thin coating on the surface. If the coating is too thin, it will get burnt out. If it is too thick, it will be trapped as bubbles in-between, and bonding is decreased. In the case of metal ceramics, the excess flux cause discolouration, and debonding.

Antifluxes

Before brazing procedure the flux is heated, melted and flowed to wet the surface area of brazing. This fluxed area helps molten brazing filler to flow, to this entire area. **To prevent the molten brazing alloys flowing to unwanted regions, antifluxes are** used. Demarking lines are drawn by **lead pencil**, or application of **suspension of rouge (Fe_2O_3)** or **whiting ($CaCO_3$),** to the areas to be protected, prevents the molten brazing filler, crossing into this region. Hence, before brazing, first apply the flux to the surface and then antiflux coating to the unwanted areas (Fig. 23.2).

Casting fluxes: The borax fluxes in powder form can be sprinkled over the alloy, while melting by a gas flame. Flux helps to melt the alloy easily, keeps the liquid alloy surface clean from oxides and protect the liquid from oxidation during casting procedure.

Fluxes used in GIC powder: Sodium, potassium or calcium fluorides are used to lower the fusion temperatures of glass ionomer (or silicate) cement powder components during the manufacturing process by fritting method.

Heat Sources for Melting Brazing Fillers

Various types of mixtures of air-gas flames, electrical heaters, infrared sources, etc. are used.

Gas brazing: Special types of gas torches with adjustments for gas-air (oxygen) mixing and reducing narrow pencil-like flame are available.

The melting of brazing filler becomes easier and faster if a suitable gas is mixed with air or oxygen. The gases should have **high flame temperature** as well as **high heat contents or calorific values.**

From Table 23.3, the **propane gas fuel appears** to be the most suitable due to its high flame temperature and calorific values.

Butane gas has similar properties and has become more popular as it is suitable for gas welding of **high fusing palladium alloys.**

Oxyacetylene gas flame has the highest temperature and large heat content. But the temperature distribution in the flame is inhomogeneous. The gas also is chemically unstable. Carbon released is added to Ni and Pd containing alloys, **decreasing their** mechanical properties. Also hydrogen gas released cause **porosity** in Pd-alloy casting.

Natural gas + air flame is suited for low fusing **HN and N alloys** and is less dangerous than others.

Hydrogen gas has low heat content and is not entirely suitable. (It takes longer times to melt the brazing fillers.)

Note: Draw the diagram of various combustion zones of a gas flame and label them, as air gas mixing, combustion, reducing and oxidizing outer zones (Fig. 23.3b, page 281 for details).

Table 23.3	Flame temperature and heat content of gas flames	
Fuel gas + O_2	Flame temperature	Calorific values kcal/m³
Acetylene gas	3140°C	12884
Propane gas	2850°C	**21221**
Natural gas	2680°C	8898
Hydrogen gas	2660°C	2362
Butane gas	Nearly similar values as propane flame	

Other Methods

1. **Electric furnace (oven) brazing**
   Heat is produced by electric current passed through the filaments in the furnace. The joining parts are well cleaned and applied with flux paste and placed in it. The substrate is heated until the brazing filler melts and flows well into the gap. Temperature can be properly controlled.

2. **Infrared brazing**
   The equipment has a **1000 watt tungsten filament quartz-iodine bulb** situated at the primary focal

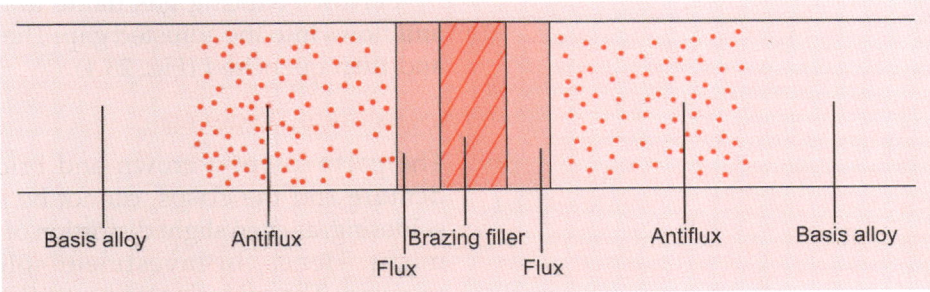

Fig. 23.2: Use of antiflux, flux and brazing filler to basis metal

point F_1 of a gold plated elliptical mirror M. The infra-red rays focus at the secondary focal point F_2. The heat rays should focus exactly on the substrate only. The brazing filler melts and flows into the earlier fluxed gap. The method can be used for brazing porcelain fused to metal articles, at about 1150°C. **It is difficult to locate F_2 exactly** (Fig. 23.3a).

3. **Modified electric spot welding** equipment can also be used for soldering orthodontic wires.

Technical Considerations for Soldering (Brazing)

The two methods commonly used are **free hand soldering** and **investment soldering** with a suitable gas torches.

Preliminaries
- **Cleanliness of surfaces:** Surfaces of soldering are polished and well cleaned for better wetting and flow of solder liquid.
- **Gap distance:** The optimum gap between the soldering parts should be about **0.1 to 0.3 mm.**

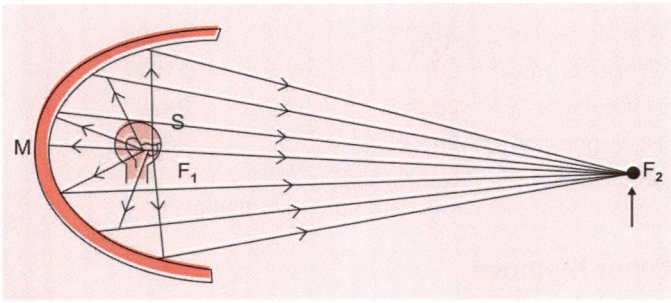

Fig. 23.3a: Infrared—heat rays focussing at conjugate focus F_2

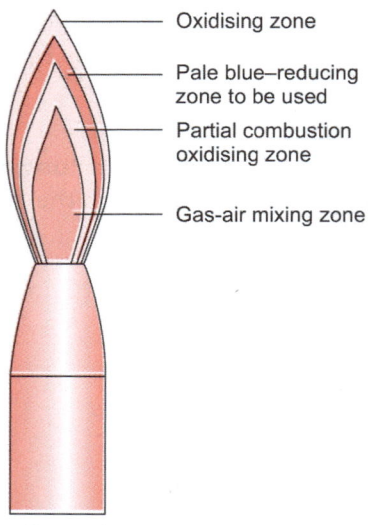

- Oxidising zone
- Pale blue—reducing zone to be used
- Partial combustion oxidising zone
- Gas-air mixing zone

Gas + air

Fig. 23.3b: Combustion zones of gas-flame

Smaller gap decreases the strength due to
- Incomplete flow into the gap
- Trapping of air
- Trapping of fluxes.

Larger gap also decreases the strength equal to that of the weaker solder material. The contraction of a large amount of solder in the gap cause distortion.

- **Fluxes:** Flux must be properly **selected,** and applied carefully on the surface, after applying antiflux.
- **Selection of gas fuel:** Should be done according to their heat content and temperatures.
- **Adjustment of gas flame: The blue coloured reducing flame** has to be applied. This part is just under the outermost oxidizing part of the flame. The flame is adjusted to have a **narrow tip** and held in contact with the substrate (article) until the soldering operation is over. Solder melts and flows into the gap. **Reducing flame protects** the surface from oxidation. The flame should not be **removed or moved** away during the soldering procedure.
- The **temperature** of the flame should be **minimum,** just that required to melt the solder. Higher temperatures may cause diffusion of liquid, volatilize some of the components of solder, Cd, Zn which produce **pitting.**
- **Time of soldering:** The flame should be held in contact until the solder melts and flows completely. Heating should be continued for **little more time** just to allow the oxides and molten flux to come out of the solder joints. Prolonged heating causes diffusion of solder-liquid into the substrate **forming a new alloy phase, which is weaker near the margins.**

METHODS OF SOLDERING

Free Hand Soldering

Usually employed for **quick soldering** of orthodontic wires, brackets, and sometimes **repairing the perforated castings.** One part, say the thicker wire is held in a vice or clamp support. Flux and antifluxes are applied. A drop of molten solder is placed at the required place on the thicker part. The thinner wire to be soldered is applied with the flux and is held in hand in contact with the solder. The two wire parts are heated by narrow reducing gas flame until the solder melts and flows into the adjusted gap. The assembly is cooled and then quenched (Fig. 23.4).

Investment Soldering

The parts say of a crown and bridge or cast partial denture and the clasps, cannot be joined by freehand soldering, as even slight distortion of the assembly cause misfit. Hence, in investment soldering method is required. The soldering parts are first assembled on the cast and joined with **sticky wax.**

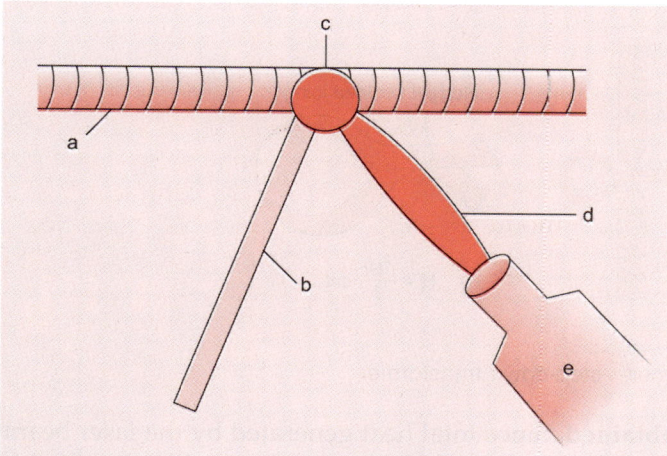

Fig. 23.4: Free hand soldering. a. Thicker part, b. thinner wire, c. drop of solder, d. reducing gas flame, e. gas torch

Suitable investment material quartz-gypsum-bonded or phosphate-bonded investment material is mixed with water and poured on a glass plate or a tile. The assembly is carefully transferred to this soldering investment mix, which is allowed to set. This investment material should have a **minimum setting and thermal expansions,** which may otherwise cause separation of parts, and distortions. Sticky wax is removed by flushing with boiling water. Apply the antiflux and fluxes properly and place the solder in the gap. The parts are heated by **reducing gas-flame** until the solder liquid flows into the gap. It is then cooled, devested, polished and delivered (Fig. 23.5).

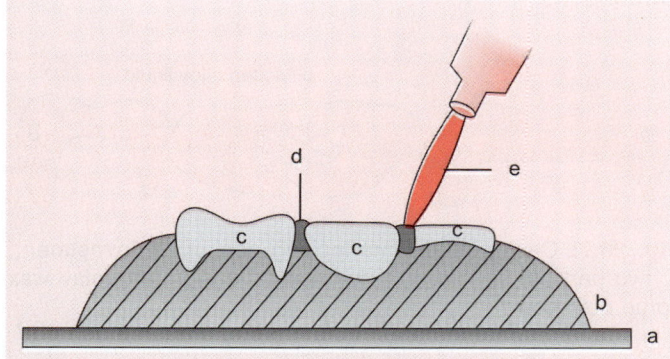

Fig. 23.5: a. Glazed ceramic tile, b. Investment, c. basis metals, d. solder, e. gas flame

Pitted Solder Joints

Overheating and prolonged heating of solders may absorb gases like H_2, N_2 and volatilize some of the low boiling points components (like tin, zinc, cadmium, etc.) of the solders. These vapours or gases get trapped inside, causing porosities, or escape through the liquid during solidification forming pits on the surface. The pits are usually observed while polishing. **Pits collect food debris** and undergo **crevice or concentration cell** corrosion. Pits can be reduced by suitable control of the temperature of the flame, time of soldering and avoiding excessive fluxing, since trapping of flux also can cause pitting.

Applications of soldering in dentistry

• Joining the various components of the cast appliances, crowns, bridges, partial dentures, etc.
• Repairing and reassembling distorted bridges
• Joining clasps to removable cast partial dentures
• Sealing the perforations in the crowns, etc.
• Improving the fittings of castings
• Joining wires and bands in orthodontic appliances
• Assembling space maintainers.

PRE-BRAZING AND POST-BRAZING

Pre-brazing: Process of brazing of two or more metal components of a prosthesis **before a ceramic veneer is fired** or **hot pressed** on the structure.

Post-brazing: Brazing of two or more metal components of a prosthesis **after the structure has been veneered** or hot pressed with porcelain on the structure. Suitable solder and soldering temperatures are to be considered.

WELDING

This is the process of fusing two or more metal parts through the application of heat, pressure, or both, with or without a filler metal to produce a localized union across the interface between the parts. In direct filling gold (pure gold) this union can be brought about only by pressure.

During welding, the temperature should be high enough to **locally melt** the metal parts, and make the atoms diffuse into each other to form a union.

The method is used for welding wrought wires, clasps to partial denture frameworks, orthodontic bands, etc.

According to melting (heating) techniques, there are different methods of welding.
1. Gas welding—in industries for brass, stainless steel, etc.
2. Arc welding—for stainless steel, base metal alloys
3. Electric resistance—spot welding in dentistry, for stainless steel, orthodontic bands, etc.
4. Laser welding titanium and its alloys, crown and bridges of noble or base metal alloy castings.

ELECTRICAL RESISTANCE OR SPOT WELDING

The instrument consists of a step-down transformer, similar to the one used in industries for arc-welding, to supply large current (i Amps) through two thick **copper electrodes** C_1 and C_2 (Fig. 23.6) (*see* Colour Plate 35, Fig. 23.3).

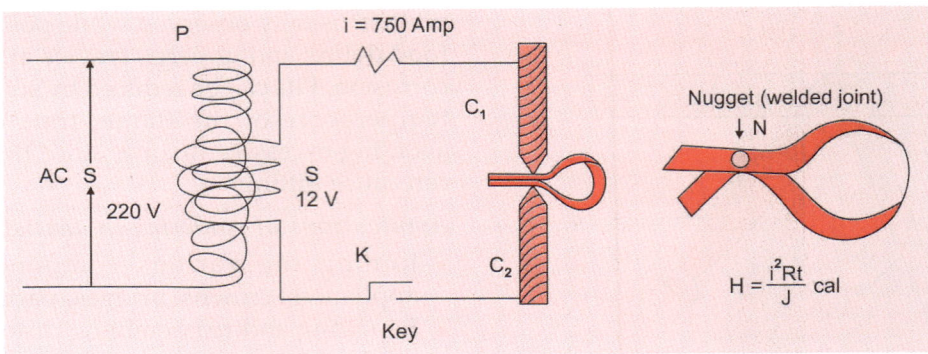

Fig. 23.6: Electric spot welding circuit—step-down transformer

The article to be welded (say matrix band), is held under pressure between the two electrodes.

Large AC or DC of about **750 amperes** is passed for a short time $1/_{50}$ sec, through C_1 and C_2 by just pressing and releasing key K. As all other metals like stainless steel have higher resistance 'R' compared to thick copper rods C_1 and C_2, large heat produced raises the temperature and melts the parts momentarily at the contact point, forming a **nugget.**

Weld-decay: Spot welding method is very simple, quick and it is very convenient to use in dentistry in case of stainless steel bands. As the parts melt, at about 1250°C, it loses corrosion resistance by sensitization at the **nugget. The welded parts gradually decay** and finally fail. This is **weld decay.** This can be minimized by reducing the time of welding or using stabilized stainless steels containing **niobium or titanium plus tantalum about six times of carbon.** Welded joints also can decay due to **stress** concentration at the nugget and inhomogeneous composition.

Note: For short notes on weld decay, nugget, passivation, sensitization and stabilization of stainless steel, the answer is nearly the same and should include all these phenomena.

LASER WELDING

A very **narrow laser beam**, carrying intense heat is used very conveniently for welding oral appliances. For example the cast parts of crown and bridge, etc. can be **welded directly on the cast itself** as the rest of the parts are not heated. This is also quite simple and investment technique is not required. Welding the parts, directly on the cast, reduces the chances of distortion.

Laser and plasma weldings are applicable for cpTi appliances. Ti forms titanium oxide corrosion-resistant film. But at higher temperatures, the oxide film becomes thicker and get debonded, at 850°C or higher temperatures.

Laser and plasma welding **cpTi in argon atmosphere** prevents oxide formations. The basis and molten materials diffuse and **integrated part is obtained.** Since total heat generated by the laser beam is negligible the welding parts can be held in hands also (*see* Colour Plate 35, Fig. 23.2).

CAST JOINING TECHNIQUE

It is the method of joining two components of a fixed cast partial denture by **casting the molten metal** into an **interlocking region** between the invested components (Fig. 23.7). Weiss and Munyon (1980) proposed this alternate method to the conventional soldering which had resulted in different properties at soldered joints are leading to corrosion and decay.

Mechanical interlocking **undercuts** are made at the joining parts. The gaps are filled with type II hard inlay wax, a sprue is attached and invested in a large casting ring. It is then dewaxed, and the molten alloy of **same basis metal is cast** into the gap, cooled, and recovered. This reduces the chance of corrosion and weakening joints.

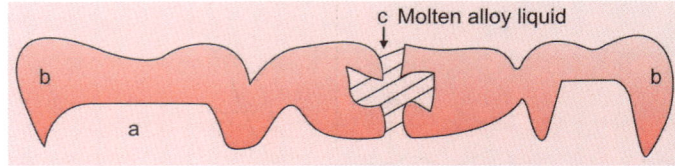

Fig. 23.7: Cast joining—interlocking design. a. Investment, b. two parts to be joined, c. interlocked design and inlay wax sprue not shown

CASTING TO EMBEDDED ALLOYS

If required, it is possible to embed a wrought or cast, preformed structure, like a clasp or a wire, into the appliance. The cast clasp or wire is placed, and the wax pattern is formed **including this.** After attaching sprue, it is invested, wax eliminated and casting of the alloy of **lower fusion temperature** is performed. During this procedure the **investment should not be overheated.**

This technique gives better mechanical properties than brazing.

LASERS IN DENTISTRY

Laser refers to light amplification of stimulated emission of radiation. Laser has become a powerful tool in various engineering, medical, dental and research areas. Very fine collimated powerful beams of monochromatic light of particular wavelengths are produced and delivered through flexible, mirrors laid, tubes or optic fibers to microsized sites. The light is absorbed and converted into large intense thermal energy at the site.

The basic components of laser equipment are:

1. Visible light source producing relevant spectra, surrounding the active medium. The photons of a particular energy, hυ, collide with the atoms of the active medium. The electron of the outermost orbit absorbs the particular photons and go to the higher excited state. Immediately it jumps back to the ground state re-emitting the photon of the same energy. This photon collides with other atoms similarly producing many photons.

2. Common active media and corresponding laser wavelengths.

   a. Gaseous-argon (λ = 488 and 514 nm) carbon dioxide (λ = 10,600 nm)

   b. Solid crystals like ruby (λ = 964 nm)

   c. Solid-state semiconductors diode wafers with multiple layers of metals like Al, Ga, In, As, etc. (λ = 800–980 nm)

   d. Neodymium with yttrium, aluminum, garnet, i.e. neodymium YAG (λ = 1064 nm)

   e. Holmium YAG (λ = 2100 nm)

   f. Erbium–chromium YSGG (λ = 2100)

   g. Erbium YAG (λ = 2940 nm)

3. Two plane mirrors, one being semitransparent is kept parallel to each other to reflect a large number of photons back and forth several times and collimate them into very narrow powerful coherent beams, which come out (or drained) through the semitransparent mirror.

When this falls on the target point of the media, it is absorbed and converted into heat energy rising the temperature instantaneously. The heat produced depends on the nature of the target material, and the depth of penetration is quite small only up to about 2.5 mm, the intensity remains almost constant and does not decrease as per inverse square law.

Applications

1. Microsurgeries in ophthalmology and other medical fields.

2. Spot welding of high fusing alloys in dentistry, like titanium, alloys of titanium, and predominantly base metal alloys.

3. In dental clinical specialities it is indicated for the following:
   - Gingivectomy, gingivoplasty
   - Gingival depigmentation
   - Frenectomy and frenotomy
   - Gingival troughing for crown impressions
   - Soft tissue crown toughening
   - Removal of gingival hypertrophy
   - Leukoplakia
   - Oral pepillectomies
   - Pulpotomy
   - Pulpotomy as an adjunct to RCT
   - Treatment of few ulcers of the oral mucosa
   - Vestibuloplasty
   - Implant recoveries
   - Excisional and incisional biopsies
   - Haemostasis and coagulation
   - Fibroma removal
   - Exposure of unerupted teeth
   - Promotion of wound healing
   - Oral ulcerations
   - Curing of composite restorations
   - Etching tooth enamel surfaces
   - Bleaching

Advantages

1. Dry and bloodless surgery
2. Minimum postoperative pain and swelling
3. Instant sterilization of the surgical site
4. Low mechanical trauma
5. No pain, no injections
6. Minimum discomfort to the patients.

MODEL QUESTIONS

I. Long Essay   (20 minutes)

1. Define the terms **soldering, brazing and welding**. Give the requirements of brazing fillers. Explain methods of brazing and welding in dentistry.

II. Short Essays   (10 minutes each)

1. Gold solders
2. Brazing fluxes
3. Freehand and investment brazing
4. Gas brazing
5. Technical considerations for brazing
6. Welding

III. Brief Answers   (5 minutes each)

1. Easy flow and free flow of solders
2. Antifluxes
3. Fluoride fluxes for brazing
4. Infrared brazing
5. Oven brazing
6. Soldering gap distance
7. Pre-soldering and post-soldering
8. Microstructure of brazed joints
9. Pitted solder joints
10. Spot welding
11. Laser welding
12. Cast joining technique
13. Weld decay (or nugget)
14. Zones of soldering gas flame
15. Reducing fluxes

Tarnish and Corrosion

The oral environment is **very hostile** to any artificial restorative foreign materials and appliances introduced into the oral cavity. Fluctuations in the pH values and temperatures during intake of food and drinks, large dynamic masticating forces acting very often, many times, abrasive properties of materials, etc. affect these foreign materials, causing:

- Tarnish and corrosion of metallic appliances
- Discolouration of the tooth and restorative materials
- Degradation of polymeric resins, composite resins, ceramics, etc.
- Attrition
- Fracture and fatigue failures
- The decay of teeth, etc.

TARNISH

Discolouration of the surface of metallic appliances due to chemical action forming a thin surface film is known as tarnish. Due to this the surface gloss, luster and finish decrease and aesthetics qualities are lost. The colour parameters, hue, chroma and values change. If tarnish is allowed to continue further, it results in corrosion or loss of material from the surface.

CAUSES FOR TARNISH

1. **Deposits on the tooth:** Hard deposits like calculus, soft deposits like plaque and thin surface films, promote the growth of microorganisms and mucin.

These release certain acids, when the carbohydrates are formed by the food debris, which attack the metallic surfaces. Pigment producing bacteria also cause tarnish.

2. **Stains:** Some food materials containing sulphur or chlorides, drinks like coffee, tea, alcohol, etc. tobacco, drugs containing mercury, iron, etc. may react with the metal and tarnish. Some of these cause discolouration of aesthetic restorations and tooth structures also.

3. **Surface films:** Thin surface films are formed due to oxidation and such other chemical reactions on the metal surfaces. This causes discolouration of the entire restoration, like stain. The surface can be protected by forming oxide films, strongly adhering to the substrate, like the **passivation of Cr, Ti, Al.**

The surface material is not lost in tarnishing. However, this is a **forerunner of corrosions.**

The discolourations produced can be observed and **compared by a visual method.** Optical instruments like **densitometers, spectrophotometers, etc.** can be used for measuring the amount of light reflected or scattered, with respect to time, which can be used for comparative studies.

CORROSION

This can be defined as the **loss of material from the surface by chemical attacks on the surface particles.** The **corrosion products are loosely bonded to the**

substrate, and can dissolve in the oral fluids or electrolytes. **Corrosion is a continuation of tarnish with the loss of surface material**. A good example is the rusting of iron or carbon steels, due to exposure to moisture. The reaction products Fe_2O_3 or $Fe(OH)_3$ becomes a thick layer of brittle material, which easily gets debonded from the iron substrate.

Corrosion results in a rough surface, which collects food debris, become unhygienic and continue to corrode further. Loss of surface finish results in poor aesthetics.

CLASSIFICATION OF CORROSIONS

- Dry chemical corrosion
- Wet electrochemical corrosion

Dry Corrosion

The chemical reactions take place between the metals and the oral environment or atmosphere, in the absence of water, saliva or electrolytes. The thin films formed on the surface of metals like silver, copper, tin, etc. due to oxidation, sulphurization or halogenation, increase in thickness. These can get detached and dissolve in solution. This results in **loss of material** from the surface. Except for noble metals, almost all others undergo these reactions and get corroded.

Applications

- Gold alloys containing, silver, copper, etc. undergo slow corrosion when exposed to the atmosphere.
- Silver, copper, tin containing alloy powder of silver amalgams undergo these reactions when exposed to the atmosphere. **The oxide films developed, prevent the wetting of mercury** and hence amalgamation reaction without trituration, cannot take place.
- The oxide films, formed by Cr, Ti and Al, adhere very strongly to the substrate and prevent further dry corrosion (this resistance developed to corrosion is **passivation**).

Dry corrosion also can be detected by visual methods. This chemical corrosion is very rarely isolated from the wet electrochemical corrosion.

Wet Electrochemical Corrosion

This refers to the loss of materials from the surface due to chemical reactions in **wet conditions** that is, in contact with water, saliva or ionic solutions. This is also accompanied by the liberation of the ions or atoms of the metal (anode), during the passage of electric charges, through the electrolyte. Hence, it is known as **electrochemical corrosion** (Fig. 24.1).

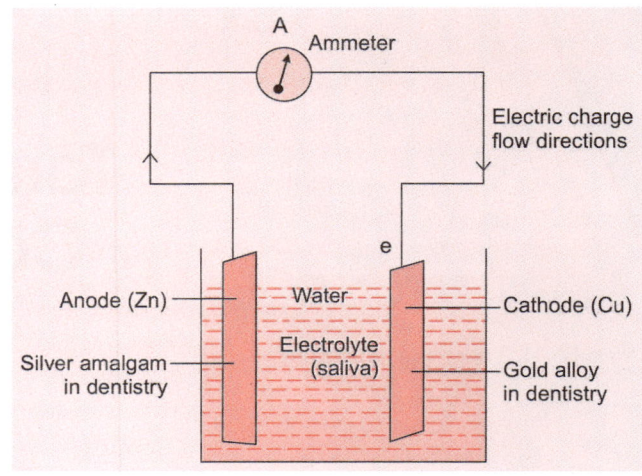

Fig. 24.1: Electrochemical cell

Theory

When two dissimilar metals, say zinc and copper, are placed (or separated) in an electrolyte, an ionic solution like water, saliva or dilute acids, they drive a small electric current through the electrolyte, due to the liberation of electrons from the anode (zinc). The positive zinc + ion goes to the solution and gets neutralized. When the electrodes are connected by an external conductor (circuit), a small potential difference is developed due to the difference in the electrode potentials. The **electromotive force** (difference in electrode potentials) is responsible for driving a current in the circuit. Depending on this difference in the electrode potentials or EMF the anodic metal (zinc) undergoes dissolution, by the passage of electric current. The rate of dissolution or corrosion of anodic metals depends on the difference in the electrode potentials of metals. Electrode potentials arise due to the free electron densities. The electrode potentials of few metals, used in dentistry show, gold has the highest positive value (+ 1.50 V), hydrogen is considered as at zero potential, and potassium has the highest negative value (–2.92 volts). When zinc (–0.76 V) is connected to copper (+0.47 V) through the electrolyte, the EMF produced is = 0.47 V – (–0.76 V) = 1.23 volts. The zinc is anodic, which undergoes electrochemical corrosion, with the zinc atoms (ions) carried to the solution. The rate of corrosion depends upon the electrode potential differences (EMFs) between the anode and the cathode, as per the electromotive series (Table 24.1).

Accordingly the following types of electrochemical corrosions can take place.

1. Galvanic Corrosion

When the two dissimilar metallic or alloy restorations come into contact through the electrolytes or

Table 24.1	Electrode potentials of some metals used in dentistry (electromotive series)	
Metal	*Ion*	*Electrode potential volts*
Gold	Au^+	+1.5
Platinum	Pt^{2+}	+0.86
Palladium	Pd^{2+}	+0.82
Mercury	Hg^{2+}	+0.80
Silver	Ag^+	+0.80
Copper	Cu^+	+0.47
Hydrogen	H^+	0.00
Tin	Sn^{2+}	−0.14
Nickel	Ni^{2+}	−0.23
Cadmium	Cd^{2+}	−0.40 +ve
Iron	Fe^{2+}	−0.44 1.23 volts −ve
Chromium	Cr^{2+}	−0.56
Zinc	Zn^{2+}	−0.76
Aluminium	Al^{3+}	−1.70
Sodium	Na^+	−2.71
Calcium	Ca^{2+}	−2.87
Potassium	K^+	−2.92

separated in the ionic medium like saliva, dentinal fluids, blood, etc. a potential difference is developed, between the two. This drives a small direct electric current through saliva, tissue fluid, dentinal fluid and pulp, completing the electrical circuit (Fig. 24.2).

This galvanic current however small produces severe pains when passes through the pulp. This is known as **galvanic shock.** For example, when a gold alloy restoration and silver amalgam restoration are opposing, the silver amalgam becomes the anode and undergoes galvanic corrosion. Here gold alloy acts as a cathode, silver amalgam—anode and saliva or dentinal fluid as the electrolytes.

Note: When high copper and low copper amalgam restorations are in the opposing teeth the high copper becomes the anode and undergoes corrosion.

The remedies are either to avoid such dissimilar metals opposing restorations or provide a good insulating base, which protects the pulp from galvanic shock.

2. Heterogeneous Composition Corrosion (Fig. 24. 3a)

This takes place one way or other in almost all alloys. The various component metals have different electrode potentials. When these come into contact through ionic oral fluids like saliva, small local voltaic cells are formed which drive small electric currents causing dissolution of anodic metals zinc with respect to copper, silver or gold.

Some of the situations for corrosion due to inhomogeneous compositions are:

• Multiphase alloys (e.g. silver amalgam, γ, $γ_1$, $γ_2$, n, Hg)
• Cored structures in single phase alloys
• Grain boundaries in homogenized alloys

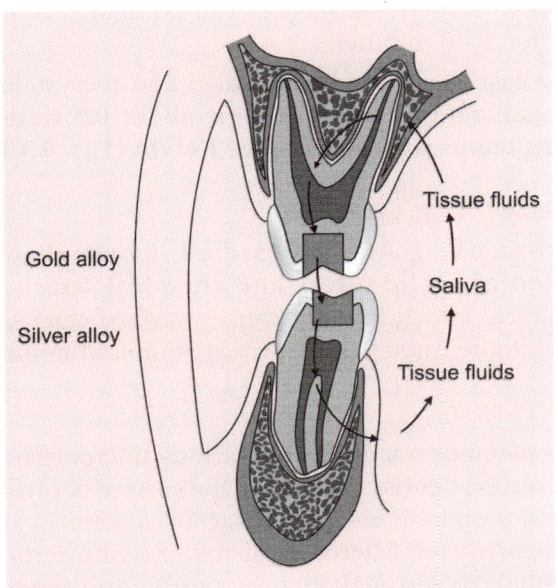

Fig. 24.2: Possible path of a galvanic current in the mouth

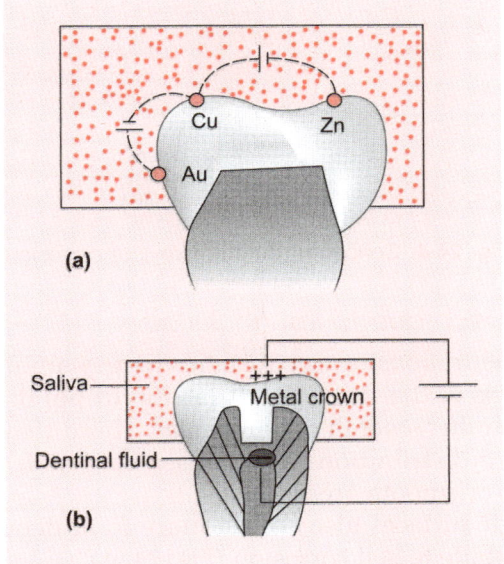

Figs 24.3a and b: Corrosion due to (a) Heterogeneous composition, (b) different ionic liquids in different surfaces

- Soldered and welded joints
- Single metallic alloy restoration with different electrolytes, of different ionic concentrations, in opposite sides of restorations in contact with saliva on one side, and dentinal fluids or pulp on the other side (Fig. 24.3b).

Electroplating of the alloy restorations with gold or applying **insulating bases** are the remedies.

3. Concentration Cell (Crevice) Corrosion
(Fig. 24.4)

Small pits on the surfaces or the crevices at the margins of metallic restorations, collect food debris or electrolytic (ionic) solutions or saliva. Concentration of oxygen ions is least at the bottom and is higher at the surface. Hence, the bottom of the pits become anodic and the corrosion takes place more, making the metals dissolve. The crevice or pit depths gradually increase.

If food debris is left at the margins of the restorations at the interproximal areas, the oxygen ion concentration becomes less than saliva. Again corrosion takes place similarly. The corrosions of rough surfaces of the restorations, takes place more, as there are many pits. This corrosion can be reduced by:

- **Polishing** the surface very well to remove all the pits.
- Minimizing the absorption of air by the molten alloy, before casting which reduces the surface, air trapping porosity (or pits).

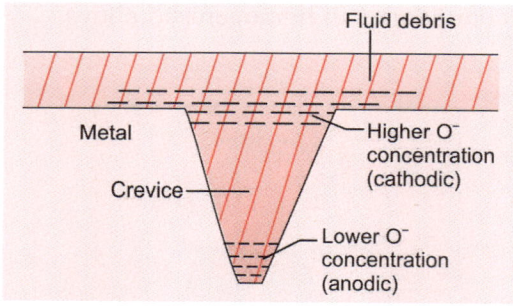

Fig. 24.4: Concentration cell (crevice) corrosion

4. Corrosion due to Rough Surface

Concentrations of electrostatic charges are more at the tips of the sharp points (**action of points**), than at the other smooth or blunt areas. This difference of charge distributions also causes corrosion, at the blunt or smooth areas.

Rough surfaces also collect more food debris and contribute to cell corrosion (Fig. 24.5).

The remedy, in this case, is also polishing the surface as smooth as possible.

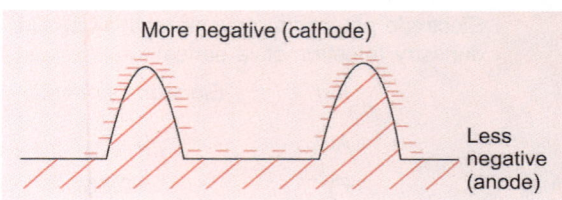

Fig. 24.5: Corrosion at the rough surface

5. Stress Corrosion

All the dental and other equipment undergo **work (strain) hardening in service**. Similarly, the fabrications of orthodontic active or passive appliances, cause maximum work hardening at the more severely worked regions. This causes an **increase in the energies at the grain** boundaries and interdendritic regions. These undergo corrosion much faster as the chemical reaction is faster at these highly **stressed** regions.

Examples

- Corrosion takes place much faster at the **severely deformed** regions, of say a sharply bent iron wire, when exposed to moisture or water or any acid.
- Orthodontic appliances get corroded at the severely deformed or bent parts of the wires.
- The instruments used in clinics also can get corroded more at the severely deformed areas, at the sharp edges and tips.

Remedy

The instruments or appliances should be subjected to **stress relief** or recovery heat treatments.

For example, the austenitic stainless steel instruments and prepared wire appliances can be treated at about 480°C for 7–10 minutes.

The cast alloys can be annealed and recrystallized. Recrystallization temperature is about **0.3 times its melting temperatures in degree Kelvin ($T_R = 0.3\ T°K$)**.

6. Corrosion Fatigue

Corrosion fatigue takes place due to the **simultaneous action of cyclic forces and chemical attack**. The chemical attack initially causes surface cracks, and the fatigue causes crack propagation and failure.

7. Biocorrosion

The metabolic activities of various microorganisms in the food debris collected on the surface or proximal areas of metallic restorations, cause chemical attack and corrosion. Microorganisms growing with and without oxygen are known as **aerobic and anaerobic** respectively.

Remedy

Maintain proper hygiene, by cleaning the food debris each time, after taking food.

Note: The electrochemical corrosion is not limited to a single mode. It is quite complex with most of the above types of corrosions taking place simultaneously.

Measurement of Corrosion

- By visual methods
- By comparing the electrical resistance of the specimen, initially and after corrosion using potentiostats
- Electrochemical linear polarization technique
- **Coupon test:** Specimen of standard size is placed in the corroding medium for a long time (1–3 months) and the **percentage loss of the material** is measured.

Methods to Minimize Corrosions

- Wherever possible use highly corrosion-resistant metals like **noble metals** or passivated base metals. Electroplating the alloys with gold or noble metals prevents inhomogeneous surface corrosions.
- The surface must be very **well polished** to remove pits, crevices and surface roughness. This resist crevice or cell corrosion and also microbiological corrosions.
- Base metal alloys can be **passivated** with Cr, Ti (or Al), and also electropolished.
- **Avoid dissimilar metals** or alloy restorations coming into contact.
- **Avoid overheating** of base metal alloys to retain the passivating effect.
- **Minimize** the number of soldering joints to reduce inhomogeneous composition corrosions.
- **Welding** is to be done very **quickly** and try to avoid welding of base metals.

- Base metals should not come into contact with hypochlorite solution.
- **Work hardened materials:** Orthodontic appliances, should be properly annealed, to minimize intergranular corrosions. The **recovery** heat treatment is given, as per manufacturers instructions.
- Surgical and clinical instruments should be **sterilized at low** temperatures.

MODEL QUESTIONS

I. Long Essays (20 minutes each)

1. Describe tarnish and corrosion. Explain dry corrosion, galvanic corrosions and remedies.
2. Describe the term corrosion. Explain the various types of corrosion and possible remedies.

II. Short Essays (10 minutes each)

1. Dry corrosion
2. Wet corrosion
3. Galvanic corrosion
4. Heterogeneous surface corrosion
5. Crevice, or concentration cell corrosion
6. Methods to minimize corrosion

III. Brief Answers (5 minutes each)

1. Tarnish
2. Stress corrosion
3. Biocorrosion
4. Measurement of tarnish and corrosions
5. Recovery heat treatments
6. Corrosion fatigue

Dental Implant Materials

Dental implantology is a fast developing specialized complex field. This branch is incorporated in many other specialities like oral surgery, prosthodontics, periodontics, etc. This is concerned with the replacement of missing teeth with the help of support, implanted in the jaws or on the tissues.

An implant may be defined as a medical device prepared from one or more biomaterials, which are placed intentionally within the body either totally or partially inserted in the epithelial surface which assists normal functioning of the body. The biomaterials should interact with the biological system, without producing any harmful biohazardous effects.

A dental implant can be defined as a foreign biomaterial, anchored to the jaw, to reproduce an entire tooth, either as a single restoration, or as a support for removable or fixed partial dentures.

INDICATIONS FOR DENTAL IMPLANTATIONS

There should be an adequate bone structure with sufficient height, length, and contour to support the implants of the suitable types, i.e. **subperiosteal, transosteal or endosseous.**

CONTRAINDICATIONS

- The impossibility of prosthesis reconstructions
- Patients sensitivity to implant component materials

- Debility and uncontrollable diseases
- Pregnancy
- Conditions, diseases or treatments which may affect or retard the healing (like radiation therapy)
- Poor oral hygiene
- Patient's poor motivation
- Unrealistic, too high expectations of the patient
- Inadequate training of dental practitioners.

IDEAL REQUIREMENTS OF IMPLANT MATERIALS

- **Bioactivity:** It is the ability to undergo osseointegration. When the living bone and biomaterials come into contact, a **biocompatible interface** of **fibrous connective tissues** is formed. This interface grows into direct contact and bonds them together. This is known as **osseointegration.**
- High corrosion resistance and chemical stability
- Biocompatible, nontoxic and nonallergic
- Suitable modulus of elasticity, resilience and proportional limit, **similar to bone**, to transmit biomechanical forces to the tissues.
- Low density to reduce weight.
- Thermal properties should be similar to bone structure, i.e. the same coefficient of thermal expansion and good insulating properties.
- Ability to form a **strong osseointegrating film**.

SHAPES, DESIGNS AND COMPONENTS

Components of implants are supplied in different sizes, shapes or designs such as **frameworks, staples, blades, spirals, screws, hollow cylinders, cones, etc**.

Three basic components of implants (Fig. 25.1)
- Fixtures
- Abutments
- Actual prosthesis

1. **Fixtures:** These have different surface designs, like **perforated, grooved, threaded, etc. which are plasma coated or hydroxyapatite (HA) or tricalcium phosphate (TCP) coated.** Selection is made according to the particular situation. The increased surface area provides better osseointegration, cortex engagement and bondings. The **endopores** have a very large number of semispherical structures on the surface which can increase the surface area by many times to improve bond strength.

2. **Abutments:** This is a transmucosal arrangement to provide a strong connection between the fixture and prosthesis. **The abutment** is connected to the fixture by means of **screwing, cementation or swagging**. Abutments can also be connected to the fixtures through **internal or external hexagonal structures with the anti-rotation system.**

3. **Prosthesis:** Suitable prostheses are fabricated and attached to the abutments by means of screws and attachments as in the case of **Branemark hybrid overdentures.**

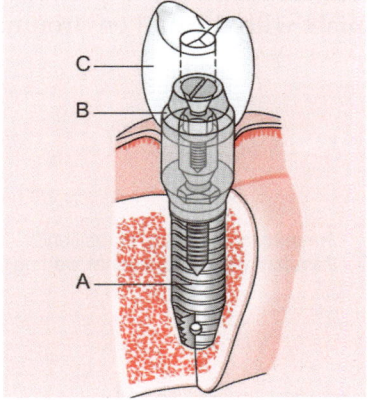

Fig. 25.1: Implant components. a. Fixtures, b. abutments, c. actual prosthesis (*see* Colour Plate 36, Fig. 25.3)

IMPLANT DESIGNS (TYPES)

There are mainly four varieties of implants:
1. Subperiosteal
2. Endosteal (endosseous)
3. Transosteal
4. Epithelial

1. **Subperiosteal implants**
This has, an implant structure and a superstructure. The cast framework is placed under the periosteum over the bony cortex. This can be used when the bone structure is inadequate for endosseous implants. However, this has not become popular due to many disadvantages (Fig. 25.2a).

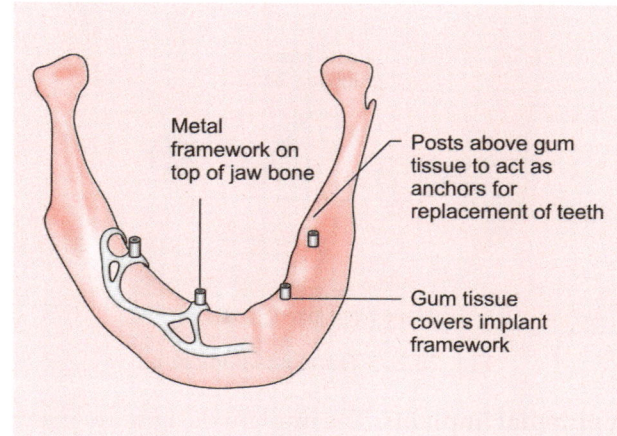

Metal framework on top of jaw bone

Posts above gum tissue to act as anchors for replacement of teeth

Gum tissue covers implant framework

Fig. 25.2a: Subperiosteal implants

2. **Endosteal (endosseous) implants**
This is the most commonly used method. The devices are placed in the alveolar or basal bones of the mandible (or maxilla) **partially submerged.** These are supplied as **thin blades, screws and cylindrical cones,** which can be used in all areas of the mouth. These act as fixtures and abutments. The **root forms endosteal implant is used to initiate the functions of the tooth root,** for proper positioning of the prosthesis and also the distribution of the forces (Fig. 25.2b).

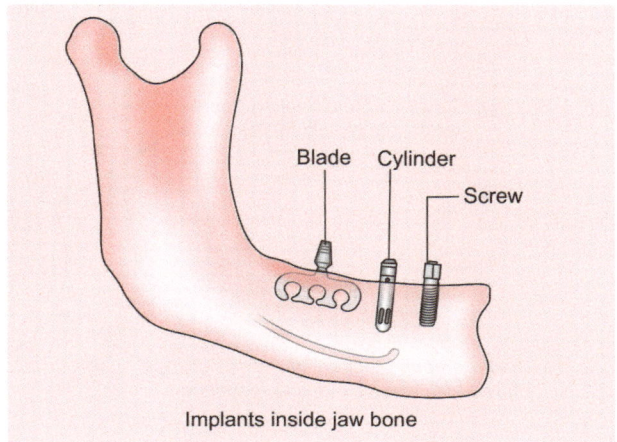

Blade   Cylinder

Screw

Implants inside jaw bone

Fig. 25.2b: Endosteal implants

3. **Transosteal (transosseous):** Combines the subperiosteal, and endosteal, with the implants passing through the **entire thickness of the alveolar bones.**

This is usually prescribed or restricted only to the **anterior** area of the mandible. This includes **transmandibular implant (TMI), staple bone implant and mandibular staple implants** (Fig. 25.2c).

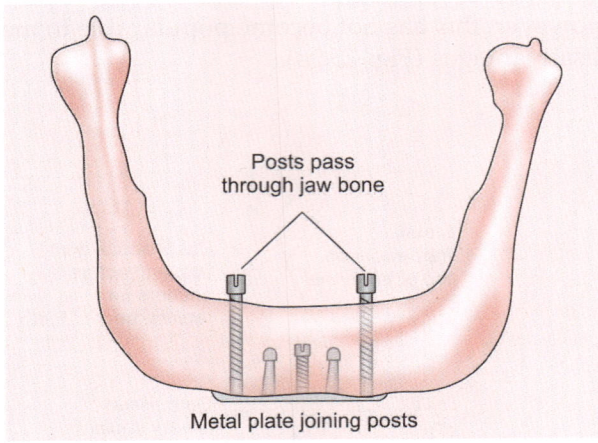

Fig. 25.2c: Transosteal implants

4. **Epithelial implants:** The implant designs are inserted into the oral mucosa with simple surgical techniques. This also has not become popular due to painful healing, etc.

BIOMECHANISM

Implants of various designs are fixed in a complicated manner, to the complex bone structures. Large dynamic masticating forces may cause stress concentrations at various points on the implant system. These unequal, differently oriented force distributions may cause **shifting, movements or displacements (micro motions)** of the implants. Long span prosthesis will have more complex mechanisms, **like bending, shearing,** etc. For absorption and distribution of these damaging forces and energies, **intra-mobile implants (IMZ)** have been developed. **This can accommodate movement of periodontal ligaments and act as shock-absorber.**

Interdependent factors for implantations (Fig. 25.3).

BRIEF OUTLINE OF IMPLANT PLACEMENT

Selection: The initial study of the clinical conditions of the patient is to be assessed thoroughly using radiographic diagnostic methods, medical and dental examinations for the selection of the line of procedure, type of the implants, materials and of proper designs.

Implantation: The next stage involves the **surgical procedure** in which the actual implant design is placed or fitted. After this, an interval of **3 months for mandibular and 6 months for maxillary implantation is required** for healing, osseointegration of the implant, and **to form a stable, immobile fixture component.**

A small secondary surgery is then conducted to uncover the part of the implant to be exposed to oral environment and a **healing cap** is fixed.

Restoration: Fixing the abutment is followed by the fabrication of the prosthesis fixed or removable partial denture, overdenture, or a single tooth. These prostheses are suitably fitted to the abutments.

Some implantation systems require only **one surgical intervention and the implant is immediately loaded** in contact with the oral environment.

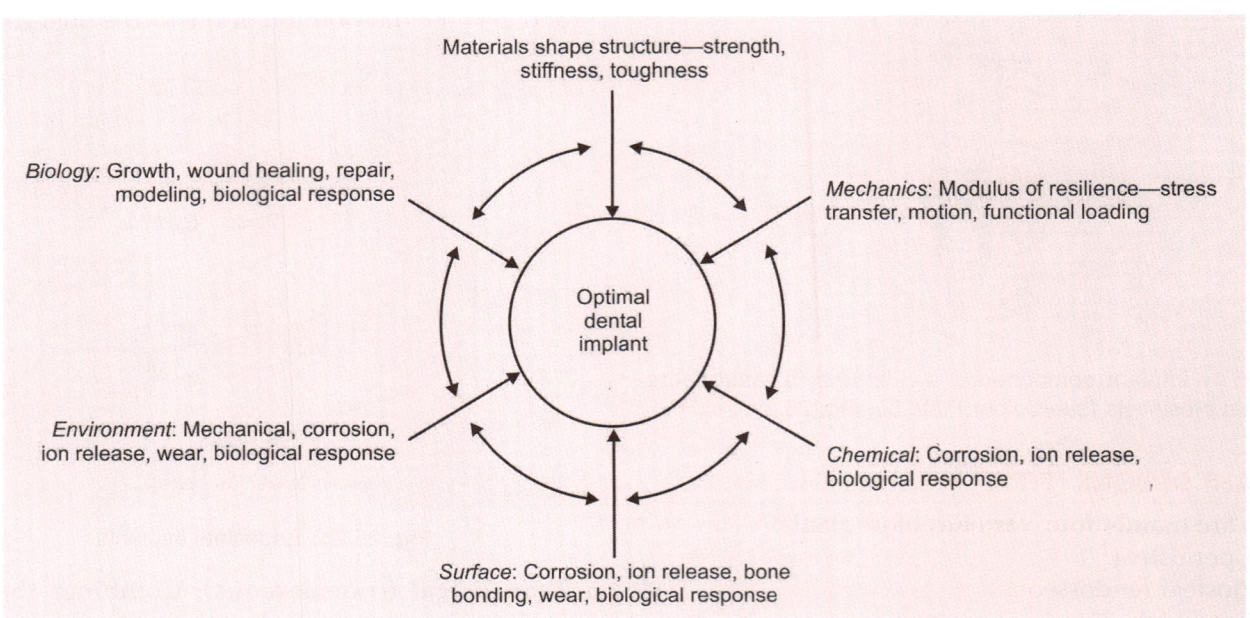

Fig. 25.3: Interdependent factors for successful implantation

MATERIALS USED FOR DENTAL IMPLANTS

Many metals, nonmetals (ceramics and resins) are used with certain surface modifications to get the desired properties.

Classification of Implant Materials

A. **Metallic:** Titanium alloys, special 18-8 stainless steel, cobalt–chromium alloys and gold alloys.

B. Surface modified or coated implants with HA or TCP

C. **Nonmetallic**
- Polymers and composites
- Inert ceramics—alumina, zirconia, and graphite.
- Bioactive ceramics—hydroxyapatite (HA), tricalcium phosphate (TCP) and bioglass.

A. Metallic Implant Materials

1. **Titanium and its alloys**
   Commercially pure titanium has four gradings: I, II, III, and IV, according to the oxygen and iron impurities. This is a metal of **low density**, 4.5 gm/cc, and high melting point (1668°C). To obtain better mechanical properties, CP-Ti is alloyed with Al, V, Mo, Zr, Nb, etc. to retain the allotropic ($\alpha + \beta$) phases. Titanium has a large oxygen affinity and forms the stable TiO_2-atomic layer on the surface. This **passivation imparts excellent corrosion resistance and bioactivity. Its low density, low modulus of elasticity and high yield strengths are the required properties for implant materials.** The **Ti-6Al-4V,** i.e. Ti (90%) + Al (6%) + V(4%) alloy, is one of the most suitable alloys. The recent titanium alloys have compositions of Ti + Nb (13%), + Zr (13%) and Ti + Mo (15%) + Nb (2.8%). Many other compositions also have been tried.

   The surface modifications can be done by increasing the area of the surface by several methods, like perforations, screw structures, anodizing, ion implantation, texturing and plasma coatings. These improve the interface strength by osseointegration. The mechanical properties, biocompatibility, corrosion resistance of titanium alloys are most suitable.

   Even though the casting procedure is very complex, the titanium alloys have **become the materials of choice.**

2. **Surgical grade 18-8 stainless steel.** This has a very low percentage of carbon (0.03%), which minimizes the sensitizations. The corrosion resistance is quite satisfactory. This does not form osseointegration and requires plasma or ceramic coatings. But as it contains 8% nickel, it is contraindicated in patients allergic to nickel.

3. **Chromium–cobalt alloys** are more stiffer than the 18-8 stainless steel. The alloy may contain, chromium about 17–30%, cobalt 60–65%, molybdenum ~ (5–10%) and a few trace materials.

   This has better mechanical properties, good corrosion resistance, and biocompatibility, but low ductility and malleability. The bioactivity is not satisfactory.

4. Many other alloys like gold alloys, palladium alloys are rarely used nowadays.

B. Surface Modified Implant Materials

To improve the biocompatibility, bioactivity, osseo-integrations and hence to form stronger **metal bone–tissue interface and greater stability of implants,** following methods are used:

- **Passivation:** A hard and **thicker** oxide layer on the base metal alloys improves the biocompatibility, as it prevents leaching of metal ions. This is done by:
  - **Immersing** the article in **40% nitric acid** for some time to form a thin oxide layer.
  - **Anodization,** i.e. bypassing electric current through the metal (as an anode). This gives better, thicker oxide layer.
  - **Ion implantation:** By bombarding high energy ions, which form the **Ti-N surface layer.**

- **Surface texturing:** Area of the surface of forming osseointegration is increased for better bond strength by:
  - Screw type design
  - Increasing surface roughness by sandblasting or such methods. The **endopore implants** have the large surface area, by producing large number of semispherical microstructures (*see* Colour Plate 36, Fig. 25.1).
  - **Surface coatings:** These are done by plasma spraying or coating with a thin layer of bioactive materials like tricalcium phosphate (TCP), hydroxyapatite (HA) to improve the osseointegration, i.e. bioactivity.

C. Nonmetallic Implant Materials

Ceramic implant materials
Ceramics are chemically inert materials of high compressive strength, low tensile and shear strengths and are very brittle. **Three varieties used in implants are inert ceramics, bioactive ceramics and bioglasses.**

Inert ceramics
Alumina (Al_2O_3) does not cause any release of ions as it is a very inert ceramic. This is used as a **gold standard** in implants. It has **high flexure strength (500 MPa) and**

rigidity. Modulus of elasticity is about 380,000 MPa and tensile strength 220 MPa. Similarly, **zirconia (ZrO₂)** also is very inert and has excellent flexure (700 MPa) and tensile strengths. These are highly biocompatible, **but not bioactive.**

Graphite: Carbon and its compound, silicon carbides is chemically inert and mechanical properties similar to dentin or bone. These help the transmission of biomechanical forces to the bone tissues. **It is used for metallic and ceramic implant coatings** (Table 25.1).

Bioactive ceramics

These undergo biointegration with the bone structure. Biointegration can be defined as the **benign acceptance of a foreign object by the living tissues**.

Hydroxyapatite (HA) and tricalcium phosphates (TCP): These are used as **bone-graft materials in granular or block forms,** which act as a skeleton for the formation of new bone structures. These HA and TCP or other forms of calcium phosphates, release Ca^{++} and PO_4^{+++} ions to the surrounding tissues, which cause biointegration to bone. But the strengths of bonds formed are much below, that of Al_2O_3.

The bond strength of coatings HA and TCP to other metals depends upon the amounts of the crystalline structure of the coating. The main purpose of coatings of this HA and TCP on metals like titanium alloys is to stimulate the adaptation to the bones by osseointegrations.

Bioglasses

This is a dense ceramic material containing **SiO_2, CaO, Na_2O, P_2O_5, MgO. The mechanism of bonding with bones** are complicated and can be explained in the following steps:

- The outer region of the bioglass dissolves releasing Ca, PO₄, Si and Na ions.
- Silica gel is formed on the surface, with large amounts of calcium and phosphorus ions released from bioglass and tissues.
  Once there is a sufficient concentration of phosphorus at the surface, osteoblasts begin to proliferate, thereby producing collagen fibrils.
- The collagen fibrils develop and get incorporated in the calcium phosphorus gel.
- **Calcium-phosphorus surface crystallizes locking the collagen fibrils.**

As bioglasses are very **brittle materials,** they are used as grafting materials for **ridge augmentation or bone defects** and not used in the case of stress bearing implants. It is also not used for coating metal implants.

Polymers and Composites—Implant Materials

These are quite tough materials and are fabricated as porous and solid structures. These are used **for**

Table 25.1 Mechanical properties of some implant materials

Implant materials	Condition	Density gm/cc	Compressive yield strength in MPa	Elongation %	Tensile strength MPa	Modulus of elasticity GPa
CP titanium	Grade 1	4.5	170	24	240	102
CP titanium	Grade 2	4.5	275	20	345	102
CP titanium	Grade 3	4.5	380	18	450	102
CP titanium	Grade 4	4.5	480	15	550	104
Ti-6Al-4V	–	4.4	860	10	930	113
Co-Cr-Mo	As-cast	8.0	450	8	700	240
18-8 Stainless steel	Annealed	8.0	190	40	490	200
	Cold worked	8.0	690	12	860	200
Al_2O_3	Polycrystalline	3.96	>400–550 (flexure)	0.1	220	380
ZrO_2	Y_2O_3-yttria stabilized	6.0	1,200 (flexure)	0.1	350	200
Cortical bone	–	0.7	–	1.0	140	18
Dentin	–	2.2	130	0.0	52	18.3
Enamel	–	2.8	250	0.0	10	84

augmentation, tissue attachments and coatings. These are also used as connectors inside implants to act as **shock absorbers**.

Polymethyl methacrylate resins were used as temporary implants to preserve the dissected space to receive the cobalt–chromium implant at a later stage. There were no adverse tissue reactions.

The use of polymers is now limited only to components. The intramobile (IMZ) implants are either plasma sprayed or hydroxyapatite-coated and incorporate **polyoxymethylene as intramobile element (IME).** This is placed in-between the implant and prosthesis **for stress relief and shock absorption.** This also initiates the biomechanical functions imitating the natural tooth structure, periodontal ligament and alveolar bone (Fig. 25.4).

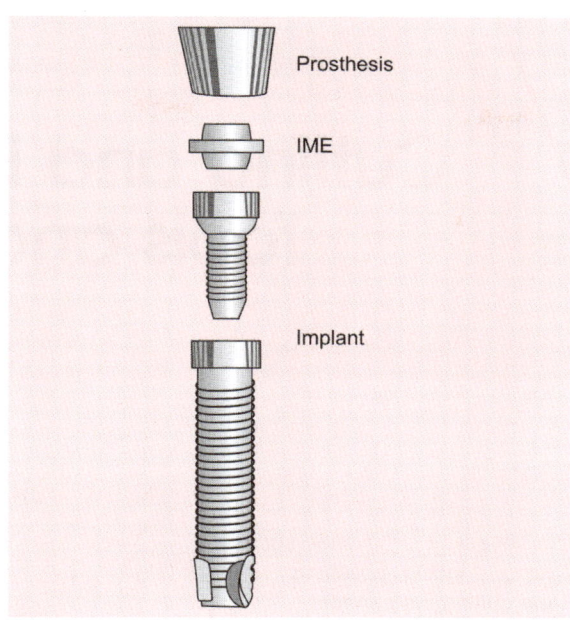

Fig. 25.4: Intramobile element shock absorber—components of the implants (*see* Colour Plate 36, Fig. 25.2)

MODEL QUESTIONS

I. Long Essays   (20 minutes each)

1. Describe the varieties of dental implants and the metallic implant materials used.
2. What is meant by dental implants? Give their requirements. Write a note on ceramic implant materials.

II. Short Essays   (10 minutes each)

1. Bioactivity of implant materials
2. Implant varieties and basic components
3. Metallic implant materials
4. Surface modifications of implants
5. Ceramic implant materials

III. Brief Answers   (5 minutes each)

1. Requirements of implant materials
2. Implant components
3. Implant varieties
4. Titanium implants
5. 18-8 stainless steel implants
6. Osseointegration
7. Polymer–composite implants
8. Coated implants
9. Bioglasses
10. Bioactive ceramics

CHAPTER 26

Cutting and Finishing Mechanics: Tools and Materials used

NECESSITY FOR FINISHING

Metallic and nonmetallic oral appliances and tooth restorations, including tooth structures, require suitable **finishing and polishing to obtain smooth glossy surfaces of minimum area** for:

- Maintaining better **oral hygiene**, by reducing the adhesion or collection of food debris and pathological bacteria, on the appliances and tooth surfaces.
- **Obtaining higher resistance to corrosion** of metallic appliances, and tooth decay by removing small pits and surface inhomogeneities (*refer* to Tarnish and Corrosion, Chapter 24).
- Obtaining higher fracture resistance, fatigue strength and service period.
- Reducing the irritations and abrasions of soft and hard tissues.
- Improving aesthetic qualities.

To obtain such surface qualities, **a series of operations or procedural steps** are to be conducted. The terms used for these are: **Bulk reduction, cutting, grinding (abrasion), polishing and finishing.** These are not well-defined, even though, the purpose is to get an excellent surface finish. The materials used should have higher hardness and toughness, than the cutting and abrasive surface of the work. Many sophisticated techniques are involved in the process.

The sequence of the procedural steps are, bulk reduction cutting, grinding (abrasion), polishing, and finishing to get desired shapes, sizes and smooth surfaces.

- The **bulk reduction** is the removal of unwanted large portion or material of the tooth or appliances, quickly. This is done by cutting and grinding instruments, like diamond points (and discs), carbide burs (and stones), steel burs and bonded other abrasives.
- **Cutting:** Removal of unwanted material for shaping is done by using **regularly shaped** instruments with sharp-edged blades.
- **Grinding:** Removal of unwanted material by wearing (or abrasion) using **irregularly shaped,** hard particles (abrasives) of various sizes, bonded in large numbers to rotating instruments, plane grinders, or emery papers.
- **Polishing and finishing:** Obtaining smooth glossy surface by minimum removal of material, by using very fine polishing agents, electropolishing, glazing or burnishing methods.

MECHANICS OF CUTTING, GRINDING AND POLISHING

- **Cutting:** Cutting is performed by **regular shaped, sharp bladed instruments** like chisels. When the blade is pressed hard into the surface of work or substrate material, producing stress more than elastic limit, nonelastic permanent notch (groove or scratching) is produced. If the blade is then sheared, the material in front of it fractures (as shear resistance is lower than compressive strengths) and then removed (Fig. 26.1a). At the same time, equal and opposite reactions act on the instrument blades, which therefore must have a higher elastic limit, strengths and abrasion resistance for longer service. Cutting instruments remove **small shavings** of surface material, when they operate at large speed, e.g. dental steel burs, saw-teeth, knife, blades, etc.

- **Grinding, abrading, wearing and corroding:** This is also breaking and removing unwanted material from the surface. The grinders (or abrasives) have large number of irregularly shaped hard particles (abrasives) with many sharp cutting edges, bonded or glued to papers, plastics, clothes or rotating instruments or sometimes lose powders as in sand blasting air abrasion. When the particles impinge, they break the surface structures and the fragments are removed (Figs 26.1b and c). Like cutting mechanism, grinding and abrasion operation is also unidirectional.

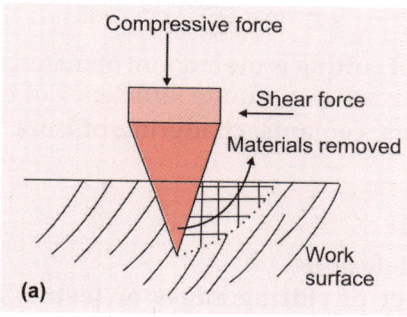

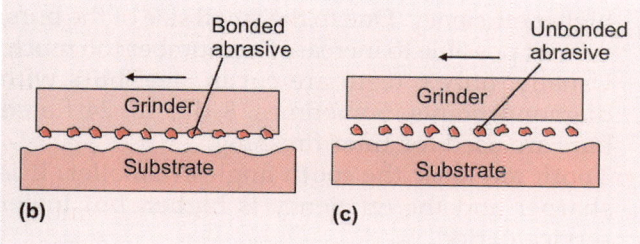

Figs 26.1a to c: (a) Cutting, (b) two body abrasions, (c) three body abrasions

- **Polishing (finishing):** Procedure of removal of fine grooves or scratches, left behind, on the surface during cutting and grinding steps. The very fine dust of hard materials (denoted as 0,00,000 or F, FF, FFF, etc.) are pressed and moved or rubbed on the surface to remove the crests of the scratches and fill the troughs left behind. This forms **microcrystalline (Beilby, Fig. 26.7)** layer, having glossy, smooth light reflecting surface.

Polishing procedure is **multidirectional and minimum material is removed from the surface.**

OTHER FINISHING METHODS

1. **Electropolishing:** As base metal, alloy castings have very hard surface, polishing is quite tedious. Also, it is quite difficult to polish the irregular surfaces of cast RPDs and FPDs. In such cases, the electropolishing method is preferred. The finished article is suspended in an electrolyte like a sulphuric acid solution, as the anode and a copper plate as the cathode. A small current of 2–5 Amps is passed through it for 1 or 2 hours. The projecting particles of the surface, get detached due to the higher potential difference and the surface become smooth and glossy.

2. **Glazing:** It is not possible to polish ceramic articles and composite resins easily. **Self-glazing** and **add-on glazing** techniques are used for ceramics. The glazed articles have better **surface integrity** (and no surface cracks), which improves its flexure strength from about 78 MPa (unglazed) to about 138 MPa. BisGMA composite resin matrix without or with small amounts of microfine fillers are applied on the composite resin restoration to obtain glazed surface.

BULK REDUCTION BY CUTTING

- **Hand cutting instruments:** These have one, two or more regular shaped sharp cutting edges or points at one or both ends of stainless steel shafts. The cutting blades have different shapes, sizes and fixed at different angles at the neck of shafts. These are denoted by instrument numbering methods. These are used for, removing carious debris, damaged enamel, cutting and leveling enamel surfaces, producing cavosurface bevels, etc. during cavity preparations. These are excavators, chisels, hoes, enamel hatchets, gingival marginal trimmers, scalars to remove calculus deposits, etc.

1st number—blade width in a tenth of mm
2nd number—blade length in mm
3rd number—the angle of the blade to the axis of the handle in 1/100 circle
4th number—the angle of the edge of the blade with shaft in 1/100 circle

These instruments are to be maintained, sterilized and properly sharpened conditions before use.

- **Rotary cutting instruments:** These are known as dental burs, which have small regular shaped sharp multiple cutting edges at the bur-head. This is connected through the neck (shank) to the steel shaft of the bur. The other end is connected through latch or friction grip to the rotating mechanisms such as mechanical gears, electrical and air pressure (air-rotor) systems, e.g. steel and carbide burs. Diamond points and separating wheels also can be called cutting instruments (Fig. 26.2).

Rotary grinding instruments do not have regular shaped cutting edges, but a large number of irregular shaped bonded abrasives of sharp cutting edges, such as diamond points, carbide, and stone grinders.

Classification of dental burs can be done according to

- Bur head material—diamond, tungsten carbide, silicon carbide, alumina, hardened steel.
- Bur head designs—number of teeth, rake angles positive, zero or negative.
- Bur head shapes—round, fissure (many shapes), inverted cone, end cutting, etc.
- Bur sizes—bur head diameters (mm)
- Attachments—straight (HP), contra-angle (RA), handpieces with latch or friction grips.
- Rotating mechanisms—electrical motor, compressed air-turbine system, with or without cooling water or air jets.
- Rotation speeds—low, medium, high, ultra-high, according to the substrate or cutting materials.
- Clinical uses—for cavity preparations, tooth preparation for crowns and bridges, removal of old amalgam restorations, finishing of restorations, trimming and finishing acrylic dentures, endodontic access opening reamers and files, oral surgery, implant procedures, etc.

Dental Steel Burs: Designs and Functions

These are prepared by shaping and cutting a steel blank using fine diamond points. Three parts of the burs are head, neck, and shank. Since the head size of bur is small, only 6, 8, 10 or 12 sharp blades (teeth) are designed as per **ADA specification No. 23**. The bur heads have mainly, **round, fissure and inverted cone shapes**. Other shapes are, **flame, peer, straight fissure, tapered fissure, cross cut fissures, end cutting,** etc. Round shaped bur is to cut a cylindrical cavity first, then fissure bur increases the cavity width and inverted cone flattens the floor and creates undercuts. Other shapes are chosen suitably for **adjusting cavo surface angles, etc**. The shank is connected to straight or contrangle hand pieces, through a **notch or latch fixing** or friction grip (*see* Colour Plate 37, Figs 26.1a and b).

The handpieces are connected to devices, to rotate the burs in the clockwise direction with controlled speed and load (pressure). These have small electric motors or compressed air turbines. Sometimes arrangements are provided for spraying or jets of water, air, or water + air mixture, to cool the cutting sites and remove the debris or clogging of bur heads (*see* colour plate 37, Figs 26.1a and b).

Terms and Definitions

1. **Tooth angle:** It is the angle between the front and flank or back of the tooth.
2. **Rake angle:** It is the angle between the radial line and the front of the tooth.
   If the radial line falls outside the tooth, i.e. radial line ahead of the front, rake angle is positive. If the radial line lies within the tooth (radial line behind the front), rake angle is negative, and when the radial line coincides with the front, rake angle is zero (Figs 26.2 and 26.3a to c).
3. **Clearance angle:** It is the angle between the flank and work surface.
4. The **flute** is the chip space in-between the adjacent teeth, i.e. back of one tooth and the front of the next tooth.
5. The **speed of cutting** is represented as linear speed of the tip of cutting edge of the bur, V cm/sec, or angular velocity ω radians/sec, or a number of rotations per second, n, i.e. 60 n rpm. These can be connected to the radius (r) of bur head as

$$V = r\omega = \frac{2\pi rn}{60} \text{ cm/sec}$$

6. The **rate of cutting** is the amount of material removed from the work per minute (efficiency of cutting).
7. **Lubricants, coolants, chattering of burs.**

FACTORS AFFECTING THE RATE OF CUTTING (EFFICIENCY)

1. **Bur head designs**
   - **Number of cutting edges or teeth:** Greater the number of teeth, faster is the rate of cutting, i.e. higher efficiency. Due to the small size of the burs, it is not possible to increase this number too much. Usually, only 6 teeth are cut in steel burs with diamond points. Sometimes, 8, 12, 16, 24 fluted burs are used for **finer** finishing.
   - **Tooth angle:** If the tooth angle is smaller, it is sharper and the efficiency is higher, but lower service period.
   - **Rake angle:** Positive rake angle reduces the tooth angle and increases efficiency. However, it has **shorter life** and also higher temperature rise (as the mass of the bur head becomes smaller). Zero rake angled bur has lower efficiency. Negative rake angle bur has the least efficiency. In industries, drills of positive rake angles are used. In dentistry negative rake angle burs are frequently used due to the following advantages:
     - Longer service period
     - Lower temperature rise, i.e. less damage to teeth

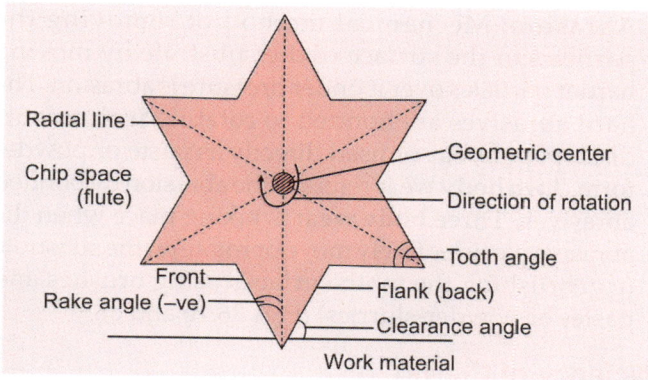

Fig. 26.2: Cross-section of bur head

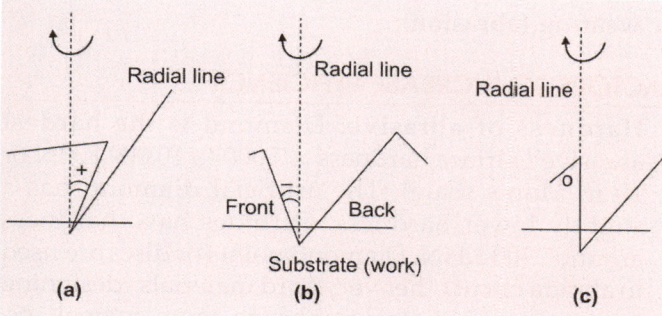

Figs 26.3a to c: (a) Positive, (b) negative, (c) zero rake angles

- Less clogging or blinding
- Easier to design

- **Clearance angle:** If the clearance angle is large, more debris get collected in the chip space, i.e **greater clogging or blinding** which decreases the efficiency of cutting. But if the clearance angle is too small, during rotation, back of teeth will rub the work, decreasing the speed and efficiency. Hence, the clearance angle should have some **optimum value** (Figs 26.2 and 26.4).

- **Run out:** If the different teeth have different lengths, their cutting edges will not lie in the circumference of the particular circle. Only a few teeth take part in cutting. Efficiency decreases and **chattering** vibration noise occurs (Fig. 26.5a).

- **Eccentricity:** If the center of rotation (CR) of bur head and the geometric center (G) do not **coincide** the bur will cut a bigger hole. The vibrations or **chattering** of bur takes place and efficiency decreases, and the bur will cut holes bigger than its diameter, causing chattering by eccentricity and seen-out (Fig. 26.5b).

2. The **speed of the bur:** As the speed of rotation increases, the rate of cutting or efficiency should increase. But as the speed increases the effectiveness of applied load decreases. Hence, above a certain speed, efficiency will not increase. For different cutting burs, e.g. diamond, carbides, steel, etc. the **optimum** speeds are different which also depend upon the material of the substrate, like alloys, enamel, dentists, etc.

3. **Load or pressure:** The efficiency should increase at higher loads or pressures. But when **pressure increases, the speed of rotation automatically decreases.** Hence, the efficiency becomes maximum only at a certain load or pressure. Different optimum loads are prescribed for different cutting instruments, substrate, materials and speeds.

4. **Removal of the debris** collected in the flute or chip-space of the burs will increase efficiency. A fine jet of water, air or their mixture is continuously sprayed to the site of cutting which removes clogging. This water spray also acts as a **coolant, reducing the temperature rise and protect the tooth.**

5. **Maintenance of the instrument:** Frequent application of suitable **lubricants, truing of bur, and conducting cutting intermittently** (not continuously) helps to increase the efficiency, life of the burs and reduce damage to the tooth structure.

WEARING, EROSIONS AND ABRASIONS

Wearing and abrasions are the procedures of removal of surface particles of substrate materials by physical and chemical attacks. Mainly these are done by:
1. Chemical erosion
2. Hard particle erosion
3. Abrasions

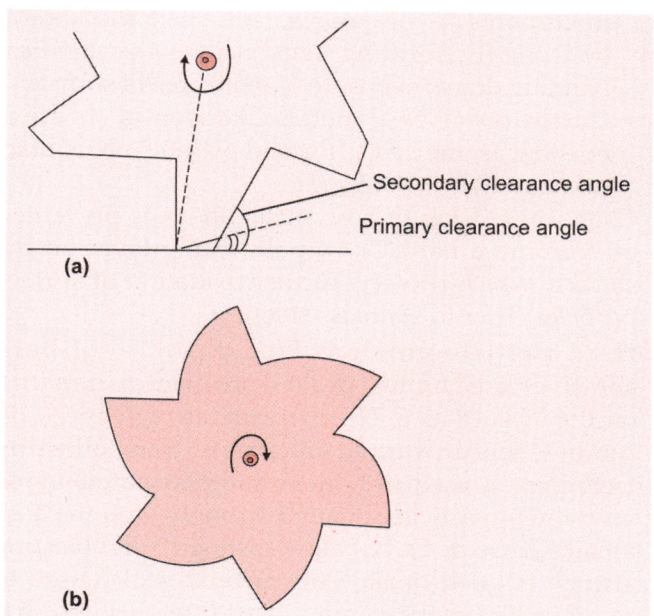

Figs 26.4a and b: (a) Bur with land, (b) bur with radial or zero clearance angle

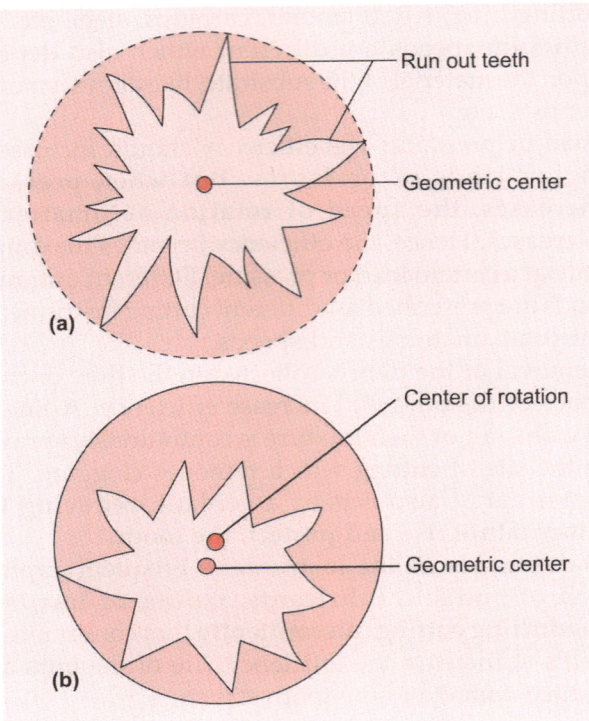

Figs 26.5a and b: (a) Run out structure, (b) eccentric rotation

1. **Chemical erosion:** Removal of material from the surface of the substrate by chemical reaction is known as chemical erosion. For example:
   - **Acid etching technique:** Phosphoric acid solution of about 10 to 37% is applied on the tooth enamel surface for a few seconds. The reaction products calcium phosphates can easily be flushed out leaving **micropores** on the surface. These help mechanical bonding (by forming 'tags') as well as chemical bonding due to exposure of more area of surface.
   - **Corrosion of** base metals like iron is chemical erosion, as, the Fe_2O_3, formed by moisture contact do not adhere to substrate.

   Chemical erosion of base metal alloys is prevented by forming a hard Cr_2O_3 passivating layer on the surface, which protects further oxidation of surface particles (*refer* to stainless steel).

2. **Hard particle erosion:** Fine particles of hard abrasives like alumina or sand are made to impinge on the surface as a jet or stream, at high speed; to remove the unwanted materials. Sand blasting technique is used to remove the phospate-bonded investment particles, bonded strongly with the base metal (Cr-Co or Cr-Ni) alloy castings. Sand blasting also gives good finish. This method is also used to roughen the metal-ceramic bonding surfaces. **Air abrasion technique** is used in the tooth cavity preparations. Attrition of teeth is also an example.

3. **Abrasion:** Mechanical method of removing the particles of the surface of the substrate by moving harder particles over it under pressure is abrasion. The hard abrasives are bonded to rotating instruments discs, papers, etc. or used directly as paste or powder form. **Two body wear** refers to the abrasion by bonded abrasives. **Three body wear** is taking place when the abrasive particles freely move or rotate on the substrate (e.g. brushing the tooth surfaces using brushes and pastes or powder-slurries) (Figs 26.1b and c).

Efficiency of Cutting

The efficiency of cutting or abrasion refers to the rate of removal of unwanted material from work by cutting or wearing (abrasion).

FACTORS TO INCREASE EFFICIENCY

- **Hardness of abrasive:** Diamond is the hardest abrasive (surface hardness = 7,000 to 10,000 KHN or 10 in Moh's scale). The artificial diamond has a slightly lower hardness. Carbides have hardness around 2500 KHN. Diamond points or discs are used to abrade or cut other very hard materials, designing tungsten carbide, steel bur heads, tooth enamel, etc.
- **Sharpness of the cutting edges:** During abrasion if the brittle abrasives fracture, more new particles of sharper cutting edges are formed which increase the efficiency.
- The **larger particle size** of abrasives increases efficiency
- **Attrition resistance** of abrasives should be higher
- **Nature of the surface** of the substrate: Brittle and softer materials can be abraded easily.
- **Speed and pressure** applied by abrasive, increase the rate of abrasion up to certain higher values. Too high speed, reduces pressure, and too high pressure reduces speed automatically and thereby decreasing efficiency.
- **Clogging or blinding** of the surface of the abrasive tools, by a collection of debris in-between the abrasive particles decrease the efficiency. Removal of the debris, by using **truing stones or water-air sprays** can increase efficiency.
- **Bond strength** of abrasives to abrasive tools, should be higher to reduce the dislodging of abrasive particles and increase the life of instruments.
- Proper maintenance of rotary instruments, by frequent lubrication, increases their efficiency.

ABRASIVE MATERIALS: PARTICLE SIZE—GRIT NUMBERS

The abrasive materials are crushed and selected according to their particle size or grits. The powder is passed through sieve meshes of definite sizes. For example, particles are said to be of 100 grit if they pass through a mesh with 100 spacing per inch length and are stopped from passing through the next number, i.e. 120 meshes/inch, i.e. average particle sizes are quoted sometimes. Usually, grit number varies from 40 (very coarse abrasive particles) even up to 2000 for very fine particle size, i.e. particle size about 0.6 mm down to 1 or 2 microns. They are graded as **super coarse, coarse, medium, fine, super fine, ultrafine (polishing pastes),** etc. These gradings are different for different abrasives, diamond, SiC, Al_2O_3, garnet, etc. and also vary according to the manufacturers. Approximate grit numbers for diamond abrasives are given in Table 26.1.

Abrasive Materials and Tools

Refer to appendix Table 14d, page 351. These hard abrasive materials are crushed into small sharp-edged irregularly shaped particles and bonded to abrasive tools of different types rotary and sometimes hand instruments. Some are available in nature, and some are synthetically prepared. Following are some of the **important abrasives and corresponding tools**.

1. **Diamond:** Naturally occurring diamond is the **hardest material,** with surface hardness, 7000–10000 KHN and number 10 in the Moh's scale. Synthetic diamond chips are prepared by heating graphite (in the presence of a catalyst) at high pressure (90 K bars) and high temperatures, about 2000°C. This has hardness slightly less than the natural diamond and **does not undergo attrition** during cutting any other materials.

Diamond points

The diamond chips are bonded through heat **resistant polyamide resinoids,** to metal shafts, **to form diamond points** of different shapes and sizes, wheels, separating thin metal discs fixed to rotating mandrill, or as fine metal polishing powder. The particles are dispersed, layer by layer on the steel shaft in decreasing sizes, to get maximum exposure. For better retention, these are **electroplated** with **nickel and also titanium nitride.**

Table 26.1	Approximate grit and particle size (microns) of diamond abrasives	
Grading	Grit numbers	Particle size microns (approx)
Extra coarse	150–100	120–180
Normal coarse	180–150	80–120
Fine	320–240	50–60
Superfine	600–400	15–40
Ultrafine	800–600	10–15
Polishing	9000–800	1–10

Different shapes are, round, barrel, flat end, beveled end, tapered, rounded end, tapered peer, donut, wheel, disc, etc.

Diamond points cut excellently and are used for brittle and hard materials like tooth enamel, base metal alloys, cutting and forming tungsten carbide and steel burs. The bur heads are properly ground for correct shapes and sizes, using truing stones, which also removes clogging. Diamond burs easily get clogged while cutting dentin.

Applications

- Grinding and shaping of base metal alloy castings (FPD, RPD), enamel cavities, cutting carbide and steel bur heads, etc.
- Finishing of ceramics before glazing, composite resins, glass ionomer cements, silver amalgam, etc.

2. **Carbides:** These are also **synthetically prepared hard abrasives** next to artificial diamonds.

Tungsten carbide is prepared by heating tungsten with carbon at high pressure and temperatures around 1500°C. The abrasive powder is **sintered and hot pressed** on the metal shaft, and the head is cut and shaped, with regular cutting edges like steel burs, into different shapes and sizes.

Tungsten carbide burs are used in case of very hard base metal and other alloy castings, reducing silver amalgam and composite resin restorations, etc.

Silicon carbide, carborundum grinding stones are very frequently used. Silicon carbide has a high hardness about 2400 KHN and prepared synthetically. This is bonded to metal shafts, rotating wheels (grinding stones), etc. through **vitreous glass-ceramic bonding.** The abrasive particles are mixed with ceramics powder slurry with water (or water-soluble glycerine) and **cold pressed** into a metal shanks to form different shapes and sizes such as round, cylindrical, barrel, pear, flame, inverted cone, discs, etc. Then it is fired, to fuse the ceramics. Sometimes the stones prepared are also rubber bonded to the shafts. These have green, grey or black colours. Silicon carbide abrasives bonded to, plastic or metal discs and even paper or cloth sheets (like sandpapers) are even available. These can be fitted to rotating mandrills.

3. **Aluminum oxide abrasives:** Fused alumina, i.e. pure Al_2O_3 is synthetically prepared by different processes and has high hardness 2100 KHN. White powder of different grit 120 to 2000 or particle sizes 1–50 microns are, vitreous ceramic bonded to shafts (white stones, and wheels), air-propelled grit (sandblasting) for cavity preparation and polishing as well

as coated abrasive. Finer particles of size 1–10 microns are used for polishing metals, and base metal alloys. The white stones are used for trimming hard base metal alloys, stainless steel, restorations, acrylic dentures, etc.

Vitreous bonded pink and ruby, coloured by adding chromium salts grinding stones of different particle sizes—coarse, medium, fine and superfine are also available.

Corundum is natural Al_2O_3 mineral abrasive used as stones, coated abrasives like **black emery paper.** It has a hardness about 2000 KHN.

The alumina abrasives may contaminate the metal alloys during abrasion or polishing. **Levigated alumina** is abrasive in the prophylaxis pastes used during scaling (removal of hard calculus deposits on the teeth). But this hard abrasive is **contra-indicated for dentifrices**.

4. **Garnet:** It is a mineral abrasive, **double silicate of aluminum and one of the metals** Fe, Co, Mg or Mn. It is quite hard (surface hardness, 1300 KHN) and brittle. When fractured, it breaks and forms chisel shaped sharp-edged new particles which increase efficiencies. This is used as coated abrasive on cloth or paper discs. This dark-coloured abrasive is used for grinding metal alloys or acrylic dentures.

5. **Zirconium silicate—zirconia** has a hardness about 1200 KHN. The white powder is used in coated abrasive discs or strips for tooth polishing (prophylaxis), polishing metals, restorations, etc.

6. **Silica abrasives:** Silica and quartz are commonly coated abrasives, **sandpapers** of different particle sizes. The grit size refers to the number of spaces per inch of a sieve mesh through which it passes. Sandpaper of 100 number refers to the average particle sizes which pass through the mesh having 100 spaces and do not pass through next, i.e. 120 numbers. These have a hardness about **800–820 KHN**, and are used for abrasion of softer metal alloys, acrylic dentures, alloy appliances, etc.

7. **Pumice and Tripoli:** These are abrasives as well as polishing agents. Pumice is a siliceous material of volcanic origin, and Tripoli is a kind of **porous rock.** These are powdered and used directly or as coated abrasives for metals and polishing agents for composite resins and acrylics. Their hardness is about 800–820 KHN, similar to sand.

8. **Kieselguhr** is also **siliceous remains of minute aquatic plants, diatoms**. Its hardness is about 800 KHN and is used as a mild abrasive. Larger particles—diatomaceous earth are used as fillers in hydrocolloid alginate impression materials.

9. **Cuttlebone or cuttlefish:** White-coloured **calcareous powder** obtained from the pulverized inner shell of a marine, **molluscs**. It is a coated abrasive used for polishing metals and amalgam restorations.

10. **Rouge:** Red iron oxide, incorporated into wax used for polishing soft metal alloys specially for **gold alloy** restorations.

11. **Chalk-French Chalk-calcite-whitening ($CaCO_3$):** This is a very mild polishing agent of low surface hardness about 130 KHN. Good polishing paste for final finishing direct filling gold, tooth enamel, amalgam and acrylics.

Abrasive Tools

The hard abrasive particles of different grits are used mainly in the following manner as:
- Bonded abrasives
- Coated abrasives
- Non-bonded abrasives
- Grinding stones and truing stones.

Bonded Abrasives

Hard abrasive particles of different sizes (coarse, medium, fine, superfine) are selected and bonded to the abrasive tools, like rotating wheels, separating discs, grinding stones of various sizes and shapes for easier applications. **During the use, abrasive particles should not be plucked out or undergo attrition.** Hence, extremely **strong bonding** is required to retain them. The following bonding methods are used.

- **Sintering:** The abrasive particles are heated to certain high temperatures, just below their melting points and **hot pressed** on abrasive tools, to form required shapes and sizes. The hot pressed powder, form a rigid solid structure (powder metallurgy technology). This is sometimes soldered to the rotating shaft. Tungsten carbide burs are sintered type and have the strongest bonding. These are cut and shaped as required later by using diamond points.

- **Vitreous bonding:** The abrasive particles are mixed with glass ceramic powder and binding liquid or water and **cold pressed** on the end of the shaft. It is then **fired** to fuse the glass-ceramic for bonding.

- **Resinoid bonding:** Abrasive particles like synthetic diamonds are bonded through heat resistant **resinoids like polyamides**. These are cold pressed and cured. The matrix is electroplated with **nickel and again with titanium nitride** for better retention.

- **Rubber bonding:** Abrasive particles are impregnated into latex or silicone rubbers cold or hot pressed into the shaft and cured. Rubber discs, cups, cylindrical, flame, bullet, etc. shaped rubber polishing tools are available for polishing composite resins, silver amalgam, etc. (*see* Colour Plate 39, Figs 26.7 and 26.8).

Coated Abrasives

Abrasive particles of various grits are mixed with **suitable adhesives and coated** to flexible metal discs, mylar cellulose, plastic discs or strips, papers or cloth sheets. Silicon carbide, emery papers, sandpapers, etc. are coated abrasives. Particle sizes are indicated by the grit size 40, 60, 80, 100, 120, etc. These can be fitted or attached to different types of mandrills and applied using lathes or handpieces for abrasion.

Nonbonded Abrasives

These are supplied in the powder form. Coarse and fine alumina or sand abrasives, propelled by air are used in sandblasting technique and sometimes for cavity preparations. Finer abrasive powders of diamond, alumina are used directly through paste or slurries in water or water-soluble glycerine for metal polishing. Pumice, Tripoli, zinc oxide, tin oxide, etc. are applied in this manner. Rouge (Fe_2O_3) is embedded in certain waxes and supplied in blocks for polishing the alloy appliances. This is convenient in the hygienic point of view, as there is no danger of inhaling **airborne silicon** particle (which may lead to **silicosis**).

Truing Stones

Very hard abrasives in the form of blocks (silicon carbides) are used as **truing or dressing stones**. It is used for shaping of grinding stones and **removes the clogging of debris**, specially in diamond burs. Arkansas stone is a hard abrasive sedimentary siliceous rock (from **Arkansas**). Its pieces are ground to small regular shapes and used for grinding.

Air Abrasion Technology

Precisely controlled high-pressure stream of Al_2O_3 (of particle size 25–30 microns) is delivered to remove the tooth enamel, dentin or unwanted restorations, **without producing heat or vibrations**. This method is becoming popular, instead of rotary devices, for, cavity preparations, removal of composite resins, stains, cleaning of teeth for adhesive bonding, roughening of surfaces for bonding, etc. in a shorter time (Fig. 26.6).

Application of Abrasive Tools

Gross reduction is first done using hand or rotary cutting instruments, like diamond discs, carbide burs or steel burs. The large unwanted portion is removed. **Next,** apply extra coarse-bonded abrasives for suitable shaping. **Next** use other bonded abrasives of suitable

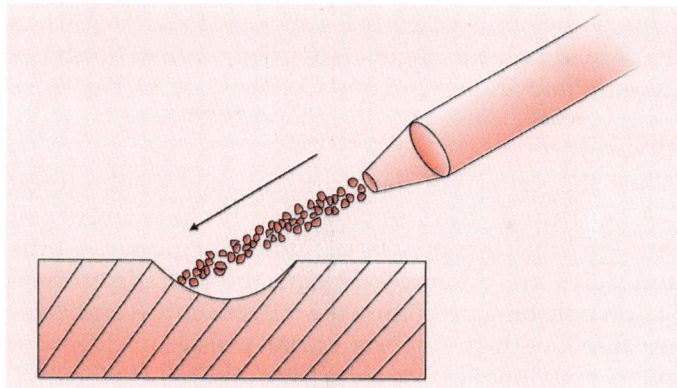

Fig. 26.6: Air abrasion

shape and grit or particle sizes one after the other, with decreasing sizes, coarse, medium, fine, etc.

Precautions to be observed are

- Selection of proper tools (size, shape).
- Selection of abrasives according to hardness and grit. Too hard or too coarse abrasives should not be used.
- **Unidirectional movement** or rotation of abrasives, rotary, or plane instruments.
- The directions of movement or rotation of abrasive tools must be away from the operator.
- Use mouth guards and vacuum suction type lathes to prevent inhaling the fine airborne silica abrasives (which may cause **silicosis**).
- Diamond tools are used with **water spray** for retention of diamond particles in the tool, remove clogging and to act as a coolant.
- Eccentrically mounted or burs with run-outs should not be used.
- **Application of high pressure or force, should not be done**, as the deep scratches produced once, cannot be easily removed during the succeeding polishing procedure.

POLISHING

The process of smoothening the surface of the substrate, after finishing with very fine abrasive tools, 24 or 32 fluted burs, without or with minimum removal of the surface material.

Very fine polishing agents (numbered as 0, 00, 000, or F, FF, FFF, etc.) are made into thick slurries in water or water-soluble glycerine. This is then applied on the work through cotton, felt, chamois leather, etc. or rotating cotton or felt buffs. Polishing is done by **multidirectional** movement of polishing agents.

The sequence of polishing is, first using fine powder of harder polishing agent. Work is then washed and polished with finer polishing powder. Again washed to remove the abrasive particles sticking to surface. Then finest mild polishing agent is applied for final finish (*see* Colour Plate 37, Fig. 26.2 and Colour Plate 39, Fig. 26.9).

Microcrystalline: Beilby Layer

When the surface of the work, finished by the finest (24, 30 fluted) burs or abrasive tools is observed through a microscope, a large number of grooves—**hills and dales** are observed. During the multidirectional (vales) polishing procedure the hills are cut off and dales are filled with the debris under pressure to form a microcrystalline surface layer (first observed by Beilby). This glossy surface can reflect incident light like a mirror (Fig. 26.7).

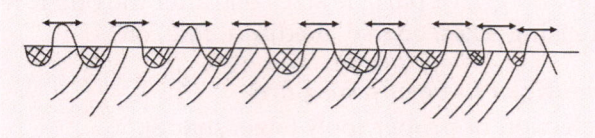

Fig. 26.7: Polishing—microcyrstalline layer

Applications

- Very fine diamond or alumina powders of particle size 1 to 5 microns are used for metal polishing.
- Rouge (Fe_2O_3) powder, embedded in wax is the best polishing agent for gold alloys as well as chrome cobalt alloy castings.
- Zirconium silicate, pumice, etc. are used for polishing composite resins, and silver amalgam. ZnO, SnO, etc. are also used for polishing amalgam restorations.
- Acrylic dentures can be first polished with pumice and finally with French chalk.
- Dentifrices should contain only mild abrasive or polishing agents.

GLAZING

It is another method of final finishing to obtain glossy, light reflecting shining surfaces of ceramic restorations. **Self and add-on glazing technics** are used. The finished article is heated quickly (or coated with thin layer of low fusing ceramic), so that surface layer melts, spreads and forms glazed surface. Ceramics have very low flexture strength (78–80 MPa), which becomes almost double (140 MPa) on glazing due to the removal of surface microcracks. Glaze composites without or with small amounts of micro fillers are applied on large particle composite restorations, to obtain better aesthetics.

FINISHING AND POLISHING OF RESTORATIONS

1. **Composite resin:** This has hard silica filler particles embedded in a much softer resin matrix. Any attempt to abrade or polish will **pluck out hard fillers** and

easily wear out the soft matrix. Even though it has surface hardness ranging from about 25 to 60 KHN, it undergoes abrasion and wears, easily, if the particle sizes are bigger. Only the microfilled composites can be polished. Hence, selection of abrasives and polishing agents and the sequential procedures should be carefully followed:
   - **Contouring** is done with 12 fluted carbide burs or diamond points
   - **Finishing** is done with 16–32 fluted carbide burs
   - **Polishing** is done with polishing pastes of alumina or diamond
   - Final polishing is done with extra-fine diamond or alumina pastes, silicon carbide incorporated rubber polishing discs or cups.
   - In case of large particle or hybrid composites, after contouring **glaze composites** can be applied. The glaze composite has no or very fine fillers of small amounts.

2. **Silver amalgam**
   - **After hardening** sufficiently, carefully carving is done without pulling from the margin, using diamond, Wartz or Hollenbeck carvers to obtain the occlusal anatomy.
   - Careful burnishing is done with ball burnisher without shifting mercury rich thin-mix to margins.
   - Smoothening is done with cotton pledget or rubber polishing cups.
   - Final polishing is delayed by 24 hours in case of low copper alloys and 1 or 2 hours for high copper single composition alloys. Zinc oxide, pumice, rouge, etc. very fine polishing powder are made into a thick slurry and applied. Dry powder should not be used as it may raise the temperature.

   Note: Very fine shining smooth surface has no better advantages.

3. **Gold alloys:** Heat treatments can increase the surface hardness, above **120 KHN** even up to **240 or 300 KHN**. Initial contouring is done with silicon carbide green stones, finishing with pink alumina stone, rubber cups, wheels or points.

   Final polishing is done with rouge (Fe_2O_3) cake or pumice paste.

4. **Acrylics:** These have comparatively low surface hardness, e.g. 16–20 KHN and can easily be abraded and polished with mild abrasives.
   - Contouring with carbide burs or sandpaper
   - Remove the scratches with rubber points
   - Polish with pumice paste using the felt wheel or prophy cups
   - Final polishing with French chalk paste in alcohol or water.

During the procedure, if the temperature rises, it may disturb and damage polymer structure.

5. **Ceramics:** Surface hardness is about **460 KHN.** Since it is very brittle material, careful finishing is required to remove surface cracks and pores before glazing.
   - Contouring is done with diamond points and discs of silicon carbide (heatless) green stones
   - Finishing with white alumina stones, or abrasive impregnated rubber discs, cups or points
   - Polishing is done with fine abrasives incorporated rubber discs or cups or diamond pastes
   - Self or overglazing is done finally.

During the procedures, temperature rise should be reduced by **intermittent operation in the presence of water coolant spray.**

DENTIFRICES

These teeth cleaning materials are supplied as a **powder, paste or gel forms.** These are applied on the teeth surface, through nylon bristle brushes for the **following purposes:**
- Removal of food debris, plaque, and stained pellicles by abrasives, with the aid of surface tension reducing agents.
- Polishing the enamel for better aesthetics.
- Removal of microorganisms and stains to reduce caries.
- Application of therapeutic materials, like, fluorides, tartar controlling agents, desensitizing agents, etc.

POWDER SYSTEM

This has not become popular as it is difficult to apply to all the areas, such as the interdental spaces. The powder mainly contains mild abrasives, calcium phosphate, sodium bicarbonate, hydrated alumina or silica, etc. In addition, it has detergents (1–6%) and small amounts colouring and flavouring materials.

PASTE OR GEL SYSTEMS

These contain the following ingredients (Table 26.2).

ABRASIVITY OF DENTIFRICES

This can be defined as its ability to clean the tooth surface by removing the debris. Standard method of measuring abrasivity of dentifrices is suggested by ADA and ISO. This is done by brushing dentin or enamel specimens irradiated by radioactive phosphorous ^{32}P with the particular abrasives, at definite pressure, speed and time or frequency of brushing rate. The amount of radioactive ^{32}P released was measured by particle counters and multiplied by 1000. The number should be between 200 and 250 and should not exceed for dentin.

Tooth enamel, dentin, cementum and hard deposit (calculus) have surface hardnesses of about 350, 70, 40 and 80 KHN respectively. Accordingly, the enamel has highest abrasive resistance. Dentifrices, therefore, **should not contain very hard abrasives like levigated or hydrated alumina or silica** as there is a danger of abrasion of tooth materials.

Factors affecting the dentifrice abrasivity are

- **Extra oral factors**
  - Hardness and size of abrasive particles
  - Percentage of abrasive content
  - Type of toothbrushes, brushing methods and frequency of brushing
- **Intraoral factors**
  - Nature of saliva and its content
  - Hygienic condition, i.e. presence of hard deposits
  - Presence of restorative materials, orthodontic and prosthetic appliances
  - Xerostomia induced by drugs, radiation therapy and salivary gland pathology
  - Exposure of dentin and dental root surfaces.

- **Effect of toothbrushes:** Even though bristle stiffness has no much effect, the flexible bristles have been found to be more effective in cleaning. This is perhaps due to flexibility and ability to reach and carry the dentifrices to the interdental surfaces. **More importance is to be laid in the selection of dentifrices, method and frequency of brushing for maintaining hygiene.**

Prophylactic Materials

Some hard deposits such as calculus, and soft deposits in the interdental spaces are formed on the tooth surface, due to the adhesion of food debris, and gradually increase. These cannot be removed by the usual dentifrice brushing methods, as the ordinary dentifrices contain only mild abrasives. Harder abrasives are contraindicated for dentifrices.

The prophylactic pastes or powders contain harder abrasives, like levigated **alumina, zirconium silicate, fine silica, or pumice.** These are applied by a trained dental hygienist (after scaling procedure) through rubber cups or bristle brushes, connected to rotary instruments, once in few months according to the clinical conditions. These remove all hard deposits and polish the teeth to reduce further adhesion by a rough surface.

This also can be done by air abrasion method. Fine abrasive prophy powders, like silica, sodium carbonate, etc. are carried through a stream of air or water jet in EVA systems prophy jet, very carefully. The jet has to impinge, at about 45° to the surface (Fig. 26.6).

Table 26.2	The composition of dentifrices—paste or gel forms		
Ingredients	Compositions wt%	Materials	Functions
Abrasives	20–55	CaCO₃, CaH₂PO₄ (2H₂O), NaHCO₃, hydrated alumina or silica or mixture of these	Removal of debris, plaque, calculus and polishing
Detergent	1–2	Sodium lauryl sulphate	Reduces surface tension for assisting the removal of debris
Humectant	20–35	Sorbitol, glycerine	To retain moisture content
Water	15–25	Deionized water	Paste former
Binder	3	Carrageenan	Binder of liquid and solid parts to get homogeneity
Tartar control agent	0–1	Disodium pyrophosphate, tetrasodium potassium pyrophosphate	Prevents calculus formation
Fluorides	0–1	NaF, SnF, NaF (PO₄)	Prevent caries
Desensitizers	0–5	Potassium nitrate, strontium chloride	Prevents occlusion of dentinal tubules
Colour and flavours	Small amounts		Appearance and flavour

This method is also indicated to remove the hard stains due to certain drugs, tobacco, caffeine, tea, etc. But a little careless application may injure the soft tissues and cause inflammations.

MODEL QUESTIONS

I. Long Essays   (20 minutes each)

1. Explain the mechanisms of cutting, grinding and polishing. Describe the various factors affecting the rate of cutting of steel burs.
2. Distinguish between abrasion and polishing. Explain bonded and nonbonded abrasives with examples and applications. Write a note on the efficiency of abrasive agents.

II. Short Essays   (10 minutes each)

1. Steel bur designs, functions and the efficiency of cutting

2. Dentifrices
3. Diamond points and discs
4. Carbide burs
5. Polishing
6. Finishing of dental restorations
7. Abrasive agents

III. Brief Answers   (5 minutes each)

1. Rake angles and clearance angles
2. Speed and load of steel burs
3. Dental abrasive stones
4. Truing stone
5. Finishing of amalgam restorations
6. Polishing of acrylic dentures
7. Microcrystalline (Beilby) layer
8. Air abrasion technology
9. Prophylactic paste
10. Instrument numbering

Appendix

Contents	Page numbers

ADA SPECIFICATION NUMBERS

(American National Standards Institute (ANSI) on dental materials, instruments and equipment. Date of specification or latest revision, addendum or reafirmation

No.	Title	Year	No.	Title	Year
1	Alloy for dental amalgam	1993	48.	Dental activator, disclosing and transillumination devices	1989
2	Gypsum-bonded casting investment for dental gold alloy	1995	49*	Analgesia equipment	—
3	Dental impression compound	1994	53*	Crown and bridge plastics	—
4	Dental inlay casting wax	1994	54	Double-pointed, parenteral, single use needles in dentistry	1986
5	Dental casting alloys	1988	55	Dispensers of alloy and mercury for dental amalgam	1992
6	Dental mercury	1995	57	Endodontic filling materials	1993
7	Dental wrought gold wire alloy	1989	58	Root canal files, type H (Hedstrom)	1988
8	Zinc phosphate cement	1935	59	Portable steam sterilizers for use in dentistry	1992
11	Dental agar impression material	1995	62*	Dental abrasive pastes	—
12	Denture base resins	1987	63	Rasps and barbed broaches	1989
13	Denture cold-curing repair resin	1897	64	Dental explorers	1994
14	Dental base metal casting alloys	1989	65	Low speed hand pieces	—
15	Synthetic resin teeth	1992	69	Dental ceramic	1991
16	Dental impression paste	1989	70*	Dental X-ray protective aprons and accessory devices	—
17	Denture base temporary relining resin	1990	71	Root canal filling condensers and spreaders	1995
18	Dental alginate impression material	1992	73	Dental absorbent points	1993
19	Elastomeric dental impression material	1993	74*	Dental stools	—
20	Dental duplicating material	1995	75*	Resilient denture liners	—
22	Intraoral dental radiographic film	1972	76	Non-sterile latex gloves for dentistry	1991
23	Dental excavating burs	1993	77*	Stiffness of tuffed area of tooth brushes	—
24	Dental baseplate wax	1991	78	Dental obturating points	1994
25	Dental gypsum products	1989	79*	Dental vacuum pumps	—
26	Dental X-ray equipment and accessory devices	1991	80	Color stability test procedure	1989
27	Direct filling resins	1993	81*	Magnets and keepers used for intraoral and extraoral retainers for prosthetic restorations	—
28	Endodontic files and reamers	1996	82*	Combined reversible/irreversible hydrocolloid impression materials	—
29	Hand instruments	1994			
30	Zinc oxide eugenol and non-eugenol cements	1996	85*	Prophy angles	—
32	Orthodontic wires not containing precious metals	1989	87*	Impression trays	—
33	Dental terminologies	1990	88*	Dental brazing alloys	—
34	Aspirating syringes	1987	89*	Dental operating lights	—
35*	High speed air-driven hand pieces		90*	Dental rubber dam	—
36*	Diamond rotary cutting instruments		91*	Ethyl silicate investments	—
37	Dental abrasive powders	1994	92*	Refractory die materials	—
38	Metal-ceramic systems	1991	93*	Soldering investments	—
39	Pit and fissure sealants	1992	94*	Dental compressed air quality	—
40A*	Unalloyed titanium for dental implants	—	95	Root canal enlargers	1996
40B*	Cast cobalt-chromium-molybdenum alloys for dental implants	—	96	Dental water-based cements	1994
41	Recommended standard practices for biological evaluation of dental materials	1989	97*	Corrosion	—
			98*	Designation system for teeth and areas of the oral cavity	—
42*	Phosphate-bonded investments	—	99*	Athletic mouth protector materials	—
43	Electricity powered dental amalgamators	1995			
44	Dental electrosurgical equipment	1986			
45*	Dental porcelain teeth	—			
46	Dental chairs	1996			
47	Dental units	1996			

* Year not specified

Table 1: Periodic chart of elements

Category labels: Light metals · Heavy metals · Nonmetals · Inert gases · High melting · Brittle · Ductile · Low melting · Noble

Period	1	2	3	4	5	6	7	8	9	10	11	12	13	14	15	16	17	18
1	1 H 1.00794																	2 He 4.002602
2	3 Li 6.941	4 Be 9.012182											5 B 10.811	6 C 12.011	7 N 14.00674	8 O 15.9994	9 F 18.984032	10 Ne 20.1797
3	11 Na 22.989768	12 Mg 24.3050											13 Al 26.981539	14 Si 28.0855	15 P 30.973762	16 S 32.066	17 Cl 35.4527	18 Ar 39.948
4	19 J 39.0983	20 Ca 40.078	21 Sc 44.955910	22 Ti 47.88	23 V 50.9415	24 Cr 51.9961	25 Mn 54.93805	26 Fe 55.847	27 Co 58.93320	28 Ni 58.6934	29 Cu 63.546	30 Zn 65.39	31 Ga 59.72	32 Ge 72.61	33 As 74.92159	34 Se 78.96	35 Gr 79.904	36 Kr 83.80
5	37 Rb 85.4678	38 Sr 87.62	39 Y 88.90585	40 Zr 91.224	41 Nb 92.90638	42 Mo 95.94	43 Tc (98.9063)	44 Ru 101.107	45 Rh 102.90550	46 Pd 106.42	47 Ag 107.8682	48 Cd 112.411	49 In 114.818	50 Sn 118.710	51 Sb 121.757	52 Te 127.60	53 I 126.90447	54 Xe 131.29
6	55 Cs 132.90543	56 Ba 137.327	57 La 138.9055	72 Hf 178.49	73 Ta 180.9479	74 W 183.84	75 Re 186.207	76 Os 190.23	77 Ir 192.22	78 Pt 195.08	79 Au 196.96654	80 Hg 200.59	81 Tl 204.3833	82 Pb 207.2	83 Bi 208.98037	84 Po (209.9828)	85 At (209.9871)[a]	86 Rn (222.0176)[a]
7	87 Fr (223.0197)[b]	88 Ra (226.0254)[b]	89 ÷Ac (227.0278)[a]	104 ?[b] (261)[a]	105 Ha[b] (262.114)[a]													

Rare earth elements — * Lanthanoid series

58 Ce 140.115	59 Pr 140.90765	60 Nd 144.24	61 Pm 144.9127	62 Sm 150.36	63 Eu 151.965	64 Gd 157.25	65 Tb 158.92534	66 Dy 162.50	67 Ho 164.93032	68 Er 167.26	69 Tm 168.93421	70 Yb 173.04	71 Lu 174.967

Radioactive elements — * Actinoid series

90 Th 232.0381	91 Pa (231.03588)[a]	92 U 238.0508	93 Np (237.0482)[a]	94 Pu (244.0642)[a]	95 Am (243.0614)[a]	96 Cm (247.0703)[a]	97 Bk (247.0703)[a]	98 Cf (251.0796)[a]	99 Es (252.083)[a]	100 Fm (257.0951)[a]	101 Md (256.094)[a]	102 No (259.1009)[a]	103 Lr (260.11)

Table 2: Physical constants of alloy forming elements in dentistry

Element	Unit cell	Symbol	Atomic weight	Melting point (°C)	Boiling point (°C)	Density (g/cm³)	Linear coefficient of thermal expansion (ppm/°C)
Aluminium	FCC	Al	26.98	660.2	2450	2.70	23.6
Antimony	–	Sb	121.75	630.5	1380	6.62	10.8
Bismuth	Rhombo-hedral	Bi	208.98	271.3	1560	9.80	13.3
Cadmium	HCP	Cd	112.40	320.9	765	8.37	29.3
Carbon		C	12.01	3700.0	4830	2.22	6.0
Chromium	BCC	Cr	52.00	1875.0	2665	7.19	6.2
Cobalt	BCC	Co	58.93	1495.0	2900	8.85	13.8
Copper	FCC	Cu	63.54	1083.0	2595	8.96	16.5
Gold	FCC	Au	196.97	1063.0	2970	19.32	14.2
Indium	Tetra-gonal	In	114.82	156.2	2000	7.31	33.0
Iridium	FCC	Ir	192.2	2454.0	5300	22.5	6.8
Iron	BCC	Fe	55.85	1527.0	3000	7.87	12.3
Lead	FCC	Pb	207.19	327.4	1725	11.34	29.3
Magnesium	HCP	Mg	24.31	650.0	1107	1.74	25.2
Mercury	Rhombo-hedral	Hg	200.59	−38.87	357	13.55	40.0
Molybdenum	BCC	Mo	95.94	2610.0	5560	10.22	4.9
Nickel	FCC	Ni	58.71	1453.0	2730	8.90	13.3
Palladium	FCC	Pd	106.4	1552.0	3980	12.02	11.8
Platinum	FCC	Pt	195.09	1769.0	4530	21.45	8.9
Rhodium	FCC	Rh	102.91	1966.0	4500	12.44	8.3
Silicon	Cubic	Si	28.09	1410.0	2480	2.33	7.3
Silver	FCC	Ag	107.87	960.8	2216	10.49	19.7
Tantalum	BCC	Ta	180.95	2996.0	5425	16.6	6.5
Tin	FCC, BCT	Sn	118.69	231.9	2270	7.298	23.0
Titanium	HCP	Ti	47.90	1668.0	3260	4.51	8.5
Tungsten	BCC	W	183.85	3410.0	5930	19.3	4.6
Zinc	HCP	Zn	65.37	420.0	906	7.133	39.7

Table 3: Bond strengths

Bond strength is measured by the shear or tensile stresses required to debond the adhesive from the substrate (enamel or dentin) or the adherend restorations

Substrate	Adhesive bonding agent	Adherend restorative	Shear bond strength in MPa
Enamel	Enamel bonding system	Composite	18–22
Enamel	Enamel bonding system	Orthodontic bracket	18–20
Enamel	Amalgam bond system	Composite	10–12
Enamel	Amalgam bond system	Amalgam	2–6
Enamel	No smear layer	Traditional GIC	8–12
Dentin	Dentin bonding system	composite	22–35
Dentin	BPDM	VLC glass ionomer	28
Dentin	No smear layer	VLC glass ionomer	10–12

Substrate	Adhesive bonding agent restorations	Adherend	Tensile bond strength in MPa
Enamel (etched)	HEMA/BisGMA	Fine composite resins	23
Enamel (etched)	—	Fine composite resins	17–20
Enamel (etched)	—	Microfine composite	10
Enamel (etched)	—	Adhesive resin cement	15
Enamel (etched)	—	Conventional resin cement	10
Enamel		Glass ionomer	5
Dentin	Polyurethane	Composite resins	1–6
Dentin	Polyacrylic acid	Composite resins	2–4
Dentin	Organic phosphonates	Composite resins	3–10
Dentin	4-META	Composite resins	3–7
Dentin	HEMA + Glutaraldehyde	Composite resins	11–18
Dentin	NPG + GMA/PMDM	Composite resins	2–12
Dentin	Maleic acid/HEMA + HEMA/BisGMA	Composite resins	23
Dentin	—	Glass ionomer	4
Dentin	—	Zinc polycarboxylate	1–4
Dentin	—	Adhesive resin cement	4
Dentin	—	Conventional resin cement	0

Table 4: Contact angles

It is the angle made by the tangent drawn at the point of contact between the solid-liquid, and the solid surface. Lower the value, better is the wettability and adhesion.

Contact materials		Angle of
Solid phase	Liquid phase	contact in degrees (°)
Impression materials		
Polysulphides	Water	42
Polysulphides	Stone mix	76–82
Polyethers	Water	42–44
Polyethers	Stone mix	50–90
Polysilicones (condn)	Water	80–102
Polysilicones	Stone mix	90
Polysilicones (addn) (hydrophobic)	Water	60–104
"	Stone mix	70–98
Polysilicone hydrophilic	Water	53
Polymer resins		
Polymethyl methacrylate	Water	62–73
Polymethyl cyanoacrylate	Water	57
Polystyrene	Water	66
Teflon	Water	110
Paraffin wax	Water	109
Denture resins		
PMMA (acrylic)	Water	75
PMMA (acrylic)	**Saliva**	**73**
PMMA (acrylic)	Alcohol	0
Polystyrene	Water	86
	Saliva	**79**
Restoratives		
Amalgam	Water	77
Acrylic Type I	Water	38
Composite resins	Water	51
Silicate cement	Water	12
Glass	Water	14
Tooth enamel	Bonding agents	0
Tooth enamel	Fluoride solutions	0
Tooth enamel	Fluoride gels	30–38
Tooth enamel	Pit and fissure sealants	0–28
Mercury		
Silver amalgam alloy g	Mercury	145°
Silver-Cu eutectic	Mercury	138
Disperse alloy	Mercury	145
Silver oxides	Mercury	130–135
Tin oxides	Mercury	107–130
Glass	Mercury	132
Metal alloys of PFM	**Porcelain liquids**	**125–140**

Table 5: Critical surface tension (Tc)

It is the surface tension of a liquid which would completely wet the given solid surface. Higher values indicate better wettability.

Materials	Product	Tc (dynes/cm)
Impression materials		
Polyether	Impregum	28
Polysilicone (condn)	Xentopren	14
Polysilicone (addn)	Express (hydrophilic)	54
	President	21
	Provil	20
Polymer resins		
Polymethyl methacrylate	—	39
Polytetrafluoroethylene	Teflon	18
Polystyrene	—	33–43
Polyethylene	—	31–33
Polyurethane	—	20–35
Paraffin	—	22–26
Metals and alloys		
Silver amalgam	—	48
Co-Cr-Mo (polished)	Vitallium	22
Co-Cr-Mo (plasma cleaned)	Vitallium	>72
Gold		57
Glass	Pyrex	170
Tooth enamel at 23°C, 50% relative humidity		**38–40**
Tooth enamel at 37°C, 100% relative humidity		**31–5**

Table 6: Ductility: Elongation percent

It is the property of a material to undergo permanent deformation by tensile stressing and is measured by the percentage elongation per unit length, when a specimen of 5 cm, gauge length is fractured by tensile force.

Materials		Ductility%/Percentage elongation	
Casting alloys	High noble	Noble	ADA Spn No. 5 elongation%
Type I	36	38	>18
Type II	38	30	>10
Type III softened	39	30	>5
Type III hardened	19	13	—
Type IV softened	35	10	>3
Type IV hardened	7	6	—

Other materials	Elongation%	Other materials	Elongation%
Metals and alloys		**Impression materials**	
HN metal-ceramics	20	Agar	
N metal-ceramics	10–34	Alginate (impression)	38
Pd-based alloys	6–30	**Resilient liners**	
Ag-based alloys	8–25	Silicones	325
Cp titanium (β)	13	**Polyphosphozene**	
Ti + 6Al + 4V	5	Fluoroelastomer	240
Co-Cr-M	1–6	**Maxillofacial**	
Ni-Cr	4–30	Silicon rubber	130–580
Fe-Cr	8–10	Polyurethane	224
18-8 stainless steel (annealed)	40	**Mouth protector**	
18-8 stainless steel (cold worked)	12	Polyvinyl acetate-polyethylene (PVA-PE) 1000	
PGP wire	14–15		
PSC wire	16–24		
Pure gold 99.94%	60		
Nickel	8–20		
Cobalt	6–15		
cpTi (α)	10–20		

Table 7: Dynamic elastic modulus (ED)

It is the ratio of stress to strain to small cyclic deformations at a given frequency at a particular stress in the static stress–strain graph.

	Product	ED in MPa	Measured at temperature T°C
Maxillofacial material			
Polyurethane	Dermathane	3.06	37°C
Polyvinyl chloride	Sartomer resin	2.51	37°C
Polysilicone rubber	Silastic (382)	3.00	37°C
Polysilicone rubber	Silastic (399)	3.82	37°C
Restorative composite resins			
Anterior	Silver	2569	40°C
Anterior	Silver	2562	40°C
Posterior	P10	8396	40°C
	P15	9645	40°C
	Profile	7911	40°C
	Profile TLC	8786	40°C
Mouth protector material	Proform	21.2	37°C
Polyvinyl acetate-polyethylene	Sta-guard	9.39	37°C

Table 8: Elastic Modulus (E, Q, Y)

Modulus of elasticity: Young's modulus of elasticity is the rigidity or resistance to tensile or compressive deformations measured as the ratio of stress/strain within the elastic limit. Units MPa, GPa, Psi, 1 GPa = 10^3 MPa = 10^9 Pa, 1 MPa = 145 Psi.

Materials	Modulus of elasticity (E) GPa	Materials	Modulus of elasticity (E) GPa
Tooth structure		**(e) Resins**	
Enamel	84	Composite resins, anterior	7–20
Dentin mineralised	14.7	Composite resins, posterior	11–25
Dentin demineralised	0.26	All purpose	9–25
Human bones cortical	14.7	Crown and bridge resins	
Human bones femur	17.2	Polymethyl methacrylate	2.5
Human bones humerus	17.2	Polyester	1.84
Radius	18.2	Polyester polyvinyl acetate	2.83
Tibia	18.1	**(f) Maxillofacial**	
Hydroxyapatite	34	Silicone	2.53 MPa
Fluoroapatite mineral	148	**(g) Impression materials**	
Restorative materials		Agar agar (impression)	1.38 MPa
(a) Liners: Ca (OH)$_2$	0.6–2.2	Agar agar (duplication)	0.48 MPa
Resins	1.7–2.6	Alginate (at 6 min)	0.26 MPa
GIC III	0.16–0.42	Polysulphides	0.013–0.12 MPa
Ketabond	0.69	Polysilicones (condensation)	0.09–0.26 MPa
(b) Luting cements		Polysilicones (addition)	0.31–0.35 MPa
ZOE—EBA + Al$_2$O$_3$	3–5.4	Polyether	0.35–0.41 MPa
ZOE—Polymer-modified	1.2–3.0	Die stone type IV	14.5 GPa
ZOE—Non-euginol	0.18	**(h) Metals and alloys**	in GPa
Zinc phosphate	8–14	Casting gold alloys	80–100 GPa
Zinc polycarboxylate cement	2.4–4.4	Casting Ag-Pd alloys	105–115
GIC (I)	4–9.8	Casting Pd-Ag alloys	110–130
Gutta-percha	0.186	Nickel-chromium alloys	145–200
(c) Restoratives and bases		Cobalt-chromium alloys	150–210
Ca(OH)$_2$	1-3	Iron-chromium alloys	180–200
ZnPO$_4$	20-25	Titanium (α)	117
Zinc polycarboxylate cement	5	Titanium (β)	70–80
GIC II	5-13	TAV (titanium alloys)	71.4
Metal reinforced GIC	4.3	Nickel-titanium	41
(d) Ceramics		Elgiloy (Cr-Co-Ni-Fe)	210
Feldspathic	60-69	18-8 stainless steel	190–200
Whisker reinforced	69	PGP wires	110
Leucite	63	PSC wires	105
Castable	74	Alumina (recrystallised)	360–420
Alumina reinforced	107		

Table 9: Latent Heat of Fusion

It is the quantity of heat in calories required to convert one gram of a material from the solid to its liquid state, at its normal melting temperature, i.e. at one atmosphere pressure.

Units: Cal/gm (or joules/gm)

Materials	Latent heat of fusion—Cals/gm	Temperature in°C
Pure metals		
Mercury	2.8	−38
Chromium	96	1875
Copper	50.6	1083
Gold	16.1	1063
Nickel	73.8	1453
Palladium	34.2	1552
Platinum	26.9	1769
Silver	25	961
Zinc	24.09	420
Waxes		
Beeswax	42.8	62.8
Carnauba wax	45.5	82.8
Inlay wax	45.9	60.0
Paraffin wax	42.4	52.0
Gutta-percha (pure)	45.2	74
Ice	79.7	0

Table 10: Proportional Limit

It is the maximum stress a material can withstand without deviating from the law of proportionality, or maximum stress up to which, stress is directly proportional to strain (S = quenched, H = heat hardened).

Material (under tension)	Proportional limit in MPa (tension)	Materials	Proportional limit in MPa (tension)
Tooth enamel (cusp)		Au-Ag-Pd (S)	440
(under compression)	240–350	Au-Ag-Pd (H)	580
Tooth dentin		PFM gold alloy	420
(under compression)	120–160	Nickel-chromium	190
Gold alloys		Ni-Cr-(PFM alloy)	545
Type I	70	18-8 stainless steel	1020–1200
Type II	190		
Type III (S)	220		
Type III (H)	260		
Gold alloy type IV (S)	285		
Gold alloy type V (H)	570		

Table 11: Shear strengths

This is the maximum shear stress, a material can withstand under shearing deformations as tested by pushout or punch test method.

Materials	Shear strength (MPa)	Materials	Shear strength (MPa)
Tooth enamel	90	Porcelain, feldspathic	128
Tooth dentin vital	138	Porcelain, aluminous	165
Tooth dentin non-vital	102	Copper	220
Amalgam	188	Iron	290
Acrylic denture (PMMA) resin	122	Nickel	480
		BeO (tension)	280
Resin bonded ZOE (base)	13	SiC (tension)	170
Resin bonded ZOE luting	12.5		
Unmodified ZOE luting	4.0		
Zinc phosphate	13		
Zinc polycarboxylate cement	27–31		

Table 12: Free surface energies

Free surface energy is the amount of work required to increase the surface area by unity (1 cm^2) or it is the energy stored in one square cm area of the free surface. units = ergs/cm^2, this same dimensions of surface tension, i.e. dynes/cm.

Materials	Free surface energy ergs/cm^2
Tooth structure	
Enamel	84–87
Dentin	92
Bacteria (responsible for caries)	
A. Odontolyticus A7-1	106
A. viscosus C7-4	111
S. mutans C7-3	128
S. salivarius B3-4	113
S. sanguis C7-2	99
Polymers	
Polymethyl methacrylate	37
Polyethylene	34
Polystyrene	38
Polytetrafluoroethylene (Teflon)	24
Wax: Paraffin	25

Table 13: Surface tension

Surface tension is the unbalanced force acting at right angles on one cm length of a line imagined on the free surface of a liquid. *Units = force/length = dyns/cm or N/m.*

Materials	ST dynes/cm	Measured at temperature (T°C)
Water	76	0°C
	72.8	20°C
	68	50°C
	59	100°C
Water + 0.02% sodium oleate (detergent, surfactant)	35.3	20°C
Benzene	29	20°C
Alcohol	22	20°C
Ether	17	20°C
Mercury	465	20°C
Porcelain	365	1038°C
Blood	56–61	37°C
Saliva	53	37°C
Polymer resins	24–34	25°C

Table 14a: Surface Hardness

Surface hardness is defined as the resistance of the surface to scratching (abrasion), indentation or penetration.

14a. Moh's scale, 14b. Brinnel (BHN), 14c. Vickers (VHN, DPH)

14d. Knoop (KHN), 14e. Shore-A-Durometer

Moh's scratch test—hardness number			
Materials number	Hardness	Materials number	Hardness
Tooth structure		Pumice	6–7
Enamel	5–6	(porcelain)	6–7
Dentin	3–4	Tin oxide	6–7
Others		Sand, quartz, cuttle	7
Talc	1	Zirconium silicate	7–5
Gypsum	2	Emery	7–9
Denture base (acrylic)	2–3	Garnet	8–9
Calcite	3	Coundum	9
Rouge (Fe_2O_3)	5–6	Silicon carbide	9–10
Microfilled composite	5–7	Tungsten carbide	9–10
Hybrid composite	5–7	Diamond	10
Abrasives			
Tripoli	6		

Table 14b: Surface hardness (BHN, RHN)

Brinnel hardness number

Materials	BHN measured with steel ball of diameter 1.6 mm/ load 123 kg	Materials	BHN measured with steel ball of diameter 1.6 mm/load 123 kg
Pure gold	24	Silver based casting alloys	130–170
Condensed mat gold	40	Palladium based casting alloys	200–250
Condensed powdered gold	46	Stainless steel	150
Condensed foil gold	69	Nickel chromium	210
Coin gold	85	Gold solders	100–200
Gold alloys: Type I (S)	45	Martensite	230–600
Type II (S)	95	**(c) Rockwell hardness number**	
Type III (S)	110	**Materials**	RHN
Type III (H)	120	Dental stone III	62
Type IV (S)	160	Die stone IV	82
Type IV (H)	220 (140–265)	Die stone V	90

Table 14c: Micro-surface hardness (VHN & KHN)

Micro-surface hardness testing is done with Vicker's square-based diamond point indentor of 136° and Knoop's diamond point rhombic based indentor of 130° and 172.5° angles.

Vicker's hardness number (VHN)

Materials	VHN (DPH) kg/mm²	Materials	VHN
Tooth enamel	300–400	Co-Cr alloys	350–390
Tooth dentin	57–60	Elgiloy	700
Alloys (casting)		**Ceramic (porcelain)**	
Ag-amalgam Sn-Hg phase	15	Castable ceramic glass	450
Ag-amalgam Ag-Hg phase	120	Feldspathic porcelain	650–700
Gold alloys		Whisker reinforced	660
Type I (soft)	55	Leucite reinforced	700
Type II (medium)	105	**PFM alloys**	
Type III (soft)	120–180	High gold	182
Type III (hard)	135–250	Au-Pd	220
Type IV (soft)	150–194	Au-Pd-Ag	218
Type IV (hard)	250–280	Pd-Cu	425
Cast 24 kt gold	28	Pd-Ag	242
Cast 22 kt gold	60	Ni-Cr	257
Condensed gold foil	60	Ni-Cr-Be	357
DFG		**Restoratives**	
Ag-based casting alloy	140–180	Glass-ionomer cements	50–90
Pd-based casting alloy	220–360	Composite resins (anterior)	40–160
CpTi	210	Composite resins (posterior)	60–150
Ti-6Al-4V alloy	320	Composite resins (all purpose)	50–150
Ni-Cr alloys	270–390		

Table 14d: Micro-surface hardness

Knoop's hardness numbers—KHN (kg/mm^2)

Materials	KHN
1. Tooth structure	
Enamel	340–430
Enamel (softened)	150–180
Enamel (etched)	90–170
Dentin	67–70
Cementum	40
Calculus	80–86
2. Restoratives	
Ca (OH)$_2$ Dycal	24
ZnPO$_4$ luting	30–40
ZnPO$_4$ base	40–55
Zinc polycarboxylate cement (luting)	25–30
Zinc polycarboxylate cement (base)	30–40
Silicate	80
Zinc silicophosphate	64
GIC	2–16
GIC II (restoration)	20–40
GIC ketac silver	25–30
GIC miracle mix	20–30
Compomer	20–50
Composite resins	25–60
Porcelain teeth	460–500
Silver amalgam (γ phase)	150–175
Silver amalgam	90–110
3. Resins	
Acrylic denture base	
Heat cure PMMA	16–18
Cold cure PMMA	12–15
Polyvinyl chloride	15
Acrylic teeth	20
4. Metals and alloys	
Pure gold (99.99%)	25
Condensed mat gold	52–62
Condensed powder gold	55–64
Condensed foil gold	69
Condensed mat-foil gold	70–75
Au-Pd alloy as cast	206
Au-Pd alloy heat treated	226
Pd based casting alloys	220–370
Ni-Cr alloy (as cast)	200–335
Co-Cr alloys (as cast)	350–415
Fe-Cr alloys (as cast)	330
Martensite steel	1100
18-8 steel	250–350
Pearlite (eutectoid steel)	350
Type IV gold alloys (soft)	220 (S)
Type in gold alloys (hard)	460 (H)

Materials	KHN
5. Abrasives and polishing agents	
Diamond (natural)	7000–10,000
Diamond (artificial–industrial)	4,000–6,000
Diamond Bort (defective crystal)	4,000–6500
Boron nitride (BN), borazon	4,700
Silicon carbide SiC (carborundum)	2500
Tungsten carbide	1900–2400
Crystalline pure Al$_2$O$_3$	2100
Corundum impure Al$_2$O$_3$	2000
Emery impure Al$_2$O$_3$	2000
Fused alumina (alumdum)	2000
Garnet (Al, Co, Fe, Mg, Mn, silicates)	1350
Arakansas stone	900–1000
Quartz, silica, Tripoli	820
Sand, Keiselguhr	800
Zr silicate, Cr$_2$O$_3$, Sno, cuttle	600–700
Rouge (Fe$_2$O$_3$)	500–600
Pumice	460–560
Flint glass-ceramics	350–560
French chalk, porcelain	400–520
Calcite (CaCO$_3$)	135

Hardness

Table 14e: Shore-A-Durometer

The durometer reads 100 when the depth of penetrometer is zero and zero when it penetrates completely. Hardness of different products: L = light, M = medium, H = heavy, P = putty elastomers are compared, with different loads.

Materials

Denture resilient liners: Silicones 43

Polyphosphazene fluoroelastomer = 50

Maxillofacial materials

Polyurethanes	*47*
Polysilicone rubbers	*30–50*
Mouth protectors	*65–82*

Impression materials

Polysulphides (L, M, N) 30, 30, 35

Cond. polysilicones (L, P) 15–30, 50–65

Add. polysilicones (L, M, H, P) 35, 50, 60, 50–75

Polyethers (L, M, M + thinner, P) 35–40, 35–60, 30–50, 40–50

Table 15: Tear strength and tear energy

Tear strength is the force required to initiate tearing of a crescent shaped specimen of 1 cm thickness with a 90° notch. Units gm/cm or kN/meter.

Tear energy is the work done or energy required to form a new surface area by tearing a trouser-shaped specimen of 1 cm thickness through 1 cm length.

Unit: ergs/cm^2, J/m^2, 1000 ergs/cm^2.

Materials	Tear strength gm/cm	Tear energy ergs/cm^2	Materials	Tear strength gm/cm	Tear energy ergs/cm^2
Impression materials			**Denture liners**		
Agar (duplicating)	250	66	Silicon rubbers	6,000	1,400
Agar tray	1000	1000	Polyphosphazene fluoroelastomer	9,700	23,000
Alginate	470–550	60–530	**Maxillofacial materials**		
Polysulphide (L, M, consistencies)	2,500–7000	700–2000	Polyurethanes	8100	1800
Polysilicones (conden) (L,P)	2300–2600	500–1000	Polyvinyl chloride	4,000–20,000	11,000
Polysilicones (addn) (LMH)	1500–4300	700–1500	Silicon rubbers	1200	650
Polyether (L, M, M + thinner, H)	1800–4800	400–850			

Table 16: Thermal conductivity

Coefficient of thermal conduction or thermal conductivity (K) is the amount of heat in calories per second passing through a body of 1 cm thickness, through one square cm area, when the temperature difference between hot and cold sides is 1°C. Units of K are cal per sec per unit area per unit temperature gradient, cal/sec/cm/°C or 4.2 joules/sec/m/°C.

Material	K in cal/sec/cm/°C × 10^3	Materials	K in cal/sec/cm/°C × 10^3	Materials	K in cal/sec/cm/°C × 10^3
Tooth enamel	2.2	Polystyrene	0.22	Platinum	165
Tooth dentin	1.6	Composite resins	2.5–3.2	Silver	1000
Bones	1.4	**Impression materials**		Titanium	10
Restoratives		Polysulphide	1.0–1.5	zinc	270
Hydroxyapatite	3.0	Polysilicones	0.7–1.4	**Others**	
Calcium hydroxide	1.5	Polyethers	2–3	Gypsum products	3.0–3.5
ZnOE (base)	1.1,1.4	**Metals**		Water	1.42
ZnPO$_4$ (base)	3.1			Beeswax	0.09
GIC II	1.6	Mercury	20		
GIC (ketac silver)	1.5	Chromium	160		
Porcelain	2.4	Copper	940		
Silver amalgam	54.0	Gold	710		
Resins		Nickel	220		
PMMA	0.37–0.5	Palladium	1680		

Table 17: Thermal Diffusivity

Thermal diffusivity is the property of the material to diffuse (flow) heat from the hot to cold regions of a body $D = K/sd$ mm^2/sec (where K = thermal conductivity, d = density and s = specific heat).

Materials	$\triangle = \dfrac{K}{sd} \ \dfrac{mm^2}{sec}$	Materials	$\triangle = \dfrac{K}{sd} \ \dfrac{mm^2}{sec}$
Tooth enamel	**0.469**	*Resins*	
Dentin	**0.18–0.26**	Acrylic resins	0.124
Bones	0.5	Composite resins	0.2–0.72
Hydroxyapatite	0.6	*Impression materials*	
		Impression compound	0.226
Restoratives		Polysulphide	0.30
Calcium hydroxide	0.18 - 0.24	Polysilicone (M)	0.32 –0.38
ZnOE unmodified	0.39 –0.47	Polysilicone (H)	0.22
ZnOE cavitec	0.086	Polyether	0.43
ZnPO$_4$	0.29 –0.308	*Others*	
Zinc polycarboxylate cement	0.332	Water	1.40
GIC fuji II	0.216	Gold	119
GIC fuji II (improved)	0.228	Amalgam	9.80
GIC ketac silver	0.516		
GIC miracle mix	0.407		
Zn-silicophosphate	0.245		
Porcelain	0.64		

Table 18: Thermal Expansion

Coefficient of (linear) thermal expansion is the change in length per unit length for 1°C change in temperature. COTE = 10^{-6}/°C or a $\times 10^6$/°C, i.e. ppm/°C.

Materials	COTE ppm/°C	Materials	COTE ppm/°C		COTE ppm/°C
Tooth enamel	**11.4**	Composite resins	17–50	Silver	19.2
Tooth dentin	**8.6**	Pit and fissure sealants	71–94	Platinum	8.9
Bones (average)	9.2	Silver amalgam	22–28	Palladium	11.8
Hydroxyapatite	9–10	Porcelain	12–14	Copper	16.8
				Chromium	6.2
Restoratives		*Impression materials*		CpTi	8.5
Calcium hydroxide		Impression compound	300–500		
Zinc oxide eugenol	35	Polysulphides	140	*Alloys*	
Zinc phosphate		Polysilicones	210	Gold alloys	14–15.5
Zinc silicophosphate		Polyether	170	Chrom-cobalt	14.7
GIC type I	10.5	Inlay waxes	350–450	Chrom-nickel	14–15
GIC type II	10.2–11.4	Acrylic resins	80–120	Pd-based alloys	14.3–15.2
Gutta percha	55			Ag-based	14.5–15.5
PMMA	80–120	*Metals*		Ti-6Al-4V	12.43
Polystyrene	65–85	Mercury	60		
Polyvinyl chloride	70	Gold	14.4		

Table 19: Transverse (flexure) strengths

It is the maximum transverse or flexure stress a material can withstand under flexure $= 3Pl/2bd^2$ for a rectangular bar of length $= l$, breadth $= b$, thickness $= d$, with load P in the middle.

Materials	Transverse strength $\left.\right\} = \dfrac{3Pl}{2bd^2}$ MPa
Alumina (recrystallised)	380
Silver-amalgam, lathe-cut	124
Silver-amalgam, admix	135
Silver-amalgam, spherical	120–140
Condensed DFG mat	160
Condensed DFG powdered	170
Condensed DFG mat foil	210
Condensed gold foil	290
Gypsum product: High strength stone	1.6–17
Investments: Silicate bonded (23–1000°C)	0.5
Investments: Gypsum bonded (23°C, 600°C)	2.5, 0.1
Phosphate bonded (23°C, 1000°C)	2.65–7.5
Porcelain: Feldspathic (less glazed)	55–65
Feldspathic glazed	140
Leucite reinforced	105
Al_2O_3 reinforced	130–140
Castable glass	125
Magnesia core (unglazed)	130
Magnesia core (glazed)	270
(IPS) Empress	350–450
Inceram zircona (ICZ)	700
Vitreous carbon	150
Restorative materials	
Calcium hydroxide	2.5–4.0
Glass ionomers: Luting	12.0–18.00
Restorative	11.0–25
Composite resins	70.0–140
Denture resin	80.0–85

Table 20: Ultimate compressive and tensile strength

1. The ultimate compressive strength is the maximum stress that a material can withstand before failure in compression.
2. The ultimate tensile strength is the maximum stress that a material can withstand before failure in tension.

[Note: (1) Approximate values: With rate of loading, i.e. load cell speed 2 mm/min (2) *Diametral tensile strength testing method.

Materials	Product	Ultimate strength	
		Compressive MPa	Tensile MPa
Human tooth structure			
Enamel		380 (cusp)	10
Dentin		300	50–105
Human bones			
Femur		167	121
Humerus		132	130
Radius		114	149
Tibia		159	140
Vertebra—cervical		10	3.0
Lumbar		5	3.7
Cements (base—24 hrs)			
Resin bonded ZOE	BQT	38	3.0*
Zinc phosphate	Zn cement improved	161	8.3
Zinc polycarboxylate cement	Durelon	80	16*
PCA	PCA	69	1.00*
Cements (luting—24 hrs)			
EBA—alumina ZOE	Optow	64–66	7*
GIC—alumina ZOE	Fuji I	120	5.5*
	Ketac-cem	122	4.5*
Non-eugenol ZOE	Nogeno-1	4.5	1.0*
Polymer modified ZOE	Fynal	35–50	4*
Resin	Panavia Ex	178	45*
Zinc phosphate	Flecks	62	9.30
	Modern tenacin	77.5	9.50
Zinc polycarboxylate cement	Durelon	67.4	15
	Shofu	55	11
Zinc silicophosphate	kryptase improved	171	-
Cement liners			
Calcium hydroxide	Dycal	14.5	2.3*
	Life	38	2.4*
Glass ionomer—VLC	Fuji lining L/CL	170	14.0*
	Vitrabond	131	12.5*
	XR ionomer	64	7.5*
	Zionomer	46	3.8*
Glass ionomer self-cured	Baseline	66.5	6.0*
	Baseline in (caps)	138	10.5*
	GC lining cement	58	4.0*
	Ketac bond	117	6*
	Ketac bond (caps)	142	11.0*
	3 M glass ionomer liner	65.1	2.5*
GIC resin	Time line	153	14.0*

Contd...

Table 20: Ultimate compressive and tensile strength *(Contd...)*

Materials	Product	Ultimate strength Compressive MPa	Ultimate strength Tensile MPa
Unmodified ZOE	Cavitec	5.5	0.5*
Crown and bridge resins acrylics	Biotone	81	—
Crown and bridge resins polyester	Mer-don	59.6	—
Crown and bridge resins polyvinyl acrylic	Luxene	83	84.5
Denture resins acrylic	Kallodent	80	80.4
Gypsum products			
Gypsum plaster II	Calspar	23	4.0*
Dental stone III	Calastone	60	6*
Improved stone IV	Velmixes	81	7.0*
Impression materials			
Impression agar-agar	Surgident	0.76	-
Impression alginate	Jeltrate	0.82	0.25*
Impression polysulphide	Caflex	1.93	1.14
Impression add. polisilicone	-	1.2–2.3	
Polymers PMMA		74	58.5*
Polyether urethane area	Pellethane	-	50*
Polyether urethane area	Biomer	-	58.5*
Porcelains feldspathic	Trubyte bioform	149	24.8*
Fused to metal	Ceramco-opaque	150	58*
Restorative materials			
Composite resins	Many products	250–450	40–55*
All purpose	Many products		
Anterior	Many products	280–450	40–55*
Posterior	Many products	320–390	37–62*
Glass ionomer II		150–160	9–14*
Metal reinforced		115–130	9–13*
Glass ionomers	Miracle mix	129	9.2*
Alumina	(recrystallised)	2180	120
Silver amalgam (24 hrs)			
Low copper (lathe-cut	Caulk fine cut	310	~ 45
Low copper (spherical)	Sybralloy	360	~ 45
Low copper (spherical)	Indilloy	410	~ 45
High copper (admix)	Dispers alloy	420	48
High copper (single compression)		430–500	50

Table 21: Yield Strength

This is the stress (compressive, tensile, shear or flexure) at which the material shows a specified limiting deviation of say 0.1% or 0.2% strain from the proportionality of stress to strain (yield stress or proof stress and offset values are the terms used), or it is the stress required to initiate a measurable specific permanent or nonrecoverable strain.

Cast metal alloys	Yield strengths (MPa)	Ultimate tensile strengths (MPa)
Pure gold (condensed)	——————	150–290 (Transverse strength)
Gold alloys		
HN (soft)	103,186, 207,275, (372)	220–450
HN (hard)	——, —, 275,493, (720)	450–750
Noble (Pd based)	—, —, 241(586 H) 434(586 H)	700–1140
Noble (Ag based)	262(S), (323 H)	600–900
Chromium cobalt	470–535	600–850
Chromium nickel	250–500	500–800
Wrought orthodontic wires		
18-8 Stainless steel	1200–1600	2250
Elgiloy	1930	2100–2540
Nickel titanium	430	1500–2500
CpTi (Grades—1, 2, 3, 4)	170,275,300,483.	1200–1300
Beta-titanium (Ti-6Al-4V)	860–930	960–1000
Pd-Au-Pt (PGP)—oven cooled	550–1030	860–1340
Pd-Ag-Cu (PSC)—oven cooled	690–790	960–1070

Table 22: Viscosity

Viscosity is the resistance of a liquid (fluid) to flow under shear stress and is measured as a ratio of shear stress and shear strain rate (in stream-lined flow). This refers to consistency and flow.

Coefficient of viscosity (η) is defined as the shear resistance (force) acting between two adjacent layers of a fluid of unit area to maintain unit velocity gradient in stream-lined flow (page 37) Units: 1 Pas (Pascal-sec) = 1 Poise = 100 centi-Poise, cP.

Materials	Measured at time	Viscosity η cP	At temp°C
Cements (luting)			
Zinc phosphate	45 sec after mixing	43,000	18
Zinc phosphate	45 sec after mixing	95,000	25
Zinc polycarboxylate	45 sec after mixing	101000	18
Zinc polycarboxylate	45 sec after mixing	109000	25
Impression materials			
Poly sulphides (light)	45 sec after mixing	60,000	37
Poly sulphides (medium)	45 sec after mixing	110000	37
Poly sulphides (high)	45 sec after mixing	450000	37
Condensation polysilicones (light)	45 sec after mixing	70000	37
Addition polysilicones (syringe)		95000	37
Addition polysilicones (medium)		150,000	37
Addition polysilicones (heavy)		690,000	37
Polyether (medium)		130,000	37
Agar-agar		280,000	45
Alginate	1.5 min after mixing	250,000	37
Impression plaster	1.5 min after mixing	23,000	37
Zinc oxide eugenol	1.5 min after mixing	100000	
Others			
Water		**1.000**	25
Mercury		1.554	25
Methyl methacrylate		0.52	25
Ethylene glycol DMA		3.4	25
Triethylene glycol DMA		7.5	25
Blood			37
Blood plasma (healthy person)		2.6–0.35	25
Blood serum (healthy person)		1.4–1.8	25
Blood serum (symptomatic)		5.0–10.0	25
Saliva (normal)			
Parotid glands		1.5	37
Sub-maxillary glands		3.4	37
Sub-lingual glands		13.4	37s

Index